Pocket Guide
to Evaluations
of Drug Interactions

NOTICE

This publication does not purport to include all reported drug interactions. All expressions of opinion and statements presented in this publication concerning the incidents and severity of possible drug interactions, as well as recognition, side effects, and treatment of such interactions, represent the consensus of the staff and consultants of First Data-Bank–St. Louis and the American Pharmaceutical Association Scientific Review Panel.

This book is intended for use by health professionals, and it should not be used by anyone who does not have such specialized training. The book can serve to assist the practitioner, but it is not a substitute for professional knowledge, judgment, training, and experience.

The inclusion in this publication of the drug in respect to which patent or trademark rights may exist shall not be deemed, and is not intended as, a grant of, or authority to exercise, any right or privilege protected by such patent or trademark. All such rights and privileges are vested in the patent or trademark owner, and no other person may exercise the same without express permission, authority, or license secured from such patent or trademark owner.

Pocket Guide to Evaluations of Drug Interactions

Editors
Frederic J. Zucchero, M.A., R.Ph.
Mark J. Hogan, Pharm.D.
Christine D. Schultz, Pharm.D.

THIRD EDITION
AMERICAN PHARMACEUTICAL ASSOCIATION
WASHINGTON, D.C.

Managing Editor: Susan Kendall
Abstractors: Daniel H. Albrant, Pharm.D., Jeann Lee
Gillespie, Pharm.D., and Susan K. Moss, R.Ph.
Production Coordinator: Mary Jane Hickey
Graphic Artist: Pamela S. Cooper
Proofreader: Nancy Burkhart

ISBN 0-917330-93-5

ISSN 1521-8392

Printed and bound in Canada by Webcom Inc.

How to Order This Book

By phone: **800-878-0729** (802-862-0095 from outside the United States)–VISA®, MasterCard®, and American Express® cards accepted.

Table of Contents

Evaluations of Drug Interactions Directory vi

How to Use *Pocket Guide to Evaluations of Drug Interactions* . . . vii

Chapter One
    Analgesic drug interactions: narcotics, nonnarcotics, non-
    steroidal anti-inflammatory agents, and agents for gout 1

Chapter Two
    Anesthetic and neuromuscular blocking agents'
    drug interactions 23

Chapter Three
    Antiarrhythmic drug interactions. 44

Chapter Four
    Anticoagulant drug interactions 68

Chapter Five
    Anticonvulsant drug interactions 102

Chapter Six
    Antidepressant drug interactions 134

Chapter Seven
    Antihypertensive drug interactions 155

Chapter Eight
    Anti-infective drug interactions. 172

Chapter Nine
    Antineoplastic drug interactions. 210

Chapter Ten
    Antipsychotic and antianxiety drug interactions 223

Chapter Eleven
    Beta-adrenergic blocking agents' drug interactions 252

Chapter Twelve
    Cardiac glycoside drug interactions. 266

Chapter Thirteen
    Diuretic drug interactions. 285

Chapter Fourteen
    Hypoglycemic drug interactions. 295

Chapter Fifteen
    Sedative-hypnotic drug interactions 309

Chapter Sixteen
    Vitamin/nutrient/food drug interactions 319

Chapter Seventeen
    Xanthine drug interactions 326

Chapter Eighteen
    Miscellaneous drug interactions. 345

Appendices
    A. Related drugs 372
    B. Code 1 interactions 380

Index 383

Evaluations of Drug Interactions Directory

Editors

Frederic J. Zucchero, M.A., R.Ph.
Clinical Assistant Professor of Pharmacy Practice
St. Louis College of Pharmacy
Medical Director
First DataBank–St. Louis
rick_zucchero@firstdatabank.com

Mark J. Hogan, Pharm.D.
Clinical Assistant Professor of Pharmacy Practice
St. Louis College of Pharmacy
Vice President/General Manager
First DataBank–St. Louis
mark_hogan@firstdatabank.com

Christine D. Schultz, Pharm.D.
Clinical Instructor of Pharmacy Practice
St. Louis College of Pharmacy
Assistant Director, Medical Affairs
First DataBank–St. Louis
christine_schultz@firstdatabank.com

Consulting Contributors

Bruce Alexander, Pharm.D.; Jerry L. Bauman, Pharm.D.;
Rebecca S. Finley, Pharm.D., M.S.; Jerry L. Frazier,
Pharm.D.; William R. Garnett, Pharm.D.; Pamela D. Garzone,
Ph.D.; Norman L. Katz, Ph.D., R.Ph.; John Loomis, Pharm.D.;
David L. Lourwood Jr., Pharm.D., BCPS; Kenneth Rockwell
Jr., Pharm.D., M.S.; Philip J. Rogers, BPharm, Ph.D.,
MRPharmS, ACPP; Terrence L. Schwinghammer, Pharm.D.;
Jon J. Tanja, M.S., FASCP; Stanley S. Weber, Pharm.D.,
FASCP, BCPP.

American Pharmaceutical Association Scientific Review Panel

Daniel H. Albrant, Pharm.D.; Ann B. Amerson, Pharm.D.;
Connie Lee Barnes, Pharm.D.; Ruth Ann Calloway, R.Ph.,
M.S.; Mark W. Todd, Pharm. D., FASHP; Candy Tsourounis,
Pharm.D.

How to Use Pocket Guide to Evaluations of Drug Interactions

Chapter Assignments

Each monograph is assigned a chapter based upon classification and pharmacologic effect. The first drug listed in the monograph heading is the drug whose pharmacologic effect was altered by the second drug. If the affected drug is not assigned a chapter, the monograph is placed in the therapeutic chapter of the other agent. For drug interactions in which neither of the two involved agents has an assigned chapter, the monographs are listed in Chapter 18 (Miscellaneous Drug Interactions) and alphabetized by the drug whose pharmacologic action is altered.

Drug Interaction Monographs

Most monographs contain eight concise pieces of information:
1. The **title** of the monograph by generic name of the interacting drugs
2. A **significance code** based on the interaction's potential harm to the patient and its frequency and predictability
3. A statement on the interaction's **potential effects***
4. Patient management **recommendations** for the healthcare professional to consider with respect to the interaction
5. A **summary** of studies in the literature
6. A discussion of pharmacologically, pharmacokinetically, or chemically **related drugs** to either of the interacting drugs (see Appendix for a complete list of the agents in a specific related drug class)
7. A comment on the postulated **mechanism** for the drug interaction
8. A cross reference to the more **detailed information** found in *Evaluations of Drug Interactions*, which is paginated by section, followed by page, followed by subpage (e.g., 5/40.05 refers to section 5, page 40, subpage 05).

Significance Codes

Each drug-drug interaction monograph has been assigned a significance code based on three major factors: potential harm to the patient, frequency and predictability of occurrence, and degree and quality of documentation. The significance code is to be considered applicable only to the agents that appear in the monograph title. The related drugs that are mentioned are not given a significance code.

Code 1.
  Highly clinically significant—Drug interactions that are of great potential harm to the patient, that are predictable or frequent, and that are well documented (see Appendix B for list of Code 1 interactions)

---

* Older monographs in *Evaluations of Drug Interactions* lack this statement, and so it is missing in the corresponding monographs of the *Pocket Guide.*

Code 2.

Moderately clinically significant—Drug interactions that are of moderate potential harm to the patient, that are less predictable or frequent, and that lack complete documentation

Code 3.

Minimally clinically significant—Drug interactions that are of little potential harm to the patient, that have variable predictability or occur infrequently, and that have little documentation

Code 4.

Not clinically significant—Drug interactions in which documentation may be based on theoretical considerations, the effects are not clinically significant, and no adverse effects are expected

Chapter One

Analgesic
Drug Interactions:

Narcotics, Nonnarcotics, Nonsteroidal Anti-inflammatory Agents, and Agents for Gout

Acetaminophen-Alcohol, Ethyl

Significance: 3—minimally clinically significant

Potential Effects: Chronic alcohol ingestion may potentiate acetaminophen toxicity.

Recommendations: Chronic alcohol abusers should be cautioned about enhancement of acetaminophen toxicity by alcohol.

Summary: The risk of acetaminophen-induced hepatotoxicity may be potentiated by chronic, heavy alcohol consumption; however, contrasting data are available. An acute ingestion of alcohol and chronic alcohol intake may protect against hepatotoxicity.

Related Drugs: There are no drugs related to acetaminophen or alcohol.

Mechanism: Acetaminophen is metabolized and oxidized to a reactive toxic metabolite, inactivated by conjugation with glutathione. Alcohol may deplete glutathione stores.

Detailed Information: See *EDI,* 1/0.01

Acetaminophen-Charcoal

Significance: 3—minimally clinically significant

Recommendations: Activated charcoal should be given as soon as possible after an acute acetaminophen overdose to reduce the absorption of acetaminophen. However, if charcoal is not used for acetaminophen overdose, the administration of these agents should be separated by as much time as possible.

Summary: There are data to show that activated charcoal significantly reduces the absorption of acetaminophen.

Related Drugs: There are no drugs related to acetaminophen.

Mechanism: Activated charcoal adsorbs acetaminophen in the gastrointestinal tract, limiting its absorption.

Detailed Information: See *EDI,* 1/0.10

Acetaminophen-Isoniazid

Significance: 3—minimally clinically significant

Potential Effects: Isoniazid decreased the clearance of acetaminophen which may lead to hepatotoxicity.

Recommendations: The use of concurrent isoniazid and acetaminophen should be approached with caution. Hepatic function should be monitored for signs of acetaminophen hepatotoxicity.

Summary: Isoniazid decreases the clearance of acetaminophen and can cause severe hepatoxicity.

Related Drugs: There are no drugs related to acetaminophen or isoniazid.

Mechanism: With large doses of acetaminophen, the metabolic pathways become saturated, leading to the formation of a toxic intermediate. A hepatic enzyme has been shown to catalyze this toxic intermediate and this enzyme is induced by isoniazid.

Detailed Information: See *EDI,* 1/0.15

Acetaminophen-Oral Contraceptive Agents

Significance: 3—minimally clinically significant

Potential Effects: Oral contraceptive agents may increase the metabolism of acetaminophen.

Recommendations: It is not known if larger doses of acetaminophen would be required in women receiving oral contraceptive agents.

Summary: Oral contraceptive agents have been shown to increase the metabolism of acetaminophen.

Related Drugs: There were no differences found in the pharmacokinetics of acetaminophen with women taking conjugated estrogens. There are no drugs related to acetaminophen.

Mechanism: The acetaminophen glucuronide metabolite was increased in women taking oral contraceptive agents.

Detailed Information: See *EDI*, 1/0.21

Acetaminophen-Phenobarbital

Significance: 3—minimally clinically significant

Potential Effects: Phenobarbital enhances the metabolism of acetaminophen. This enhancement may lead to increased acetaminophen induced hepatic damage because of the depletion of enzymes that inactivate the toxic metabolite.

Recommendations: The concurrent use of these agents need not be avoided. However, some patients may be at a greater risk of developing hepatotoxicity.

Summary: The concurrent administration of acetaminophen and phenobarbital may result in an increased risk of hepatotoxicity and hepatic necrosis. However, conflicting data are available.

Related Drugs: Primidone has shown to increase the clearance of acetaminophen and decrease its half-life and area-under-curve. A similar interaction may be expected to occur between acetaminophen and other barbiturates. There are no drugs related to acetaminophen.

Mechanism: Phenobarbital may increase the formation of acetaminophen's toxic metabolite, normally inactivated by conjugation with glutathione. Excessive metabolite formation may deplete glutathione.

Detailed Information: See *EDI*, 1/0.23

Acetaminophen-Phenytoin

Significance: 3—minimally clinically significant

Potential Effects: Concurrent use may result in increased acetaminophen clearance. This may result in depletion of glutathione stores, leading to potential acetaminophen toxicity.

Recommendations: No specific precautions are required; however, patients may be at a greater risk of developing hepatotoxicity should acetaminophen overdose occur.

Summary: There are data to show that the concurrent administration of acetaminophen and phenytoin results in an increased clearance and a reduced bioavailability of acetaminophen; however, conflicting data are available.

Related Drugs: A similar interaction may occur between acetaminophen and other hydantoin anticonvulsants. There are no drugs related to acetaminophen.

Mechanism: Phenytoin may increase the formation of acetaminophen's toxic metabolite, normally inactivated by conjugation with glutathione. Excessive metabolite formation may deplete glutathione.

Detailed Information: See *EDI*, 1/0.30

Acetaminophen-Propranolol

Significance: 3—minimally clinically significant

Potential Effects: Propranolol may decrease the metabolism of acetaminophen leading to increased levels.

Recommendations: The concurrent use of these agents need not be avoided in patients with normal hepatic function. Patients with decreased hepatic function should be carefully monitored for increased acetaminophen levels if these agents are used concurrently.

Summary: There are data to show that acetaminophen concentrations were increased with concurrent propranolol. However, contrasting data have shown propranolol to have no significant effect on acetaminophen metabolism.

Related Drugs: Other beta-blocking agents that are hepatically metabolized may be expected to interact with acetaminophen. There are no drugs related to acetaminophen.

Mechanism: Propranolol may inhibit the oxidation and glucuronidation pathways in the liver, leading to the reduction in the clearance of acetaminophen.

Detailed Information: See *EDI*, 1/0.35

Acetaminophen-Sulfinpyrazone

Significance: 3—minimally clinically significant

Potential Effects: Sulfinpyrazone may increase the toxic effects of acetaminophen on the liver, especially in cases of acetaminophen overdose.

Recommendations: Avoid using these agents together. If they are used together, liver function should be monitored.

Summary: Sulfinpyrazone has been reported to increase the clearance of acetaminophen and reduce its half-life. The increased clearance may lead to a depletion of hepatic glutathione, leading to hepatic necrosis.

Related Drugs: Probenecid reduces the hepatic formation of acetaminophen glucuronide. There are no drugs related to acetaminophen.

Mechanism: Sulfinpyrazone enhances the elimination of acetaminophen, leading to the formation of acetaminophen's toxic metabolite, normally inactivated by conjugation with glutathione. Excessive metabolite formation may deplete glutathione.

Detailed Information: See *EDI*, 1/0.50

Acetaminophen-Terfenadine

Significance: 2—moderately clinically significant

Potential Effects: Concurrent administration of terfenadine with high dose acetaminophen administration may result in increased terfenadine levels and cardiotoxicity.

Recommendations: Concurrent use of terfenadine and large doses of acetaminophen should be approached with caution.

Summary: In a single case report, concomitant administration of terfenadine and acetaminophen resulted in Torsades de Pointes, a serious ventricular arrhythmia.

Related Drugs: Although documentation is lacking, a similar reaction would be expected to occur between large doses of acetaminophen and astemizole. Increased serum levels of loratadine may also be expected; however, elevated levels of loratadine have not been shown to produce Torsades de Pointes. Cetirizine is excreted mostly as unchanged drug; lack of metabolism suggests that this agent is unlikely to interact like terfenadine or astemizole.

Mechanism: The formation of the N-acetyl-p-aminobenzoquinone imine from acetaminophen has been shown to inhibit the cytochrome $P450_{3A4}$ isozyme. It is postulated that high dose acetaminophen administration resulted in accumulation of terfenadine and Torsades de Pointes.

Detailed Information: See *EDI*, 1/0.63

Alfentanil-Erythromycin

Significance: 2—moderately clinically significant

Potential Effects: Erythromycin inhibits the metabolism of alfentanil, resulting in increased levels.

Recommendations: Caution should be used if alfentanil is administered to patients maintained on erythromycin. The dose of alfentanil may need to be decreased or the use of alfentanil may need to be avoided.

Summary: A study has shown that the clearance of alfentanil is decreased by erythromycin.

Related Drugs: A like interaction may occur between alfentanil and other macrolide antibiotics. Whether an interaction would occur between erythromycin and narcotic analgesics is unknown.

Mechanism: This interaction may occur as a result of competitive inhibition of alfentanil by erythromycin.

Detailed Information: See *EDI*, 1/0.65

Allopurinol-Aluminum Hydroxide

Significance: 3—minimally clinically significant

Potential Effects: Aluminum hydroxide may decrease the absorption of allopurinol. This may lead to a decrease in allopurinol action, resulting in increased uric acid levels.

Recommendations: Patients should be advised to take aluminum hydroxide at least three hours after taking allopurinol because this was shown to circumvent the interaction.

Summary: Receiving concurrent allopurinol and aluminum hydroxide for high uric acid and phosphate concentrations will not decrease uric acid levels. When administration times were separated, uric acid levels were shown to decrease.

Related Drugs: All antacids may alter the pharmacokinetics of allopurinol. There are no drugs related to allopurinol.

Mechanism: Aluminum hydroxide may decrease the gastrointestinal absorption of allopurinol by changing gastrointestinal transit time or pH, or by binding or chelating allopurinol.

Detailed Information: See *EDI*, 1/0.70

Allopurinol-Probenecid

Significance: 3—minimally clinically significant

Recommendations: The concurrent administration of allopurinol and probenecid need not be avoided. However, this regimen should be used cautiously in patients with impaired renal function because of the danger of urate or urate precursors forming in the kidney. Fluid intake should be maintained at a level of 3L/day in all patients taking these drugs. Alkalinization of the urine may also be desirable as a means of promoting and ensuring adequate uric acid clearance through the kidney.

Summary: Concurrent use of allopurinol and probenecid may decrease the effectiveness of allopurinol.

Related Drugs: A similar interaction can expect to occur with sulfinpyrazone. There are no drugs related to allopurinol.

Mechanism: Allopurinol may inhibit the metabolism of probenecid and probenecid may increase the renal excretion of oxypurinol (alloxanthine), resulting in a decrease in the inhibition of uric acid production.

Detailed Information: See *EDI*, 1/1.00

Aspirin-Acetazolamide

Significance: 2—moderately clinically significant

Potential Effects: The concurrent use of these agents may result in acetazolamide or salicylate toxicity.

Recommendations: If concomitant administration is necessary, patients should be monitored for increased acetazolamide and/or salicylate serum levels or toxicity. One or both agents may need to be discontinued.

Summary: Concurrent administration of aspirin and acetazolamide leads to a decrease in clearance and plasma protein binding, and an increase in unbound acetazolamide. There are also reports of severe salicylate intoxication and the development of severe acid base imbalance.

Related Drugs: The concurrent administration of aspirin and dichlorphenamide may result in salicylate intoxication. An interaction may be expected to occur between acetazolamide and other salicylates. An interaction may not occur with aspirin and methazolamide.

Mechanism: Aspirin may inhibit the plasma protein binding of acetazolamide, inhibiting its renal tubular secretion. For salicylate intoxication, the interaction may result from metabolic acidemia, increasing the salicylate available.

Detailed Information: See *EDI*, 1/2.10

Aspirin-Alcohol, Ethyl

Significance: 2—moderately clinically significant

Recommendations: The combination of alcohol and aspirin should be avoided in patients predisposed to gastrointestinal disease. Concurrent use does not appear to present a significant problem in normal subjects. Predisposed patients requiring an analgesic may use acetaminophen or buffered aspirin. Patients receiving aspirin for its hematologic (antiplatelet) effects should be cautioned about the potential hazards of concurrent alcohol use.

Summary: Aspirin or alcohol alone will disrupt the gastric mucosal barrier. Alcohol potentiates the erosive effects of aspirin resulting in increased fecal blood loss and may prolong bleeding time.

Related Drugs: A similar interaction does not occur with buffered salicylate products, choline salicylate and diflunisal. Other salicylates have been found to effect clotting factor synthesis and are irritating to the gastric mucosa.

Mechanism: Aspirin breaks down the normal gastric mucosal barrier, resulting in injury and irritation to the gastrointestinal mucosa. Aspirin effects hemostasis and potentiates the prolonged bleeding time associated with aspirin therapy.

Detailed Information: See *EDI*, 1/3.00

Aspirin-Aluminum Hydroxide, Magnesium Hydroxide

Significance: 2—moderately clinically significant

Recommendations: Patients should be counseled before initiating, switching, or discontinuing antacid use while on high dose salicylate therapy, since different antacids affect salicylate levels to varying degrees because of differing extents of urinary alkalinization. Patients using enteric-coated products should be advised not to ingest antacids simultaneously to avoid premature drug release from this particular dosage form.

Summary: Salicylate levels decrease following the concurrent administration of an antacid preparation containing aluminum hydroxide and magnesium hydroxide.

Related Drugs: A similar interaction is expected to occur with magnesium trisilicate, sodium bicarbonate, calcium carbonate, and salicylate preparations. There is conflicting data regarding the levels of salicylates with diflunisal.

Mechanism: The decreased serum salicylate concentration is attributed to an increase in urine alkalinity and an increase in gastric pH, effecting the delivery of the salicylate to the gastric area or a decreased gastric transit time.

Detailed Information: See *EDI,* 1/5.00

Aspirin-Charcoal

Significance: 3—minimally clinically significant

Recommendations: Because of aspirin's rapid absorption, it has been recommended that activated charcoal be given as soon as possible in an acute aspirin overdose. A 10:1 ratio of activated charcoal to aspirin has also been recommended. However, if charcoal is not used for aspirin overdose, it may be advisable to separate the administration of aspirin and charcoal by as much time as possible.

Summary: Concomitant administration of activated charcoal and aspirin significantly reduces the gastrointestinal absorption of aspirin.

Related Drugs: A like interaction is expected with other salicylates.

Mechanism: Activated charcoal adsorbs aspirin in the gastrointestinal tract, limiting its absorption.

Detailed Information: See *EDI,* 1/6.10

Aspirin-Dipyridamole

Significance: 3—minimally clinically significant

Potential Effects: Dipyridamole may decrease the metabolism of aspirin resulting in increased levels.

Recommendations: The clinical significance of this interaction has not been determined. Aspirin levels may need to be monitored during concurrent therapy with dipyridamole.

Summary: There are data to show that dipyridamole causes an increase in the peak concentration and area-under-curve of unchanged aspirin.

Related Drugs: It is not known if dipyridamole would interact with other salicylates. There are no drugs related to dipyridamole.

Mechanism: Dipyridamole may decrease the deacetylation of aspirin, resulting in increased levels.

Detailed Information: See *EDI,* 1/6.30

Aspirin-Ginkgo

Significance: 3—minimally clinically significant

Potential Effects: The addition of *Ginkgo biloba* to the therapy of a patient maintained on aspirin may result in increased bleeding times and possible hemorrhagic complications.

Recommendations: Caution should be observed if *Ginkgo biloba* is added to the therapy of a patient maintained on aspirin. Patients should be monitored for increased bleeding times and hemorrhagic complications.

Summary: The addition of *Ginkgo biloba* extract to the regimen of a patient maintained on aspirin may result in spontaneous bleeding and hemorrhagic complications.

Related Drugs: It is not known whether an interaction would occur between the other platelet aggregation inhibitors and *Ginkgo biloba* extract.

Mechanism: Although the mechanism of this interaction is not known, the terpenoid ginkgolide B, a component of *Ginkgo biloba,* has been shown to be a potent inhibitor of platelet-activating factor which is necessary for platelet aggregation. The long-term use of this extract was associated with subdural hematomas and increased bleeding time.

Detailed Information: See *EDI,* 1/6.50

Aspirin-Griseofulvin

Significance: 3—minimally clinically significant

Potential Effects: The addition of griseofulvin to an aspirin regimen may result in decreased plasma salicylate levels.

Recommendations: It is recommended that an alternative non-steroidal anti-inflammatory agent be used if possible. However, if concurrent aspirin and griseofulvin therapy is necessitated, the doses of griseofulvin and aspirin could be staggered and the salicylate serum concentration should be carefully monitored. The dose of aspirin may need to be adjusted.

Summary: There are data to show concurrent administration of aspirin and griseofulvin resulted in a marked decrease in the salicylate serum concentrations.

Related Drugs: It is unknown whether an interaction would occur between griseofulvin and other salicylates. There are no drugs related to griseofulvin.

Mechanism: The mechanism of this interaction is not known; however, the most probable mechanism involves the interference of aspirin absorption by griseofulvin.

Detailed Information: See *EDI,* 1/6.60

Aspirin-Methylprednisolone

Significance: 2—moderately clinically significant

Potential Effects: Methylprednisolone may decrease salicylate levels, possibly by increasing the glomerular filtration rate.

Recommendations: Although serum salicylate levels may decrease with concurrent methylprednisolone therapy, the decrease appears to be transient. However, salicylate levels should be closely monitored since an increased dosage of aspirin may be necessary if the decrease in levels persists. Also, it is important to be aware of significantly increased salicylate levels when the corticosteroid dosage is decreased or discontinued.

Summary: There are data to show that plasma concentrations of salicylate decrease and clearance increases with concomitant methylprednisolone or prednisone. This may lead to unwarranted increases in the dosage of aspirin.

Related Drugs: A similar interaction is expected with dexamethasone, triamcinolone, methylprednisolone and other corticosteroids.

Mechanism: Corticosteroids have been shown to increase the glomerular filtration rate, and the decreased salicylate concentrations may be the result of an increase in salicylate clearance induced by prednisone.

Detailed Information: See *EDI,* 1/7.00

Aspirin-Nitroglycerin

Significance: 3—minimally clinically significant

Recommendations: Although the clinical effects of the interaction may not be significant, physicians should be aware that nitroglycerin's vasodilatory and hemodynamic effects may be altered by the concomitant administration of aspirin.

Summary: There are data to show that aspirin increases the amount of nitroglycerin absorbed and the peak concentration of nitroglycerin.

Related Drugs: A similar interaction is expected with aspirin and other salicylates and with nitroglycerin and other nitrate derivatives.

Mechanism: Aspirin may increase the amount of nitroglycerin absorbed through vasodilation or it may modify the effect of nitroglycerin.

Detailed Information: See *EDI,* 1/8.10

Aspirin-Oral Contraceptive Agents

Significance: 3—minimally clinically significant

Potential Effects: The effect of aspirin may be decreased by the short-term use of oral contraceptive agents.

Recommendations: Patients on chronic aspirin therapy who are taking oral contraceptive agents for a short time may require a temporary increase in the aspirin dosage.

Summary: There are data to show that a low dose estrogen contraceptive agent significantly reduces the pharmacokinetics of aspirin.

Related Drugs: A similar interaction may be expected to occur between oral contraceptive agents and other salicylates.

Mechanism: Oral contraceptive agents may induce the metabolism of aspirin.

Detailed Information: See *EDI,* 1/8.21

Diclofenac-Cyclosporine

Significance: 2—moderately clinically significant

Potential Effects: The concurrent use of these agents may result in a decreased renal function.

Recommendations: Monitor renal function closely if these agents are used together. Diclofenac may need to be discontinued.

Summary: Decreased renal function resulted when diclofenac was added to the therapy of a patient maintained on cyclosporine. Renal function did not respond to lowering the cyclosporine dose.

Related Drugs: Sulindac, ketoprofen, mefanamic acid, naproxen and piroxicam have been reported to cause a similar interaction with cyclosporine. Although documentation is lacking, a similar interaction may be expected to occur between cyclosporine and the other nonsteroidal anti-inflammatory agents based on pharmacologic similarity and the proposed mechanism. It is unknown if there is a similar interaction between tacrolimus and nonsteroidal anti-inflammatory agents.

Mechanism: It has been suggested that nonsteroidal anti-inflammatory drugs may enhance cyclosporine nephrotoxicity by inhibiting prostaglandin synthesis. It has been postulated that nonsteroidal anti-inflammatory drugs may enhance the toxic effects of cyclosporine independent of any change in cyclosporine level.

Detailed Information: See *EDI*, 1/8.25

Fenoprofen-Phenobarbital

Significance: 3—minimally clinically significant

Potential Effects: Phenobarbital may increase the metabolism of fenoprofen, resulting in decreased effects.

Recommendations: Although the concurrent use of these agents need not be avoided, it is prudent to be aware of the possibility of this interaction as the dose of fenoprofen may need to be increased.

Summary: There are data to show that phenobarbital decreases the area-under-curve and increases the elimination rate constant of fenoprofen.

Related Drugs: A similar interaction may occur between phenobarbital and other NSAIAs and between fenoprofen and other barbiturates. The concurrent use of phenylbutazone and phenobarbital may reduce the half-life of phenylbutazone.

Mechanism: Phenobarbital may increase the metabolism of fenoprofen by inducing the hepatic microsomal enzymes responsible for its metabolism.

Detailed Information: See *EDI*, 1/8.30

Fentanyl-Propranolol

Significance: 3—minimally clinically significant

Potential Effects: Propranolol decreases the first pass extraction of fentanyl by the lungs, resulting in increased systemic availability.

Recommendations: Monitor patients for increased effects of fentanyl if coadministered with propranolol.

Summary: There are data to show that coadministration of propranolol and fentanyl may lead to an increased entry of fentanyl into the systemic circulation.

Related Drugs: It is not known whether an interaction would occur between propranolol and other narcotic analgesics or between fentanyl and other beta blocking agents.

Mechanism: The mechanism for this interaction is not known. Data are available to show that propranolol can alter the amount of fentanyl which accumulates in the lungs.

Detailed Information: See *EDI*, 1/8.35

Gold Sodium Thiomalate-Naproxen

Significance: 2—moderately clinically significant

Potential Effects: Concurrent use of these agents may result in pneumonitis.

Recommendations: One or both agents should be discontinued if pneumonitis develops.

Summary: There are data to show that concurrent gold sodium thiomalate and naproxen have resulted in toxic pneumonitis.

Related Drugs: It is not known whether an interaction would occur between gold sodium thiomalate and other NSAIAs. A similar interaction may be expected between naproxen and other gold compounds.

Mechanism: Gold sodium thiomalate inhibits the lymphocyte proliferation and naproxen may cause additional immunosuppressive effects. Gold compounds may have an inhibitory effect on cell-mediated immune response and naproxen may have an additive effect.

Detailed Information: See *EDI*, 1/8.37

Gold Sodium Thiomalate-Tobacco

Significance: 3—minimally clinically significant

Recommendations: Further studies are needed to determine whether there is a similar effect on the uptake of gold by other cells, particularly monocytes, since the effect of gold on the function of the monocytes appears to be an important aspect of the antirheumatic activity of gold complexes. Therefore, no special precautions appear necessary at this time.

Summary: There are data to show that tobacco-smoking patients using gold sodium thiomalate have higher erythrocyte gold concentrations and lower plasma gold concentrations than non-smokers.

Related Drugs: Evidence shows that tobacco smoking raised erythrocyte gold concentrations in patients receiving auranofin. A similar interaction may occur between tobacco smoking and the injectable gold compound, aurothioglucose.

Mechanism: Tobacco smokers have elevated concentrations of thiocyanate and cyanide which form complexes with gold. Gold also binds to albumin and in erythrocytes.

Detailed Information: See *EDI*, 1/8.41

Ibuprofen-Baclofen

Significance: 3—minimally clinically significant

Potential Effects: Ibuprofen may cause a decrease in the clearance of baclofen, leading to toxicity.

Recommendations: Patients should be monitored for acute renal insufficiency and signs of baclofen toxicity (e.g., confusion, disorientation, bradycardia, hypothermia) when baclofen is administered with ibuprofen.

Summary: There are data to show that ibuprofen potentiates baclofen toxicity and increases serum blood urea nitrogen and creatinine levels.

Related Drugs: A similar interaction may occur between baclofen and other NSAIAs. There are no drugs related to baclofen.

Mechanism: Acute renal insufficiency secondary to ibuprofen therapy may result in a decreased clearance of baclofen and baclofen toxicity.

Detailed Information: See *EDI*, 1/8.43

Indomethacin-Aluminum Hydroxide

Significance: 3—minimally clinically significant

Potential Effects: Aluminum hydroxide may reduce the rate and extent of indomethacin absorption.

Recommendations: Although the concurrent use of these agents need not be avoided, it may be best to separate their administration by as much time as possible.

Summary: Aluminum hydroxide may reduce the rate and extent of indomethacin absorption.

Related Drugs: Due to conflicting results, it is difficult to determine if an interaction would occur between indomethacin and other antacids or between aluminum hydroxide and other NSAIAs.

Mechanism: Aluminum hydroxide may adsorb indomethacin or indomethacin may form an insoluble aluminum salt.

Detailed Information: See *EDI,* 1/8.50

Indomethacin-Aspirin

Significance: 3—minimally clinically significant

Recommendations: Because concurrent administration of these agents offers no therapeutic advantage over higher doses of either drug alone, concurrent use is not recommended. However, the clinical significance of this interaction appears to be minimal, and concomitant use need not be avoided.

Summary: There are data to show that large doses of aspirin may decrease the serum levels of indomethacin.

Related Drugs: Sodium salicylate has been shown to interact with other NSAIAs. Documentation is lacking regarding an interaction between indomethacin and other salicylates.

Mechanism: The mechanism is not fully known; however, aspirin decreases the bioavailability of oral indomethacin.

Detailed Information: See *EDI,* 1/9.00

Indomethacin-Cimetidine

Significance: 3—minimally clinically significant

Potential Effects: Cimetidine may decrease indomethacin levels.

Recommendations: Indomethacin and cimetidine may be given together since the therapeutic effectiveness of indomethacin was not shown to be affected.

Summary: There are data to show that patients who receive indomethacin and cimetidine have a decreased plasma concentration, urinary excretion and metabolites of indomethacin.

Related Drugs: Because of conflicting data, it is difficult to determine if an interaction would occur between cimetidine and other NSAIAs or between indomethacin and other H_2-receptor antagonists.

Mechanism: Cimetidine may decrease the absorption of indomethacin.

Detailed Information: See *EDI,* 1/10.01

Indomethacin-Nitroglycerin

Significance: 3—minimally clinically significant

Recommendations: When administered orally, indomethacin does not appear to adversely alter the beneficial effect of nitroglycerin on exercise tolerance in patients with stable angina of effort. Currently no information is available concerning the concomitant administration of these drugs in patients with unstable angina or myocardial infarction. If the drugs are coadministered, these latter patients should be observed for a possible reduction in anginal threshold and/or myocardial ischemia.

Summary: There are data to show that indomethacin reduces the vasodilator effect of nitroglycerin. However, all data do not support this.

Related Drugs: A similar interaction may occur between indomethacin and other nitrate derivatives and between nitroglycerin and other NSAIAs.

Mechanism: Nitroglycerin may stimulate the synthesis and release of prostacyclin and other prostaglandins which may be responsible for its vasodilatory effect. Indomethacin inhibits prostaglandin synthesis.

Detailed Information: See *EDI,* 1/10.10

Indomethacin-Phenylpropanolamine

Significance: 2—moderately clinically significant

Recommendations: If indomethacin and phenylpropanolamine are to be used together, the patient's blood pressure should be monitored frequently within the first hour after both agents are administered. If a hypertensive episode should occur, phentolamine has been used to successfully reduce the blood pressure.

Summary: There are data to show that taking a preparation containing phenylpropanolamine may lead to the development of serious hypertension.

Related Drugs: There are no documented reports involving phenylpropanolamine and other NSAIAs. It may be possible that other sympathomimetics and other NSAIAs may interact similarly.

Mechanism: Phenylpropanolamine is an indirect-acting sympathomimetic possessing vasoconstrictive activity, and indomethacin may suppress the synthesis of the prostaglandins which normally reduces blood pressure by vasodilatation.

Detailed Information: See *EDI,* 1/11.00

Indomethacin-Probenecid

Significance: 2—moderately clinically significant

Potential Effects: Probenecid may increase indomethacin levels, which may lead to an increase in side effects.

Recommendations: The use of these agents together need not be avoided. However, if increased side effects occur, the indomethacin dose may need to be decreased.

Summary: The administration of probenecid can reduce the plasma clearance and elevate the plasma levels of indomethacin.

Related Drugs: A similar interaction has been shown to occur between probenecid and ketoprofen and probenecid and naproxen and may be expected to occur between probenecid and other NSAIAs. It is unknown whether sulfinpyrazone interacts similarly with indomethacin.

Mechanism: Probenecid reduces nonrenal and possibly the biliary clearance of indomethacin. Probenecid may inhibit the glucuronidation of ketoprofen and renal excretion of ketoprofen conjugates.

Detailed Information: See *EDI*, 1/13.00

Meperidine-Chlorpromazine

Significance: 2—moderately clinically significant

Recommendations: The combination of meperidine and chlorpromazine is widely used as an operative premedicant. The dose of meperidine should be reduced by 25% to 50% when given with phenothiazines.

Summary: Chlorpromazine potentiates the sedative, hypotensive, and respiratory depressant effects of meperidine.

Related Drugs: Other phenothiazines, thioxanthenes, butyrophenones, dihydroindolones, and dibenzoxazepines may interact with meperidine. Fentanyl, hydromorphone and oxymorphone have been shown to interact with other phenothiazines. A similar interaction may occur with other narcotics.

Mechanism: Chlorpromazine increases the rate of appearance of normeperidine, a toxic metabolite of meperidine. Promethazine decreases the metabolism and prolongs the half-life of narcotic analgesics.

Detailed Information: See *EDI*, 1/15.00

Meperidine-Phenelzine

Significance: 1—highly clinically significant

Potential Effects: Concurrent use of these agents may result in potentially fatal CNS excitation or depression.

Recommendations: Concurrent use of these agents should be avoided. If the interaction occurs, IV corticosteroids may be beneficial. This interaction may occur several days after phenelzine is discontinued.

Summary: Concomitant use of meperidine and phenelzine may result in excitatory and depressant effects on the CNS leading to deep coma and death.

Related Drugs: Pargyline, tranylcypromine, isocarboxazid, furazolidone and procarbazine have been reported to interact with meperidine. Dextromethorphan has interacted with phenelzine resulting in death. The administration of propoxyphene with phenelzine has resulted in sedation and somnolence. Nalorphine has reportedly enhanced depression. All narcotics should be used cautiously in the presence of MAO inhibitors.

Mechanism: Although the mechanism is not specifically known, the combination of meperidine and MAO inhibitors has been shown to increase serotonin. MAO inhibitors also act as enzyme inhibitors, allowing accumulation of toxic levels of the agent.

Detailed Information: See *EDI*, 1/17.00

Meperidine-Phenobarbital

Significance: 3—minimally clinically significant

Recommendations: If increased sedation occurs or analgesic efficacy decreases following concurrent administration of phenobarbital and meperidine, the dosage of one or both agents should be adjusted accordingly.

Summary: The use of phenobarbital causes an increase in the clearance of meperidine, an increase in the cumulative excretion of normeperidine, and a decrease in the cumulative urinary excretion of meperidine.

Related Drugs: A similar interaction has been shown to occur with methadone and phenobarbital. The administration of propoxyphene has resulted in an increase in phenobarbital levels. Due to conflicting data, it is difficult to determine if an interaction would occur between phenobarbital and other narcotic analgesics. A similar interaction may be expected to occur between meperidine and other barbiturates.

Mechanism: Phenobarbital induces the hepatic metabolism of meperidine, resulting in an increased formation of normeperidine.

Detailed Information: See *EDI*, 1/18.10

Meperidine-Phenytoin

Significance: 3—minimally clinically significant

Recommendations: Oral doses of meperidine generate greater amounts of normeperidine than equal analgesic IV doses. Therefore, IV doses may be preferable to oral dosing in those receiving phenytoin. Also, to gain satisfactory analgesia, patients on long-term phenytoin therapy may require more frequent and larger doses of meperidine when phenytoin is being used concurrently.

Summary: The use of phenytoin may result in an increased clearance and plasma concentration of meperidine and a decreased elimination half-life and bioavailability.

Related Drugs: A similar interaction may occur between meperidine and other hydantoin anticonvulsants. An interaction may occur with other narcotic analgesics.

Mechanism: The probable mechanism of the increased elimination of meperidine may be due to the enhanced metabolism by phenytoin.

Detailed Information: See *EDI*, 1/19.00

Methadone-Ammonium Chloride

Significance: 3—minimally clinically significant

Recommendations: It may be best to measure steady-state plasma levels in patients complaining of withdrawal symptoms during concurrent ammonium chloride. This interaction may be useful in the treatment of methadone intoxication, since the total body clearance of methadone can be increased by approximately 50% by lowering urinary pH to 5.1.

Summary: There are data to show that concurrent administration of methadone and ammonium chloride causes an increase in the renal clearance of methadone.

Related Drugs: Since all narcotics are excreted unchanged to some extent, an interaction between ammonium chloride and the other narcotics is expected to occur. Other agents that acidify the urine may also interact with methadone.

Mechanism: The renal clearance of methadone is highly influenced by urinary pH and the clearance will increase as the pH decreases. Above a pH of 6, metabolism is the main route of elimination.

Detailed Information: See *EDI*, 1/20.10

Methadone-Diazepam

Significance: 3—minimally clinically significant

Potential Effects: Diazepam may increase the effects of methadone.

Recommendations: The concurrent use of methadone and diazepam need not be avoided; however, patients should be monitored for possible enhancement of methadone effects and respiratory depression when receiving concurrent diazepam.

Summary: There are data to show that the concurrent use of methadone and diazepam has resulted in an increase in pupillary constriction and scores on a subjective opioid effects rating scale.

Related Drugs: Propoxyphene has been shown to alter the pharmacokinetics of agents related to diazepam. There are data to show that meperidine given with diazepam or diazepam's related agents has resulted in a depressed respiratory rate. It is difficult to determine whether a similar effect would occur with diazepam and other narcotic analgesics or between methadone and other benzodiazepines.

Mechanism: The mechanism of this interaction is unknown; however, coadministration of methadone and diazepam does not result in altered pharmacokinetics of either agent.

Detailed Information: See *EDI,* 1/21.00

Methadone-Rifampin

Significance: 2—moderately clinically significant

Potential Effects: The addition of rifampin to the therapy of a patient maintained on methadone may result in an increase in methadone oral clearance and decreased serum levels, resulting in withdrawal symptoms.

Recommendations: In those patients receiving methadone, antituberculosis therapy with isoniazid should be well tolerated. However, rifampin alone or rifampin plus isoniazid may offer desirable therapeutic benefits. In those cases, methadone dosage may need to be increased within several days of beginning cotherapy.

Summary: Patients maintained on methadone in a maintenance program for addiction may experience withdrawal symptoms when rifampin therapy is instituted. Methadone plasma concentrations may be decreased by 33% to 68% in patients receiving concomitant rifampin compared with patients on nonrifampin regimens.

Related Drugs: Although documentation is lacking regarding a similar interaction with the other narcotics or between methadone and rifabutin, because of pharmacologic similarity an interaction may be expected to occur.

Mechanism: Rifampin decreased methadone plasma concentrations, increased the urinary excretion of methadone's major metabolite, and increased the oral clearance of methadone by fourfold. These results suggest that rifampin induces the hepatic metabolism of methadone. However, there was no consistent change in the methadone half-life, indicating that other mechanisms may be involved.

Detailed Information: See *EDI,* 1/23.00

Morphine-Amitriptyline

Significance: 3—minimally clinically significant

Potential Effects: Concurrent use of these agents may result in enhanced analgesia.

Recommendations: Concurrent use of these agents may increase morphine levels, and this may be beneficial in some patients, although not consistently. Choice of a tricyclic antidepressant should be based on clinical evaluation.

Summary: There are data to show that amitriptyline significantly increases the bioavailability of morphine. Amitriptyline and other tricyclic antidepressants may enhance the analgesic effect of morphine. However, there are contrasting data to show that tricyclic antidepressants do not produce analgesia.

Related Drugs: Because of conflicting results, it is difficult to determine if an interaction would occur between amitriptyline and other narcotics or between morphine and other tricyclic antidepressants.

Mechanism: The increased analgesic effect may be due to the synergy produced by the two agents in a common neural circuit. The metabolism of desipramine may also be inhibited by methadone.

Detailed Information: See *EDI,* 1/24.10

Morphine-Cimetidine

Significance: 2—moderately clinically significant

Recommendations: A severe interaction may occur with the concurrent use of these agents. If respiratory depression or other CNS side effects develop, the narcotic dose may need to be decreased or the drug may need to be discontinued. In one report, naloxone successfully reversed the CNS effects. However, no cause and effect relationship for an interaction has been established, and these agents need not be routinely avoided.

Summary: There are data to show that the administration of cimetidine and morphine have led to serious CNS side effects. This interaction may be exacerbated in patients with pre-existing breathing disorders.

Related Drugs: A similar interaction may occur between cimetidine and other narcotic analgesics. Documentation is lacking regarding an interaction between morphine and other H_2-receptor antagonists.

Mechanism: Cimetidine may potentially exaggerate the effect of morphine by competitive inhibition, by reducing hepatic clearance and blood flow, or by preventing hepatic microsomal oxidation.

Detailed Information: See *EDI,* 1/25.00

Morphine-Metoclopramide

Significance: 3—minimally clinically significant

Potential Effects: Metoclopramide may increase the sedation effects of oral extended release morphine.

Recommendations: Metoclopramide may increase the sedation and decrease the time to onset of sedation of morphine. Patients should be monitored for increased sedation when administering these agents concurrently.

Summary: There are data to show that the administration of morphine and metoclopramide may lead to a faster onset of action of morphine and increased levels of sedation.

Related Drugs: It is not known if a similar interaction would occur between metoclopramide and other narcotics. There are no drugs related to metoclopramide.

Mechanism: Metoclopramide increases gastric emptying; therefore, the rate of morphine absorbed may be increased and the time to peak concentration decreased.

Detailed Information: See *EDI,* 1/26.10

Naproxen-Cholestyramine

Significance: 3—minimally clinically significant

Potential Effects: Cholestyramine may delay the absorption of naproxen.

Recommendations: Any potential interaction may be avoided by administering naproxen two hours prior to or four to six hours after cholestyramine.

Summary: There are data to show that cholestyramine delays the absorption of naproxen and there may be a delay in pain relief before steady-state concentrations of naproxen are achieved.

Related Drugs: The half-life of tenoxicam and piroxicam were reduced when coadministered with cholestyramine. Phenylbutazone absorption was shown to be delayed by cholestyramine. Cholestyramine has been shown to delay the absorption of acidic drugs. A similar interaction may occur between naproxen and other anion exchange resins.

Mechanism: As the pH of the surrounding fluid becomes more basic, more naproxen is adsorbed to the resin and the resin slows the rate of absorption of naproxen.

Detailed Information: See *EDI*, 1/27.00

Oxyphenbutazone-Methandrostenolone

Significance: 3—minimally clinically significant

Recommendations: When oxyphenbutazone is administered concurrently with methandrostenolone, and possibly other anabolic steroids, the resulting increased serum oxyphenbutazone levels may increase the risk of adverse reactions. Patients receiving both agents should be monitored closely for oxyphenbutazone-induced toxicity.

Summary: When oxyphenbutazone and methandrostenolone are concurrently administered, serum oxyphenbutazone levels may be elevated.

Related Drugs: Because of conflicting results, it is difficult to determine whether an interaction would occur between sulfinpyrazone and methandrostenolone. A similar interaction may occur with other anabolic steroids and oxyphenbutazone.

Mechanism: Inhibition of oxyphenbutazone metabolism and the displacement of oxyphenbutazone from its binding site on serum albumin are the proposed mechanisms in this interaction.

Detailed Information: See *EDI*, 1/29.00

Phenylbutazone-Charcoal

Significance: 3—minimally clinically significant

Recommendations: It has been recommended that activated charcoal be administered as soon as possible after an acute phenylbutazone overdose to significantly reduce the absorption of phenylbutazone. However, if charcoal is not being used for phenylbutazone overdose, it may be advisable to separate the administration of phenylbutazone and charcoal by as much time as possible.

Summary: The absorption of phenylbutazone was greatly reduced with the concurrent administration of phenylbutazone.

Related Drugs: Oxyphenbutazone may interact similarly with activated charcoal. There are no drugs related to charcoal.

Mechanism: Charcoal adsorbs phenylbutazone and prevents its absorption.

Detailed Information: See *EDI*, 1/30.10

Phenylbutazone-Desipramine

Significance: 3—minimally clinically significant

Recommendations: Data on the clinical effects of this interaction are not available. Since both drugs are normally administered on a long-term basis and since only the rate, rather than the extent, of phenylbutazone absorption seems to be affected, the clinical significance may be minor. Patients may be monitored for possible decreased phenylbutazone effect if concurrent tricyclic antidepressant therapy is indicated.

Summary: Concurrent administration of phenylbutazone and desipramine has resulted in reduced plasma levels of phenylbutazone. This may lead to a diminished therapeutic effect of phenylbutazone.

Related Drugs: Oxyphenbutazone absorption is decreased by desipramine. Imipramine has been shown to decrease phenylbutazone absorption. It is unknown whether other tricyclic antidepressants or tetracyclic antidepressants will produce the same effect, but agents with significant anticholinergic effect may be expected to exert a similar effect.

Mechanism: Gastrointestinal absorption of phenylbutazone is inhibited or delayed from an anticholinergic inhibition of gastric emptying.

Detailed Information: See *EDI*, 1/31.00

Phenylbutazone-Misoprostol

Significance: 3—minimally clinically significant

Potential Effects: Enhanced phenylbutazone-induced neurological side effects may result.

Recommendations: Neurological side effects should be monitored with concurrent administration of phenylbutazone and misoprostol. Phenylbutazone may need to be discontinued.

Summary: There are data to show that the concurrent administration of phenylbutazone and misoprostol results in enhanced neurological side effects.

Related Drugs: There are no drugs related to misoprostol. It is not known whether an interaction would occur between misoprostol and other NSAIAs.

Mechanism: The mechanism of this interaction is unknown.

Detailed Information: See *EDI*, 1/33.00

Probenecid-Clofibrate

Significance: 3—minimally clinically significant

Recommendations: Although the clinical significance was not determined, it is important to monitor patients and use a lower dose of clofibrate when necessary.

Summary: The concurrent use of probenecid and clofibrate has been shown to cause a reduction in renal and metabolic clearance of clofibric acid (metabolite of clofibrate), leading to an increase in the therapeutic and toxic effects of clofibrate.

Related Drugs: There are no drugs related to clofibrate. An interaction may occur between clofibrate and sulfinpyrazone.

Mechanism: The decrease in clofibric acid binding may be caused by direct displacement from plasma protein binding sites. Through competitive inhibition, probenecid may inhibit the formation of clofibric acid glucuronide, leading to accumulation of the glucuronide in the plasma with subsequent hydrolysis to clofibric acid.

Detailed Information: See *EDI*, 1/35.00

Probenecid-Penicillamine

Significance: 3—minimally clinically significant

Recommendations: The concurrent use of these agents is con-traindicated in hyperuricemic cystinuric patients. However, the clinical significance of this interaction was not determined in patients receiving penicillamine for reasons other than cystinuria. Therefore, these patients should be observed for a decreased effect of penicillamine.

Summary: There are data to show that the coadministration of these agents has resulted in increased cystine excretion and decreased cystine-penicillamine mixed disulfide excretion in the urine, reducing the beneficial effects of penicillamine.

Related Drugs: There are no drugs related to penicillamine. It is not known if sulfinpyrazone would interact with penicillamine.

Mechanism: The mechanism of the interaction is unknown.

Detailed Information: See *EDI*, 1/36.10

Propoxyphene-Alcohol, Ethyl

Significance: 2—moderately clinically significant

Recommendations: It is unlikely that moderate amounts of alcohol and the usual doses of propoxyphene will result in a serious adverse reaction. However, patients should be advised about the dangers associated with concurrent ingestion of therapeutic doses of propoxyphene and large amounts of alcohol or exces-sive amounts of propoxyphene with any amount of alcohol. Naloxone has been used successfully to reverse propoxyphene-induced respiratory depression.

Summary: Concurrent ingestion of propoxyphene and alcohol may result in dangerous respiratory and CNS depression.

Related Drugs: An interaction may occur between alcohol and other narcotic analgesics.

Mechanism: Alcohol has been shown to increase the systemic avail-ability of propoxyphene and lower the minimum lethal blood con-centration of propoxyphene.

Detailed Information: See *EDI*, 1/37.00

Propoxyphene-Amphetamine

Significance: 3—minimally clinically significant

Recommendations: The use of amphetamines and other indirect acting sympathomimetics for the treatment of propoxyphene-induced CNS depression is not recommended. Naloxone, a nar-cotic antagonist, has been shown to be effective in controlling both respiratory depression and convulsive seizures following propoxyphene overdoses and has not been shown to have pro-convulsant activity.

Summary: Amphetamines, which may be used to treat propoxyphene-induced CNS depression, may increase the seizure potential of propoxyphene.

Related Drugs: A similar interaction is expected to occur with other indirect-acting sympathomimetics and propoxyphene. A like interaction is expected to occur with other narcotic analgesics and amphetamines.

Mechanism: Amphetamines produce CNS stimulation by indirectly increasing the release of norepinephrine and by impeding its neuronal reuptake.

Detailed Information: See *EDI*, 1/39.00

Propoxyphene-Charcoal
Significance: 3—minimally clinically significant
Recommendations: It has been recommended that activated charcoal be used as adjunct therapy in an acute propoxyphene overdose to adsorb any propoxyphene remaining in the stomach. A specific narcotic antagonist such as naloxone should be administered to counteract any respiratory depression or convulsions caused by an overdose of propoxyphene. However, if charcoal is not being used for propoxyphene overdose, the administration of the two agents should be separated by as much time as possible.
Summary: There are data to show that activated charcoal significantly reduces plasma levels of propoxyphene.
Related Drugs: Documentation is lacking regarding a similar interaction between charcoal and other narcotic analgesics.
Mechanism: Activated charcoal adsorbs propoxyphene in the gastrointestinal tract, limiting its absorption.
Detailed Information: See *EDI*, 1/40.10

Propoxyphene-Orphenadrine
Significance: 4—not clinically significant
Recommendations: Although it may be prudent to be aware of a possible interaction, the concurrent use of these agents need not be avoided. If CNS effects do occur, they are probably caused by either agent alone or by an additive effect and may require a reduction in the dose or discontinuation of one or both agents.
Summary: An alleged interaction with the concurrent use of these agents cannot be substantiated. The CNS effects observed were similar to those reported for either agent alone.
Related Drugs: A lack of interaction may be expected between orphenadrine and other narcotic analgesics, as well as between propoxyphene and other anti-parkinsonian anticholinergics.
Mechanism: The mechanism is unknown, but may be due to the combined effect on the central nervous system by both drugs.
Detailed Information: See *EDI*, 1/41.00

Sulfinpyrazone-Aspirin
Significance: 2—moderately clinically significant
Recommendations: Aspirin and other salicylates, especially in high doses, should be avoided in patients taking sulfinpyrazone for its uricosuric effect.
Summary: There are data to show that aspirin antagonizes the uricosuric activity of sulfinpyrazone and sulfinpyrazone-induced uric acid excretion may be significantly inhibited by large doses of aspirin. However, contrasting data have shown that aspirin significantly increases the plasma clearance of sulfinpyrazone.
Related Drugs: Sodium salicylate has been shown to interact in a similar manner with sulfinpyrazone. A like interaction is expected to occur with other salicylates. Phenylbutazone has been shown to block the uricosuric action of large amounts of aspirin and vice versa. Oxyphenbutazone and probenecid may interact with aspirin.
Mechanism: Sulfinpyrazone and salicylates compete for common binding sites on plasma proteins and prevent sulfinpyrazone from reaching its site of action.
Detailed Information: See *EDI*, 1/43.00

Sulfinpyrazone-Niacin

Significance: 3—minimally clinically significant

Recommendations: Patients should be monitored for a possible decrease in the uricosuric activity of sulfinpyrazone. Niacin may need to be discontinued if this occurs.

Summary: The concurrent use of sulfinpyrazone and niacin may inhibit the uricosuric action of sulfinpyrazone.

Related Drugs: There are no drugs related to niacin. An interaction may occur between niacin and probenecid.

Mechanism: It is not known if niacin interferes with the mechanism of action of sulfinpyrazone or if it is from the hyperuricemia that is a common side effect of niacin.

Detailed Information: See *EDI*, 1/45.00

Sulfinpyrazone-Probenecid

Significance: 4—not clinically significant

Recommendations: The data concerning this drug interaction are inconclusive; therefore, no particular action need be taken. However, concurrent use might be avoided because the possible benefits of such therapy would be negligible.

Summary: There are data to show that the concurrent use of sulfinpyrazone and probenecid may produce an increase in uric acid secretion.

Related Drugs: There is no documentation of a similar interaction between probenecid and phenylbutazone or its metabolite oxyphenbutazone.

Mechanism: Probenecid blocks the renal tubular secretion of sulfinpyrazone and its major active metabolite.

Detailed Information: See *EDI*, 1/47.00

Chapter Two

Anesthetic and Neuromuscular Blocking Agents' Drug Interactions

Bupivacaine-Diazepam

Significance: 3—minimally clinically significant

Potential Effects: Administration of diazepam prior to bupivacaine administration may result in increased serum levels of bupivacaine.

Recommendations: Patients receiving diazepam premedication prior to use of epidural bupivacaine should be closely monitored for an increase in the pharmacologic effects of bupivacaine. The dose of bupivacaine may have to be adjusted.

Summary: There are data to indicate that administration of diazepam will alter bupivacaine pharmacokinetics, resulting in increased levels of bupivacaine.

Related Drugs: An interaction may occur between bupivacaine and the other benzodiazepines, which undergo phase I metabolism. The other local anesthetics would be expected to interact similarly with diazepam.

Mechanism: Diazepam may inhibit the metabolism of bupivacaine, which has the same route of metabolism.

Detailed Information: See *EDI,* 2/0.01

Bupivacaine-Ritodrine

Significance: 2—moderately clinically significant

Potential Effects: Concurrent use of these agents may result in beta adrenergic stimulation of the heart, resulting in hypotension and tachycardia.

Recommendations: Caution should be used with patients who have received ritodrine for preterm labor when an anesthetic is to be used during cesarean section. Anesthesia may have to be deferred to allow the betamimetic effects of ritodrine to subside. Patient's cardiac status should be closely monitored.

Summary: There are data to show that coadministration of bupivacaine and ritodrine has resulted in ventricular tachycardia, fibrillation and hypotension, necessitating cardiopulmonary resuscitation.

Related Drugs: A similar interaction can be expected to occur with other local anesthetic agents and ritodrine. There are no drugs related to ritodrine.

Mechanism: While the mechanism of this interaction is unknown, it is thought that unopposed beta-adrenergic stimulation of the heart occurred as a result of the residual effects of ritodrine and the sympathetic blockade of bupivacaine.

Detailed Information: See *EDI,* 2/0.03

Enflurane-Isoniazid

Significance: 3—minimally clinically significant

Recommendations: If a patient receiving isoniazid is given enflurane anesthesia, renal function should be monitored, since enflurane induced nephrotoxicity may occur as a result of elevated serum fluoride levels induced by isoniazid in some patients.

Summary: There are data to show that administration of isoniazid and the use of enflurane anesthesia resulted in significantly elevated serum fluoride levels with transient polyuria.

Related Drugs: A similar interaction may be expected to occur between isoniazid and other fluorinated inhalation anesthetics. There is evidence that isoniazid treatment increased the hepatic microsomal defluorination of isoflurane, methoxyflurane and enflurane. There are no drugs related to isoniazid.

Mechanism: Isoniazid may increase the metabolism of enflurane by enzyme induction.

Detailed Information: See *EDI,* 2/0.10

Ether-Neomycin

Significance: 1—highly clinically significant

Recommendations: It is important to be prepared to treat the neuromuscular and respiratory depression that is frequently produced by this interaction, particularly if the aminoglycoside is administered intraperitoneally. If neuromuscular blockade and respiratory depression are encountered, the intravenous use of neostigmine (0.2 to 2.5mg), calcium (1G), and possibly sodium bicarbonate (dose not reported), either alone or concurrently, may be helpful in reversing the blockade in some but not all patients. The administration of analeptic agents (e.g., doxapram and nikethamide) is of no value. Supportive care and ventilatory assistance should be administered and continued until the neuromuscular blockade has passed. Vital signs should be monitored because secondary circulatory collapse may occur, and volume replacement should be administered as necessary.

Summary: Depression of neuromuscular transmission can be produced independently with ether or neomycin. There are data to show that the coadministration of these drugs may enhance respiratory depression or may prolong neuromuscular blockade.

Related Drugs: Inhalation anesthetic agents such as cyclopropane, halothane, methoxyflurane, and nitrous oxide have been reported to interact with neomycin. A similar interaction may occur with other inhalation anesthetics and neomycin. Other aminoglycoside antibiotics are known to interact with ether. A similar interaction is expected to occur between ether and the other aminoglycosides, as well as the nonaminoglycoside antibiotics.

Mechanism: This interaction may be from a synergistic effect of the neuromuscular blocking properties of both agents due to reduced sensitivity of the postjunctional membrane and interference of transmitter release.

Detailed Information: See *EDI*, 2/1.00

Etomidate-Verapamil

Significance: 3—minimally clinically significant

Potential Effects: Concurrent use of verapamil and etomidate may result in prolonged action of etomidate.

Recommendations: The concurrent use of verapamil and etomidate may result in a prolongation of anesthesia and Cheynes-Stokes respirations. Respiratory function should be monitored, and additional ventilatory support may be required.

Summary: The coadministration of verapamil may prolong the duration of action of etomidate anesthesia, leading to classic Cheynes-Stokes respirations and necessitating ventilatory assistance.

Related Drugs: It is not known whether an interaction would occur between etomidate and other calcium channel blocking agents. There are no drugs related to etomidate.

Mechanism: The mechanism of this interaction is not known.

Detailed Information: See *EDI*, 2/2.50

Gallamine-Diazepam

Significance: 3—minimally clinically significant

Potential Effects: Diazepam may potentiate the neuromuscular blockade of gallamine.

Recommendations: The use of these agents together need not be avoided. However, patients should be monitored for an increased neuromuscular blockade when gallamine is given with diazepam.

Summary: There are data to show that administration of diazepam increased the magnitude of the neuromuscular blockade of gallamine and caused respiratory depression. However, contrasting data indicate that there is no interaction between these agents.

Related Drugs: No interaction was shown to occur between diazepam and tubocurarine or pancuronium. Because of conflicting results, it is difficult to determine if an interaction would occur between diazepam and other neuromuscular blocking agents. Diazepam was shown to reduce the neuromuscular blocking activity of the depolarizing agent succinylcholine; however, conflicting data are available. Because of conflicting results, it is not known if an interaction would occur between gallamine and other benzodiazepines.

Mechanism: The mechanism of this interaction is unknown. Diazepam may exert a peripheral action involving direct muscle depression and/or limit the release of acetylcholine, prolonging the neuromuscular blockade produced by gallamine.

Detailed Information: See *EDI,* 2/3.00

Halothane-Epinephrine

Significance: 1—highly clinically significant

Potential Effects: The administration of these agents together may result in ventricular arrhythmias.

Recommendations: Avoid the use of these agents together. If IV epinephrine is necessary, the use of nitrous oxide should be considered.

Summary: There are data to indicate that administration of epinephrine during halothane anesthesia may lead to serious ventricular arrhythmias.

Related Drugs: Norepinephrine has been shown to interact with halothane in a manner similar to epinephrine. A similar interaction is expected to occur with isoproterenol, terbutaline, the other direct-acting sympathomimetics, the indirect-acting sympathomimetics or the mixed-acting sympathomimetics when coadministered with halothane. Chloroform, methoxyflurane, or enflurane when coadministered with epinephrine will increase the incidence of arrhythmias. A similar interaction is expected to occur between epinephrine and other inhalation anesthetics.

Mechanism: Although the exact mechanism for this interaction is unknown, the anesthetics' ability to precipitate arrhythmias is enhanced by events that stimulate the release of endogenous catecholamines.

Detailed Information: See *EDI,* 2/5.00

Halothane-Phenytoin

Significance: 3—minimally clinically significant

Recommendations: Since it is not clear that phenytoin increases the likelihood of halothane-induced toxicity, no additional precautions are warranted. However, if patients receiving phenytoin show signs of hepatitis (fever, elevated transaminase levels, etc.), close monitoring of serum phenytoin concentrations and clinical signs of phenytoin toxicity (e.g., nystagmus, blurring of vision, ataxia) is indicated, and appropriate changes in doses should be made.

Summary: There are data to show that phenytoin may increase the likelihood of halothane-induced hepatotoxicity and the hepatic dysfunction may reduce the clearance of phenytoin, resulting in toxicity.

Related Drugs: Phenytoin and phenobarbital have been implicated in a patient's fatal fluroxene-induced hepatotoxicity. The hepatotoxicity is usually not seen with the other halogenated anesthetic agents; therefore, a similar interaction is not expected to occur. The other hydantoin anticonvulsants may interact with halothane similar to phenytoin.

Mechanism: Hepatotoxicity following halothane anesthesia is expected. Phenytoin metabolism is dependent on the liver microsomal system, and injury to the microsomal system from any source would be expected to inhibit phenytoin metabolism.

Detailed Information: See *EDI,* 2/7.00

Halothane-Rifampin

Significance: 2—moderately clinically significant

Recommendations: Although a cause and effect relationship was never clearly established, these agents should be used with caution and only when necessary.

Summary: There are data to show that coadministration of rifampin and isoniazid may lead to serious hepatotoxicity.

Related Drugs: There are no drugs related to rifampin. A similar interaction is not expected to occur between rifampin and other halogenated inhalation anesthetics since hepatotoxicity is usually not observed with these agents.

Mechanism: The mechanism is unknown. However, it has been suggested that the interaction is from the combined effects of the two agents on the liver.

Detailed Information: See *EDI,* 2/9.00

Ketamine-Diazepam

Significance: 2—moderately clinically significant

Recommendations: The clinician should be aware of this interaction, since a patient pretreated with diazepam may need a lower dose of ketamine.

Summary: There are data to show that when diazepam and ketamine were coadministered, patients experienced less initial tachycardia and hypertension. Patients also required a significantly lower dose of ketamine.

Related Drugs: Documentation is lacking regarding a similar interaction between ketamine and other benzodiazepines. There are no drugs related to ketamine.

Mechanism: The mechanism of this interaction is unknown.

Detailed Information: See *EDI,* 2/11.00

Ketamine-Halothane

Significance: 2—moderately clinically significant

Recommendations: When halothane anesthesia is used, ketamine should be administered with caution. The patient's blood pressure should be carefully monitored, because the hypotension has been severe enough in some reports to necessitate the use of a vasopressor.

Summary: There are data to show that during halothane anesthesia, the concurrent use of ketamine caused a rapid increase in arteriolar peripheral resistance and a decrease in cardiac output, stroke volume and blood pressure.

Related Drugs: Similar effects were seen when ketamine was used with enflurane. A similar interaction is expected to occur with other halogenated inhalation anesthetics.

Mechanism: It is possible that halothane, acting as a sympatholytic, uncovers the direct negative inotropic effects of ketamine, resulting in significant hypotension.

Detailed Information: See *EDI,* 2/13.00

Ketamine-Thyroid

Significance: 3—minimally clinically significant

Recommendations: Until further clinical studies are done, the concurrent use of these agents need not be avoided. However, if this interaction does occur, propranolol may be useful since it has been shown to control both the heart rate and the increase in blood pressure.

Summary: There are data to show that coadministration of thyroid replacement and ketamine resulted in hypertension and tachycardia.

Related Drugs: There are no drugs related to ketamine. A similar interaction is expected to occur between ketamine and other thyroid drugs.

Mechanism: The mechanism of this interaction is unknown. Ketamine produces hypertension and tachycardia, although less severely. Therefore, it is believed that thyroid replacement is the offender in this interaction.

Detailed Information: See *EDI,* 2/15.00

Methoxyflurane-Secobarbital

Significance: 2—moderately clinically significant

Recommendations: Methoxyflurane should be avoided in patients who are receiving barbiturates. If the use of methoxyflurane is necessary, the barbiturate should be discontinued well in advance of administering this anesthetic.

Summary: There are data to show that coadministration of methoxyflurane and secobarbital will lead to renal insufficiency.

Related Drugs: A similar interaction has been documented with pentobarbital and methoxyflurane. A similar interaction between secobarbital and other halogenated anesthetic agents would not be expected. A similar interaction is expected to occur between methoxyflurane and other barbiturates.

Mechanism: Barbiturates, which induce hepatic microsomal enzymes, lead to an increased production of toxic metabolites, increasing the incidence of nephrotoxicity.

Detailed Information: See *EDI,* 2/17.00

Methoxyflurane-Tetracycline

Significance: 2—moderately clinically significant

Recommendations: Until more is known concerning the possible effects of concurrent tetracycline and methoxyflurane administration on renal function, these drugs should not be used together. When alternate therapy is not possible, renal status should be carefully monitored. Concurrent administration of methoxyflurane and other antibiotics known to be nephrotoxic (e.g., aminoglycosides, polymyxin) should be avoided.

Summary: There are data to show that the concurrent administration of tetracycline and methoxyflurane may result in severe nephrotoxicity.

Related Drugs: Methoxyflurane is expected to interact with the other tetracyclines. Doxycycline may not exhibit a similar toxicity. Methoxyflurane is the only general anesthetic implicated as a causative agent of renal toxicity.

Mechanism: The concurrent administration of tetracycline and methoxyflurane may result in additive nephrotoxic effects or create a synergistic basis for the toxicity.

Detailed Information: See *EDI*, 2/19.00

Metocurine-Phenytoin

Significance: 2—moderately clinically significant

Potential Effects: Phenytoin may decrease the extent and length of neuromuscular blockade produced by metocurine.

Recommendations: Patients receiving phenytoin should be monitored for a decreased response to metocurine when it is administered concurrently. The metocurine dose may need to be increased. Atracurium may be considered as an alternative agent to metocurine.

Summary: There are data to show that administration of phenytoin with metocurine may decrease the extent of neuromuscular blockade and higher metocurine plasma concentrations were required to obtain neuromuscular blockade.

Related Drugs: A comparable interaction was shown to occur between pancuronium, vecuronium or atracurium with phenytoin; however, all data did not support this. Because of conflicting results, it is difficult to determine if an interaction would occur between phenytoin and other nondepolarizing neuromuscular blocking agents or depolarizing agents. A similar interaction is expected to occur between metocurine and other hydantoin anticonvulsants.

Mechanism: Phenytoin may increase anticholinesterase activity, resulting in a higher acetylcholine concentration at the neuromuscular junction.

Detailed Information: See *EDI*, 2/20.10

Nitric Oxide-Alcohol, Ethyl

Significance: 2—moderately clinically significant

Potential Effects: A lower motor neuron disorder may result when nitric oxide is administered to a patient with chronic ethanol exposure.

Recommendations: Caution should be exercised when administering nitric oxide to patients with a history of chronic ethanol exposure.

Summary: Nitric oxide may have caused extensive lower motor neuron disorder in a patient with chronic ethanol exposure.

Related Drugs: There are no drugs related to nitric oxide, and it is not known if nitric oxide will react with other alcohols or glycols.

Mechanism: It is postulated that nitric oxide may mediate excitotoxicity generated by chronic alcohol use, resulting in neuronal disturbances.

Detailed Information: See *EDI,* 2/20.50

Pancuronium-Aminophylline

Significance: 2—moderately clinically significant

Recommendations: Patients should be monitored during concurrent use of these agents, and the dose of the neuromuscular blocking agent may need to be increased.

Summary: There are data to show that the concurrent use of pancuronium and aminophylline causes resistance to the neuromuscular blockade, possibly leading to supraventricular tachycardia.

Related Drugs: There is a lack of documentation regarding a similar interaction between pancuronium and other theophylline derivatives, as well as an interaction between theophylline derivatives and other neuromuscular blocking agents.

Mechanism: The mechanism of this interaction is unknown.

Detailed Information: See *EDI,* 2/21.00

Pancuronium-Azathioprine

Significance: 3—minimally clinically significant

Recommendations: Concurrent use or subsequent use of azathioprine following pancuronium administration should be avoided if neuromuscular blockade is desired. If concomitant use is necessary, the dose of pancuronium may need to be increased.

Summary: There are data to show that the administration of azathioprine antagonized the neuromuscular blocking action of pancuronium.

Related Drugs: There is evidence of azathioprine and gallamine reversing the neuromuscular blockade produced by tubocurarine. A similar interaction is expected to occur with other nondepolarizing neuromuscular blocking agents. The effects of succinylcholine have been shown to be potentiated by azathioprine. Documentation is lacking on whether the other thiopurine antineoplastic agents interact similarly with pancuronium.

Mechanism: Azathioprine allows cyclic AMP to accumulate. This prolongs the time of depolarization, causing a generation of repetitive activity, and increases transmitter release.

Detailed Information: See *EDI,* 2/23.00

Pancuronium-Carbamazepine

Significance: 3—minimally clinically significant

Potential Effects: Carbamazepine decreases the recovery time from pancuronium neuromuscular blockade.

Recommendations: Patients receiving carbamazepine should be monitored for a more rapid recovery from neuromuscular blockade when pancuronium is administered. The dose of pancuronium may need to be adjusted.

Summary: There are data to show that coadministration of carbamazepine and pancuronium leads to a shorter recovery from neuromuscular blockade.

Related Drugs: It is not known if a similar interaction would occur between carbamazepine and other nondepolarizing neuromuscular blocking agents or the depolarizing neuromuscular blocking agents. There are no drugs related to carbamazepine.

Mechanism: The mechanism of this interaction is not known.

Detailed Information: See *EDI*, 2/24.10

Pancuronium-Clindamycin

Significance: 2—moderately clinically significant

Recommendations: These agents should be used concurrently with caution and only if concomitant use is necessary. It is important to be aware of prolonged neuromuscular blockade, and ventilatory assistance should be available if necessary.

Summary: There are data to show that clindamycin prolongs the neuromuscular blockade produced by pancuronium.

Related Drugs: A similar interaction with clindamycin or lincomycin and two nondepolarizing neuromuscular blocking agents has been documented. A similar interaction may be expected to occur with the other nondepolarizing neuromuscular blocking agents. Succinylcholine has also been reported to be enhanced by clindamycin.

Mechanism: There may be an additive or synergistic pharmacologic activity with these agents.

Detailed Information: See *EDI*, 2/25.00

Pancuronium-Cyclosporine

Significance: 2—moderately clinically significant

Potential Effects: Cyclosporine may prolong the neuromuscular blocking effects of pancuronium.

Recommendations: Monitor patients carefully for prolonged neuromuscular blockade when these agents are used concurrently. Atracurium may be an alternative to pancuronium; however, studies are lacking.

Summary: There are data to show that coadministration of cyclosporine may prolong the neuromuscular blocking effects of pancuronium, leading to muscle paralysis, increased respiratory distress, blood pressure, heart rate, and respiratory rate.

Related Drugs: A similar interaction has been reported between cyclosporine and vecuronium. A similar interaction is expected to occur with other nondepolarizing neuromuscular blocking agents and cyclosporine. Succinylcholine is expected to interact to a lesser extent with cyclosporine. There are no drugs related to cyclosporine.

Mechanism: A nonionic surfactant used as a vehicle in cyclosporine may interfere with pancuronium, increasing the concentration at the neuromuscular junction.

Detailed Information: See *EDI*, 2/26.50

Pancuronium-Furosemide

Significance: 3—minimally clinically significant

Potential Effects: Furosemide may prolong the neuromuscular blockade of pancuronium because of hypokalemia.

Recommendations: Avoiding hypokalemia can reduce the potential risks of this interaction in a patient receiving diuretic therapy who will be given pancuronium. The serum potassium level should be determined and corrected if necessary to avoid the possibility of prolonged neuromuscular blockade from a hypokalemic state.

Summary: There are data to show that administration of furosemide with pancuronium causes an increase in recovery times.

Related Drugs: Theoretically, an enhanced neuromuscular blockade can be predicted to arise from potassium-depleting diuretics and d-tubocurarine. A similar interaction can occur between tubocurarine and other potassium-depleting diuretics and thiazide-related diuretics, as well as with other neuromuscular blocking agents and furosemide.

Mechanism: The neuromuscular function is potassium dependent and the disruption of extracellular potassium levels by furosemide could enhance actions of pancuronium.

Detailed Information: See *EDI,* 2/26.70

Pancuronium-Hydrocortisone

Significance: 3—minimally clinically significant

Recommendations: If the patient is receiving corticosteroids, or if corticosteroids may be used during surgery, the dose of the neuromuscular blocking agent may need to be increased.

Summary: There are data to show that following hydrocortisone administration, there was a partial recovery from the neuromuscular blockade produced by pancuronium.

Related Drugs: There is evidence to show that prednisone may decrease the neuromuscular blockade. A similar interaction is expected to occur between pancuronium and other corticosteroids or between hydrocortisone and other neuromuscular blocking agents.

Mechanism: This interaction may involve competition at the myoneural junction, altered protein binding, or induction of hepatic biotransformation.

Detailed Information: See *EDI,* 2/27.00

Pancuronium-Lithium Carbonate

Significance: 3—minimally clinically significant

Recommendations: Pancuronium or other neuromuscular blocking agents should be used with caution in patients taking lithium carbonate. Patients should be closely monitored, and ventilatory assistance should be provided as necessary.

Summary: There are data to show that lithium carbonate enhanced and prolonged the neuromuscular blockade actions of pancuronium. However, there are conflicting data that did not find similar results.

Related Drugs: There are no drugs related to lithium carbonate. There is evidence that lithium and succinylcholine administration has led to prolonged apnea; however, this has been disputed with other data. The effect of lithium on gallamine and tubocurarine is not clear. The neuromuscular blockade of succinylcholine and pancuronium was prolonged by lithium. Because of conflicting results, it is difficult to determine whether an interaction would occur between lithium carbonate and other nondepolarizing neuromuscular blocking agents.

Mechanism: Although the mechanism of this interaction is unknown, it has been suggested that it may be caused by the changes in electrolyte balance induced by lithium and the reduction of acetylcholine.

Detailed Information: See *EDI,* 2/29.00

Pancuronium-Nitroglycerin

Significance: 3—minimally clinically significant

Recommendations: Until further clinical studies are performed in humans, it is important to be aware of the possible prolongation of neuromuscular blockade. If nitroglycerin is to be used, it may be advisable to use a noninteracting neuromuscular blocking agent. Alternatively, neostigmine has been shown to rapidly and completely reverse muscle paralysis, even during the prolongation produced by nitroglycerin.

Summary: There are animal data to show that nitroglycerin used prior to pancuronium administration increases the duration and depth of neuromuscular blockade.

Related Drugs: The neuromuscular blockade produced by tubocurarine, succinylcholine, and gallamine was not prolonged by nitroglycerin. Due to conflicting reports, it is difficult to determine whether an interaction would occur between nitroglycerin and other nondepolarizing neuromuscular blocking agents, or between pancuronium and other nitrates.

Mechanism: The mechanism of this interaction is unknown. However, this interaction is not caused by an altered plasma clearance of pancuronium, circulatory changes, or changes in the acid-base or electrolyte balance.

Detailed Information: See *EDI,* 2/31.00

Pancuronium-Thiotepa (Triethylene Thiophosphoramide)

Significance: 3—minimally clinically significant

Recommendations: The concurrent use of these agents should be used with caution, and ventilatory assistance should be available.

Summary: There are data to show that administration of pancuronium followed by thiotepa may lead to rapid and prolonged respiratory depression.

Related Drugs: Documentation is lacking of a similar interaction between other neuromuscular blocking agents and other antineoplastic alkylating agents.

Mechanism: The mechanism of this interaction is unknown. However, it has been suggested that the presence of myasthenia gravis may be a predisposing and critical factor.

Detailed Information: See *EDI,* 2/33.00

Propofol-Aminophylline

Significance: 3—minimally clinically significant

Potential Effects: Aminophylline may increase dosage requirements for propofol.

Recommendations: Until additional studies are forthcoming, the patient should be monitored and the dose of propofol should be adjusted as necessary for the required effect.

Summary: There are data to show that the propofol dosage required for sedation was increased by concomitant aminophylline.

Related Drugs: It is not known whether an interaction would occur between propofol and other theophylline derivatives. There are no drugs related to propofol.

Mechanism: The mechanism of this interaction is not known.

Detailed Information: See *EDI,* 2/34.07

Propofol-Diazepam

Significance: 3—minimally clinically significant

Potential Effects: Concurrent use of diazepam and propofol may result in prolonged recovery time.

Recommendations: The patient should be monitored for the possibility of prolonged recovery time with concurrent use of propofol and diazepam.

Summary: There are data to show that the effects of propofol may be increased with concomitant diazepam and cause prolonged recovery time. However, all data do not support this.

Related Drugs: It is not known whether an interaction would occur between propofol and other benzodiazepines. There are no drugs related to propofol.

Mechanism: The mechanism of this interaction is not known, although the possibility exists that Cremophor® (a nonionic emulsifying agent in propofol) may be a factor leading to prolonged recovery time.

Detailed Information: See *EDI*, 2/34.05

Succinylcholine-Cimetidine

Significance: 2—moderately clinically significant

Potential Effects: Cimetidine may prolong the neuromuscular blockade of succinylcholine.

Recommendations: Patients receiving cimetidine should be observed for an increased duration of action of succinylcholine. Ventilatory assistance should be provided if necessary. Ranitidine may be an alternative to cimetidine in some cases.

Summary: There are data to show that the duration of action of succinylcholine significantly increased with concurrent cimetidine. However, all data do not support this.

Related Drugs: There is documentation of a similar interaction with ranitidine and vecuronium. Because the mechanism of the interaction is not known, it is not known if a similar interaction would occur between succinylcholine and other H_2-receptor antagonists or between cimetidine and other nondepolarizing neuromuscular blocking agents.

Mechanism: The mechanism of this interaction is not known.

Detailed Information: See *EDI*, 2/34.10

Succinylcholine-Cyclophosphamide

Significance: 2—moderately clinically significant

Recommendations: Although the information concerning an interaction between the two drugs is limited, it would be prudent to either determine pseudocholinesterase levels before administering these drugs concurrently in a patient on cyclophosphamide therapy, or avoid the concomitant use of these agents. Alternatively, a neuromuscular blocking agent other than succinylcholine could be used with cyclophosphamide.

Summary: There are data to show that cyclophosphamide may potentiate the neuromuscular blockade produced by succinylcholine by inhibiting its metabolism leading to prolonged respiratory depression.

Related Drugs: The nondepolarizing neuromuscular blocking agents would not be expected to interact with cyclophosphamide. Other cytotoxic drugs that inhibit pseudocholinesterase would be expected to interact in a similar manner with succinylcholine.

Mechanism: Cyclophosphamide decreases pseudocholinesterase activity and this decrease may prolong the neuromuscular blockade produced by succinylcholine.

Detailed Information: See *EDI,* 2/35.00

Succinylcholine-Dexpanthenol

Significance: 4—not clinically significant

Recommendations: The possibility of an interaction between succinylcholine and dexpanthenol at usual doses appears to be unlikely. Therefore, no additional precautions are necessary when these compounds are used concurrently.

Summary: There are data to show that dexpanthenol prolonged the respiratory depression induced by succinylcholine; however, contrasting data are available.

Related Drugs: There are no reports of this interaction occurring with the nondepolarizing neuromuscular blocking agents.

Mechanism: The excess acetylcholine produced by dexpanthenol may saturate its enzymatic metabolic pathway and then compete with succinylcholine for metabolism.

Detailed Information: See *EDI,* 2/37.00

Succinylcholine-Diethylstilbestrol

Significance: 2—moderately clinically significant

Recommendations: It may be advisable to measure plasma cholinesterase levels before administration of succinylcholine in patients receiving estrogens or oral contraceptive agents containing estrogens.

Summary: There are data to show that the use of succinylcholine with diethylstilbestrol may result in prolonged ventilatory inadequacy secondary to severe depression of plasma cholinesterase.

Related Drugs: Oral contraceptive agents containing estrogens can significantly reduce plasma cholinesterase levels. A similar interaction is expected to occur with other estrogens. A similar interaction with diethylstilbestrol would not be expected to occur with the nondepolarizing neuromuscular blocking agents.

Mechanism: It has been suggested that estrogens reduce the synthesis or release of cholinesterase in the liver, resulting in a decreased succinylcholine degradation.

Detailed Information: See *EDI,* 2/38.10

Succinylcholine-Echothiophate

Significance: 2—moderately clinically significant

Recommendations: If a patient is receiving echothiophate, it would be prudent to determine pseudocholinesterase activity before administering succinylcholine. It may be best to decrease the dose of succinylcholine or use a nondepolarizing neuromuscular blocking agent.

Summary: There are data to show that the effect of succinylcholine may be prolonged in patients receiving echothiophate ophthalmic preparations, resulting in prolonged neuromuscular blockade and apnea.

Related Drugs: A similar interaction may occur between succinylcholine and other ophthalmic cholinesterase inhibitors. It is not known to what extent demecarium and physostigmine would interact with succinylcholine. The nondepolarizing neuromuscular blocking agents would not be expected to interact with echothiophate in a similar manner.

Mechanism: Concurrent echothiophate may prevent the metabolism of succinylcholine.

Detailed Information: See *EDI*, 2/38.30

Succinylcholine-Isoflurane

Significance: 2—moderately clinically significant

Potential Effects: Isoflurane may increase succinylcholine phase II neuromuscular blockade.

Recommendations: Patients should be closely observed during concurrent use of these agents because a decreased succinylcholine dose may be necessary.

Summary: There are data to show that isoflurane potentiated the neuromuscular blockade produced by succinylcholine leading to tachyphylaxis.

Related Drugs: Enflurane and halothane have been shown to have a comparable interaction when administered with succinylcholine. Documentation is lacking for a similar interaction between succinylcholine and other halogenated inhalation anesthetics. Prolonged duration of action was observed for pipecuronium, atracurium and pancuronium when given immediately after enflurane. The effects of atracurium are potentiated by halothane. A similar interaction is expected to occur with the nondepolarizing neuromuscular blocking agents and isoflurane. Enflurane potentiates the neuromuscular blockade of tubocurarine and halothane and decreases the ED50 of tubocurarine and pancuronium.

Mechanism: The mechanism of this interaction is not fully known. An increase in muscle blood flow induced by isoflurane may be an explanation. The potentiation of the neuromuscular blocking agents is likely to be caused by decreased acetylcholine at the neuromuscular junction.

Detailed Information: See *EDI*, 2/39.00

Succinylcholine-Lidocaine

Significance: 2—moderately clinically significant

Recommendations: Patients who receive lidocaine, especially in large intravenous doses concomitantly with succinylcholine, should be observed closely to determine the need for artificial ventilation.

Summary: There are data to show that lidocaine may prolong and intensify the neuromuscular blocking effect and duration of apnea produced by succinylcholine.

Related Drugs: Tubocurarine interacts with lidocaine in a manner similar to succinylcholine. A similar interaction is expected to occur with other nondepolarizing neuromuscular blocking agents. Local anesthetics have been reported to interact similarly with succinylcholine.

Mechanism: The mechanism of this interaction has not been fully established. Lidocaine may produce neuromuscular blockade; it displaces succinylcholine from plasma protein and pseudocholinesterase, resulting in greater amounts of succinylcholine. The respiratory depression is probably through a CNS effect.

Detailed Information: See *EDI*, 2/41.00

Succinylcholine-Metoclopramide

Significance: 3—minimally clinically significant

Potential Effects: Metoclopramide may prolong the neuromuscular blockade of succinylcholine.

Recommendations: The dosage of succinylcholine may need to be reduced when coadministered with metoclopramide.

Summary: There are data to show that a prolongation of succinyl-choline neuromuscular blockade occurred with concurrent meto-clopramide.

Related Drugs: It is not known whether an interaction would occur between metoclopramide and other nondepolarizing neuromuscular blocking agents. There are no drugs related to metoclopramide.

Mechanism: The mechanism of this interaction is unknown. The effect is thought to be related to the prolongation of the neuromuscular blockade induced by succinylcholine.

Detailed Information: See *EDI*, 2/46.10

Succinylcholine-Neostigmine

Significance: 2—moderately clinically significant

Recommendations: The concurrent use of succinylcholine and an anticholinesterase agent should be avoided during the depolarizing phase of the neuromuscular blockade and should only be used with great caution, if at all, in the desensitizing phase. If concomitant use is necessary, closely monitor the patient and provide ventilatory assistance if necessary.

Summary: There are data to show that neostigmine may antagonize or enhance the neuromuscular blocking effect of succinylcholine.

Related Drugs: Edrophonium and pyridostigmine prolonged the neuromuscular blockade produced by succinylcholine. A similar interaction is expected to occur between succinylcholine and other anticholinesterases. The nondepolarizing neuromuscular blocking agents would not be expected to interact in a similar manner; however, documentation is lacking.

Mechanism: The action of neostigmine effectively increases the concentration of acetylcholine at the neuromuscular junction by decreasing its rate of hydrolysis.

Detailed Information: See *EDI*, 2/43.00

Succinylcholine-Procainamide

Significance: 3—minimally clinically significant

Recommendations: Patients receiving succinylcholine and procainamide concurrently should be observed for signs of neuromuscular blockade, especially prolonged apnea. Artificial ventilation may be required for a longer time in such patients.

Summary: There are data to show that procainamide may prolong and intensify the neuromuscular blockade produced by succinylcholine.

Related Drugs: The same interaction with succinylcholine has been demonstrated with procaine and quinidine. No documentation exists regarding an interaction between procainamide and the nondepolarizing neuromuscular blocking agents.

Mechanism: Procainamide may displace succinylcholine from the cholinesterase system or inhibit plasma cholinesterase, leading to a greater concentration of succinylcholine.

Detailed Information: See *EDI*, 2/45.00

Succinylcholine-Promazine

Significance: 2—moderately clinically significant

Recommendations: Promazine should be used with caution in patients receiving succinylcholine, and ventilatory assistance should be made available. In a study, edrophonium successfully treated the prolonged apnea.

Summary: There are data to show that promazine followed by succinylcholine has resulted in total muscle relaxation, prolonged apnea and cyanosis.

Related Drugs: A similar interaction is expected to occur with other phenothiazines and succinylcholine. A similar interaction is not expected to occur between promazine and the nondepolarizing neuromuscular blocking agents.

Mechanism: The mechanism is not fully known; however, it has been suggested that promazine may lower serum cholinesterase levels, resulting in succinylcholine remaining at the site of action for a prolonged period of time.

Detailed Information: See *EDI,* 2/47.00

Succinylcholine-Thiopental

Significance: 2—moderately clinically significant

Potential Effects: Concurrent use of these agents in the same IV line may result in anaphylaxis and death.

Recommendations: If these agents are to be used together, care should be taken to avoid physical mixing during the administration process.

Summary: There are data to show that concurrent use of succinylcholine and thiopental has caused bradycardia, severe bronchospasm, hypotension and cardiac arrest resulting in anaphylaxis and death.

Related Drugs: It is not known whether an interaction would occur between thiopental and other neuromuscular blocking agents or between succinylcholine and other barbiturates.

Mechanism: The mechanism of this interaction is not known.

Detailed Information: See *EDI,* 2/48.10

Succinylcholine-Trimethaphan

Significance: 2—moderately clinically significant

Recommendations: Trimethaphan and any neuromuscular blocking agent should be used concurrently with caution. If concomitant use is necessary, ventilatory assistance should be available.

Summary: There are data to show that patients on trimethaphan and succinylcholine have exhibited prolonged apnea, indicating an increased neuromuscular blocking effect.

Related Drugs: Tubocurarine and trimethaphan may increase the neuromuscular blocking effect of tubocurarine. If trimethaphan causes a neuromuscular blockade, a similar interaction between trimethaphan and other nondepolarizing neuromuscular blocking agents can occur. There are no drugs related to trimethaphan.

Mechanism: Trimethaphan can inhibit pseudocholinesterase, which metabolizes succinylcholine.

Detailed Information: See *EDI,* 2/49.00

Thiopental-Morphine

Significance: 2—moderately clinically significant

Recommendations: Patients should be closely monitored during concurrent use of these agents. If the dose of the narcotic cannot be lowered, it is important to be prepared for ventilatory assistance.

Summary: There are data to show that concurrent use of thiopental and morphine may lead to an increased respiratory depression.

Related Drugs: Thiopental and meperidine exhibited a similar interaction. A similar interaction may occur with other narcotics and other barbiturate anesthetics.

Mechanism: Although the mechanism is not fully known, since each agent produces respiratory depression on its own, an additive synergistic effect may be involved.

Detailed Information: See *EDI,* 2/51.00

Thiopental-Probenecid

Significance: 3—minimally clinically significant

Recommendations: It is important to be aware of the possibility of prolonged anesthesia after concurrent use of thiopental and probenecid. Probenecid may need to be discontinued prior to the use of thiopental if this effect is not desired.

Summary: There are data to show that thiopental anesthesia is prolonged after probenecid administration.

Related Drugs: A similar interaction is expected to occur between probenecid and other barbiturate anesthetics. There is no documentation regarding a similar interaction between thiopental and other uricosuric agents.

Mechanism: The mechanism of this interaction is unknown.

Detailed Information: See *EDI,* 2/53.00

Thiopental-Reserpine

Significance: 2—moderately clinically significant

Recommendations: Withdrawal of reserpine prior to surgery is not mandatory; however, it is important to be aware that hypotension and bradycardia may occur. If reserpine is not withdrawn prior to surgery and if hypotension does occur, an exacerbated effect may be noticed since the endogenous catecholamines have already been chronically depleted by reserpine. Therefore, the use of an indirect-acting sympathomimetic agent would be ineffective, and a direct-acting sympathomimetic agent would be required to treat the hypotension.

Summary: There are data to show that reserpine may enhance the CNS depression caused by thiopental, resulting in hypotension and bradycardia.

Related Drugs: Pentobarbital and thiamylal are reported to interact with reserpine in animals. A similar interaction is expected to occur with other barbiturates and reserpine. All other rauwolfia alkaloids have a potential for interacting with thiopental or other barbiturates.

Mechanism: The mechanism for this interaction is unknown. However, reserpine causes a depletion of catecholamines and serotonin in the central and peripheral nervous systems and cardiovascular tissue.

Detailed Information: See *EDI,* 2/55.00

Thiopental-Sulfisoxazole

Significance: 2—moderately clinically significant

Recommendations: When thiopental is used during long-term oral sulfisoxazole therapy, the thiopental dosage may have to be adjusted to provide smaller, more frequent doses in order to compensate for the effect of concomitant sulfisoxazole administration.

Summary: There are data to show that sulfisoxazole reduces the amount of thiopental required for anesthesia and shortens the awakening time.

Related Drugs: A similar interaction is expected to occur with other ultrashort-acting barbiturate anesthetics. The effect of using longer-acting barbiturates with other sulfonamides is not known.

Mechanism: Sulfisoxazole displaces thiopental from plasma protein binding sites, increasing the amount of free thiopental available to exert an anesthetic effect.

Detailed Information: See *EDI,* 2/57.00

Tubocurarine-Gentamicin

Significance: 1—highly clinically significant

Potential Effects: Concurrent use of these agents may prolong the neuromuscular blockade.

Recommendations: Concurrent use should be avoided. Other antibiotics should be considered. Atracurium could possibly be used in place of tubocurarine.

Summary: Aminoglycosides have been shown to produce a neuromuscular blockade, prolonging the respiratory depressant and muscle relaxant effects of tubocurarine and other neuromuscular depressant drugs.

Related Drugs: All aminoglycosides have been shown experimentally to produce neuromuscular blockade. Potentiation of neuromuscular blocking agents has been reported with all currently available aminoglycosides. The neuromuscular blockade produced by pancuronium, gallamine, vecuronium, succinylcholine and atracurium may be potentiated by these antibiotics.

Mechanism: The antibiotics produce neuromuscular blockade by inhibiting acetylcholine release presynaptically and by reducing the sensitivity of the postjunctional membrane.

Detailed Information: See *EDI,* 2/61.00

Tubocurarine-Ketamine

Significance: 2—moderately clinically significant

Recommendations: These agents should be used concurrently with caution. Patients should be closely monitored throughout anesthesia when ketamine and a neuromuscular blocking agent are used concurrently.

Summary: There are data to show that ketamine augments the neuromuscular blocking properties of tubocurarine.

Related Drugs: There are no drugs related to ketamine. There are conflicting data concerning the potentiation of ketamine by succinylcholine or pancuronium. Because of this, it is difficult to determine whether an interaction would occur between ketamine and other nondepolarizing neuromuscular blocking agents.

Mechanism: Several mechanisms have been suggested. Ketamine may decrease motor end-plate sensitivity, potentiating tubocurarine, or it may interfere with protein binding, making more tubocurarine available.

Detailed Information: See *EDI,* 2/65.00

Tubocurarine-Morphine

Significance: 2—moderately clinically significant

Recommendations: If morphine is given to a patient recovering from tubocurarine blockade or to one in whom the blockade has been antagonized recently by neostigmine, ventilation should be monitored and controlled so that the partial pressure of carbon dioxide in the arterial blood does not increase. If it does increase, tubocurarine blockade may reappear or recovery may be delayed. Administration of morphine (5mg/70Kg) and tubocurarine (9mg/Kg) in small intermittent doses rather than large bolus injections should minimize hypotension.

Summary: The administration of morphine augments the neuro-muscular blockade produced by tubocurarine. Tubocurarine and morphine both reduce blood pressure and may produce hypotension if used concurrently.

Related Drugs: A similar interaction is expected to occur between morphine and other neuromuscular blocking agents. A similar interaction is expected to occur between tubocurarine and other narcotics.

Mechanism: Morphine may augment the neuromuscular blockade of tubocurarine and reduce neostigmine's ability to antagonize tubocurarine blockade.

Detailed Information: See *EDI*, 2/67.00

Tubocurarine-Propranolol

Significance: 2—moderately clinically significant

Potential Effects: The concurrent use of these agents may result in prolonged neuromuscular blockade or hypotension.

Recommendations: Patients receiving these agents concurrently should be monitored for prolonged neuromuscular blockade or hypotension. Excessive bradycardia may also occur. If prolonged neuromuscular blockade occurs, neostigmine (1 to 3mg) with atropine (0.6 to 1.2mg) may be given.

Summary: There are data to show that tubocurarine produced a pro-longed neuromuscular blockade in patients receiving propranolol.

Related Drugs: The depolarizing neuromuscular blocking agent succinylcholine has been shown to interact with propranolol sim-ilar to tubocurarine. The other nondepolarizing neuromuscular blocking agents might also interact with propranolol. Any of the other beta blocking agents may potentially interact with tubocu-rarine as well.

Mechanism: Propranolol depresses post-tetanic repetitive activity and may depress the motor nerve terminal activity of tubocu-rarine. Propranolol may render the postjunctional membrane insensitive to acetylcholine, as well as enhance the duration of neuromuscular blockade.

Detailed Information: See *EDI*, 2/69.00

Tubocurarine-Quinidine

Significance: 2—moderately clinically significant

Potential Effects: Concurrent use of these agents may result in additive neuromuscular blockade.

Recommendations: Monitor patients closely for prolonged neuro-muscular blockade when these agents are used together. Neostigmine (1 to 3mg IV) with atropine sulfate (0.6 to 1.2 mg IV) may be used to antagonize the action of the tubocurarine. How-ever, this was not effective in one case, and should not be used with succinylcholine.

Summary: Quinidine, administered simultaneously with tubocu-rarine, may cause recurrent neuromuscular effects of tubocu-rarine, resulting in intensified respiratory depression and apnea.

Related Drugs: Gallamine has been shown to interact with quinidine in animals. A similar interaction is expected to occur with other nondepolarizing neuromuscular blocking agents and quinidine and between tubocurarine and other cinchona alkaloids.

Mechanism: The interaction with the neuromuscular blocking agents is caused by an additive pharmacologic effect of quinidine and the neuromuscular blocking agents on skeletal muscle.

Detailed Information: See *EDI*, 2/71.00

Vecuronium-Dantrolene

Significance: 3—minimally clinically significant

Potential Effects: Dantrolene may prolong the neuromuscular blocking effects of vecuronium.

Recommendations: Patients receiving dantrolene prior to vecuronium should be observed for prolonged neuromuscular blockade.

Summary: There are data to show that dantrolene administered with vecuronium caused an increase in recovery time from the neuromuscular blockade produced by vecuronium.

Related Drugs: A similar interaction is expected to occur between dantrolene and other nondepolarizing neuromuscular blocking agents and the depolarizing neuromuscular blocking agent, succinylcholine. There are no drugs related to dantrolene.

Mechanism: The prolonged neuromuscular blockade of vecuronium is related to a dantrolene-induced decrease of transmitter mobilization at the neuromuscular junction.

Detailed Information: See *EDI*, 2/72.01

Vecuronium-Magnesium Sulfate

Significance: 2—moderately clinically significant

Potential Effects: Vecuronium's action may be potentiated by magnesium sulfate.

Recommendations: When these agents are administered together, vecuronium should be carefully titrated to twitch response. Patients should be closely monitored.

Summary: There are data to show that magnesium sulfate potentiates the neuromuscular blockade caused by vecuronium.

Related Drugs: Pancuronium and atracurium exhibited comparable interactions. A similar interaction may be expected to occur between magnesium sulfate and other nondepolarizing neuromuscular blocking agents. It is not known if a similar interaction would occur with the use of the oral magnesium salts.

Mechanism: Increases in plasma magnesium potentiate the activity of nondepolarizing and depolarizing neuromuscular blocking agents, reduce end-plate sensitivity, decrease muscle fiber excitability and suppress peripheral neuromuscular function.

Detailed Information: See *EDI*, 2/72.10

Vecuronium-Piperacillin

Significance: 2—moderately clinically significant

Potential Effects: Piperacillin may prolong vecuronium's neuromuscular blockade.

Recommendations: If vecuronium is used for neuromuscular blockade, the patient should be monitored for a prolonged duration of action of vecuronium if piperacillin is administered. Additional ventilatory support may be required.

Summary: Piperacillin may prolong the duration of action of vecuronium.

Related Drugs: Vecuronium was prolonged by mezlocillin and azlocillin. It is not known whether an interaction would occur between vecuronium and the nonacylaminopenicillins or between piperacillin and other nondepolarizing neuromuscular blocking agents.

Mechanism: The mechanism of this interaction is not known, but the speculated site of action is prejunctional.

Detailed Information: See *EDI*, 2/72.25

Vecuronium-Testosterone

Significance: 3—minimally clinically significant

Potential Effects: Testosterone administration may result in resistance to vecuronium.

Recommendations: Caution should be used when administering vecuronium to a patient maintained on testosterone.

Summary: There are data to show that patients maintained on testosterone will exhibit resistance to the muscle relaxation effects of vecuronium.

Related Drugs: A similar resistance has been demonstrated with succinylcholine. An interaction may occur between testosterone and other nondepolarizing neuromuscular blocking agents. It is not known whether an interaction would occur between vecuronium and other androgen derivatives.

Mechanism: This interaction involves a combination of factors. The increased volume of distribution may explain the initial resistance. Testosterone may simulate hormones and/or corticosteroids in enhancing neuromuscular transmission and may augment an increased number of acetylcholine receptors from increased skeletal muscle mass.

Detailed Information: See *EDI*, 2/72.30

Vecuronium-Verapamil

Significance: 2—moderately clinically significant

Potential Effects: Verapamil can prolong the neuromuscular blockade produced by vecuronium.

Recommendations: Patients taking verapamil should be administered conservative doses of neuromuscular blocking agents. If reversal of the blockade is not obtained, the use of edrophonium should be considered.

Summary: There are data to show that verapamil causes difficulty with the reversal of the neuromuscular blockade caused by vecuronium.

Related Drugs: Pancuronium, tubocurarine and succinylcholine have demonstrated similar interactions with the coadministration of verapamil. A similar interaction may occur between verapamil and other nondepolarizing neuromuscular blocking agents. Documentation is lacking regarding an interaction between vecuronium and other calcium channel blockers.

Mechanism: Verapamil may reduce the mobilization or release of the transmitter acetylcholine and therefore reduces prejunctional stimulus.

Detailed Information: See *EDI*, 2/73.00

Chapter Three

Antiarrhythmic Drug Interactions

Amiodarone-Cholestyramine

Significance: 3—minimally clinically significant

Potential Effects: Cholestyramine may reduce the enterohepatic circulation of amiodarone, leading to an increased elimination of the amiodarone.

Recommendations: Cholestyramine may be administered to patients with dose-dependent amiodarone side effects. In other patients, amiodarone levels and effects should be closely monitored. The dose of amiodarone may need to be increased.

Summary: There are data to show that amiodarone followed by cholestyramine administration significantly decreases the mean serum level and elimination half-life of amiodarone.

Related Drugs: A similar interaction may be expected to occur between amiodarone and other anion exchange resins. There are no drugs related to amiodarone.

Mechanism: Cholestyramine significantly reduces the enterohepatic circulation of amiodarone, enhancing its elimination.

Detailed Information: See *EDI,* 3/0.01

Amiodarone-Cyclosporine

Significance: 2—moderately clinically significant

Potential Effects: The addition of amiodarone to a cyclosporine regimen may result in increased cyclosporine levels and toxicity.

Recommendations: Patients should be carefully monitored for changes in cyclosporine levels and clearance with the concurrent use of these agents. The dose of cyclosporine may need to be adjusted to maintain cyclosporine serum levels within the therapeutic range.

Summary: Concurrent amiodarone and cyclosporine resulted in decreased cyclosporine clearance, leading to increased levels and potential nephrotoxicity.

Related Drugs: There are no drugs related to cyclosporine or amiodarone.

Mechanism: Although the mechanism of this interaction is not known, the interaction with cyclosporine may occur in the adipose tissue throughout the body.

Detailed Information: See *EDI,* 3/0.02

Amiodarone-Diltiazem

Significance: 2—moderately clinically significant

Potential Effects: Use of these agents together may cause a decrease in cardiac function.

Recommendations: Patients should be monitored for decreased cardiac function when using these agents together. One or both drugs may need to be discontinued.

Summary: There are data to show that coadministration of diltiazem and amiodarone may lead to sinus arrest and severe, low cardiac output with oliguria.

Related Drugs: A similar interaction may occur between amiodarone and other calcium channel blockers. There are no drugs related to amiodarone.

Mechanism: It has been suggested that the interaction was the result of additive hemodynamic and electrophysiologic effects.

Detailed Information: See *EDI,* 3/0.03

Amiodarone-Lidocaine

Significance: 2—moderately clinically significant

Potential Effects: Use of these agents together has resulted in adverse cardiac effects.

Recommendations: Use these agents together with caution. Monitor the patient's cardiac status.

Summary: There are data to show that receiving amiodarone with 2% lidocaine may cause severe sinus bradycardia and sinoatrial arrest.

Related Drugs: A similar interaction is expected to occur between amiodarone and tocainide or mexiletine, or the oral antiarrhythmic agents related to lidocaine. There are no drugs related to amiodarone.

Mechanism: Lidocaine and amiodarone are known to depress the sinus node; the interaction may be due to an additive effect of the two agents on the sinus node.

Detailed Information: See *EDI*, 3/0.05

Diltiazem-Cisapride

Significance: 2—moderately clinically significant

Potential Effects: The concurrent administration of cisapride and diltiazem may result in prolongation of the rate corrected QT interval (QT_c).

Recommendations: The concurrent administration of cisapride and diltiazem should be approached with caution. The manufacturer of cisapride states that an electrocardiogram should be considered prior to the initiation of therapy with cisapride.

Summary: The concurrent administration of cisapride and diltiazem may have resulted in prolongation of the QT_c interval in a single case report. When metoclopramide was substituted for cisapride, the patient's QT_c interval was normal (QT_c of 440 msec) within two months.

Related Drugs: Although nifedipine plasma concentrations were significantly increased when given with cisapride, no detrimental hypotensive effects occurred. It is not known whether an interaction would occur between cisapride and the other calcium channel blocking agents. However, information concerning a possible interaction between cisapride and bepridil (a calcium channel blocking agent not chemically related to the dihydropyridine or the tetralol calcium channel blocking agents) has been mentioned.

Mechanism: It is postulated that diltiazem may inhibit the metabolism of cisapride at the $P450_{3A4}$ isozyme. Cisapride is metabolized at the $P450_{3A4}$ isozyme and elevated levels of cisapride have been shown to result in QT prolongation, torsades de pointes, cardiac arrest, and sudden death.

Detailed Information: See *EDI*, 3/0.06

Diltiazem-Cyclosporine

Significance: 1—highly clinically significant

Potential Effects: Diltiazem may increase cyclosporine levels, resulting in decreased renal function.

Recommendations: Patients should be closely monitored for increased cyclosporine and serum creatinine levels during concurrent therapy with diltiazem. The dose of cyclosporine may need to be adjusted.

Summary: Concurrent administration of cyclosporine and diltiazem resulted in increased cyclosporine levels to as high as 1100ng/ml as well as increased serum creatinine levels.

Related Drugs: Concomitant administration of verapamil or nicardipine with cyclosporine also has resulted in significant increases in cyclosporine levels. Several studies have reported that concurrent isradipine had either no effect on cyclosporine kinetics or a beneficial nephroprotective effect. Conversely, one case report documents a threefold increase in trough cyclosporine concentration with concurrent isradipine. Although one study reported a significant increase in plasma cyclosporine levels following a single dose of felodipine, there was an increase in glomerular filtration rate, renal plasma flow, and urinary sodium excretion, suggesting that a single dose of felodipine may have beneficial effects on renal hemodynamics in renal transplant patients. It is difficult to determine whether an interaction would occur between cyclosporine and the other calcium channel blocking agents. There are no drugs related to cyclosporine.

Mechanism: It has been suggested that diltiazem interferes with the hepatic metabolism of cyclosporine.

Detailed Information: See *EDI,* 3/0.07

Disopyramide-Alcohol, Ethyl

Significance: 3—minimally clinically significant

Recommendations: Until further clinical studies are done, the concurrent use of these agents need not be avoided. However, if disopyramide levels increase, the dose of disopyramide may need to be adjusted or the discontinuation of alcohol should be encouraged.

Summary: The concurrent use of disopyramide and alcohol has led to a significant reduction in the apparent metabolic clearance of disopyramide.

Related Drugs: There are no drugs related to disopyramide.

Mechanism: Alcohol may have an inhibitory effect on disopyramide metabolism.

Detailed Information: See *EDI,* 3/0.10

Disopyramide-Atenolol

Significance: 3—minimally clinically significant

Recommendations: The concurrent use of disopyramide and atenolol need not be avoided. However, since the clearance of disopyramide decreased while the concentration of the metabolite of disopyramide (which has some antiarrhythmic activity) did not change, patients should be monitored for an increased antiarrhythmic effect. During concomitant atenolol therapy the dose of disopyramide may need to be adjusted.

Summary: There are data to show that administration of atenolol and disopyramide significantly reduces the clearance of disopyramide, while its other pharmacokinetic parameters remain unchanged.

Related Drugs: There are data to show that propranolol does not cause any change in the concentration of disopyramide; however, all data do not support this. Because of conflicting results, it is difficult to determine if an interaction would occur between disopyramide and other beta-blocking agents. There are no drugs related to disopyramide.

Mechanism: The effect of atenolol on a small metabolized fraction of disopyramide may account for the change in the elimination of disopyramide. However, a hepatic or renal blood flow cause cannot be excluded.

Detailed Information: See *EDI*, 3/0.30

Disopyramide-Charcoal

Significance: 2—moderately clinically significant

Potential Effects: Charcoal adsorbs disopyramide, leading to a decrease in disopyramide absorption.

Recommendations: Charcoal may be useful in the treatment of disopyramide overdosage. If charcoal is being used for other reasons, the administration of these agents should be separated by as much time as possible.

Summary: Charcoal significantly decreases the bioavailability and serum concentration of disopyramide.

Related Drugs: There are no drugs related to disopyramide.

Mechanism: Charcoal adsorbs disopyramide when both drugs are given concurrently.

Detailed Information: See *EDI*, 3/0.50

Disopyramide-Cyclosporine

Significance: 3—minimally clinically significant

Potential Effects: Cyclosporine may lead to increases in disopyramide levels, leading to pronounced anticholinergic side effects.

Recommendations: Monitor the patient for increases in serum creatinine or disopyramide toxicity during concurrent use of these agents.

Summary: There are data to show that coadministration of disopyramide and cyclosporine caused serum creatinine levels to increase and potentiate disopyramide-induced anticholinergic side effects.

Related Drugs: There are no drugs related to disopyramide or cyclosporine.

Mechanism: The exact mechanism of this interaction is unknown, but cyclosporine may have caused nephrotoxicity or a change in the metabolism of disopyramide.

Detailed Information: See *EDI*, 3/0.65

Disopyramide-Erythromycin

Significance: 2—moderately clinically significant

Potential Effects: Erythromycin may decrease the metabolism of disopyramide, resulting in increased disopyramide levels and possible toxicity.

Recommendations: Patients maintained on disopyramide should be closely monitored for changes in cardiac status if erythromycin is added to their drug regimen. The dose of disopyramide may need to be adjusted.

Summary: There are data to show that coadministration of disopyramide and erythromycin can increase serum creatinine levels and potentiate cardiac complications, necessitating electrical cardioversion.

Related Drugs: A similar interaction may be expected to occur between disopyramide and other macrolide antibiotics. There are no drugs related to disopyramide.

Mechanism: It has been suggested that erythromycin interferes with hepatic enzymes used to metabolize disopyramide, causing an increase in the disopyramide level.

Detailed Information: See *EDI,* 3/0.67

Disopyramide-Isosorbide Dinitrate

Significance: 2—moderately clinically significant

Potential Effects: The occurrence of dry mouth that may be associated with disopyramide therapy because of its anticholinergic side effects may prevent the dissolution of sublingual isosorbide dinitrate tablets, resulting in ineffective therapy.

Recommendations: Attempts at increasing salivation (e.g., chewing gum, artificial saliva products) may prove useful in increasing the effectiveness of sublingual isosorbide dinitrate in some patients. If the ineffectiveness of the sublingual isosorbide dinitrate continues, the use of oral, topical, or translingual spray forms of the nitrates, or the substitution of another appropriate antiarrhythmic agent, may need to be considered.

Summary: There are data to show that disopyramide can cause dry mouth, making the absorption of a sublingual isosorbide dinitrate tablet difficult.

Related Drugs: A similar interaction may occur between disopyramide and other sublingual nitrate tablets. There are no drugs related to disopyramide.

Mechanism: Dry mouth is a common side effect of disopyramide therapy because of its anticholinergic effects.

Detailed Information: See *EDI,* 3/0.70

Disopyramide-Phenytoin

Significance: 2—moderately clinically significant

Potential Effects: Phenytoin increases the hepatic metabolism of disopyramide, resulting in decreased disopyramide plasma levels and possibly a decrease in its efficacy. Increased anticholinergic side effects may also occur.

Recommendations: Although the metabolite of disopyramide has some antiarrhythmic activity, patients receiving these agents concurrently should be monitored for decreased antiarrhythmic control and increased anticholinergic side effects.

Summary: There are data to show that concurrent phenytoin and disopyramide can result in a decrease in the plasma concentration and efficacy of disopyramide.

Related Drugs: A similar interaction is expected to occur between disopyramide and other hydantoin anticonvulsants. There are no drugs related to disopyramide.

Mechanism: Phenytoin may increase the hepatic metabolism of disopyramide.

Detailed Information: See *EDI,* 3/1.00

Disopyramide-Quinidine

Significance: 3—minimally clinically significant

Recommendations: The concurrent use of these agents need not be avoided. However, a longer interval between the last dose of disopyramide and the first dose of quinidine may be warranted. Patients on high dose disopyramide therapy should be closely monitored.

Summary: There are data to show that the concurrent use of disopyramide and quinidine has led to an increase in disopyramide serum concentration and a decrease in quinidine serum concentration.

Related Drugs: There are no drugs related to disopyramide. Documentation is lacking regarding a similar interaction between disopyramide and other cinchona alkaloids.

Mechanism: The mechanism of this interaction is unknown.

Detailed Information: See *EDI*, 3/3.00

Disopyramide-Rifampin

Significance: 3—minimally clinically significant

Recommendations: Although the patients were taking other drugs that could have a role in this interaction, rifampin is still strongly suspected because of its known induction properties. Because the metabolite of disopyramide has some antiarrhythmic activity, the increased rate of metabolism of disopyramide cannot be equated with a shorter duration of response. Therefore, patients should be monitored for a loss of antiarrhythmic effect.

Summary: Disopyramide metabolism may be significantly increased with concomitant rifampin. It is not certain if disopyramide will alter the disposition of rifampin.

Related Drugs: There are no drugs related to rifampin or disopyramide.

Mechanism: Rifampin accelerated disopyramide metabolism by enzyme induction.

Detailed Information: See *EDI*, 3/5.00

Felodipine-Erythromycin

Significance: 3—minimally clinically significant

Potential Effects: The addition of erythromycin to felodipine may result in elevated plasma felodipine concentrations and increased incidence of adverse events.

Recommendations: Patients receiving concurrent therapy should be monitored for an increase in the clinical effects of felodipine. The dosage of felodipine may need to be decreased, or erythromycin may need to be discontinued.

Summary: The addition of erythromycin to felodipine may result in elevated plasma felodipine concentrations and increased incidence of adverse events including palpitations, flushing, and lower extremity edema.

Related Drugs: *In vitro*, clarithromycin, erythromycin, and rokitamycin did not inhibit the formation of the nifedipine M-1 metabolite when added to nifedipine, although pretreatment with either clarithromycin or erythromycin did inhibit its formation. Only erythromycin inhibited the formation of the nifedipine M-2 metabolite. Erythromycin and roxithromycin appear to be weak inhibitors of nifedipine oxidation. Azithromycin does not produce hepatic cytochrome P450 induction or inactivation as erythromycin estolate does; therefore, an interaction would not be expected to occur between azithromycin and felodipine or nifedipine. An interaction would likely occur between erythromycin and other dihydropyridine calcium channel blocking agents. An interaction may be expected to occur between felodipine and the other macrolide antibiotics.

Mechanism: It is hypothesized that erythromycin inhibits the primary metabolic pathway for felodipine. Felodipine is believed to undergo CYP3A4 metabolism both in the gut and the liver, accounting for its low bioavailability.

Detailed Information: See *EDI,* 3/5.50

Flecainide-Amiodarone

Significance: 2—moderately clinically significant

Recommendations: Plasma flecainide levels should be closely monitored in patients receiving concurrent flecainide and amiodarone. Because amiodarone has a long half-life, it is important to monitor patients closely for several weeks. When amiodarone is added to flecainide therapy, it may be advisable to decrease the dose of flecainide by one third to one half, and a further dosage reduction may be required.

Summary: There are data to show that amiodarone causes an increase in flecainide plasma levels.

Related Drugs: Flecainide is unrelated to the Class IB antiarrhythmic agents. There are no drugs related to amiodarone.

Mechanism: It was suggested that amiodarone inhibits the hepatic metabolism of flecainide.

Detailed Information: See *EDI,* 3/6.01

Flecainide-Ammonium Chloride

Significance: 2—moderately clinically significant

Potential Effects: Ammonium chloride, by acidifying the urine, increases flecainide elimination.

Recommendations: Patients should be carefully monitored if flecainide and ammonium chloride are used concurrently. The dose of flecainide may need to be increased. Attempts to acidify the urine could be considered as a therapeutic measure in patients with high serum levels of flecainide, but this requires further study.

Summary: The renal clearance and urinary elimination of flecainide were increased with decreasing urinary pH caused by ammonium chloride.

Related Drugs: A similar interaction may occur between flecainide and other urinary acidifiers. It is not known if a similar interaction would occur between ammonium chloride and the other Class IC antiarrhythmic, encainide.

Mechanism: The increased elimination half-life of flecainide may be a result of a change in the degree of ionization of the drug at the adsorption site.

Detailed Information: See *EDI,* 3/6.07

Flecainide-Charcoal

Significance: 3—minimally clinically significant

Potential Effects: Charcoal adsorbs flecainide, leading to decreased levels.

Recommendations: The interaction may be useful in some patients in the case of flecainide intoxication. The administration of charcoal may be useful even after some delay. However, if charcoal is being used for other medical reasons, the administration of these agents should be separated by as much time as possible.

Summary: There are data to show that charcoal causes a significant decrease in flecainide plasma levels.

Related Drugs: It is not known if a similar interaction would occur with the other Class IC antiarrhythmic agent, encainide. There are no drugs related to charcoal.

Mechanism: Charcoal adsorbs flecainide when both drugs are given concurrently, reducing the absorption of flecainide in the gastrointestinal tract.

Detailed Information: See *EDI,* 3/6.03

Flecainide-Cimetidine

Significance: 2—moderately clinically significant

Potential Effects: Cimetidine may increase flecainide levels.

Recommendations: Monitor for increased flecainide levels when these agents are used together. The dose of flecainide may need to be decreased.

Summary: Cimetidine causes an increase in the peak concentration of flecainide and the amount of flecainide excreted in the urine.

Related Drugs: Similar interactions have been documented with cimetidine and encainide or propafenone. A similar interaction may be expected to occur between cimetidine and the other Class IC antiarrhythmic agent, indecainide. The other H_2-receptor antagonists would not be expected to interact with flecainide, if the mechanism is caused by flecainide's metabolism by cimetidine.

Mechanism: Cimetidine may inhibit the hepatic microsomal enzymes responsible for the metabolism of flecainide.

Detailed Information: See *EDI,* 3/6.05

Flecainide-Isoproterenol

Significance: 2—moderately clinically significant

Potential Effects: Isoproterenol may decrease the effectiveness of flecainide.

Recommendations: Use these agents together with caution. If loss of antiarrhythmic activity occurs, isoproterenol should be discontinued, and the use of a beta-blocking agent may be necessary.

Summary: There are data to show that coadministration of flecainide and isoproterenol causes a loss of antiarrhythmic activity of flecainide.

Related Drugs: A similar interaction may occur between flecainide and other beta agonist-sympathomimetics. It is not known to what extent the sympathomimetics with both alpha and beta agonist activity would interact with flecainide. Flecainide is unrelated to the Class IB antiarrhythmic agents.

Mechanism: Isoproterenol may shorten the refractory period of the accessory pathway through its beta-adrenergic stimulation, resulting in a loss of flecainide's efficacy.

Detailed Information: See *EDI,* 3/6.10

Flecainide-Quinine

Significance: 3—minimally clinically significant

Potential Effects: The addition of quinine to a flecainide regimen may increase flecainide serum levels.

Recommendations: Patients should be monitored if quinine is added to the therapy of a patient maintained on flecainide. The dose of flecainide may need to be adjusted.

Summary: Quinine decreased the clearance and increased the half-life of flecainide.

Related Drugs: Encainide was shown to similarly interact with quinine. Mexiletine and encainide increased quinidine sulfate serum concentrations, whereas concurrent flecainide and tocainide did not. There is no documentation for an interaction between quinine and other antiarrhythmic agents.

Mechanism: The inhibition of cytochrome P-450 isozymes by quinine is likely to be responsible for the inhibition of flecainide metabolism.

Detailed Information: See *EDI,* 3/6.25

Flecainide-Sodium Bicarbonate

Significance: 2—moderately clinically significant

Potential Effects: Sodium bicarbonate alkalinizes the urine, resulting in decreased flecainide elimination and possible toxicity.

Recommendations: The patient should be carefully monitored if these agents are used concurrently. The dose of flecainide may need to be decreased.

Summary: The renal clearance and urinary elimination of flecainide were decreased with increasing urinary pH caused by sodium bicarbonate.

Related Drugs: A similar interaction may occur between flecainide and other urinary alkalinizers. It is not known if a similar interaction would occur between sodium bicarbonate and the other Class IC antiarrhythmic, encainide.

Mechanism: A prolonged elimination half-life of flecainide may be the result of a higher degree of renal tubular reabsorption of un-ionized flecainide molecules at an alkaline pH.

Detailed Information: See *EDI,* 3/6.30

Lidocaine-Cimetidine

Significance: 1—highly clinically significant

Potential Effects: Cimetidine increases lidocaine levels, possibly resulting in lidocaine toxicity.

Recommendations: If these agents are given together, monitor lidocaine levels. The dose of lidocaine may need to be decreased, or ranitidine or possibly famotidine may be used instead of cimetidine.

Summary: There are data to show that the concurrent administration of cimetidine and lidocaine has resulted in increased lidocaine serum concentrations; however, contrasting data are available.

Related Drugs: Ranitidine has shown comparable results when administered with lidocaine. Lidocaine would not be expected to interact with the other H_2-receptor antagonists. Mexiletine was shown to react similarly to lidocaine when administered with cimetidine.

Mechanism: Cimetidine may inhibit the microsomal enzymes involved in the metabolism of lidocaine and may induce a reduction in hepatic blood flow, reducing the hepatic clearance of lidocaine.

Detailed Information: See *EDI,* 3/7.00

Lidocaine-Phenobarbital

Significance: 3—minimally clinically significant

Recommendations: It is recommended that lidocaine plasma levels be monitored to assure that they are in the therapeutic range. However, since induction of metabolism may result in increased levels of pharmacologically active metabolites, the clinical significance of this interaction requires further investigation.

Summary: There are data to show that plasma levels of lidocaine may be decreased during concurrent administration of phenobarbital.

Related Drugs: A similar interaction is expected to occur with other barbiturates and lidocaine. The elimination of tocainide was not influenced by pretreatment with phenobarbital.

Mechanism: The induction of lidocaine metabolism by phenobarbital is most likely responsible for this interaction.

Detailed Information: See *EDI,* 3/9.00

Lidocaine-Procainamide

Significance: 3—minimally clinically significant

Recommendations: Until further clinical studies are performed, the concurrent use of these agents need not be avoided. However, it is important to be aware of a possible interaction, and if CNS symptoms occur, discontinuing lidocaine appears to be beneficial.

Summary: There are data to show that the coadministration of procainamide and lidocaine has resulted in restlessness, visual disturbances, and delirium. These symptoms may have been caused by CNS toxicity.

Related Drugs: Documentation is lacking regarding a similar interaction between procainamide and tocainide. There are no drugs related to procainamide.

Mechanism: The mechanism of this interaction is not fully known; however, the two drugs may have a synergistic effect on the CNS.

Detailed Information: See *EDI,* 3/10.10

Lidocaine-Propranolol

Significance: 2—moderately clinically significant

Recommendations: Since lidocaine has a narrow therapeutic index, concurrent administration with a beta-blocking agent may require the dosage or infusion rate of lidocaine to be reduced. Lidocaine serum levels should be monitored with appropriate dosage adjustments.

Summary: The concurrent administration of propranolol and lidocaine significantly decreased the metabolic clearance of lidocaine.

Related Drugs: Pindolol, metoprolol and atenolol did not significantly affect lidocaine metabolism. Nadolol was found to increase lidocaine plasma levels and decrease clearance. Because of conflicting data, it is not known whether the other beta-adrenergic blocking agents would interact with lidocaine. When tocainide and propranolol were administered, severe paranoia and confusion resulted. Tocainide and metoprolol showed no influence on hemodynamic parameters.

Mechanism: Propranolol decreases the cardiac output and hepatic blood flow, decreasing the metabolic clearance of lidocaine. Propranolol may also influence the hepatic drug-metabolizing capacity.

Detailed Information: See *EDI,* 3/11.00

Mexiletine-Aluminum Hydroxide, Magnesium Hydroxide

Significance: 3—minimally clinically significant

Potential Effects: The aluminum hydroxide component may prolong the gastric emptying time, which may prolong the time to reach peak concentration of mexiletine.

Recommendations: The concomitant use of these agents need not be avoided since the bioavailability of mexiletine was not altered. However, further studies are necessary.

Summary: Administration of an antacid with mexiletine was found to increase mexiletine's peak plasma concentration.

Related Drugs: Antacids increased tocainide's area-under-curve and decreased the clearance and maximum plasma concentration. A similar interaction is expected between mexiletine and other antacids; however, only aluminum-containing antacids may interact.

Mechanism: The aluminum hydroxide component of the antacid may decrease the gastric emptying rate, prolonging the time to reach peak concentration of mexiletine.

Detailed Information: See *EDI,* 3/12.01

Mexiletine-Ammonium Chloride

Significance: 3—minimally clinically significant

Potential Effects: Ammonium chloride acidifies the urine, which increases the excretion of mexiletine.

Recommendations: Monitor mexiletine serum levels and clinical response when these agents are used together.

Summary: There are data to show that administration of mexiletine with ammonium chloride acidifies the urine, increasing the excretion of mexiletine.

Related Drugs: Other agents that acidify the urine may interact with mexiletine. It is not known if an interaction would occur between ammonium chloride and other antiarrhythmic agents related to mexiletine.

Mechanism: As the urine pH decreases, the tubular reabsorption of the ionized mexiletine also decreases, resulting in an increased excretion of unchanged drug.

Detailed Information: See *EDI,* 3/12.03

Mexiletine-Atropine

Significance: 3—minimally clinically significant

Potential Effects: Atropine decreases the gastric emptying rate, which may lead to a decrease in the rate of mexiletine absorption.

Recommendations: The use of these agents concurrently need not be avoided. This interaction may be of significance only when initiating mexiletine therapy.

Summary: Administration of atropine reduces the maximum plasma concentration and elimination half-life of mexiletine.

Related Drugs: It is not known if a similar interaction would occur between atropine and the other Class IB antiarrhythmic agent, tocainide. A similar interaction may be expected to occur between mexiletine and other anticholinergics.

Mechanism: Atropine decreases the rate of mexiletine absorption because of a decrease in the gastric emptying rate.

Detailed Information: See *EDI,* 3/12.05

Mexiletine-Metoclopramide

Significance: 3—minimally clinically significant

Potential Effects: Metoclopramide increases the gastric emptying rate, which may result in an increase in the absorption of mexiletine.

Recommendations: The concomitant use of these agents need not be avoided. However, this interaction may be of some significance when initiating mexiletine therapy.

Summary: Metoclopramide increases the gastric emptying rate, resulting in an increased absorption of mexiletine.

Related Drugs: It is not known if a similar interaction would occur between metoclopramide and the other Class IB antiarrhythmic agent, tocainide. There are no drugs related to metoclopramide.

Mechanism: Metoclopramide may enhance the rate of mexiletine absorption because of an increase in the gastric emptying rate.

Detailed Information: See *EDI,* 3/12.07

Mexiletine-Phenytoin

Significance: 3—minimally clinically significant

Potential Effects: Phenytoin may decrease plasma levels of mexiletine.

Recommendations: Monitor the patient's cardiac status and levels of mexiletine when these agents are used together. The dose of mexiletine may need to be increased.

Summary: Phenytoin has been shown to decrease area-under-curve, mean elimination half-life and plasma levels of mexiletine.

Related Drugs: Phenytoin has been shown to reduce the bioavailability and increase the clearance of lidocaine. Phenytoin may also interact with tocainide. A similar interaction is expected to occur between mexiletine and other hydantoin anticonvulsants.

Mechanism: Phenytoin may induce the hepatic enzymes responsible for the metabolism of mexiletine.

Detailed Information: See *EDI,* 3/12.09

Mexiletine-Rifampin

Significance: 3—minimally clinically significant

Potential Effects: Rifampin may increase the metabolism of mexiletine.

Recommendations: Monitor the patient's cardiac status and mexiletine levels when these agents are used together.

Summary: Rifampin has been shown to cause a decrease in the elimination half-life of mexiletine and an increase in its metabolism and nonrenal clearance. There were no pharmacokinetic changes with mexiletine.

Related Drugs: Tocainide administered with rifampin has shown altered tocainide pharmacokinetics. Lidocaine may interact similarly with rifampin based on metabolism. There are no drugs related to rifampin.

Mechanism: Rifampin induces the hepatic microsomal enzymes responsible for the metabolism of mexiletine.

Detailed Information: See *EDI,* 3/12.11

Mexiletine-Tobacco

Significance: 3—minimally clinically significant

Potential Effects: Cigarette smoking increases the elimination of mexiletine.

Recommendations: Patients stabilized on mexiletine who start or stop smoking should be observed for a change in the therapeutic effects of mexiletine.

Summary: There are data to show that cigarette smoking significantly increases the elimination of mexiletine. The effect on the clearance of mexiletine was less marked and the other pharmacokinetic parameters were unaffected.

Related Drugs: A similar interaction may be expected to occur with other Class IB antiarrhythmic agents related to mexiletine.

Mechanism: Cigarette smoking increases the rate of conjugation of mexiletine with glucuronic acid and induces its aliphatic hydroxylation.

Detailed Information: See *EDI*, 3/12.13

Moricizine-Cimetidine

Significance: 3—minimally clinically significant

Potential Effects: Cimetidine may decrease the metabolism of moricizine, leading to increased levels.

Recommendations: Monitor patients closely during concurrent cimetidine and moricizine administration. The dose of moricizine may need to be decreased.

Summary: Cimetidine has been shown to decrease the clearance and to increase the elimination half-life and area-under-curve of moricizine.

Related Drugs: Moricizine is not chemically related to the other antiarrhythmic agents. It is not known whether the other H_2-receptor antagonists would interact with moricizine.

Mechanism: The mechanism of this interaction is not known; however, it has been suggested that cimetidine inhibits the hepatic metabolism of moricizine.

Detailed Information: See *EDI*, 3/12.17

Nifedipine-Cimetidine

Significance: 2—moderately clinically significant

Potential Effects: Cimetidine inhibits the metabolism of nifedipine, resulting in increased levels and pharmacologic activity.

Recommendations: Until further studies are performed, patients should be monitored for increased nifedipine effects during concurrent use of nifedine and cimetidine. Ranitidine, nizatidine, or famotidine may be alternatives to cimetidine.

Summary: Cimetidine caused a rise in maximal plasma levels and area-under-curve of nifedipine. Patients also experienced a significant reduction in arterial blood pressure.

Related Drugs: Ranitidine was shown to exhibit a similar interaction when administered with nifedipine. Cimetidine caused an increase in the elimination half-life and a reduction in clearance of verapamil.

Mechanism: Cimetidine inhibits the hepatic drug metabolizing enzymes by binding to cytochrome P450. It is not known how cimetidine influenced the decreased blood pressure.

Detailed Information: See *EDI*, 3/12.20

Nifedipine-Ethanol

Significance: 3—minimally clinically significant

Potential Effects: Concurrent nifedipine and ethanol may result in increased nifedipine levels and cardiac effects.

Recommendations: Patients maintained on nifedipine should be monitored for potentiation of nifedipine effects if ethanol is given concurrently.

Summary: Concurrent nifedipine and ethanol administration resulted in an increase in nifedipine area-under-curve.

Related Drugs: Verapamil exhibited a similar interaction when administered with ethanol. Felodipine and ethanol significantly decreased blood pressures. Nifedipine exaggerated the ethanol-induced motor incoordination. A similar interaction is expected between ethanol and other calcium channel blocking agents, if the mechanism involves the inhibition of cytochrome P450 isozymes.

Mechanism: Ethanol inhibits nifedipine metabolism, possibly because both agents are metabolized by dehydrogenation.

Detailed Information: See *EDI*, 3/12.25

Nifedipine-Halothane

Significance: 3—minimally clinically significant

Recommendations: It is important to be aware of a possible interaction between nifedipine and halothane and to use these agents with caution, especially in patients with decreased left ventricular function.

Summary: The concurrent use of nifedipine under halothane anesthesia has led to myocardial depression.

Related Drugs: Halothane and verapamil have been shown to have an additive negative inotropic effect. A similar interaction is expected to occur between halothane and other calcium channel blockers. Documentation is lacking regarding an interaction between nifedipine and the other halogenated inhalation anesthetics.

Mechanism: Halothane and calcium channel blocking agents have a pronounced independent negative inotropic effects, and an additive effect may explain the mechanism.

Detailed Information: See *EDI*, 3/12.30

Nifedipine-Magnesium Sulfate

Significance: 3—minimally clinically significant

Potential Effects: Concurrent use of these agents may result in marked hypotension.

Recommendations: Concurrent administration of magnesium sulfate and nifedipine should be approached with caution. Blood pressure should be carefully monitored when these agents are used together.

Summary: Administration of nifedipine with magnesium sulfate resulted in marked hypotension.

Related Drugs: A similar interaction is expected to occur between magnesium sulfate and other calcium-channel blocking agents, if the hypotensive response is related to magnesium sulfate and nifedipine. There are no drugs related to magnesium sulfate.

Mechanism: Although the mechanism is not known, the marked hypotension is because of an interaction between magnesium sulfate and nifedipine.

Detailed Information: See *EDI*, 3/12.40

Procainamide-Alcohol, Ethyl

Significance: 3—minimally clinically significant

Recommendations: Procainamide and N-acetylprocainamide levels should be monitored in patients concurrently ingesting alcohol while on procainamide therapy. The dosage of procainamide may need to be adjusted.

Summary: The concurrent ingestion of alcohol with procainamide resulted in a significant reduction in procainamide half-life and an increase in the elimination half-life and total clearance.

Related Drugs: There are no drugs related to procainamide.

Mechanism: Alcohol may affect the acetylation of procainamide.

Detailed Information: See *EDI*, 3/13.00

Procainamide-Amiodarone

Significance: 2—moderately clinically significant

Potential Effects: Amiodarone may cause an increase in procainamide and NAPA levels.

Recommendations: Monitor procainamide and NAPA levels when these agents are used together. The dose of procainamide may need to be decreased by 20% to 50%.

Summary: There are data to show that administration of procainamide with amiodarone increases procainamide serum levels, resulting in procainamide toxicity.

Related Drugs: There are no drugs related to procainamide or amiodarone.

Mechanism: This interaction may be due to a decrease in procainamide tissue binding, releasing procainamide into the serum.

Detailed Information: See *EDI*, 3/14.01

Procainamide-Cimetidine

Significance: 2—moderately clinically significant

Potential Effects: Cimetidine may cause an increase in procainamide and NAPA levels.

Recommendations: Monitor procainamide and NAPA levels when cimetidine is administered concurrently. The dose of procainamide may need to be decreased.

Summary: There are data to show that cimetidine increases procainamide serum levels, resulting in procainamide toxicity.

Related Drugs: Ranitidine has been shown to cause increases in procainamide serum levels; however, all data do not support this. There are no drugs related to procainamide.

Mechanism: It has been suggested that this interaction is a cimetidine-induced reduction in renal blood flow, competing for active tubular secretion.

Detailed Information: See *EDI*, 3/14.10

Procainamide–Para-Aminobenzoic Acid

Significance: 3—minimally clinically significant

Potential Effects: Administration of PABA to patients receiving procainamide may decrease the NAPA/procainamide serum level ratio. This may lead to an increased antiarrhythmic activity of procainamide.

Recommendations: Monitor the NAPA and procainamide levels if these agents are used concomitantly.

Summary: There are data to show that coadministration of PABA and procainamide may decrease the NAPA/procainamide serum ratio, leading to an increased antiarrhythmic activity of procainamide.

Related Drugs: There are no drugs related to procainamide or PABA.

Mechanism: PABA competitively inhibits the acetylation of procainamide, resulting in a decrease in the NAPA/procainamide ratio.

Detailed Information: See *EDI,* 3/14.21

Procainamide-Propranolol

Significance: 3—minimally clinically significant

Recommendations: Until further clinical studies are done, the concurrent use of these agents need not be avoided; however, procainamide and NAPA levels should be routinely monitored.

Summary: Propranolol has been shown to decrease the plasma clearance of procainamide and increase the elimination half-life; however, all data do not support this.

Related Drugs: Metoprolol and procainamide had no effect on the clearance and elimination half-life of procainamide. Because of conflicting results, it is difficult to determine if an interaction would occur between procainamide and other beta-blocking agents. There are no drugs related to procainamide.

Mechanism: The mechanism of the interaction is unknown.

Detailed Information: See *EDI,* 3/14.30

Procainamide-Quinidine

Significance: 3—minimally clinically significant

Potential Effects: Quinidine may increase the plasma level and half-life of procainamide and its active metabolite.

Recommendations: Concurrent use of quinidine and procainamide may be beneficial in certain circumstances. However, high dose procainamide should be used with caution with quinidine. Monitor patients' procainamide and NAPA levels.

Summary: The concurrent use of quinidine and procainamide resulted in increased levels of both procainamide and NAPA, an active metabolite.

Related Drugs: It is not know if procainamide would interact similarly with quinine. There are no drugs related to procainamide.

Mechanism: Quinidine may interfere with the renal elimination of procainamide by interfering with glomerular filtration, proximal tubular secretion, or reabsorption in the distal tubule.

Detailed Information: See *EDI,* 3/14.50

Procainamide-Trimethoprim

Significance: 3—minimally clinically significant

Potential Effects: Concurrent trimethoprim and procainamide therapy may result in an increase in procainamide and NAPA levels because of competition for excretion of procainamide by trimethoprim.

Recommendations: Monitor procainamide and NAPA levels when using procainamide and trimethoprim together.

Summary: Trimethoprim decreased the renal clearance of procainamide and of NAPA, an active metabolite of procainamide, and increased serum concentrations were observed.

Related Drugs: There are no drugs related to procainamide or trimethoprim.

Mechanism: Trimethoprim increases procainamide and NAPA serum concentrations by competing for tubular secretion.

Detailed Information: See *EDI*, 3/14.70

Propafenone-Cyclosporine

Significance: 2—moderately clinically significant

Potential Effects: Propafenone may inhibit the metabolism of cyclosporine resulting in increased cyclosporine levels.

Recommendations: Caution should be used when propafenone therapy is instituted in a patient maintained on cyclosporine. Cyclosporine whole-blood levels should be monitored, and the dose of cyclosporine may need to be reduced.

Summary: The addition of propafenone to a cyclosporine regimen has been shown to result in an increase in cyclosporine whole blood levels.

Related Drugs: It is not known whether an interaction would occur between cyclosporine and other antiarrhythmic agents. There are no drugs related to cyclosporine.

Mechanism: Propafenone may inhibit the metabolism of cyclosporine.

Detailed Information: See *EDI*, 3/14.80

Propafenone-Quinidine

Significance: 2—moderately clinically significant

Potential Effects: Quinidine may increase propafenone plasma concentration and pharmacologic effects.

Recommendations: Patients receiving propafenone should be carefully monitored for cardiac function changes if quinidine is added to therapy. The dose of propafenone may need to be reduced.

Summary: Concurrent quinidine and propafenone administration has been shown to increase the propafenone plasma concentration.

Related Drugs: Quinine would be expected to interact with propafenone in a similar manner. It is not known whether an interaction would occur between quinidine and other antiarrhythmic agents.

Mechanism: Quinidine inhibits the hepatic cytochrome P450 mediated 5-hydroxylation of propafenone, resulting in a decreased clearance of propafenone.

Detailed Information: See *EDI*, 3/14.90

Quinidine-Amiodarone

Significance: 1—highly clinically significant

Potential Effects: Amiodarone can cause an increase in quinidine levels.

Recommendations: Monitor quinidine levels if these agents are used together. The dose of quinidine may need to be decreased.

Summary: Amiodarone can cause an increase in quinidine levels, causing atypical ventricular tachycardia and a prolonged QT interval.

Related Drugs: There are no drugs related to amiodarone. It is not known if a similar interaction would occur between amiodarone and quinine.

Mechanism: The most likely mechanisms include a decrease in quinidine tissue binding, releasing quinidine into the serum and effectively decreasing the volume of distribution, or decreasing the renal or hepatic clearance of quinidine.
Detailed Information: See *EDI*, 3/16.10

Quinidine-Cimetidine

Significance: 2—moderately clinically significant
Potential Effects: Cimetidine decreases the clearance of quinidine.
Recommendations: Patients taking these agents together should be monitored for signs of quinidine toxicity (e.g., cinchonism, lethargy, tachyarrhythmias, vomiting).
Summary: Concurrent administration of cimetidine and quinidine resulted in reduced quinidine clearance, increased half-life, and increased peak plasma concentration.
Related Drugs: Quinidine and ranitidine have been shown to cause dizziness, nausea, irregular heart rate, and ventricular bigeminy with ECG changes. However, all data do not support this. It is not known if an interaction would occur between quinidine and other H_2-receptor antagonists.
Mechanism: An increase in quinidine absorption with concurrent cimetidine may explain the elevated quinidine plasma concentrations.
Detailed Information: See *EDI*, 3/17.00

Quinidine-Diphenoxylate/Atropine

Significance: 3—minimally clinically significant
Potential Effects: Diphenoxylate/atropine decreases GI motility which may result in a decrease in quinidine levels.
Recommendations: Quinidine levels should be monitored and the dosage adjusted as necessary during concomitant administration of diphenoxylate with atropine and quinidine sulfate.
Summary: Concurrent administration of quinidine sulfate and diphenoxylate with atropine has been shown to result in a significant decrease in quinidine levels.
Related Drugs: A similar interaction between quinidine sulfate and difenoxin/atropine may occur. No documentation is available for an interaction between diphenoxylate and quinine.
Mechanism: The ability of diphenoxylate to decrease gastrointestinal motility may affect the absorption of quinidine.
Detailed Information: See *EDI*, 3/18.01

Quinidine-Ketoconazole

Significance: 2—moderately clinically significant
Potential Effects: Ketoconazole may decrease the clearance of quinidine, resulting in increased levels.
Recommendations: Patients maintained on quinidine sulfate should be closely monitored for changes in cardiac status or changes in quinidine serum levels if ketoconazole is added to, or withdrawn from, concurrent quinidine therapy. The dose of quinidine may need to be decreased.
Summary: Ketoconazole may decrease the clearance of quinidine, resulting in increased levels and changes in serum creatinine.
Related Drugs: Other quinidine salts may interact in a similar manner with ketoconazole. A similar interaction is expected to occur between quinine and ketoconazole.

Mechanism: The reduction of plasma quinidine concentration is most likely the result of an inhibition of hepatic enzyme activity by ketoconazole.

Detailed Information: See *EDI*, 3/18.05

Quinidine-Metoclopramide

Significance: 3—minimally clinically significant

Potential Effects: Metoclopramide may decrease the absorption of quinidine, leading to a decrease in quinidine's area-under-curve.

Recommendations: Monitor patients for a decrease in quinidine levels during cotherapy with metoclopramide. The dosage of quinidine may need to be increased.

Summary: Metoclopramide has been shown to decrease quinidine's area-under-curve and absorption.

Related Drugs: It is not known if a similar interaction would occur between metoclopramide and quinine. There are no drugs related to metoclopramide.

Mechanism: Metoclopramide may decrease the absorption of quinidine.

Detailed Information: See *EDI*, 3/18.10

Quinidine-Phenobarbital

Significance: 2—moderately clinically significant

Recommendations: Quinidine plasma levels should be monitored during concurrent use of these agents. If a loss of arrhythmia control is evident, the dose of quinidine may need to be increased. Also, if a patient is stabilized on both agents, the dose of quinidine may have to be decreased upon withdrawal of the barbiturate.

Summary: The concurrent administration of quinidine and phenobarbital has been shown to result in a reduction of the elimination half-life of quinidine and the area-under-curve.

Related Drugs: Similar changes in quinidine levels after pentobarbital administration have been documented. A similar interaction may occur between quinidine and other barbiturates. The half-life of quinine was reported to be significantly decreased in patients receiving phenobarbital, primidone or phenytoin.

Mechanism: Phenobarbital, a known enzyme inducer, may increase the metabolism of quinidine.

Detailed Information: See *EDI*, 3/19.00

Quinidine-Phenytoin

Significance: 2—moderately clinically significant

Recommendations: Combination therapy of quinidine and phenytoin will probably require an alteration in quinidine dosage to maintain therapeutic quinidine serum levels. Careful monitoring and possible readjustment of quinidine levels will be required when phenytoin therapy is begun or discontinued, as seen in one patient where decreasing the phenytoin dosage resulted in an increased quinidine level.

Summary: Quinidine serum levels may be reduced by the concurrent use of phenytoin.

Related Drugs: Other hydantoin anticonvulsants may interact with quinidine. The half-life of quinine was found to be significantly decreased in patients receiving phenobarbital, phenytoin, or primidone.

Mechanism: Phenytoin, a known enzyme inducer, may increase the metabolism of quinidine.

Detailed Information: See *EDI*, 3/21.00

Quinidine-Reserpine

Significance: 3—minimally clinically significant

Recommendations: To minimize the possible toxic effects resulting from concurrent administration of quinidine and reserpine, treatment with these agents should not be initiated simultaneously. Treatment with reserpine should be initiated first and an interval of at least 24 hours should be allowed before introducing quinidine. When quinidine is added to the regimen of a reserpine-treated patient, the dose should be increased cautiously and cardiac function should be monitored closely.

Summary: The antiarrhythmic and cardiodepressant effects of quinidine may be enhanced by the administration of reserpine.

Related Drugs: All quinidine salts may have a similar interaction with reserpine. There is no documentation regarding an interaction with quinine. A similar interaction is expected to occur with the other rauwolfia alkaloids.

Mechanism: Reserpine depletes myocardial tissue of its catecholamine stores and causes a decrease in the electrical automaticity and excitability of myocardial tissue. This effect may enhance quinidine's direct myocardial tissue depressant activity and could result in quinidine toxicity.

Detailed Information: See *EDI*, 3/23.00

Quinidine-Rifampin

Significance: 2—moderately clinically significant

Recommendations: When using rifampin concurrently with quinidine, the response to quinidine should be closely monitored and the dose increased if necessary.

Summary: The antiarrhythmic effect of quinidine was diminished when rifampin was coadministered with quinidine.

Related Drugs: A similar interaction is expected to occur with quinine. There are no drugs related to rifampin.

Mechanism: Rifampin, a known enzyme inducer, may increase the metabolism of quinidine.

Detailed Information: See *EDI*, 3/25.00

Quinidine-Sucralfate

Significance: 3—minimally clinically significant

Potential Effects: Quinidine absorption may be decreased resulting in decreased quinidine levels and effect.

Recommendations: Because of the lack of studies, it is not known whether the bioavailability of quinidine can be altered when given concomitantly with sucralfate. Since a potential has been shown for such a reaction, be cautious when using these agents together.

Summary: Concomitant quinidine and sucralfate resulted in decreased quinidine levels.

Related Drugs: Aluminum hydroxide has been shown to delay the gastrointestinal absorption of quinidine in animals. It is not known whether a similar interaction would occur between quinidine and other aluminum salts.

Mechanism: This interaction could occur in humans because of the ability of sucralfate to bind to the quinidine moiety when these two drugs are given simultaneously.

Detailed Information: See *EDI*, 3/26.50

Quinidine-Verapamil

Significance: 1—highly clinically significant

Potential Effects: Concurrent verapamil and quinidine causes an increase in quinidine levels and possible hypotension.

Recommendations: Use these agents together with caution. Quinidine levels should be monitored and dosage may have to be decreased. One or both drugs may need to be discontinued.

Summary: There are data to show that verapamil causes an increase in quinidine levels, causing hypotension and acute pulmonary edema.

Related Drugs: Nifedipine and quinidine resulted in decreased quinidine serum levels. An interaction is expected to occur between quinidine and other calcium channel blockers, but it is difficult to determine if quinidine levels would increase or decrease. Quinidine administered with nifedipine or diltiazem would result in hypotension. No documentation is available regarding an interaction between verapamil quinine.

Mechanism: Verapamil inhibits the metabolism of quinidine, which results in increased quinidine levels.

Detailed Information: See *EDI*, 3/27.00

Verapamil-Calcium Gluconate

Significance: 2—moderately clinically significant

Recommendations: Patients should be monitored for a change in their response to verapamil if calcium is added to, or withdrawn from, their therapy.

Summary: There are data to show that coadministration of verapamil and calcium may cause changes in verapamil response.

Related Drugs: A similar interaction is expected to occur between calcium gluconate and other calcium channel blockers. The other salts of calcium may be expected to interact similarly with calcium gluconate.

Mechanism: This interaction results from an antagonistic effect between the two agents.

Detailed Information: See *EDI*, 3/29.00

Verapamil-Dantrolene

Significance: 2—moderately clinically significant

Potential Effects: The concurrent use of these agents may result in hyperkalemia and myocardial depression.

Recommendations: Monitor for increased potassium levels when the agents are used concurrently. A decreased dose of dantrolene or the use of nifedipine may help circumvent or lessen the magnitude of the interaction.

Summary: The concurrent administration of verapamil and dantrolene was shown to result in hyperkalemia and myocardial depression.

Related Drugs: Nifedipine exhibits a similar interaction with dantrolene, and in an animal study, nifedipine and dantrolene resulted in hyperkalemia and cardiovascular collapse. A similar interaction is expected to occur between dantrolene and other calcium channel blockers. There are no drugs related to dantrolene.

Mechanism: The addition of verapamil may limit the compensatory mechanisms for a dantrolene-induced increases in serum potassium, resulting in a sustained elevation of potassium levels.

Detailed Information: See *EDI,* 3/30.01

Verapamil-Phenobarbital

Significance: 3—minimally clinically significant

Potential Effects: Phenobarbital may increase the metabolism of verapamil. Also the protein binding of verapamil may be decreased by phenobarbital. These two potential effects may result in an insignificant or no net change in the pharmacologically active unbound concentration of verapamil.

Recommendations: Although the concurrent administration of phenobarbital and verapamil need not be avoided, patients should be monitored for changes in verapamil serum levels. The dose of verapamil may need to be adjusted.

Summary: Phenobarbital has been shown to increase the verapamil free fraction, the total systemic clearance and the rate of elimination of verapamil.

Related Drugs: A similar interaction is expected to occur with other calcium channel blockers and phenobarbital and with other barbiturates.

Mechanism: Phenobarbital may increase the hepatic metabolism of verapamil.

Detailed Information: See *EDI,* 3/30.30

Verapamil-Propranolol

Significance: 2—moderately clinically significant

Potential Effects: Concurrent use of verapamil and propranolol may result in serious hypotension, bradycardia, and, rarely, ventricular asystole.

Recommendations: Patients undergoing concurrent therapy with verapamil and propranolol should be closely monitored for blood pressure, heart rate and clinical status, especially during the first days of concomitant therapy.

Summary: Concurrent use of verapamil and propranolol may result in serious hypotension, decreased cardiac contractility, bradycardia, and ventricular asystole.

Related Drugs: Pindolol, metoprolol or atenolol with verapamil has exhibited a similar interaction. There are many documented reports regarding an interaction between other beta-blockers and calcium channel blockers; however, much of the data are conflicting.

Mechanism: An additive cardiodepressive response may be seen with concomitant use of these agents, and the concurrent administration of propranolol may block the beta-adrenergic activity originally stimulated by verapamil.

Detailed Information: See *EDI,* 3/31.00

Verapamil-Rifampin

Significance: 2—moderately clinically significant

Potential Effects: Rifampin induces the hepatic metabolism of oral verapamil, leading to decreased serum levels and efficacy. This effect is significant only with oral verapamil.

Recommendations: Patients receiving oral verapamil should be monitored for decreased verapamil levels during concurrent rifampin therapy. If decreased levels or effects of verapamil occur during concomitant rifampin administration, the dose of verapamil may need to be increased.

Summary: Rifampin induces the hepatic metabolism of oral verapamil, leading to a decrease in serum levels and efficacy of rifampin.

Related Drugs: A similar interaction is expected to occur with other calcium channel blockers and rifampin. There are no drugs related to rifampin.

Mechanism: Rifampin decreases the bioavailability of oral verapamil by increasing its first-pass metabolism through the induction of hepatic microsomal enzymes.

Detailed Information: See *EDI,* 3/35.00

Verapamil-Sulfinpyrazone

Significance: 3—minimally clinically significant

Recommendations: Until further clinical studies are available, the concurrent use of verapamil and sulfinpyrazone need not be avoided. However, if a decreased response to verapamil is noted, the dose of verapamil may need to be increased.

Summary: There are data to show that sulfinpyrazone causes an increase in the oral plasma clearance of verapamil.

Related Drugs: A similar interaction is expected to occur between sulfinpyrazone and other calcium channel blockers. It is not known if verapamil would interact with probenecid.

Mechanism: Sulfinpyrazone decreases the bioavailability of verapamil by increasing its first-pass metabolism.

Detailed Information: See *EDI,* 3/37.00

Chapter Four

Anticoagulant
Drug Interactions

Acenocoumarol-Cetirizine

Significance: 3—minimally clinically significant

Potential Effects: The addition of cetirizine to the therapy of a patient maintained on acenocoumarol may result in an increase in international normalized ratio (INR) and anticoagulant activity.

Recommendations: Caution is advised when cetirizine is added to or removed from an acenocoumarol regimen. The patient's prothrombin time and INR should be monitored. Cetirizine may need to be discontinued.

Summary: The addition of cetirizine to acenocoumarol therapy resulted in an increase in anticoagulant activity and increased the patient's INR values from 1.5 to 14.

Related Drugs: A similar interaction would be expected to occur between cetirizine and the other coumarin oral anticoagulants. It is not known whether an interaction would occur between acenocoumarol and the other antihistamines related to cetirizine.

Mechanism: It is postulated that cetirizine competitively displaces acenocoumarol from protein binding sites because the carboxylic acid moiety on the cetirizine molecule would enable a strong protein bond. It was also speculated that the patient's renal impairment may have increased cetirizine serum levels, thus further increasing cetirizine's effect on acenocoumarol. These two factors could explain the increased anticoagulant effect noted in the patient.

Detailed Information: See *EDI*, 4/0.30

Dicumarol-Allopurinol

Significance: 1—highly clinically significant

Recommendations: Patients should be closely monitored for an increased anticoagulant response during concurrent use of dicumarol and allopurinol. If necessary, the dose of the anticoagulant may need to be decreased.

Summary: Allopurinol has been documented to significantly prolong dicumarol half-life.

Related Drugs: In patients receiving phenprocoumon, bleeding episodes have occurred after allopurinol treatment. Warfarin activity has been shown to increase with allopurinol; however, all data do not support this. Because of conflicting data, it is difficult to determine whether a similar interaction would occur with anisindione and phenindione. There are no drugs related to allopurinol.

Mechanism: Allopurinol inhibits the hepatic metabolism of dicumarol, prolonging its half-life.

Detailed Information: See *EDI*, 4/1.00

Dicumarol-Chloramphenicol

Significance: 2—moderately clinically significant

Recommendations: The concurrent use of dicumarol and chloramphenicol should be avoided. If concomitant use is necessary, frequent monitoring of prothrombin levels is required, and patients should be observed for clinical signs of dicumarol overdosage (e.g., hematuria, melena, bruising).

Summary: The anticoagulant activity of dicumarol may be enhanced by the concurrent administration of chloramphenicol. Chloramphenicol has been shown to increase the average dicumarol half-life.

Related Drugs: A similar interaction may occur with other coumarin anticoagulants and anisindione or phenindione. There are no drugs related to chloramphenicol.

Mechanism: Chloramphenicol may enhance the anticoagulant activity by reducing the availability of vitamin K, and it may interfere with the production of prothrombin.

Detailed Information: See *EDI*, 4/3.00

Dicumarol-Corticotropin

Significance: 2—moderately clinically significant

Recommendations: Clotting time tests and clinical signs of hemorrhage should be monitored closely during concurrent administration of dicumarol and corticotropin or corticosteroids. The dosage of the anticoagulant may need to be either increased or decreased based on the results of such monitoring.

Summary: Corticotropin and corticosteroids have been shown to increase and decrease the hypoprothrombinemic effect of dicumarol and other oral anticoagulants, causing hemorrhagic episodes.

Related Drugs: The activity of phenindione is enhanced by corticotropin. Increased sensitivity to warfarin was documented with prednisone administration. Phenprocoumon and anisindione may also interact with corticotropin or corticosteroid. Cortisone and prednisone may interact with dicumarol. A similar interaction is expected to occur with other cortico-steroids and dicumarol.

Mechanism: Corticosteroids have been shown to increase the coagulability of the blood, and corticotropin and corticosteroids may lower vascular integrity.

Detailed Information: See *EDI*, 4/5.00

Dicumarol-Methylphenidate

Significance: 3—minimally clinically significant

Recommendations: The concurrent use of these agents need not be avoided. However, it is prudent to be aware of a possible interaction, and prothrombin levels should be frequently monitored.

Summary: Methylphenidate has been documented to increase the half-life of dicumarol; however, all data do not support this.

Related Drugs: It is difficult to determine whether a similar interaction would occur between methylphenidate and phenprocoumon warfarin, anisindione, phenindione or the other indirect-acting sympathomimetic agents.

Mechanism: Methylphenidate may inhibit the hepatic metabolism of dicumarol.

Detailed Information: See *EDI*, 4/7.00

Dicumarol-Oral Contraceptive Agents

Significance: 2—moderately clinically significant

Recommendations: The evidence is limited, but does indicate that the blood coagulation response of some oral anticoagulant agents may be changed with concurrent oral contraceptive agents. Some adjustment in the anticoagulant dosage may be necessary.

Summary: The concurrent administration of oral contraceptive agents and dicumarol has been shown to diminish the anticoagulant response.

Related Drugs: Because of conflicting data, it is difficult to determine whether a similar interaction would occur with phenprocoumon, warfarin, anisindione or phenindione.

Mechanism: It has been suggested that the estrogenic component of the oral contraceptive agent is responsible for the alterations in blood coagulation.

Detailed Information: See *EDI*, 4/9.00

Dicumarol-Phenytoin

Significance: 2—moderately clinically significant

Recommendations: If dicumarol, warfarin, or phenprocoumon and phenytoin are coadministered, an increase in phenytoin half-life, serum levels, or side effects should occur within the first four weeks of therapy, particularly when the anticoagulant is added to the drug regimen of a patient previously stabilized on phenytoin. If signs and symptoms of phenytoin toxicity develop (e.g., nystagmus, gait ataxia, poor muscle tone, or lethargy), serum phenytoin levels should be determined and doses of phenytoin reduced to establish therapeutic levels. Similarly, prothrombin times should be monitored closely. Caution should be exercised when establishing anticoagulant doses after discontinuation of phenytoin or carbamazepine because of the possibility of a subsequent increase in anticoagulant effect, which takes approximately three weeks to develop.

Summary: Concurrent administration of dicumarol and phenytoin may result in a significant increase in the half-life and serum level of phenytoin. Phenytoin may decrease serum dicumarol levels and decrease its anticoagulant effect.

Related Drugs: Warfarin has been documented to cause phenytoin toxicity. Phenytoin has been documented to enhance warfarin's effect. Phenprocoumon has been reported to impair phenytoin metabolism, whereas phenindione had no effect. Phenytoin causes no change in the levels of phenprocoumon. It is difficult to determine whether an interaction would occur with anisindione. A similar interaction is expected to occur with other hydantoin anticonvulsants and dicumarol. Carbamazepine reduces the anticoagulant effect of warfarin.

Mechanism: Dicumarol may impair the P-hydroxylation of phenytoin, causing an increase in phenytoin half-life, accumulation, and intoxication. Phenytoin may induce dicumarol metabolism.

Detailed Information: See *EDI*, 4/11.00

Heparin-Aspirin

Significance: 1—highly clinically significant

Recommendations: Since the combination of low dose heparin and aspirin is effective prophylaxis for postoperative thromboembolism, this combination will continue to be used. Patients should be closely observed for hemorrhagic complications; however, these may not always be predicted by laboratory monitoring of coagulation status. Heparinized patients requiring antipyresis or analgesia should receive acetaminophen rather than aspirin.

Summary: The combined use of heparin and aspirin may result in serious bleeding complications. Aspirin also prevents heparin-induced platelet aggregation.

Related Drugs: No drugs are related to heparin and there are no reports of heparin interactions with other salicylates.

Mechanism: Heparin and aspirin prolong bleeding time, and heparin potentiates aspirin-induced prolongation of bleeding time. Aspirin may decrease platelet aggregation, removing a hemostatic mechanism for protection against heparin-induced bleeding.

Detailed Information: See *EDI,* 4/13.00

Heparin-Carbenicillin

Significance: 2—moderately clinically significant

Potential Effects: Carbenicillin may prolong bleeding time and may theoretically increase the effects of concurrent heparin. The prolongation of bleeding time may occur only with high doses of carbenicillin.

Recommendations: Coagulation must be monitored frequently when these agents are used concurrently.

Summary: Carbenicillin and other penicillins have been shown to prolong bleeding time.

Related Drugs: Similar effects on bleeding have been reported with penicillin G, ticarcillin, ampicillin, and methicillin. All penicillins may alter platelet function and may interact with heparin. There are no drugs related to heparin. A similar interaction between carbenicillin and dicumarol, warfarin and anisindione may occur.

Mechanism: This interaction may be due to the additive pharmacologic activities of heparin and carbenicillin.

Detailed Information: See *EDI,* 4/15.00

Heparin-Dextran

Significance: 2—moderately clinically significant

Recommendations: Data pertaining to the concurrent use of dextran 40 and heparin suggest baseline studies (thrombin time, activated prothrombin time, or the Lee White clotting time) should be performed before and intermittently during therapy until anticoagulation is achieved. Although sufficient data to formulate a conclusive recommendation for the concomitant use of dextran 70 or 75 and heparin are lacking, the two should only be used in combination when patients can be closely monitored. Limited data suggest dextran 70 or 75 may cause a greater incidence of adverse reactions and have less effect on the sludging of red blood cells than the use of dextran 40; however, a firm recommendation as to the preferred agent cannot be offered.

Summary: Use of dextran 70 or dextran 75 in combination with heparin is associated with a significantly higher incidence of bleeding. Dextran 40 has been administered with heparin without untoward effects.

Related Drugs: There are no drugs chemically related to either dextran or heparin.

Mechanism: Heparin and dextran possess independent and synergistic effects prolonging coagulation time and reducing clot strength.

Detailed Information: See *EDI,* 4/17.00

Heparin-Nitroglycerin

Significance: 2—moderately clinically significant

Potential Effects: The use of nitroglycerin may decrease the effect of heparin.

Recommendations: The effect of heparin should be frequently monitored (e.g., by the use of APTT) when these agents are used together. The dose of one or both agents may need to be adjusted.

Summary: There are data to show that the use of nitroglycerin may decrease the effect of heparin. However, one study documented that the propylene glycol vehicle in the nitroglycerin induced heparin resistance; however, all data do not support this.

Related Drugs: It is not known if a similar interaction would occur between heparin and other nitrate derivatives. There are no drugs related to heparin.

Mechanism: The mechanism of this interaction is not known; however, various theories are documented.

Detailed Information: See *EDI,* 4/18.01

Heparin-Tobacco

Significance: 3—minimally clinically significant

Recommendations: Based on limited evidence, tobacco smokers may require larger heparin dosages than nonsmokers in order to achieve adequate anticoagulation in the treatment of thromboembolic disease. Further study is needed to determine the clinical significance of this potential interaction.

Summary: There are data to show that tobacco smokers may require larger heparin dosages than nonsmokers in order to achieve anticoagulation.

Related Drugs: There are no drugs related to heparin.

Mechanism: The mechanism of this interaction has not been established.

Detailed Information: See *EDI,* 4/18.10

Phenindione-Haloperidol

Significance: 3—minimally clinically significant

Recommendations: Until further clinical studies are performed, the concurrent use of these agents need not be avoided. However, it is important to be aware of a possible interaction, and if inadequate anticoagulation occurs a decrease in the haloperidol dose or an increase in the phenindione dose may be necessary.

Summary: The concurrent use of phenindione and haloperidol may lead to a reduction in the anticoagulant effect of phenindione.

Related Drugs: There is no documentation regarding an interaction between haloperidol and dicumarol, phenprocoumon, warfarin or anisindione. Documentation is lacking regarding an interaction between phenindione and other phenothiazines, thioxanthenes, dihydroindolones or the dibenzoxazepines.

Mechanism: The mechanism of this interaction is unknown.

Detailed Information: See *EDI,* 4/19.00

Ticlopidine-Aluminum Hydroxide, Magnesium Hydroxide

Significance: 3—minimally clinically significant

Potential Effects: Concurrent administration of ticlopidine with aluminum or magnesium hydroxide may result in decreased ticlopidine blood levels.

Recommendations: Ticlopidine and antacids should not be administered at the same time.

Summary: When administered with a combination aluminum-magnesium hydroxide antacid, ticlopidine absorption decreased approximately 20%.

Related Drugs: Although documentation is lacking, based on the mechanism of action other antacids could be expected to interact in a similar fashion. There are no drugs related to ticlopidine.

Mechanism: The exact mechanism of this interaction is unknown. Both magnesium and aluminum have been shown to form insoluble chelation complexes with drugs. Direct drug adsorption and the formation of poorly soluble salt complexes have also been reported.

Detailed Information: See *EDI*, 4/20.00

Ticlopidine-Cyclosporine

Significance: 2—moderately clinically significant

Potential Effects: Ticlopidine may decrease whole-blood cyclosporine levels.

Recommendations: Caution should be used when ticlopidine is added to a cyclosporine regimen. Cyclosporine whole-blood levels may be reduced to subtherapeutic levels. The dose of cyclosporine may need to be increased or the ticlopidine discontinued.

Summary: The addition of ticlopidine to a cyclosporine regimen has been shown to decrease cyclosporine whole-blood levels.

Related Drugs: There are no drugs related to ticlopidine or cyclosporine.

Mechanism: The mechanism of this interaction is not known, but ticlopidine may decrease the cyclosporine whole-blood concentration.

Detailed Information: See *EDI*, 4/20.50

Warfarin-Acarbose

Significance: 3—minimally clinically significant

Potential Effects: The addition of acarbose to a stable warfarin regimen may result in an increased anticoagulant effect.

Recommendations: Patients should be carefully monitored for changes in international normalized ratio (INR) or anticoagulant effect when acarbose is added to or removed from the therapy of a patient maintained on warfarin. The dose of warfarin may need to be adjusted.

Summary: The addition of acarbose to a stable warfarin regimen resulted in an increased anticoagulant effect and an increase in the patient's INR value to 4.85 after two weeks of acarbose therapy.

Related Drugs: It is not known whether an interaction would occur between acarbose and the other coumarin anticoagulant agents. There are no drugs related to acarbose.

Mechanism: Since acarbose is not absorbed, it is postulated that this interaction is related to the increased absorption of warfarin, but more studies are needed to determine the precise mechanism of this interaction.

Detailed Information: See *EDI*, 4/20.70

Warfarin-Acetaminophen

Significance: 3—minimally clinically significant

Potential Effects: Concurrent warfarin and acetaminophen administration may result in a change in hypoprothrombinemic response.

Recommendations: Enhancement of warfarin's hypoprothrombinemic effect by acetaminophen appears to be controversial. The use of therapeutic dosages of acetaminophen would thus be preferable to aspirin as an antipyretic or analgesic in the patient requiring oral anticoagulants. However, the use of high doses of acetaminophen may result in an increased prothrombin time. Therefore, the need for monitoring prothrombin time is still necessary for individual patient response to acetaminophen-anticoagulant coadministration.

Summary: Concurrent warfarin and acetaminophen administration may result in a change in hypoprothrombinemic response. The risk of this interaction appears to be dose-related, with higher doses of acetaminophen more likely to increase prothrombin time and international normalized ratio values.

Related Drugs: High doses of acetaminophen (2600 to 4000mg/day) have caused significant increases in prothrombin times in patients taking coumarin derivatives, including anisindione, dicumarol, and phenprocoumon. No significant effects on prothrombin times were observed in patients taking phenprocoumon who received two 650mg doses of acetaminophen administered four hours apart. Phenindione and nicoumalone may also be expected to interact with acetaminophen in a similar manner because they are pharmacologically related to the above agents.

Mechanism: The mechanism of this interaction is unknown. More studies are needed, but the mechanism may involve a combination of acetaminophen's effect on prothrombin time and a competitive inhibition of metabolic pathways.

Detailed Information: See *EDI*, 4/21.00

Warfarin-Alcohol, Ethyl

Significance: 3—minimally clinically significant

Recommendations: No special precautions are necessary when administering warfarin to patients reporting minimal to moderate alcohol consumption as long as routine prothrombin time determinations are regularly obtained. Administration of warfarin to patients who chronically abuse alcohol may require frequent laboratory evaluation to prevent excessive warfarin anticoagulation.

Summary: The use of small or moderate amounts of alcohol is unlikely to produce a significant effect on warfarin; however, continuous, heavy alcohol consumption may significantly alter warfarin metabolism and patient response.

Related Drugs: Alcohol may be expected to interact with dicumarol, phenprocoumon, anisindione and phenindione.

Mechanism: Chronic alcohol abuse may result in exaggerated response to warfarin, possibly secondary to impaired hepatic synthesis of clotting factor precursors or impaired hepatic drug metabolism capacity.

Detailed Information: See *EDI*, 4/23.00

Warfarin-Amiodarone

Significance: 1—highly clinically significant

Potential Effects: Amiodarone causes an increase in the pharmacologic effect of warfarin.

Recommendations: The dosage of warfarin needs to be adjusted based on the prothrombin time when these agents are used together.

Summary: The concurrent administration of warfarin and amiodarone has been shown to result in an increase in the hypoprothrombinemic response to warfarin.

Related Drugs: Similar results were noted when amiodarone was administered concomitantly with acenocoumarol. A similar interaction may occur between amiodarone and dicumarol, phenprocoumon or anisindione. There are no drugs related to amiodarone.

Mechanism: Amiodarone may inhibit the hepatic metabolism of warfarin or an interaction may result from the noncompetitive inhibition of metabolism. Amiodarone may also lower the levels of vitamin K-dependent clotting factors.

Detailed Information: See *EDI*, 4/24.10

Warfarin-Ascorbic Acid

Significance: 4—not clinically significant

Recommendations: No routine adjustment of warfarin dose needs to be made during concurrent ascorbic acid therapy. However, in patients exhibiting changing (increasing) dosage requirements of warfarin during maintenance anticoagulant therapy, possible concurrent ascorbic acid ingestion should be eliminated as a causative factor.

Summary: No significant alteration of warfarin by concurrent ascorbic acid has been demonstrated in controlled clinical studies.

Related Drugs: There are no reports demonstrating a similar interaction between ascorbic acid and dicumarol, phenprocoumon, anisindione or phenindione. There are no drugs related to ascorbic acid.

Mechanism: The decrease in plasma warfarin concentration during concurrent administration of ascorbic acid may result from diarrhea.

Detailed Information: See *EDI*, 4/25.00

Warfarin-Aspirin

Significance: 1—highly clinically significant

Recommendations: Concurrent administration of warfarin and salicylate compounds, including aspirin, sodium salicylate, and diflunisal, should be avoided whenever possible. Either acetaminophen or another nonsteroidal anti-inflammatory agent that does not interact with warfarin should be substituted for aspirin according to the indication present. If warfarin and aspirin in moderate to large dosages are administered together, frequent prothrombin time determinations should be performed initially to monitor the transient increase in warfarin effect which is likely to occur.

Summary: Concurrent administration of moderate to large doses of aspirin and warfarin may potentiate the anticoagulant action of warfarin and increase the risk of warfarin-induced bleeding.

Related Drugs: Dicumarol and phenindione have been shown to not interact with low doses of aspirin. Dicumarol, phenindione, phenprocoumon and anisindione may interact with higher doses of aspirin. Sodium salicylate and diflunisal have been shown to interact with anticoagulants. A similar interaction is expected to occur with other salicylates and warfarin.

Mechanism: Aspirin and related compounds will displace warfarin from plasma protein binding sites, increasing an anticoagulant effect and decreasing total plasma warfarin concentrations. Aspirin will directly decrease platelet aggregation and prolong bleeding time, and oral salicylate administration may cause gastrointestinal bleeding.

Detailed Information: See *EDI,* 4/27.00

Warfarin-Azathioprine

Significance: 2—moderately clinically significant

Potential Effects: The addition of azathioprine to the therapy of a patient maintained on warfarin may result in a decrease in the anticoagulant effects of warfarin.

Recommendations: The anticoagulant effect of warfarin should be carefully monitored if azathioprine is added to or withdrawn from warfarin therapy.

Summary: Concurrent administration of azathioprine in a patient resulted in a decrease in the anticoagulant effects of warfarin.

Related Drugs: Mercaptopurine has been reported to have a similar interaction with warfarin. There have been no reports of an interaction between azathioprine and the other coumarin anticoagulants or the indandione derivatives, although because of pharmacologic similarity, an interaction may be expected.

Mechanism: Although the exact mechanism is unknown, mercaptopurine might induce the hepatic microsomal enzymes responsible for warfarin metabolism; but a decreased gastrointestinal absorption of warfarin cannot be ruled out. Animal experiments have suggested that synthesis or inactivation of the prothrombin complex may also be involved.

Detailed Information: See *EDI,* 4/28.05

Warfarin-Cefamandole

Significance: 2—moderately clinically significant

Recommendations: If cefamandole is added to, or withdrawn from, warfarin therapy, the prothrombin time should be monitored. An adjustment of the warfarin dose or the administration of vitamin K may be necessary.

Summary: Cefamandole was reported to increase warfarin sensitivity, resulting in increased prothrombin times and possibly severe bleeding.

Related Drugs: Coagulation abnormalities have been reported with moxalactam, cefoperazone, cefoxitin, and cefazolin; therefore, cephalosporins would be expected to interact similarly with warfarin. Cefamandole may also interact with dicumarol, phenprocoumon and anisindione.

Mechanism: Cefamandole may increase prothrombin time through prothrombin production, suppression of vitamin K-producing bacterial flora, inhibition of warfarin metabolism, and altered ribosomal function.

Detailed Information: See *EDI,* 4/28.10

Warfarin-Chloral Hydrate

Significance: 2—moderately clinically significant

Recommendations: During initial concurrent administration of warfarin and chloral hydrate, frequent prothrombin time determinations should be made to monitor possible increases in warfarin anticoagulant action. Although temporary warfarin dosage adjustments are not generally necessary, changes in warfarin therapy should be determined on an individual patient basis. For long-term sedative hypnotic therapy, a benzodiazepine is preferable to chloral hydrate (see also Warfarin-Chlordiazepoxide, below).

Summary: Concurrent administration of chloral hydrate and warfarin may be associated with a transient increase in warfarin anticoagulant action.

Related Drugs: Chloral betaine and triclofos have been shown to produce similar effects on warfarin metabolism. Dicumarol has been shown to interact with chloral hydrate, similar to warfarin. A similar interaction is expected to occur between chloral hydrate and phenprocoumon, anisindione and phenindione.

Mechanism: The major metabolite of chloral hydrate displaces warfarin from plasma protein binding sites, increasing the warfarin free fraction in plasma. This elevated free drug concentration is associated with an increased hypoprothrombinemic effect and promotes increased systemic drug clearance.

Detailed Information: See *EDI*, 4/29.00

Warfarin-Chlordiazepoxide

Significance: 4—not clinically significant

Recommendations: Warfarin therapy during concurrent chlordiazepoxide administration should be monitored in a routine fashion. Therefore, no special precautions are necessary when these drugs are given concurrently.

Summary: Concurrent administration of chlordiazepoxide and warfarin produces no clinically significant effect on warfarin.

Related Drugs: Benzodiazepines have not demonstrated any interaction with warfarin. The coumarin anticoagulant phenprocoumon has been demonstrated not to interact with nitrazepam. No data describing anisindione and phenindione have been presented. It is not possible to determine whether an interaction would occur with chlordiazepoxide.

Mechanism: The benzodiazepines may induce hepatic microsomal enzymes.

Detailed Information: See *EDI*, 4/31.00

Warfarin-Chlorthalidone

Significance: 3—minimally clinically significant

Recommendations: The concurrent use of warfarin and chlorthalidone may require a higher dose of warfarin. Prothrombin levels should be monitored and the dose of the anticoagulant adjusted as necessary.

Summary: The concurrent use of chlorthalidone and warfarin has been shown to reduce the hypoprothrombinemic response.

Related Drugs: Documentation is lacking regarding a similar interaction between other thiazide related diuretics and warfarin or between dicumarol, acenocoumarol, anisindione or phenindione and chlorthalidone. A similar interaction is expected to occur with other oral anticoagulants and thiazide related diuretics.

Mechanism: The mechanism of this interaction is not known. Chlorthalidone may improve hepatic function and increase clotting factor synthesis. The effects of warfarin may be antagonized by a decrease in plasma, which concentrates circulating clotting factors.

Detailed Information: See *EDI,* 4/32.10

Warfarin-Cholestyramine

Significance: 2—moderately clinically significant

Potential Effects: Cholestyramine may decrease the anticoagulant action of warfarin. The half-life of warfarin may be decreased and the clearance increased by cholestyramine.

Recommendations: Concurrent use of these agents should be avoided. If they must be given together, cholestyramine should be administered three to six hours after the warfarin. Prothrombin times should be carefully monitored during concomitant therapy. Colestipol may be an alternative to cholestyramine.

Summary: Concurrent administration of oral cholestyramine and warfarin may result in a significant decrease in the anticoagulant activity of warfarin.

Related Drugs: Phenprocoumon showed a similar interaction with warfarin. A similar interaction may be expected to occur between cholestyramine and dicumarol or anisindione. Colestipol has been reported not to interact with phenprocoumon or warfarin. Whether the other coumarin and indandione anticoagulants would also fail to interact with colestipol has not been established.

Mechanism: Cholestyramine binds warfarin in a pH dependent fashion, suggesting a direct interaction of the two drugs in the gut.

Detailed Information: See *EDI,* 4/33.00

Warfarin-Cimetidine

Significance: 1—highly clinically significant

Potential Effects: Cimetidine inhibits the metabolism of warfarin, leading to an increase in the hypoprothrombinemic response of warfarin, resulting in bleeding in some cases.

Recommendations: The use of cimetidine should be avoided in patients receiving warfarin. The hypoprothrombinemic response to warfarin should be closely monitored if cimetidine is added to, or withdrawn from, therapy and the warfarin dose adjusted accordingly. Ranitidine should be also be used with caution. Famotidine or nizatidine may be alternatives to cimetidine or ranitidine since they have not been shown to interact.

Summary: The concomitant administration of warfarin and cimetidine has been shown to significantly increase plasma warfarin levels and prolong the hypoprothrombinemic response of warfarin.

Related Drugs: Phenindione has been shown to react similarly with warfarin; however, phenprocoumon did not show a similar interaction. There is no documentation regarding an interaction with dicumarol or anisindione. Ranitidine did not significantly affect prothrombin time or plasma warfarin concentration; however, all data do not support this. Preliminary studies indicate that warfarin is not affected by the other H_2-receptor antagonists.

Mechanism: Cimetidine may inhibit the hepatic metabolism of warfarin and may inhibit a specific enantiomer of warfarin.

Detailed Information: See *EDI,* 4/35.00

Warfarin-Cisapride

Significance: 2—moderately clinically significant

Potential Effects: The addition of cisapride to the therapy of a patient maintained on warfarin may result in hypoprothrombinemia.

Recommendations: Patients should be carefully monitored for changes in anticoagulant effect when cisapride is added to or discontinued from the therapy of a patient maintained on warfarin.

Summary: The addition of cisapride to the therapy of a patient maintained on warfarin resulted in hypoprothrombinemia, increasing the international normalized ratio values from 2.5 to 10.7.

Related Drugs: A similar interaction would be expected to occur between cisapride and the other coumarin anticoagulants provided that the metabolism of these other agents follows a similar metabolic pathway. There are no drugs related to cisapride.

Mechanism: A decrease in warfarin metabolism may result from competitive binding with cisapride at active sites on the cytochrome $P450_{3A4}$ isoenzyme, leading to increased warfarin levels and subsequent hypoprothrombinemia.

Detailed Information: See *EDI*, 4/36.00

Warfarin-Clofibrate

Significance: 1—highly clinically significant

Recommendations: Because the concurrent use of clofibrate and warfarin may lead to excessive warfarin-induced anticoagulation and clinically significant hemorrhagic side effects, frequent prothrombin time determinations should be made during concurrent therapy. A reduction in warfarin dosage requirements should be expected, although the magnitude of clofibrate effect will vary among individual patients. Warfarin dosage in patients concurrently receiving clofibrate should be individually titrated using appropriate laboratory evaluation.

Summary: Concurrent administration of oral clofibrate and warfarin may enhance warfarin's anticoagulant action.

Related Drugs: Phenindione and dicumarol exhibit a similar interaction with warfarin. Phenprocoumon, indandione and anisindione may also interact with clofibrate.

Mechanism: Clofibrate displaces warfarin from plasma protein binding sites, competitively and noncompetitively. The enhancement of warfarin's effect in patients may be directly associated with clofibrate's hypolipidemic action.

Detailed Information: See *EDI*, 4/37.00

Warfarin-Cyclosporine

Significance: 2—moderately clinically significant

Potential Effects: Concurrent use of these agents may result in decreased levels/activity of either agent.

Recommendations: Both cyclosporine levels and warfarin activity (prothrombin time) should be monitored during concurrent therapy. The dose of one or both drugs may need to be increased.

Summary: There are data to show that the concurrent use of these agents may result in decreased levels and activity of either or both agents.

Related Drugs: It is not known if cyclosporine would interact with dicumarol or anisindione.

Mechanism: The mechanism of this interaction is not known.

Detailed Information: See *EDI*, 4/38.05

Warfarin-Diazoxide

Significance: 3—minimally clinically significant

Recommendations: Until further clinical studies are performed, the concurrent use of these agents need not be avoided. However, it is prudent to be aware of a potential interaction and to monitor prothrombin times frequently.

Summary: The concurrent administration of warfarin and diazoxide may potentiate the hypoprothrombinemic effect of warfarin.

Related Drugs: There are no drugs related to diazoxide. A similar interaction is expected to occur with dicumarol, phenprocoumon, or anisindione and warfarin. An interaction with diazoxide may also occur.

Mechanism: Diazoxide can displace warfarin from human albumin.

Detailed Information: See *EDI,* 4/38.10

Warfarin-Diphenhydramine

Significance: 4—not clinically significant

Recommendations: No specific precautions need be taken during concurrent administration of diphenhydramine and warfarin.

Summary: Concurrent administration of oral diphenhydramine and warfarin produces no clinically significant effect on warfarin.

Related Drugs: No documentation exists regarding an interaction between diphenhydramine and dicumarol, acenocoumarol, anisindione or phenindione. There is a lack of documentation of this interaction with other antihistamines.

Mechanism: Antihistamines have been shown to induce hepatic microsomal enzymes in animal studies.

Detailed Information: See *EDI,* 4/39.00

Warfarin-Disopyramide

Significance: 3—minimally clinically significant

Recommendations: The pharmacologic activity of warfarin may need to be monitored when disopyramide is added to, or deleted from, therapy.

Summary: Disopyramide may enhance the hypoprothrombinemic response to warfarin.

Related Drugs: A similar interaction is expected to occur between disopyramide and dicumarol, acenocoumarol, anisindione or phenindione, if the mechanism involves competition for the same metabolic pathways. There are no drugs related to disopyramide.

Mechanism: Disopyramide and warfarin may compete for the same hepatic metabolic pathways.

Detailed Information: See *EDI,* 4/41.00

Warfarin-Disulfiram

Significance: 1—highly clinically significant

Recommendations: The concurrent use of warfarin and disulfiram should be avoided. When these drugs must be administered concurrently, a decrease of usual dosages of warfarin may be necessary. Patient education and careful monitoring of prothrombin activity are recommended.

Summary: Concurrent administration of warfarin and disulfiram may result in elevated serum warfarin levels and an enhanced hypoprothrombinemic response.

Related Drugs: Disulfiram may interact with dicumarol, acenocoumarol, anisindione or phenindione. No drugs are related to disulfiram.

Mechanism: Inhibition of the hepatic enzyme system by disulfiram results in increased warfarin levels and an enhanced hypoprothrombinemic effect.

Detailed Information: See *EDI*, 4/43.00

Warfarin-Erythromycin

Significance: 1—highly clinically significant

Potential Effects: Erythromycin causes an increase in warfarin's effect on prothrombin time, which may lead to bleeding.

Recommendations: Avoid the concurrent use of warfarin and erythromycin. If these agents must be used together, prothrombin times should be carefully monitored.

Summary: The concurrent administration of warfarin and erythromycin may increase the hypoprothrombinemic action of warfarin, resulting in bruising and hematuria in some cases. Prothrombin times, which have been shown to significantly increase following the initiation of erythromycin to patients maintained on warfarin, returned to control values when erythromycin was discontinued.

Related Drugs: Prolonged prothrombin times have been documented in patients receiving azithromycin concurrently with warfarin and in patients receiving acenocoumarol when erythromycin ethylsuccinate or clarithromycin were added to their regimens. Ponsinomycin had no significant effects on nicoumalone pharmacokinetics. A similar interaction may be expected to occur between erythromycin and the other coumarin anticoagulants and anisindione. Other macrolide antibiotics may also be expected to interact with coumarin anticoagulants.

Mechanism: The mechanism is unknown. However, several mechanisms have been postulated, such as antibiotic-induced reduction of vitamin K-producing bacterial flora in the intestine, inhibition of warfarin metabolism, and enhanced responsiveness to warfarin as a result of altered ribosomal function. It has also been suggested that a metabolite of erythromycin inhibits drug metabolism and not erythromycin itself, since erythromycin has been shown to induce microsomal enzymes and promote its own biotransformation into metabolites that form inactive complexes with cytochrome P450.

Detailed Information: See *EDI*, 4/45.00

Warfarin-Ethacrynic Acid

Significance: 2—moderately clinically significant

Recommendations: Patients stabilized on warfarin should be monitored for prothrombin activity whenever ethacrynic acid is added to, or withdrawn from, the regimen. Furosemide or bumetanide may be suitable alternatives since some studies have reported that warfarin is unaffected by their concurrent use. Since intravenously administered ethacrynic acid has been associated with gastrointestinal bleeding, patients should also be monitored for possible hemorrhage.

Summary: Ethacrynic acid has been documented to significantly increase prothrombin time.

Related Drugs: Dicumarol, acenocoumarol, anisindione or phenindione may interact with ethacrynic acid. Other loop diuretics have no effect on warfarin.

Mechanism: Ethacrynic acid has been shown to displace warfarin from human albumin *in vitro* and enhance warfarin-induced hypoprothrombinemia in rats.

Detailed Information: See *EDI*, 4/47.00

Warfarin-Ethchlorvynol

Significance: 2—moderately clinically significant

Recommendations: Patients stabilized on dicumarol or warfarin should be monitored for prothrombin activity whenever ethchlorvynol is added to, or withdrawn from, the drug regimen. The substitution of benzodiazepine compounds as an alternative to ethchlorvynol should be considered since benzodiazepines do not significantly affect the activity of oral anticoagulants (see also Warfarin-Chlordiazepoxide, page 78).

Summary: Ethchlorvynol may significantly decrease the anticoagulant activity of warfarin when these drugs are administered concurrently.

Related Drugs: Dicumarol has been shown to interact with ethchlorvynol. Phenprocoumon, anisindione or phenindione may interact in a similar manner, if the mechanism involves induction of hepatic enzymes by ethchlorvynol.

Mechanism: Ethchlorvynol may increase warfarin metabolism by induction of hepatic microsomal enzymes.

Detailed Information: See *EDI*, 4/49.00

Warfarin-Etoposide, Vindesine

Significance: 3—minimally clinically significant

Potential Effects: Etoposide and/or vindesine may increase the anticoagulant action of warfarin.

Recommendations: Monitor prothrombin times when these agents are used together. The dose of warfarin may need to be adjusted.

Summary: There are data to show that etoposide and/or vindesine may increase the anticoagulant action of warfarin.

Related Drugs: A similar interaction is expected to occur between etoposide and vindesine with dicumarol, acenocoumarol, anisindione or phenindione. Vindesine resembles vincristine in activity; therefore, a similar interaction may occur between these agents and warfarin. A similar interaction is expected to occur with other antineoplastic agents and warfarin.

Mechanism: Etoposide may displace warfarin from its binding sites. Etoposide and/or vindesine may competitively inhibit the hepatic enzymes responsible for the metabolism of warfarin.

Detailed Information: See *EDI*, 4/50.10

Warfarin-Etretinate

Significance: 2—moderately clinically significant

Potential Effects: Warfarin's anticoagulant effect may be decreased.

Recommendations: The International Normalized Ratio should be carefully monitored in patients maintained on warfarin when etretinate is added to, or withdrawn from, therapy. The dose of warfarin needs to be adjusted.

Summary: The addition of etretinate to the therapy of patients stabilized on warfarin has been shown to result in a decrease in the anticoagulant effect of warfarin.

Related Drugs: A similar interaction is expected to occur between warfarin and other retinoic acid derivatives. It is not known whether an interaction would occur between etretinate and acenocoumarol, phenprocoumon, nicoumalone, anisindione or pheninidione.

Mechanism: Studies in animal models have found that etretinate may cause an induction of hepatic mixed function oxidase system enzymes, increasing the rate of metabolism of warfarin.

Detailed Information: See *EDI*, 4/50.60

Warfarin-Felbamate

Significance: 2—moderately clinically significant

Potential Effects: An increase in the International Normalized Ratio (INR) may occur with the addition of felbamate to the therapy of a patient maintained on warfarin.

Recommendations: Warfarin levels and INR values/prothrombin times should be carefully monitored if felbamate is added to, or withdrawn from, therapy. The dose of warfarin may need to be adjusted.

Summary: There are data to show that felbamate increases the INR in patients stabilized on warfarin.

Related Drugs: An interaction may occur between felbamate and other coumarin anticoagulant agents. It is not known whether an interaction would occur between felbamate and the indandione anticoagulant agents. An interaction may occur between warfarin and meprobamate (see page 90).

Mechanism: Felbamate may inhibit the metabolism of warfarin.

Detailed Information: See *EDI*, 4/50.65

Warfarin-Fluconazole

Significance: 2—moderately clinically significant

Potential Effects: The anticoagulation effect of warfarin may be potentiated with concurrent fluconazole and may result in bleeding episodes.

Recommendations: Patients' prothrombin times and international normalized ratios should be closely monitored during the concomitant use of these agents and when fluconazole is discontinued. The dose of warfarin may need to be adjusted or fluconazole may need to be discontinued. One set of authors recommends a step-wise approach to the reduction of warfarin dosage over the first four days of concurrent therapy by reducing warfarin to 80%, 50%, 43%, and finally 36% of the previous maintenance dosage.

Summary: Fluconazole enhances the anticoagulant effects of warfarin and may cause an increase in prothrombin time and possible bleeding episodes.

Related Drugs: Ketoconazole and itraconazole have also been shown to potentiate the effects of warfarin and cause bleeding episodes, although the data on ketoconazole are conflicting. Several case reports document the potentiation of warfarin or acenocoumarol by concurrent oral miconazole or miconazole oral gel. Prolongation of prothrombin time has also been documented in a patient after fluconazole was added to nicoumalone therapy. A similar interaction would be expected to occur between warfarin and other imidazole antifungal agents and between fluconazole and other coumarin anticoagulants. It is not known whether an interaction would occur with the indanedione derivatives.

Mechanism: It is postulated that the mechanism of this interaction involves an inhibition of the cytochrome P450 system. An *in vitro* study has demonstrated that fluconazole inhibits the metabolism of S-warfarin at the cytochrome $P450_{2C9}$ and the metabolism of R-warfarin at the cytochrome $P450_{3A4}$.

Detailed Information: See *EDI,* 4/50.70

Warfarin-Fluoxetine

Significance: 3—minimally clinically significant

Potential Effects: The addition of fluoxetine to a stable warfarin regimen may result in an increase in the effect of warfarin.

Recommendations: Patients maintained on warfarin should be carefully monitored for changes in prothrombin time if fluoxetine is added to, or removed from, therapy. The dose of one or both agents may need to be adjusted.

Summary: The addition of fluoxetine may result in an increase in the anticoagulation activity of warfarin.

Related Drugs: Paroxetine and sertraline were shown to exhibit a similar interaction with warfarin. The anticoagulant effect of nicoumalone and warfarin may be enhanced by fluvoxamine and paroxetine. It is not known whether an interaction would occur between fluoxetine and dicumarol, acenocoumarol, phenprocoumon, anisindione or phenindione.

Mechanism: The mechanism for this interaction in not known, but may involve plasma protein binding.

Detailed Information: See *EDI,* 4/50.80

Warfarin-Ginkgo

Significance: 3—minimally clinically significant

Potential Effects: The addition of *Ginkgo biloba* to the therapy of a patient maintained on warfarin may result in increased bleeding times and hemorrhagic complications.

Recommendations: Caution should be observed if *Ginkgo biloba* is added to the therapy of a patient maintained on warfarin. Patients should be monitored for increased bleeding times and hemorrhagic risk. The dose of warfarin may need to be adjusted.

Summary: The addition of *Ginkgo biloba* to the therapy of a patient maintained on warfarin may have resulted in increased bleeding times and an intracerebral hemorrhage.

Related Drugs: It is not known whether an interaction would occur between *Ginkgo biloba* and the other coumarin anticoagulant agents.

Mechanism: Spontaneous bilateral subdural hematomas have been associated with chronic *Ginkgo biloba* use. Increased bleeding and hemorrhagic complications resulted from the addition of *Ginkgo biloba* to the regimen of a patient maintained on aspirin. It has been suggested that the coadministration of two antiplatelet agents might have contributed to the risk of hemorrhage.

Detailed Information: See *EDI,* 4/50.85

Warfarin-Ginseng

Significance: 2—moderately clinically significant

Potential Effects: The addition of ginseng to the therapy of a patient maintained on a stable warfarin regimen may result in a significant decline in the international normalized ratio (INR).

Recommendations: INR values should be carefully monitored if ginseng is added to or discontinued from the regimen of a patient maintained on warfarin. The warfarin dosage may need to be adjusted or the ginseng may need to be discontinued.

Summary: The addition of ginseng to the therapy of a patient maintained on a stable warfarin regimen resulted in a significant decline in the INR from a range of 3.0–4.0 to 1.5.

Related Drugs: It is not known whether an interaction would occur between ginseng and the other coumarin or indandione anticoagulants.

Mechanism: The mechanism of this interaction is not known.

Detailed Information: See *EDI*, 4/50.90

Warfarin-Glucagon

Significance: 1—highly clinically significant

Recommendations: It has been suggested that if more than 25mg of glucagon per day is to be given for longer than one to two days, the dosage of warfarin should be reduced and prothrombin time should be monitored closely.

Summary: Administration of glucagon was shown to increase the hypoprothrombinemic effect of warfarin.

Related Drugs: A similar interaction is expected to occur between glucagon and dicumarol, acenocoumarol, anisindione or phenindione. No drugs are related to glucagon.

Mechanism: Glucagon may potentiate the hypoprothrombinemic action of warfarin by acting synergistically to depress hepatic synthesis of vitamin K-sensitive clotting proteins or by increasing the affinity of warfarin.

Detailed Information: See *EDI*, 4/51.00

Warfarin-Glutethimide

Significance: 1—highly clinically significant

Recommendations: If glutethimide is administered to patients receiving oral anticoagulants, they should be carefully monitored and the dosage of warfarin adjusted as needed, since the enzyme induction by glutethimide can occur from several days to one week after initiation of therapy. Conversely, the withdrawal of glutethimide from the drug regimen could lead to severe bleeding unless the patient is monitored and the anticoagulant dosage adjusted downward as needed. After the discontinuation of glutethimide, it may take up to four weeks for the prothrombin time to return to pretreatment levels. In patients requiring a hypnotic agent, a benzodiazepine can be used as an alternative to glutethimide since these compounds do not significantly affect the prothrombin time achieved with anticoagulants (see also Warfarin-Chlordiazepoxide, page 78).

Summary: Glutethimide stimulates the metabolism of warfarin, reducing its anticoagulant effect.

Related Drugs: Aminoglutethimide was shown to have a similar interaction with warfarin. A similar interaction is expected to occur between methyprylon and other oral anticoagulants. Glutethimide has been shown to significantly decrease dicumarol plasma levels. Phenprocoumon and anisindione may interact similarly to warfarin.

Mechanism: Glutethimide increases the activity of the hepatic microsomal enzymes involved in drug metabolism.

Detailed Information: See *EDI*, 4/53.00

Warfarin-Griseofulvin

Significance: 2—moderately clinically significant

Potential Effects: Griseofulvin increases the metabolism of warfarin, decreasing the effect on coagulation.

Recommendations: If griseofulvin is added to, or withdrawn from, warfarin therapy, the prothrombin time should be monitored and warfarin's dosage may need to be adjusted.

Summary: Coadministration of griseofulvin and warfarin has been shown to result in a decreased prothrombin time, requiring an increase in the dose of warfarin. However, data are available indicating that griseofulvin has no effect on warfarin's hypoprothrombinemic response.

Related Drugs: A similar interaction may occur between griseofulvin and dicumarol, phenprocoumon, or anisindione. There are no drugs related to griseofulvin.

Mechanism: Griseofulvin may induce liver enzymes, increase the rate of metabolic biotransformation or interfere with the absorption of warfarin, decreasing the hypoprothrombinemic effect of warfarin.

Detailed Information: See *EDI,* 4/55.00

Warfarin-Ibuprofen

Significance: 2—moderately clinically significant

Potential Effects: Although not a significant problem at recommended therapeutic doses, ibuprofen may cause some displacement of warfarin from plasma protein binding sites.

Recommendations: No specific adjustments of warfarin's maintenance dosage need to be made during concurrent therapy with ibuprofen. However, prothrombin times should be closely monitored in cases of increasing age or renal impairment if ibuprofen is added to, or withdrawn from, a patient's therapy.

Summary: Administration of therapeutic doses of ibuprofen and warfarin should not significantly affect warfarin's anticoagulant action.

Related Drugs: Fenoprofen, tolmetin, naproxen and piroxicam have been shown to have a similar interaction with warfarin. Ketoprofen resulted in increasing prothrombin time and gastrointestinal bleeding. Documentation is lacking regarding an interaction between warfarin and meclofenamate. The effects of other NSAIAs appear to be drug-specific. Phenprocoumon has been reported to not interact with ibuprofen. Documentation is lacking regarding an interaction between ibuprofen and dicumarol or anisindione.

Mechanism: The mechanism behind this interaction varies depending on the NSAIA.

Detailed Information: See *EDI,* 4/57.00

Warfarin-Ifosfamide

Significance: 2—moderately clinically significant

Potential Effects: The anticoagulant activity of warfarin may be increased.

Recommendations: Patients maintained on warfarin should be closely monitored for changes in anticoagulation activity if ifosfamide is added to, or withdrawn from, therapy. The dose of warfarin may need to be adjusted.

Summary: The anticoagulant activity of warfarin may be increased when ifosfamide is added to the therapy of a patient maintained on warfarin.

Related Drugs: Cyclophosphamide reduced the anticoagulant effect of warfarin. A similar interaction is expected to occur between ifosfamide and acenocoumarol, dicumarol, phenprocoumon, anisindione or phenindione, if the mechanism involves inhibition of hepatic metabolism.

Mechanism: Ifosfamide could displace warfarin from plasma protein binding sites, resulting in an increase in International Normalized Ratio. Ifosfamide may be inhibit the cytochrome P450 mediated metabolism of warfarin.

Detailed Information: See *EDI*, 4/58.50

Warfarin-Indomethacin

Significance: 2—moderately clinically significant

Potential Effects: Indomethacin can cause gastric ulceration and hemorrhage, and it impairs platelet function. It may also increase the effects of warfarin.

Recommendations: Patients receiving these agents concurrently should be monitored closely for changes in prothrombin time as well as for clinical signs of increased anticoagulation.

Summary: There are data to show that indomethacin can cause gastric ulceration and hemorrhage, impairing platelet function and prolonging bleeding time. Indomethacin should still be used cautiously in patients receiving oral anticoagulants.

Related Drugs: There are many NSAIAs that have interacted with warfarin to some extent. The effects of other NSAIAs on warfarin metabolism and clinical symptoms appear to be drug-specific. A similar interaction is expected to occur between indomethacin and dicumarol or anisindione. Ibuprofen has been shown to have no significant effect on the anticoagulant activity of phenprocoumon.

Mechanism: The exact mechanism of the potential interaction between indomethacin and warfarin is unknown but may be related to indomethacin-induced displacement of warfarin from plasma protein binding sites.

Detailed Information: See *EDI*, 4/59.00

Warfarin-Influenza Virus Vaccine

Significance: 3—minimally clinically significant

Potential Effects: Influenza virus vaccine may increase the anticoagulant effects of warfarin, although several studies reported no interaction between these agents.

Recommendations: Patients receiving these agents together should be closely monitored for increases in the anticoagulant effect of warfarin.

Summary: The administration of influenza virus vaccine to patients on warfarin therapy may result in an increased prothrombin time; however, all data do not support this.

Related Drugs: Documentation is lacking regarding a similar interaction between influenza virus vaccine and dicumarol, phenprocoumon or anisindione. The administration of pneumococcal vaccine did not affect the anticoagulant response.

Mechanism: The influenza virus vaccine may affect the metabolism of warfarin and the coagulation pathways.

Detailed Information: See *EDI*, 4/61.00

Warfarin-Isoniazid

Significance: 3—minimally clinically significant

Recommendations: Until further clinical studies are available, patients should be monitored for an increased anticoagulant action after isoniazid is added to warfarin therapy. The dosage of warfarin may need to be decreased.

Summary: Isoniazid causes an increase in the anticoagulant action of warfarin.

Related Drugs: There are no drugs related to isoniazid. Dicumarol increased prothrombin time and blood levels after administration of isoniazid. A similar interaction is expected to occur with phenprocoumon, anisindione or phenindione, if the mechanism of the interaction is related to inhibition of hepatic metabolism by isoniazid.

Mechanism: Isoniazid may inhibit the hepatic microsomal enzymes responsible for the metabolism of the anticoagulant.

Detailed Information: See *EDI,* 4/63.00

Warfarin-Lovastatin

Significance: 2—moderately clinically significant

Potential Effects: Concurrent use of these agents may result in an increase in the hypoprothrombinemic activity of warfarin.

Recommendations: The patient should be monitored for changes in prothrombin time if lovastatin is added to or discontinued from therapy of a patient maintained on warfarin. The dose of warfarin may need to be adjusted.

Summary: The addition of lovastatin to warfarin therapy resulted in increased prothrombin times and bleeding.

Related Drugs: Similar interactions have been reported between fluindione and pravastatin and between acenocoumarol and simvastatin. Conversely, one case reported no interaction between warfarin and simvastatin. An interaction would be expected to occur between warfarin and the other HMG-CoA reductase inhibitors. It is not known whether an interaction would occur between lovastatin and the other oral anticoagulant agents.

Mechanism: The mechanism of this interaction is not known, but it has been postulated that lovastatin may inhibit the hepatic hydroxylation of warfarin or that lovastatin, which is highly plasma protein bound, may displace warfarin from its binding site. Either of these possible mechanisms may result in a potentiation of warfarin's hypo-prothrombinemic action.

Detailed Information: See *EDI,* 4/64.50

Warfarin-Magnesium Hydroxide

Significance: 4—not clinically significant

Recommendations: No special precautions are necessary when antacids containing aluminum or magnesium hydroxide are concurrently administered with warfarin. As a routine practice, however, simultaneous administration of antacids with warfarin should not necessarily be encouraged.

Summary: Concurrent administration of warfarin with antacids containing aluminum and/or magnesium hydroxide does not produce any significant effect on warfarin.

Related Drugs: The absorption of dicumarol is slightly enhanced by the simultaneous administration of magnesium hydroxide suspension. The effects of aluminum or magnesium hydroxideproducts on phenprocoumon, anisindione or phenindione have not been evaluated.

Mechanism: Antacids increase intestinal pH, decreasing the absorption of warfarin.

Detailed Information: See *EDI*, 4/65.00

Warfarin-Meprobamate

Significance: 3—minimally clinically significant

Recommendations: Since there may be a significant decrease in the prothrombin time only in a rare patient receiving meprobamate and warfarin, it is prudent to routinely check weekly prothrombin times for the first four weeks after initiating meprobamate in warfarin-stabilized patients. The use of another anti-anxiety agent such as a benzodiazepine may be a satisfactory alternative.

Summary: Meprobamate has been reported to induce the hepatic microsomal enzymes that metabolize warfarin in animals.

Related Drugs: There is a lack of documentation of a similar interaction with the propanediol derivatives, related to meprobamate; however, an interaction may be expected if these agents also induce hepatic enzymes. A similar interaction is expected to occur between meprobamate and dicumarol, acenocoumarol, anisindione or phenindione, if the mechanism involves hepatic microsomal enzyme induction.

Mechanism: Meprobamate may accelerate the metabolic inactivation of drugs metabolized hepatic microsomal enzymes.

Detailed Information: See *EDI*, 4/69.00

Warfarin-Methyltestosterone

Significance: 1—highly clinically significant

Recommendations: It is important to monitor prothrombin times critically in patients receiving these agents concurrently. If methyltestosterone or other C-17-alkylated androgens are administered concomitantly with oral anticoagulants, the anticoagulant dosage may need to be decreased based on changes in prothrombin time.

Summary: Concurrent administration of warfarin and methyltestosterone can significantly increase the hypoprothrombinemic actions of warfarin.

Related Drugs: Oxymetholone, methandrostenolone, danazol, and stanozolol increase the hypoprothrombinemic action of warfarin, dicumarol, and phenindione. A similar interaction may be expected to occur with phenprocoumon or anisindione. Other C-17-alkylated androgen derivatives may be expected to interact similarly with warfarin.

Mechanism: The interaction may be related to an increase in the decay of clotting proteins, a decrease in vitamin K, an increase in warfarin receptor sites, or an alteration in the vitamin K-sensitive clotting factors.

Detailed Information: See *EDI*, 4/75.00

Warfarin-Metronidazole

Significance: 2—moderately clinically significant

Potential Effects: Concurrent metronidazole may enhance the hypoprothrombinemic effect of warfarin.

Recommendations: The racemic mixture is the usual commercially available warfarin. Therefore it can be anticipated that excessive hypoprothrombinemia and bleeding may occur in patients receiving concurrent metronidazole. Appropriate precautions and monitoring of prothrombin levels should be undertaken if these agents are to be used concomitantly, including a decrease in the warfarin dosage if necessary.

Summary: In two studies, metronidazole significantly enhanced the hypoprothrombinemic effect of warfarin. The onset of the interaction occurred within four to ten days and appeared as excessive bruising of the legs.

Related Drugs: Since the mechanism appears to involve a specific warfarin racemate, it is not known if a similar interaction would occur between metronidazole and the other coumarin anticoagulants and the indandione derivatives. Phenprocoumon is a racemic mixture, as is warfarin, and may be expected to interact similarly. An interaction would be expected to occur between warfarin and the other metronidazole-related antibacterial agents.

Mechanism: Studies show that metronidazole inhibits the enzymatic pathway responsible for the ring hydroxylation of S(-) warfarin. This indicates that the S(-) racemate, which is the more potent, is retained in the body whereas the R(+) racemate is unaffected.

Detailed Information: See *EDI,* 4/77.00

Warfarin-Miconazole

Significance: 2—moderately clinically significant

Potential Effects: Miconazole may increase the anticoagulant action of warfarin.

Recommendations: Patients receiving warfarin and miconazole concomitantly should be monitored for changes in the anticoagulant effect of warfarin. The dosage of warfarin may need to be initially decreased, or miconazole may need to be discontinued.

Summary: The concurrent administration of warfarin and miconazole may increase the anticoagulant effect of warfarin.

Related Drugs: A similar interaction is expected to occur between miconazole and dicumarol or anisindione, if the mechanism involves displacement of warfarin from protein binding. There are no drugs related to miconazole.

Mechanism: Miconazole displaces warfarin from plasma protein binding sites.

Detailed Information: See *EDI,* 4/79.00

Warfarin-Mitotane

Significance: 2—moderately clinically significant

Potential Effects: Mitotane may increase the metabolism of warfarin, decreasing the anticoagulant effect.

Recommendations: Monitor patients' prothrombin time frequently when mitotane is added to, or withdrawn from, warfarin therapy.

Summary: Mitotane may increase the metabolism of warfarin, decreasing the anticoagulant effect, necessitating an increase in the warfarin dosage.

Related Drugs: A similar interaction is expected to occur between mitotane and dicumarol, phenprocoumon or anisindione. There are no drugs related to mitotane.

Mechanism: Mitotane reduces the hypoprothrombinemic effect of warfarin by increasing its metabolism secondary to induction of hepatic microsomal enzymes.

Detailed Information: See *EDI,* 4/80.10

Warfarin-Moricizine

Significance: 2—moderately clinically significant

Potential Effects: Moricizine may increase the effects of warfarin.

Recommendations: Patients maintained on warfarin should be monitored for changes in prothrombin time if moricizine is added to therapy.

Summary: The addition of moricizine to the regimen of a patient maintained on warfarin resulted in increased prothrombin time and bleeding.

Related Drugs: It is not known whether an interaction would occur between moricizine and acenocoumarol, dicumarol or phenindione. There are no drugs related to moricizine.

Mechanism: Moricizine may displace warfarin from plasma protein binding sites.

Detailed Information: See *EDI*, 4/80.25

Warfarin-Nafcillin

Significance: 2—moderately clinically significant

Potential Effects: Nafcillin may induce warfarin resistance as well as increase the risk of bleeding because of platelet dysfunction.

Recommendations: Coagulation should be closely monitored during concurrent use of these agents. The warfarin dosage may need to be adjusted.

Summary: There are data to show that nafcillin may induce warfarin resistance and increase the risk of bleeding secondary to platelet dysfunction.

Related Drugs: Dicloxacillin sodium, piperacillin, azlocillin and penicillin G have been reported to prolong bleeding time. Amoxicillin and warfarin administration resulted in an embolism. Ticarcillin has been reported to decrease platelet function. Carbenicillin has been reported to decrease platelet function and inhibit fibrinogen conversion. Documentation is lacking regarding an interaction between warfarin and other penicillins and between penicillins and dicumarol, acenocoumarol, phenprocoumon, nicoumalon or anisindione.

Mechanism: The mechanism by which nafcillin would induce warfarin resistance has not been determined, but may be due to hepatic microsomal enzyme induction.

Detailed Information: See *EDI*, 4/80.30

Warfarin-Nalidixic Acid

Significance: 1—highly clinically significant

Potential Effects: Nalidixic acid may increase warfarin's anticoagulant effects, possibly by displacing warfarin from plasma albumin.

Recommendations: It is important to monitor patients for an increased anticoagulant response when warfarin and nalidixic acid or the fluoroquinolone antibiotics are used concurrently. The dosage of warfarin may need to be decreased.

Summary: There are data to show that nalidixic acid may increase warfarin's anticoagulant effects.

Related Drugs: Nicoumalone and nalidixic acid were shown to have a similar interaction with warfarin. A similar interaction is expected to occur between nalidixic acid and dicumarol or anisindione. Enoxacin did not affect the hypoprothrombinemic response of warfarin. Norfloxacin has been shown to cause a significant rise in prothrombin time; however, not all data support this. A similar interaction may occur between warfarin and other fluoroquinolones and quinolones.

Mechanism: Nalidixic acid has been shown to displace warfarin on plasma albumin *in vitro*.
Detailed Information: See *EDI,* 4/81.00

Warfarin-Neomycin

Significance: 3—minimally clinically significant
Recommendations: The possibility of a clinically significant enhancement of warfarin activity by the oral aminoglycosides may occur only in certain patients who have a dietary deficiency of vitamin K and are receiving large doses of the aminoglycoside. Nevertheless, monitoring of prothrombin activity is warranted when the two drugs are administered concurrently, as it is whenever any drug is added to, or deleted from, the regimen of a patient receiving an oral anticoagulant.
Summary: Concurrent administration of warfarin and oral neomycin may result in a slight increase in the hypoprothrombinemic effect of warfarin.
Related Drugs: The other oral aminoglycosides may interact with warfarin. A similar interaction is expected to occur between neomycin and dicumarol, phenprocoumon, anisindione or phenindione.
Mechanism: Neomycin may enhance a hypoprothrombinemic response by decreasing vitamin K availability.
Detailed Information: See *EDI,* 4/83.00

Warfarin-Nortriptyline

Significance: 4—not clinically significant
Recommendations: Avoidance of concurrent administration of these two agents does not appear necessary. However, patients should be monitored for changes in anticoagulant response when antidepressants are added to an oral anticoagulant regimen.
Summary: Nortriptyline has been reported not to interfere with warfarin pharmacokinetics.
Related Drugs: Hypoprothrombinemic effects were not reported with nortriptyline. No interaction was documented with amitriptyline or nortriptyline with dicumarol or warfarin. Because of conflicting reports, it is difficult to determine whether an interaction would occur between phenprocoumon, anisindione or phenindione with nortriptyline, or between warfarin and the other tricyclic antidepressants or tetracyclic antidepressants.
Mechanism: Nortriptyline may inhibit the metabolism of dicumarol. The tricyclic antidepressants may slow gastrointestinal motility. It has been shown that warfarin is not affected by nortriptyline.
Detailed Information: See *EDI,* 4/85.00

Warfarin-Omeprazole

Significance: 3—minimally clinically significant
Potential Effects: The anticoagulant effect of warfarin may be increased.
Recommendations: The concurrent administration of omeprazole and warfarin may result in an increase in the hypoprothrombinemic effect of warfarin. Patients receiving warfarin should be closely monitored if omeprazole is added to, or withdrawn from, therapy.
Summary: There are data to show that administration of omeprazole may increase the anticoagulation effect of warfarin.

Related Drugs: A similar interaction is expected to occur between omeprazole and dicumarol or anisindione. There are no drugs related to omeprazole.

Mechanism: Omeprazole inhibits metabolism through inhibition of the cytochrome P450 isoenzymes, and the increase in warfarin may be due to inhibition, affecting the elimination of warfarin.

Detailed Information: See *EDI*, 4/86.10

Warfarin-Phenobarbital

Significance: 1—highly clinically significant

Recommendations: If possible, it is best to avoid the concurrent use of warfarin and phenobarbital. If phenobarbital therapy is initiated in a patient stabilized on a particular dosage of warfarin, it is likely that an increase in the dosage of warfarin will be required. If phenobarbital is discontinued, the therapy should be monitored closely and the need for reducing the anticoagulant dosage must be carefully considered.

Summary: The anticoagulant effect of warfarin can be decreased by the administration of phenobarbital, and it may be necessary to increase the warfarin dose.

Related Drugs: Amobarbital, aprobarbital, barbital, butabarbital, pentobarbital, and secobarbital interact with coumarin anticoagulants. Other barbiturates may act similarly to phenobarbital. Reports indicate that warfarin or dicumarol may need dosage adjustments when administered with phenobarital. Phenprocoumon is also influenced. Caution is indicated with anisindione and phenindione because of a similar metabolic fate.

Mechanisms: Phenobarbital increases the hepatic microsomal enzymes responsible for metabolizing warfarin, resulting in a decreased anticoagulant response.

Detailed Information: See *EDI*, 4/87.00

Warfarin-Phenylbutazone

Significance: 1—highly clinically significant

Recommendations: Concurrent warfarin and phenylbutazone therapy threatens all patients with the potential for serious hemorrhage and should be avoided. If the combination must be used, close observation for bleeding is mandatory, and alternatives to phenylbutazone should be administered whenever possible. These alternatives (e.g., acetaminophen, other non-steroidal anti-inflammatory agents) are discussed in other monographs. Excessive hypoprothrombinemia can be treated with phytonadione (vitamin K, 5 to 10mg) given subcutaneously or orally and by discontinuing the anticoagulant until prothrombin levels return to the proper range. Larger doses of vitamin K do not hasten response and will make the patient resistant to subsequent warfarin therapy. Evidence of hemorrhage requires immediate return of prothrombin levels to normal ranges, attention to blood volume restoration, and other medical and surgical treatments as indicated. If hemorrhage is severe, fresh frozen plasma may be given to supply clotting factors.

Summary: Phenylbutazone enhances the hypoprothrombinemic effect of warfarin and can cause serious bleeding episodes.

Related Drugs: Phenprocoumon has been reported to interact with phenylbutazone or its analogs. Phenindione has shown a similar interaction with phenylbutazone. A similar interaction is expected to occur between dicumarol or anisindione and phenylbutazone. Oxyphenbutazone interacts with dicumarol and acenocoumarol.

Mechanism: Phenylbutazone increases the plasma concentration of unbound warfarin, inhibits the metabolism of warfarin and may cause gastric ulceration and decrease platelet aggregation.

Detailed Information: See *EDI*, 4/89.00

Warfarin-Phytonadione

Significance: 1—highly clinically significant

Recommendations: Cases of warfarin resistance and increased warfarin dosage requirements have been reported in patients receiving a variety of enteral nutrition supplements, apparently resulting from the relatively high vitamin K content in these products. Although these products have since been reformulated to provide amounts of vitamin K more consistent with the normal dietary intake of 300 to 500mg/day, one report suggests that these products may still affect the warfarin dosage required. As a result, it is prudent to monitor the prothrombin time of patients stabilized on warfarin when large quantities of tube feedings are initiated or stopped. Excessive intake of foods containing vitamin K, such as green leafy vegetables, should also be avoided in patients stabilized on warfarin. The effects of vitamin K ingestion may persist for several days after intake is stopped. On the other hand, the effectiveness of vitamin K as an antidote for warfarin overdose is well documented, with phytonadione reported to be more effective than menadione and the drug of choice for this condition.

Summary: Warfarin inhibits the vitamin K-dependent synthesis of clotting factors, and vitamin K antagonizes the inhibitory effect of warfarin.

Related Drugs: Dicumarol, phenprocoumon, anisindione and phenindione affect these agents in a similar manner. Drugs with vitamin K activity include menadione (vitamin K3), menadione sodium diphosphate and phytonadione. Vitamin K is found in green leafy vegetables and in oral nutritional supplements.

Mechanism: Coumarin anticoagulants inhibit vitamin K-dependent synthesis, and vitamin K intake in excess of normal dietary consumption may reverse or impair the anticoagulant effect of warfarin.

Detailed Information: See *EDI*, 4/91.00

Warfarin-Propafenone

Significance: 2—moderately clinically significant

Potential Effects: Concurrent propafenone may result in an enhanced warfarin anticoagulant effect.

Recommendations: The addition or removal of propafenone from the therapy of a patient maintained on warfarin should be approached with caution. The prothrombin time should be monitored for changes and the warfarin dose may need to be adjusted.

Summary: Concurrent propafenone and warfarin has been shown to result in an enhanced warfarin anticoagulant effect.

Related Drugs: Propafenone potentiated the anticoagulant effect of fluindione. A similar interaction may occur between propafenone and acenocoumarol, phenprocoumon, nicoumalone, anisindione and phenindione. It is not known if an interaction would occur between warfarin and other Class IC antiarrhythmics.

Mechanism: Both drugs are metabolized by the hepatic cytochrome P450 system, and the interaction reflects the higher binding affinity of propafenone for cytochrome P450.5

Detailed Information: See *EDI,* 4/92.50

Warfarin-Propoxyphene

Significance: 2—moderately clinically significant

Recommendations: Patients' prothrombin times should be monitored closely during concurrent use of these agents. The dose of warfarin may need to be decreased, the propoxyphene may need to be discontinued, or the use of a noninteracting analgesic may be considered.

Summary: The concurrent use of warfarin and propoxyphene may lead to decreased prothrombin levels and bleeding episodes.

Related Drugs: A similar interaction is expected to occur between warfarin and other narcotic analgesics and between propoxyphene and dicumarol, phenprocoumon, anisindione or phenindione.

Mechanism: Propoxyphene, which is metabolized by the same hepatic microsomal enzymes that hydroxylate warfarin, may compete for metabolism.

Detailed Information: See *EDI,* 4/93.00

Warfarin-Propranolol

Significance: 2—moderately clinically significant

Potential Effects: Propranolol may increase warfarin serum levels, which may lead to an increase in anticoagulation.

Recommendations: Although propranolol may increase serum warfarin concentrations, the clinical significance of this potential interaction has not been established. However, patients should be monitored for increased effects of warfarin, and prothrombin time should be monitored routinely. Acebutolol might be considered as a possible alternative therapy to propranolol in patients maintained on anticoagulation therapy.

Summary: There are data to show that propranolol may increase warfarin serum levels, leading to an increase in anticoagulation.

Related Drugs: Neither atenolol nor metoprolol altered the effects of warfarin. Acebutolol did not result in a change in prothrombin time. Esmolol did not affect warfarin plasma levels. It is difficult to determine if an interaction would occur between warfarin and other beta-blocking agents. Phenprocoumon with metoprolol increased plasma phenprocoumon levels. It is difficult to determine whether an interaction would occur between propranolol and dicumarol or anisindione.

Mechanism: Beta-blocking agents may increase serum warfarin concentrations by inhibiting the hepatic metabolism of warfarin.

Detailed Information: See *EDI,* 4/94.10

Warfarin-Quinidine

Significance: 2—moderately clinically significant

Recommendations: Concurrent administration of warfarin and quinidine is not recommended, but if necessary there should be frequent monitoring of prothrombin times as well as monitoring for clinical symptoms of warfarin overdose. Use of an alternative antiarrhythmic agent that does not interact with the anticoagulant may be preferable to the use of quinidine.

Summary: Concurrent administration of quinidine and warfarin may result in enhanced hypoprothrombinemic activity. Quinidine can inhibit the production of vitamin K-dependent clotting factors.

Related Drugs: Quinine may exert a hypoprothrombinemic effect. Dicumarol and phenindione have been reported to enhance hypoprothrombinemic activity; however, dicumarol has been reported to decrease the anticoagulant effect. A similar interaction is expected to occur between quinidine and phenprocoumon or anisindione.

Mechanism: The additive effect shown by quinidine may be related to the depressant effect on the vitamin K-dependent clotting factors. The decreased anticoagulant effects may be due to the enhanced production of prothrombin and other coagulation factors.

Detailed Information: See *EDI,* 4/95.00

Warfarin-Rifampin

Significance: 1—highly clinically significant

Potential Effects: Rifampin induces the metabolism of warfarin, decreasing warfarin's pharmacologic effects.

Recommendations: Monitor patients' prothrombin times when rifampin is added to, or withdrawn from, cotherapy with warfarin.

Summary: The administration of rifampin has been shown to result in a decreased warfarin pharmacologic effect.

Related Drugs: A similar interaction may occur between rifampin and dicumarol or anisindione. There are no drugs related to rifampin.

Mechanism: Rifampin, a known inducer of hepatic microsomal enzymes, increases the hepatic metabolism of warfarin.

Detailed Information: See *EDI,* 4/97.00

Warfarin-Spironolactone

Significance: 3—minimally clinically significant

Recommendations: The clinical significance of long-term cotherapy has not been determined. If a reduction in the hypopro-thrombinemic effect should occur with long-term administration, suitable dosage adjustments of warfarin may be indicated.

Summary: The concurrent administration of spironolactone has been shown to decrease the hypoprothrombinemic effect of warfarin.

Related Drugs: An interaction may occur between spironolactone and dicumarol, phenprocoumon, anisindione or phenindione. A similar interaction is expected between other potassium sparing diuretics and warfarin.

Mechanism: Spironolactone-induced diuresis may concentrate the blood clotting factors as a result of plasma water loss, leading to a reduced anticoagulant effect.

Detailed Information: See *EDI,* 4/99.00

Warfarin-Sucralfate

Significance: 3—minimally clinically significant

Potential Effects: Sucralfate may possibly decrease the action of warfarin.

Recommendations: Monitor the patient's prothrombin time when these agents are used together.

Summary: There are data to show that administration of sucralfate may possibly decrease the action of warfarin.

Related Drugs: There are no drugs related to sucralfate. No documentation exists concerning whether a similar interaction would occur between sucralfate and dicumarol, phenprocoumon or anisindione.

Mechanism: The mechanism of this potential interaction is unknown.

Detailed Information: See *EDI*, 4/101.00

Warfarin-Sulfamethoxazole

Significance: 1—highly clinically significant

Potential Effects: Sulfamethoxazole may be expected to enhance warfarin's anticoagulant effect.

Recommendations: Patients receiving sulfamethoxazole, either alone or as cotrimoxazole, and warfarin would be expected to display enhanced anticoagulant effects. Appropriate precautions should be taken to prevent excessive hypoprothrombinemia and bleeding.

Summary: Concurrent administration of sulfamethoxazole and trimethoprim, as cotrimoxazole, has augmented the hypoprothrombinemic effect of warfarin, significantly increasing warfarin levels.

Related Drugs: Sulfisoxazole and sulfamethazole have been shown to increase the hypoprothrombinemic activity of warfarin. A similar interaction is expected to occur between warfarin and other sulfonamides. Phenindione has been shown to not interact with cotrimoxazole. No documentation demonstrates that dicumarol, phenprocoumon or anisindione interacts similarly with sulfonamides. Proguanil was shown to potentiate the effect of warfarin. Trimethoprim would also be expected to interact with warfarin.

Mechanism: Several mechanisms have been proposed. Sulfonamides may displace plasma protein bound warfarin, the antibiotics may reduce vitamin K synthesis or the sulfonamides may inhibit warfarin metabolism.

Detailed Information: See *EDI*, 4/103.00

Warfarin-Sulfinpyrazone

Significance: 1—highly clinically significant

Potential Effects: Sulfinpyrazone decreases the metabolism of warfarin, thereby increasing warfarin's pharmacologic effect.

Recommendations: The use of these agents together should be avoided. If they are given together, the prothrombin time should be monitored and the dose of warfarin decreased as necessary.

Summary: Concomitant sulfinpyrazone and warfarin therapy significantly potentiates the hypoprothrombinemic effect of warfarin.

Related Drugs: Sulfinpyrazone has been shown to not interact with phenprocoumon. It is not known if an interaction would occur between sulfinpyrazone and dicumarol or anisindione, or between warfarin and probenecid.

Mechanism: Sulfinpyrazone inhibits certain metabolic pathways, decreases the clearance of warfarin, displaces warfarin from plasma proteins and has been shown to displace phenprocoumon.

Detailed Information: See *EDI*, 4/105.00

Warfarin-Tamoxifen

Significance: 2—moderately clinically significant

Potential Effects: Tamoxifen may increase the hypoprothrombinemic effects of warfarin. The antitumor activity of tamoxifen may also be reduced as a result of cotherapy.

Recommendations: Patients maintained on warfarin should have prothrombin times closely monitored if tamoxifen is added to, or withdrawn from, cotherapy. The dose of warfarin may need to be adjusted.

Summary: Tamoxifen may increase the hypoprothrombinemic effects of warfarin.

Related Drugs: A similar interaction may occur between tamoxifen and dicumarol or anisindione.

Mechanism: Tamoxifen and warfarin are metabolized by hepatic microsomal enzyme systems. Tamoxifen may increase the pharmacological activity of warfarin by competitive enzyme inhibition.

Detailed Information: See *EDI,* 4/107.00

Warfarin-Terbinafine

Significance: 2—moderately clinically significant

Potential Effects: The addition of terbinafine to or discontinuation from the therapy of a patient maintained on warfarin may result in changes in international normalized ratio (INR) and anticoagulant effect.

Recommendations: The addition of terbinafine to, or the discontinuation from, the therapy of a patient maintained on warfarin should be approached with caution. The patient should be carefully monitored for changes in INR and anticoagulant effect, which may take several weeks to develop. The dose of warfarin may need to be adjusted.

Summary: The addition of oral terbinafine to the therapy of a patient maintained on warfarin resulted in decreased warfarin anticoagulant effect, although another study in 16 subjects showed no interaction.

Related Drugs: It is not known whether an interaction would occur between terbinafine and the other coumarin anticoagulants. It is not known whether a similar interaction would occur with warfarin and butenafine, a benzylamine derivative with a mode of action similar to the allylamine antifungal agent terbinafine.

Mechanism: The mechanism may involve enzyme induction, but documentation is lacking.

Detailed Information: See *EDI,* 4/108.50

Warfarin-Tetracycline

Significance: 3—minimally clinically significant

Recommendations: The possibility of enhanced warfarin activity caused by tetracycline or its analogs appears to be slight when dietary intake of vitamin K is maintained at adequate levels and antibiotic clearance is normal. Nevertheless, close monitoring of prothrombin activity is warranted when the two drugs are administered concurrently or when one or the other is deleted from the regimen.

Summary: A broad spectrum antibiotic such as tetracycline can potentiate the hypoprothrombinemic effect of warfarin.

Related Drugs: Various tetracycline analogs may interact in a similar manner. Doxycycline has been implicated as the cause of an increased hypothrombinemic effect of warfarin. Dicumarol, phenprocoumon, anisindione or phenindione may interact similarly.

Mechanism: This interaction has often been considered to be inhibition of bacterial synthesis of vitamin K, resulting in an increased hypoprothrombinemic effect.

Detailed Information: See *EDI,* 4/109.00

Warfarin-Thyroid

Significance: 1—highly clinically significant

Recommendations: Initiation of thyroid replacement therapy in patients stabilized on warfarin carries a significant risk of excessive prothrombin response and hemorrhage. Conversely, warfarin therapy should be started in small doses in hyperthyroid patients, and any change of thyroid status in patients already receiving warfarin may necessitate a change in the warfarin dosage requirement. A decrease in the dosage of warfarin required for anticoagulation usually becomes necessary within one to four weeks after starting therapy with thyroid compounds. Since hyperthyroidism may increase patient sensitivity to warfarin, individuals undergoing unexplained changes in warfarin requirements should have an evaluation of thyroid function. Patients' prothrombin times should be closely monitored while they are on antithyroid therapy, since a dosage increase or discontinuation of the antithyroid drug may necessitate an increase or a decrease, respectively, of the warfarin dosage.

Summary: Thyroid compounds increase the hypoprothrombinemic effect of warfarin and other anticoagulants.

Related Drugs: Levothyroxine has exhibited a similar interaction. Dicumarol and phenindione have been shown to interact with thyroid derivatives. A similar interaction is expected to occur with phenprocoumon and anisindione. All thyroid compounds are expected to interact with the anticoagulants.

Mechanism: Hyperthyroidism may reduce serum albumin and there may be an enhanced degradation of vitamin K-dependent factors.

Detailed Information: See *EDI,* 4/111.00

Warfarin-Tobacco

Significance: 4—not clinically significant

Recommendations: Although there is a theoretical basis for an interaction between warfarin and tobacco, the limited evidence to date suggests that no special precautions are necessary when warfarin is administered to tobacco smokers. Further clinical studies designed specifically to evaluate this interaction are necessary.

Summary: There is no evidence that tobacco smokers require different maintenance doses of warfarin than nonsmokers.

Related Drugs: There is no documentation regarding an interaction between tobacco smoking and dicumarol, phenprocoumon or anisindione.

Mechanism: An increased maintenance dosage requirement in smokers could theoretically result from induction of warfarin metabolism.

Detailed Information: See *EDI,* 4/112.10

Warfarin-Trazodone

Significance: 3—minimally clinically significant

Potential Effects: Concomitant administration of trazodone with warfarin may result in decreased pharmacologic effects of the warfarin.

Recommendations: Patients receiving warfarin should be closely monitored when trazodone is added to, or withdrawn from, their therapy. A report recommends monitoring prothrombin and partial thromboplastin times three times a week, when trazodone is initiated, until the drug's effects are optimal. The dosage of warfarin may need to be adjusted.

Summary: There are data to show that concomitant administration of trazodone with warfarin may result in decreased warfarin effects.

Related Drugs: It is not known if a similar interaction would occur between trazodone and dicumarol or anisindione. Trazodone is unrelated to tricyclic, tetracyclic, or other available antidepressant agents.

Mechanism: The mechanism of this interaction is not known.

Detailed Information: See *EDI,* 4/112.30

Warfarin-Troglitazone

Significance: 3—minimally clinically significant

Potential Effects: The addition of troglitazone to the therapy of a patient maintained on warfarin may result in an increased international normalized ratio (INR) and the possible need for warfarin dosage adjustment.

Recommendations: Patients should be closely monitored for increased INR and warfarin anticoagulant effects when troglitazone is added to or removed from the therapy of a patient maintained on warfarin. The dose of warfarin may need to be adjusted.

Summary: The addition of troglitazone to the therapy of a patient maintained on warfarin resulted in an increased INR and necessitated warfarin dosage adjustment.

Related Drugs: It is not known whether an interaction would occur between troglitazone and the other coumarin anticoagulant or the indanedione anticoagulant agents. There are no drugs related to troglitazone.

Mechanism: The mechanism is thought to be due to either inhibition of the cytochrome P450 enzyme system (which would result in decreased warfarin metabolism) or displacement of warfarin from plasma protein binding sites. Either of these suggested pathways would result in increased warfarin serum levels and subsequent effects.

Detailed Information: See *EDI,* 4/112.60

Warfarin-Vitamin E

Significance: 2—moderately clinically significant

Recommendations: Until further clinical studies are reported, the concurrent use of these agents need not be avoided. However, it is prudent to monitor patients during concomitant administration, and a lower dose of warfarin may be necessary. It should be noted that the vitamin E effect can be overcome by either stopping the vitamin E or administering vitamin K.

Summary: The concurrent use of vitamin E may enhance the hypoprothrombinemic effect of warfarin.

Related Drugs: A similar interaction is expected to occur between vitamin E and phenprocoumon, anisindione or phenindione. No drugs are related to vitamin E.

Mechanism: The mechanism is unknown. Vitamin E may interfere with the oxidation of the reduced form of vitamin K.

Detailed Information: See *EDI,* 4/113.00

Chapter Five

Anticonvulsant
Drug Interactions

Carbamazepine-Charcoal

Significance: 1—highly clinically significant

Recommendations: It has been recommended that activated charcoal be administered as soon as possible after an acute carbamazepine overdose. Also, activated charcoal may significantly increase the elimination of carbamazepine if given in multiple doses thereafter. If charcoal is not used for carbamazepine overdose, it may be advisable to separate the administration of these agents by as much time as possible.

Summary: Charcoal significantly reduces carbamazepine absorption and increases elimination.

Related Drugs: There are no drugs related to carbamazepine or charcoal.

Mechanism: Charcoal adsorbs carbamazepine and prevents its absorption and may prevent enterohepatic recycling of carbamazepine, increasing its elimination.

Detailed Information: See *EDI*, 5/1.00

Carbamazepine-Cimetidine

Significance: 2—moderately clinically significant

Potential Effects: Cimetidine may increase carbamazepine levels. Monitor carbamazepine levels if cimetidine is added to, or withdrawn from, therapy.

Recommendations: Ranitidine may be used as an alternative to cimetidine.

Summary: Cimetidine has been shown to decrease the clearance of carbamazepine, resulting in increased carbamazepine plasma concentrations; however, all data do not support this.

Related Drugs: Ranitidine was documented to not change the carbamazepine area-under-curve or elimination half-life. There are no drugs related to carbamazepine.

Mechanism: Cimetidine inhibits the hepatic metabolism of carbamazepine and the autoinduction of carbamazepine.

Detailed Information: See *EDI*, 5/3.00

Carbamazepine-Danazol

Significance: 2—moderately clinically significant

Potential Effects: Danazol may inhibit the metabolism of carbamazepine, leading to increased carbamazepine levels and carbamazepine toxicity in some cases.

Recommendations: Although plasma carbamazepine levels were increased above the therapeutic range by danazol, toxicity did not occur in all patients. Therefore, the patient's clinical condition and carbamazepine serum levels should be monitored. The dosage of carbamazepine may need to be decreased or danazol may need to be discontinued.

Summary: Danazol may increase carbamazepine levels and toxicity.

Related Drugs: A similar interaction may be expected to occur between carbamazepine and other androgen derivatives. There are no drugs related to carbamazepine.

Mechanism: Danazol causes an inhibition of carbamazepine metabolism and a reduction in the clearance of carbamazepine.

Detailed Information: See *EDI*, 5/4.01

Carbamazepine-Desipramine

Significance: 3—minimally clinically significant

Recommendations: Although concurrent use of these agents need not be avoided, if desipramine is added to, or withdrawn from, carbamazepine therapy, serum carbamazepine concentrations should be monitored. Additionally, the patient should be monitored for signs of carbamazepine toxicity or lack of efficacy.

Summary: Desipramine has been shown to cause an acute episode of nausea, vomiting, visual illusions, slurred speech, and ataxia in a patient taking carbamazepine.

Related Drugs: A similar interaction is expected to occur between carbamazepine and other tricyclic antidepressants or the tetracyclic antidepressants. Nomifensine may be expected to interact with carbamazepine. There are no drugs related to carbamazepine.

Mechanism: Desipramine and carbamazepine may compete for hydroxylation by the hepatic microsomal enzyme system, increasing the carbamazepine concentration.

Detailed Information: See *EDI*, 5/4.10

Carbamazepine-Erythromycin

Significance: 1—highly clinically significant

Potential Effects: Erythromycin will cause an increase in carbamazepine levels, resulting in carbamazepine toxicity (e.g., nausea, nystagmus, ataxia).

Recommendations: Use of the agents together should be avoided. If they must be given together, patients should be monitored for increased carbamazepine levels and side effects. A decreased carbamazepine dose may be necessary.

Summary: The concurrent administration of erythromycin and carbamazepine has resulted in significant increases in plasma concentrations of carbamazepine.

Related Drugs: Administration of carbamazepine and troleandomycin has resulted in a similar interaction. Clarithromycin has been documented to double carbamazepine's concentration and dose ratio. There are no drugs related to carbamazepine.

Mechanism: Erythromycin may inhibit the hepatic metabolism of carbamazepine through competitive binding to cytochrome P450.

Detailed Information: See *EDI*, 5/5.00

Carbamazepine-Felbamate

Significance: 2—moderately clinically significant

Potential Effects: Coadministration of carbamazepine and felbamate results in decreases in both the concentration of carbamazepine plasma levels and clearance of felbamate, in addition to an increase in carbamazepine epoxide plasma levels, thus possibly leading to an increase in carbamazepine epoxide concentrations.

Recommendations: Patients should be carefully monitored for changes in seizure potential with initial concomitant use of these agents. The concurrent use of these agents may be purposeful and the dose of one or both agents may need to be adjusted.

Summary: There are data to show that coadministration of carbamazepine and felbamate results in decreases in the concentration of carbamazepine plasma levels and clearance of felbamate, in addition to an increase in carbamazepine epoxide plasma levels and concentrations.

Related Drugs: There are no related drugs to carbamazepine. It is not known whether meprobamate would interact similarly with carbamazepine.

Mechanism: The interaction between carbamazepine and felbamate occurs via an alteration in the metabolic pathway. Felbamate has been shown to induce isozymes responsible for the conversion of carbamazepine to the epoxide. Carbamazepine also causes an increase in the clearance of felbamate.

Detailed Information: See *EDI*, 5/5.50

Carbamazepine-Hydrochlorothiazide

Significance: 3—minimally clinically significant

Potential Effects: Concurrent use of these agents may result in hyponatremia as a result of a synergistic effect of both agents.

Recommendations: Patients should be monitored for hyponatremia when carbamazepine and hydrochlorothiazide are administered concurrently. One or both drugs may need to be discontinued. Also, if a patient's serum sodium levels are adequate during concurrent therapy, the levels should be monitored if the carbamazepine dose is increased.

Summary: Hyponatremia has been documented to occur when carbamazepine and hydrochlorothiazide are coadministered.

Related Drugs: Furosemide was shown to exhibit a similar interaction with carbamazepine. A similar interaction may occur between carbamazepine and other thiazide diuretics, the thiazide-related diuretics, and other loop diuretics. There are no drugs related to carbamazepine.

Mechanism: It is possible that a synergistic effect occurs between the two agents, causing hyponatremia.

Detailed Information: See *EDI*, 5/6.10

Carbamazepine-Isoniazid

Significance: 2—moderately clinically significant

Recommendations: It is important to monitor carbamazepine levels during concurrent use of these agents. It may be necessary to reduce the dose of carbamazepine if toxic symptoms appear since this has been shown to reverse toxicity.

Summary: Concurrent administration of carbamazepine and isoniazid may lead to neurologic changes secondary to elevated carbamazepine levels.

Related Drugs: There are no drugs related to carbamazepine or isoniazid.

Mechanism: Isoniazid inhibits the hepatic metabolism of carbamazepine. Isoniazid-induced hepatotoxicity has been attributed to a reactive intermediate that results in cell death, and carbamazepine may potentiate this.

Detailed Information: See *EDI*, 5/7.00

Carbamazepine-Isotretinoin

Significance: 3—minimally clinically significant

Potential Effects: Isotretinoin may cause a decrease in carbamazepine levels, resulting in loss of seizure control.

Recommendations: Patients maintained on carbamazepine should be closely monitored for decreases in carbamazepine levels or seizure control if isotretinoin is added to therapy. The dose of carbamazepine may need to be adjusted.

Summary: Isotretinoin may cause a decrease in carbamazepine and carbamazepime epoxide (CPZ-E, the active metabolite) levels, resulting in loss of seizure control.

Related Drugs: There are no drugs related to carbamazepine or isotretinoin.

Mechanism: It is suggested that isotretinoin alters the bioavailability or clearance or both of carbamazepine and CPZ-E.

Detailed Information: See *EDI*, 5/8.05

Carbamazepine-Metoclopramide

Significance: 3—minimally clinically significant

Recommendations: Patients receiving carbamazepine and metoclopramide concurrently should be monitored for signs and symptoms of neurotoxicity, and carbamazepine levels should be measured. One or both drugs may need to be discontinued, as this reduces the neurotoxic symptoms.

Summary: There are data to show that the administration of metoclopramide has led to carbamazepine-induced neurotoxicity.

Related Drugs: There are no drugs related to carbamazepine or metoclopramide.

Mechanism: The mechanism of this interaction is unknown.

Detailed Information: See *EDI*, 5/8.10

Carbamazepine-Metronidazole

Significance: 2—moderately clinically significant

Potential Effects: Concurrent carbamazepine and metronidazole may result in increased carbamazepine serum levels and signs of carbamazepine toxicity.

Recommendations: Patients on carbamazepine who begin therapy with metronidazole should be carefully monitored for increased carbamazepine levels and signs of toxicity.

Summary: In a case report, the concurrent use of carbamazepine and metronidazole resulted in increased levels of carbamazepine and symptoms of carbamazepine toxicity.

Related Drugs: There are no drugs related to carbamazepine. Although documentation is lacking, a similar interaction would be expected to occur between carbamazepine and anti-infective agents related to metronidazole based on the postulated mechanism and pharmacological and structural similarity.

Mechanism: It is postulated that the interaction is a result of selective inhibition of the aromatic hydroxylation of carbamazepine by metronidazole.

Detailed Information: See *EDI*, 5/8.25

Carbamazepine-Niacinamide

Significance: 3—minimally clinically significant

Recommendations: Carbamazepine plasma levels should be monitored in patients receiving concurrent niacinamide, especially when niacinamide is added to, or withdrawn from, therapy or the dose is changed. The dose of carbamazepine may need to be decreased. It is not known if a smaller dose of niacinamide (e.g., the amount that may be found in a multivitamin preparation) would interact with carbamazepine.

Summary: The administration of niacinamide decreased the clearance and increased the plasma levels of carbamazepine.

Related Drugs: There are no drugs related to carbamazepine. Niacin (nicotinic acid) may be expected to interact similarly with carbamazepine.

Mechanism: Niacinamide may inhibit the hepatic metabolism of carbamazepine. The decrease in carbamazepine clearance correlated highly with increasing niacinamide doses.

Detailed Information: See *EDI*, 5/8.30

Carbamazepine-Oral Contraceptive Agents

Significance: 3—minimally clinically significant

Potential Effects: Carbamazepine may induce the metabolism of ethinylestradiol, leading to decreased levels.

Recommendations: The concomitant use of oral contraceptives and carbamazepine need not be avoided. However, the potential for reduced efficacy of the oral contraceptive should be a consideration in patients receiving both drugs.

Summary: There are data to show that carbamazepine causes oral contraceptive failure; however, it is unclear if other factors such as patient compliance are responsible. The potential for reduced efficacy of oral contraceptives should be considered.

Related Drugs: There are no drugs related to carbamazepine.

Mechanism: The cytochrome P450 metabolism of ethinylestradiol may be induced by administration of carbamazepine.

Detailed Information: See *EDI*, 5/8.50

Carbamazepine-Phenobarbital

Significance: 3—minimally clinically significant

Recommendations: Carefully monitor patients receiving both phenobarbital and carbamazepine to assure that adequate therapeutic carbamazepine concentrations are maintained. The possibility of shortened carbamazepine half-life should be taken into consideration when establishing dosage frequency to prevent large fluctuations in plasma concentration. One report suggests giving carbamazepine three times a day—morning, evening, and bedtime—to keep carbamazepine plasma levels fairly constant during the day and to counteract subtherapeutic levels in the morning.

Summary: Phenobarbital has been shown to decrease serum carbamazepine half-life and plasma concentration levels when given in combination; however, all data do not support this.

Related Drugs: Carbamazepine has been reported to lower serum concentrations of primidone. Other barbiturates may interact in a manner similar to phenobarbital. There are no drugs related to carbamazepine.

Mechanism: Phenobarbital is thought to induce the metabolism of carbamazepine to its epoxide metabolite.

Detailed Information: See *EDI*, 5/9.00

Carbamazepine-Propoxyphene

Significance: 2—moderately clinically significant

Potential Effects: Propoxyphene may increase carbamazepine levels.

Recommendations: The use of these agents together should be avoided. Monitor for increased carbamazepine levels and toxicity. Propoxyphene may need to be discontinued.

Summary: Propoxyphene has been documented to increase carbamazepine levels.

Related Drugs: A similar interaction may occur between carbamazepine and other narcotic analgesics. There are no drugs related to carbamazepine.

Mechanism: Propoxyphene may inhibit the hepatic metabolism of carbamazepine, resulting in increased carbamazepine levels.

Detailed Information: See *EDI*, 5/11.00

Carbamazepine-Terfenadine

Significance: 3—minimally clinically significant

Potential Effects: Terfenadine administration may result in increased levels of free carbamazepine and toxicity.

Recommendations: Patients receiving terfenadine and carbamazepine should be closely monitored for increased serum levels of free carbamazepine and signs of carbamazepine toxicity.

Summary: The addition of terfenadine to carbamazepine therapy has resulted in increased carbamazepine adverse effects and toxicity.

Related Drugs: A similar interaction may occur between carbamazepine and other H_1-receptor antagonists. An interaction would be expected to occur between terfenadine and other tricyclic antidepressant agents. A recent study has shown that terfenadine has no effect on phenytoin (see also Phenytoin-Carbamazepine, page 113).

Mechanism: Terfenadine may displace carbamazepine from plasma proteins, leading to an increase in the toxicities associated with carbamazepine.

Detailed Information: See *EDI*, 5/12.05

Carbamazepine-Verapamil

Significance: 2—moderately clinically significant

Potential Effects: Verapamil may cause an increase in carbamazepine levels, resulting in increased side effects.

Recommendations: Monitor the patient for increased carbamazepine levels and side effects when these agents are used together.

Summary: There are data to show that verapamil causes an increase in carbamazepine levels, resulting in increased side effects and neurotoxicity.

Related Drugs: Diltiazem exhibited a similar interaction with carbamazepine. Nifedipine did not interact with carbamazepine and its levels were unaffected. Felodipine plasma levels were shown to decrease. It is not known whether an interaction would occur between carbamazepine and other calcium channel blocking agents. There are no drugs related to carbamazepine.

Mechanism: It was suggested that verapamil and diltiazem may inhibit the hepatic metabolism of carbamazepine.

Detailed Information: See *EDI*, 5/12.10

Clonazepam-Carbamazepine

Significance: 3—minimally clinically significant

Potential Effects: Carbamazepine may decrease clonazepam levels when used concurrently.

Recommendations: Monitor clonazepam levels when carbamazepine is added to, or withdrawn from, clonazepam

Summary: Concurrent carbamazepine reduced plasma clonazepam concentrations, making seizure control difficult since these agents may have an additive anticonvulsant action.

Related Drugs: Carbamazepine was shown to decrease alprazolam serum levels. A similar interaction is expected to occur with other benzodiazepines that are metabolized by phase I reactions and carbamazepine, if the mechanism involves induction of hepatic enzymes. There are no drugs related to carbamazepine.

Mechanism: Carbamazepine is known to induce hepatic enzymes, which is thought to be the mechanism responsible for the reduced clonazepam levels.

Detailed Information: See *EDI,* 5/13.00

Clonazepam-Primidone

Significance: 4—not clinically significant

Recommendations: The clinical significance of this interaction is difficult to assess. Clonazepam has exhibited therapeutic effects over a wide range of plasma concentrations, and the possible change in primidone levels may offset any decreased levels of clonazepam.

Summary: Reports concerning an interaction between primidone and clonazepam are contradictory.

Related Drugs: Nitrazepam has been reported to decrease the primidone serum concentration. Clorazepate given with primidone resulted in personality changes. A similar interaction is expected to occur with other benzodiazepines and primidone and other barbiturates with clonazepam.

Mechanism: Phenobarbital, a known inducer of microsomal enzymes, can cause an increased clearance of drugs that undergo hepatic elimination.

Detailed Information: See *EDI,* 5/15.00

Ethosuximide-Carbamazepine

Significance: 3—minimally clinically significant

Potential Effects: The concurrent use of these agents may result in decreased ethosuximide serum levels.

Recommendations: Patients should be monitored for decreased ethosuximide levels during concurrent therapy with carbamazepine. The dose of ethosuximide may need to be increased.

Summary: There are data to show that the concurrent use of these agents may result in decreased ethosuximide serum levels.

Related Drugs: A similar interaction is expected to occur between carbamazepine and other succinimide anticonvulsants. There are no drugs related to carbamazepine.

Mechanism: Carbamazepine increased the clearance and reduced the levels of ethosuximide by inducing the hepatic microsomal enzymes.

Detailed Information: See *EDI,* 5/16.01

Ethosuximide-Isoniazid

Significance: 3—minimally clinically significant

Recommendations: If gastrointestinal symptoms and psychotic behavior occur during concurrent use of these agents, ethosuximide plasma levels should be monitored. The dose of ethosuximide may need to be decreased.

Summary: There are data to show that the admintration of isoniazid and ethosuximide may induce gastrointestinal symptoms and psychotic behavior.

Related Drugs: An interaction may occur between isoniazid and other succinimides. There are no drugs related to isoniazid.

Mechanism: Isoniazid inhibits the metabolism of ethosuximide.

Detailed Information: See *EDI*, 5/16.03

Ethosuximide-Valproic Acid

Significance: 3—minimally clinically significant

Recommendations: Concomitant use of ethosuximide and valproic acid need not be avoided; however, if valproic acid is added to, or withdrawn from, therapy, the serum ethosuximide concentration should be monitored and the patient observed for signs of toxicity or lack of efficacy.

Summary: Valproic acid and ethosuximide have been shown to increase, decrease, or have no effect on serum ethosuximide concentrations, toxicity, or efficacy.

Related Drugs: Similar interactions may occur between valproic acid and other succinimide anticonvulsants. There are no drugs related to valproic acid; however, sodium valproate and divalproex sodium would be expected to interact in the same manner as valproic acid. Valproic acid has been reported to increase levels of trimethadione. There is no documentation regarding an interaction between valproic acid and paramethadione.

Mechanism: Valproic acid may inhibit the hepatic metabolism of ethosuximide. The inhibition of metabolism may be dependent upon serum valproic acid concentrations or the administration of other agents that compete for metabolism.

Detailed Information: See *EDI*, 5/16.10

Lamotrigine-Acetaminophen

Significance: 3—minimally clinically significant

Potential Effects: Acetaminophen may result in an increase in lamotrigine clearance.

Recommendations: When acetaminophen and lamotrigine are given concurrently (particularly when multiple doses of acetaminophen are necessary), patients should be monitored for a possible decrease of lamotrigine clinical effects. Although further studies are needed, the dose of lamotrigine may need to be increased.

Summary: Concurrent acetaminophen and lamotrigine may result in an increase in lamotrigine clearance and a decreased clinical effect, a study suggested.

Related Drugs: There are no drugs related to lamotrigine or acetaminophen.

Mechanism: It was suggested that acetaminophen facilitated lamotrigine removal through an unknown mechanism which may involve acetaminophen-mediated activation of a glucuronyl transferase.

Detailed Information: See *EDI*, 5/16.30

Lamotrigine-Sodium Valproate

Significance: 3—minimally clinically significant

Potential Effects: Concurrent lamotrigine and sodium valproate may result in a decrease in clearance of lamotrigine.

Recommendations: Patients receiving lamotrigine should be monitored for changes in levels and possible toxicity if sodium valproate is added to, or withdrawn from, therapy. The dosage of lamotrigine may need to be adjusted.

Summary: Concurrent sodium valproate and lamotrigine resulted in a decreased clearance of lamotrigine.

Related Drugs: Valproic acid and divalproex sodium would be expected to interact similarly with lamotrigine. There are no drugs related to lamotrigine.

Mechanism: The reduced clearance of lamotrigine by sodium valproate is as a result of impaired glucuronide formation in the liver.

Detailed Information: See *EDI*, 5/16.50

Phenobarbital-Valproic Acid

Significance: 2—moderately clinically significant

Potential Effects: The concomitant administration of these agents may result in increased phenobarbital serum levels and toxicity and/or decreased valproic acid serum levels.

Recommendations: Patients receiving these agents concurrently should be monitored for increased phenobarbital serum levels and/or decreased valproic acid serum levels. The dose of one or both agents may need to be adjusted.

Summary: The concurrent administration of phenobarbital and valproic acid has been shown to result in increased phenobarbital serum concentrations, and studies have shown decreased serum valproic acid concentrations.

Related Drugs: Valproic acid and primidone have shown significant increases in primidone concentrations; however, contrasting data exist. Mephobarbital decreased the serum level and dose ratio of valproic acid. It is difficult to determine if an interaction would occur between valproic acid and other barbiturates. Sodium valproate has been shown to increase phenobarbital levels. Divalproex sodium would be expected to interact similarly.

Mechanism: Valproic acid may inhibit the hepatic metabolism of phenobarbital. Phenobarbital may induce the hepatic metabolism of valproic acid.

Detailed Information: See *EDI*, 5/17.00

Phenytoin-Acetazolamide

Significance: 4—not clinically significant

Recommendations: The concurrent use of these agents need not be avoided. However, special attention to the early detection of osteomalacia should be given to patients receiving this combination of agents.

Summary: Use of phenytoin and acetazolamide may accelerate the osteomalacia induced by anticonvulsant therapy.

Related Drugs: An interaction between acetazolamide and other hydantoin anticonvulsants has not been documented. No reports are available regarding an interaction between hydantoins and other carbonic anhydrase inhibitors.

Mechanism: Acetazolamide enhances urinary calcium excretion and urinary phosphate excretion, causing systemic acidosis, which retards the dihydroxycholecalciferol.

Detailed Information: See *EDI*, 5/19.00

Phenytoin-Alcohol, Ethyl

Significance: 2—moderately clinically significant

Recommendations: If phenytoin is administered to patients who ingest alcohol chronically, the serum phenytoin level should be monitored to assure that they are in the therapeutic range. Conversely, in alcoholic patients whose phenytoin dose has been titrated to therapeutic levels, a decrease in serum phenytoin levels may occur when alcohol is discontinued, necessitating an increase in the phenytoin dose.

Summary: Long-term alcohol ingestion may increase the metabolism and clearance of phenytoin. However, it has been shown that long-term alcohol ingestion can inhibit phenytoin metabolism, decreasing serum phenytoin levels.

Related Drugs: The other hydantoin derivatives may interact with alcohol in a similar manner.

Mechanism: Increased phenytoin clearance during alcohol withdrawal results from an increased metabolic rate, secondary to enzyme induction by alcohol.

Detailed Information: See *EDI*, 5/21.00

Phenytoin-Allopurinol

Significance: 2—moderately clinically significant

Recommendations: Close patient attention is necessary during the concurrent administration of phenytoin and allopurinol. If phenytoin toxicity appears, the dosage may need to be adjusted downward.

Summary: Concurrent allopurinol administration has resulted in an increase in phenytoin serum concentration.

Related Drugs: A similar interaction is expected to occur between allopurinol and other hydantoin anticonvulsants. There are no drugs related to allopurinol.

Mechanism: Allopurinol inhibits the oxidative metabolism of phenytoin in the liver, resulting in an increased serum concentration.

Detailed Information: See *EDI*, 5/23.00

Phenytoin-Aluminum Hydroxide, Magnesium Trisilicate

Significance: 3—minimally clinically significant

Recommendations: There is no need to routinely avoid concurrent use of these agents. However, if loss of seizure control occurs, the administration of phenytoin and the antacid should be separated by as much time as possible and the dose of phenytoin modified as required.

Summary: A combination antacid containing aluminum hydroxide and magnesium trisilicate was shown to reduce phenytoin serum concentrations; however, data have shown no alterations in phenytoin absorption.

Related Drugs: It is not possible to determine if antacids will interact with phenytoin. Documentation is lacking regarding an interaction with other hydantoin anticonvulsants and a magnesium trisilicate-aluminum hydroxide combination antacid.

Mechanism: The aluminum hydroxide and magnesium trisilicate may adsorb phenytoin, reducing phenytoin absorption.

Detailed Information: See *EDI*, 5/24.10

Phenytoin-Amiodarone

Significance: 2—moderately clinically significant

Potential Effects: Amiodarone may cause an increase in phenytoin levels.

Recommendations: Monitor phenytoin levels when these agents are used together; the dose of phenytoin may need to be decreased.

Summary: Amiodarone increased phenytoin serum concentrations and was associated with ataxia, nystagmus, clouding of vision, and bilateral leg weakness.

Related Drugs: A similar interaction may occur between amiodarone and other hydantoin anticonvulsants. There are no drugs related to amiodarone.

Mechanism: The hepatic metabolism of phenytoin may be inhibited by amiodarone, and amiodarone may displace phenytoin from serum and tissue protein binding sites.

Detailed Information: See *EDI,* 5/24.30

Phenytoin-Aspirin

Significance: 4—not clinically significant

Recommendations: Although the patient's phenytoin levels (free and total) should be monitored closely during concurrent salicylate therapy, these agents need not be avoided.

Summary: Several studies have indicated that aspirin and other salicylates may cause a transient increase in phenytoin plasma levels.

Related Drugs: A similar interaction is expected to occur between other hydantoin anticonvulsants and other salicylates.

Mechanism: Salicylates have been shown to displace phenytoin from plasma protein binding sites; however, the metabolic clearance of phenytoin may increase, resulting in a lower total phenytoin plasma level.

Detailed Information: See *EDI,* 5/25.00

Phenytoin-Carbamazepine

Significance: 3—minimally clinically significant

Potential Effects: The concurrent use of these agents may result in increased or decreased phenytoin levels or decreased carbamazepine levels.

Recommendations: Serum concentrations of both agents should be monitored during concomitant therapy. Seizure control and serum levels should be monitored if either agent is added to, or withdrawn from, therapy.

Summary: Conflicting results have occurred when phenytoin and carbamazepine were administered concurrently. The use of these agents may result in increased or decreased phenytoin levels or decreased carbamazepine levels.

Related Drugs: A similar interaction is expected to occur between carbamazepine and other hydantoin anticonvulsants; however, it is not known which agent will be affected or if the levels will increase or decrease. There are no drugs related to carbamazepine.

Mechanism: Carbamazepine induces the hepatic metabolism of phenytoin, causing a decrease in serum levels, and inhibits the hepatic metabolism of phenytoin, causing an increase in serum levels. The decreased carbamazepine levels may occur by induction of hepatic metabolism, and phenytoin may increase the drug's biotransformation.

Detailed Information: See *EDI,* 5/27.00

Phenytoin-Carmustine, Methotrexate, Vinblastine

Significance: 2—moderately clinically significant

Potential Effects: The serum levels of phenytoin may be decreased. This may lead to loss of seizure control.

Recommendations: Monitor phenytoin levels when these agents are used together. The dosage of phenytoin may need to be adjusted.

Summary: There are data to show that administration of phenytoin and carmustine may lead to a high incidence of partial seizures.

Related Drugs: Use of vinblastine, bleomycin and cisplatin necessitated a doubling in phenytoin dosage. It is not known if a similar interaction would occur with ethotoin or mephenytoin.

Mechanism: Decreased gastrointestinal absorption of phenytoin may be the cause of this interaction, secondary to the antineoplastic agents.

Detailed Information: See *EDI*, 5/29.00

Phenytoin-Charcoal

Significance: 2—moderately clinically significant

Potential Effects: Charcoal may decrease the adsorption of phenytoin. This effect may be used to treat acute phenytoin overdose.

Recommendations: Multiple activated charcoal doses (30G in 26% sorbitol) may be given for acute phenytoin toxicity. Administer charcoal as far apart from phenytoin administration as possible. The patient should be monitored for changes in phenytoin levels.

Summary: There are data to show that administration of charcoal significantly decreases the absorption of phenytoin.

Related Drugs: Ethotoin and mephenytoin may also interact with charcoal.

Mechanism: Charcoal adsorbs phenytoin, limiting its absorption.

Detailed Information: See *EDI*, 5/31.00

Phenytoin-Chloramphenicol

Significance: 2—moderately clinically significant

Recommendations: In view of the increases in serum phenytoin concentration that have been observed after a single dose of chloramphenicol, it is recommended that frequent phenytoin levels be obtained after the initiation of chloramphenicol therapy, and that careful observation of the patient for signs and symptoms of phenytoin toxicity (e.g., ataxia, nystagmus) be undertaken with subsequent proper phenytoin dosage adjustments if needed. With regard to potential chloramphenicol toxicity, it has been recommended that a dosage of chloramphenicol no greater than 75mg/Kg/day be considered in patients receiving phenytoin concomitantly.

Summary: It has been shown that chloramphenicol has a direct inhibitory effect on the metabolism of phenytoin, decreasing the metabolic clearance and increasing the serum concentration of phenytoin; however, there are conflicting data.

Related Drugs: A similar interaction is expected to occur between other hydantoin anticonvulsants and chloramphenicol. There are no drugs related to chloramphenicol.

Mechanism: Concurrent administration of chloramphenicol may inhibit phenytoin metabolism, causing elevated serum levels. Competition for hepatic enzyme binding sites may explain the inhibition of chloramphenicol metabolism.

Detailed Information: See *EDI*, 5/33.00

Phenytoin-Chlorpheniramine

Significance: 2—moderately clinically significant

Recommendations: Although this interaction is based on isolated case reports, it is necessary to monitor phenytoin levels during concurrent use of these agents. If toxicity does occur, the dose of phenytoin may need to be decreased, or chlorpheniramine may need to be discontinued.

Summary: Phenytoin toxicity has been reported after the concurrent administration of chlorpheniramine.

Related Drugs: A similar interaction is expected to occur between phenytoin and other antihistamines. An interaction between chlorpheniramine and other hydantoin anticonvulsants may be expected.

Mechanism: Chlorpheniramine may inhibit the liver microsomal enzymes responsible for phenytoin metabolism.

Detailed Information: See *EDI,* 5/35.00

Phenytoin-Chlorpromazine

Significance: 3—minimally clinically significant

Potential Effects: The concomitant administration of these agents may result in an increase or decrease in phenytoin serum levels. This interaction is subject to individual variability.

Recommendations: Patients receiving phenytoin should be monitored for increases or decreases in their phenytoin levels when chlorpromazine is added to, or withdrawn from, their therapy. Also, epileptic patients should be monitored closely for a possible increase in seizure frequency.

Summary: There are data to show the concomitant administration of these agents may result in an increase or decrease in phenytoin serum levels, indicating that this interaction is subject to individual variability.

Related Drugs: Prochlorperazine and thioridazine have been reported to increase phenytoin levels, but inconsistent data are available. Mesoridazine has been shown to decrease phenytoin concentrations. Phenytoin decreased clozapine plasma concentrations. It is difficult to determine if an interaction would occur between phenytoin and the phenothiazines, the thioxanthenes, the dihydroinidolones or the dibenzoxazepines. Documentation is lacking regarding an interaction between chlorpromazine and other hydantoin anticonvulsants.

Mechanism: Chlorpromazine, other phenothiazines, and phenytoin probably compete for the limited metabolic capacity of the microsomal hydroxylation enzymes in the liver.

Detailed Information: See *EDI,* 5/37.00

Phenytoin-Cimetidine

Significance: 1—highly clinically significant

Potential Effects: Cimetidine inhibits the metabolism of phenytoin, leading to increased phenytoin serum levels and toxicity.

Recommendations: If these agents are used concomitantly, patients should be monitored for increased phenytoin serum levels and toxicity. Famotidine may be an alternative to cimetidine.

Summary: There are data to show that coadministration of these agents causes increased phenytoin levels and phenytoin toxicity.

Related Drugs: A similar interaction is expected to occur between cimetidine and other hydantoin anticonvulsants. Ranitidine exhibited a similar interaction; however, ranitidine has also been reported not to interact with phenytoin. The clearance of phenytoin was not affected by famotidine. It cannot be determined if an interaction would be expected to occur between other H_2-receptor antagonists and phenytoin.

Mechanism: Cimetidine inhibits hepatic microsomal enzymes and impairs the metabolism of phenytoin, resulting in increased serum phenytoin levels.

Detailed Information: See *EDI,* 5/39.00

Phenytoin-Ciprofloxacin

Significance: 3—minimally clinically significant

Potential Effects: Ciprofloxacin may decrease phenytoin levels or increase seizure frequency.

Recommendations: Patients maintained on phenytoin should be carefully monitored for changes in plasma phenytoin levels or seizure frequency if ciprofloxacin is added to or discontinued from therapy. The dose of phenytoin may need to be adjusted.

Summary: The addition of ciprofloxacin to the therapy of a patient maintained on phenytoin resulted in decreased phenytoin serum levels and an increased frequency of seizures; however, conflicting data are available.

Related Drugs: Although there is no documentation for an interaction between ciprofloxacin and the other hydantoin anticonvulsant agents, or between phenytoin and the other quinolone antibacterial agents, an interaction may be expected to occur.

Mechanism: It is postulated that the reduction in phenytoin serum concentration is due to ciprofloxacin's induction of phenytoin metabolism.

Detailed Information: See *EDI,* 5/40.50

Phenytoin-Cyclosporine

Significance: 2—moderately clinically significant

Potential Effects: Phenytoin may decrease the concentration of cyclosporine, which may lead to graft rejection.

Recommendations: Monitor cyclosporine levels when phenytoin is added to therapy. An increase in the cyclosporine dose may be necessary.

Summary: The administration of phenytoin has resulted in a reduction in the cyclosporine maximum concentration and area-under-curve and an increase in total body clearance. Decreased cyclosporine levels could lead to graft rejection.

Related Drugs: A similar interaction is expected to occur between cyclosporine and other hydantoin anticonvulsants. There are no drugs related to cyclosporine.

Mechanism: It is possible that phenytoin induces the hepatic metabolism of cyclosporine.

Detailed Information: See *EDI,* 5/41.00

Phenytoin-Dexamethasone

Significance: 2—moderately clinically significant

Recommendations: If the dexamethasone suppression test is used in patients who have been receiving phenytoin long term, the test should be interpreted with caution and a higher dose of dexamethasone may be necessary. Patients receiving both drugs concurrently should be observed for possible diminution of the therapeutic effect of dexamethasone or other corticosteroids and/or signs and symptoms of phenytoin toxicity (e.g., nystagmus, gait ataxia, poor muscle tone, or lethargy). These effects may require an increase in corticosteroid dosage, a decrease in phenytoin dose, or both, to establish therapeutic levels.

Summary: Phenytoin impairs the response to dexamethasone and may result in a decrease in the therapeutic response to dexamethasone. Administration of dexamethasone may result in a significant increase in the half-life and serum level of phenytoin.

Related Drugs: Phenytoin has been reported to increase the metabolism of hydrocortisone, methylprednisolone, prednisolone, and prednisone. A similar interaction is expected to occur with other corticosteroids and phenytoin. Primidone has increased the metabolism of dexamethasone and reduced its clinical effectiveness. A similar interaction is expected to occur with other hydantoin anticonvulsants and other anticonvulsants that cause enzyme induction.

Mechanism: Phenytoin affects corticosteroid metabolism by stimulating hepatic enzymes responsible for corticosteroid metabolism, and phenytoin and dexamethasone may compete for the metabolic capacity of these enzymes.

Detailed Information: See *EDI,* 5/43.00

Phenytoin-Diazepam

Significance: 3—minimally clinically significant

Potential Effects: Diazepam may increase or decrease phenytoin levels.

Recommendations: Monitor phenytoin levels when these agents are used together. Phenytoin dosage may need to be adjusted.

Summary: There are conflicting reports regarding the effect of diazepam on phenytoin serum concentrations. Diazepam may increase or decrease phenytoin levels.

Related Drugs: Phenytoin serum levels have been shown to be increased during administration of chlordiazepoxide, clonazepam, and nitrazepam. Phenytoin levels have been shown to be decreased with chlordiazepoxide and clonazepam. Other benzodiazepines have not been reported to alter phenytoin levels. It is difficult to determine whether an interaction would occur between diazepam and other hydantoin anticonvulsants.

Mechanism: Possible mechanisms include a benzodiazepine microsomal enzyme induction or inhibition of phenytoin metabolism. The apparent volume of distribution of phenytoin may also be affected by benzodiazepines.

Detailed Information: See *EDI,* 5/45.00

Phenytoin-Diazoxide

Significance: 2—moderately clinically significant

Recommendations: Phenytoin plasma levels should be monitored, and an increased phenytoin dosage may be necessary if loss of seizure control occurs. Also, when diazoxide is discontinued, phenytoin dosage may need to be decreased to avoid toxicity.

Summary: Phenytoin serum levels may be decreased to subtherapeutic levels by concurrent oral diazoxide.

Related Drugs: A similar interaction may occur between diazoxide and other hydantoin anticonvulsants. There are no drugs related to diazoxide.

Mechanism: Diazoxide may increase the hepatic metabolism of phenytoin and increase its clearance. Displacement from plasma protein binding sites may also play a role. The reduced effects of diazoxide may be the result of induction of diazoxide's metabolism by phenytoin.

Detailed Information: See *EDI*, 5/47.00

Phenytoin-Disulfiram

Significance: 1—highly clinically significant

Recommendations: If a patient must be treated with both drugs, a baseline phenytoin level should be drawn before disulfiram is added to the regimen. The levels should be measured again in two to four days, and once or twice weekly until a new steady-state is established. In most cases, the plateau will be reached two to three weeks after the last dosage adjustment. The patient should also be monitored clinically for signs of phenytoin toxicity (e.g., ataxia, nystagmus) since symptom severity and height of serum level usually are parallel. Both parameters may be used as guides for adjusting the phenytoin dose if necessary. In most cases, decreasing the phenytoin dose will be sufficient to avoid toxicity, but some patients may require withdrawal of the disulfiram.

Summary: Addition of disulfiram to a stable phenytoin regimen will result in decreased phenytoin metabolism and increased phenytoin levels that may lead to toxicity.

Related Drugs: A similar interaction is expected to occur with the other hydantoin anticonvulsants and disulfiram.

Mechanism: Increased phenytoin levels result from disulfiram inhibition of the major route of metabolism of phenytoin.

Detailed Information: See *EDI*, 5/49.00

Phenytoin-Dopamine

Significance: 1—highly clinically significant

Recommendations: Although this precaution is based on one report, phenytoin should be used with the greatest care, or not at all, in patients receiving dopamine to support blood pressure. If hypotension occurs, discontinue phenytoin.

Summary: The administration of dopamine and phenytoin has been shown to produce a dramatic hypotension effect, possibly causing death.

Related Drugs: There is no documentation concerning the interaction of dopamine with other hydantoin anticonvulsants. No reports are available regarding an interaction between phenytoin and other agents used to treat shock; therefore, it cannot be determined if an interaction exists between other anticonvulsants and other sympathomimetics.

Mechanism: The hypotensive effect may be due to dopamine preventing the uptake at storage sites and increasing the synthesis of norepinephrine while phenytoin exerts a greater myocardial depressant effect secondary to catecholamine depletion.

Detailed Information: See *EDI*, 5/51.00

Phenytoin-Ethosuximide

Significance: 3—minimally clinically significant

Recommendations: Patients receiving phenytoin should be closely monitored for increased serum phenytoin concentrations or signs of toxicity (e.g., ataxia, nystagmus) when ethosuximide is coadministered. Patients stabilized on both drugs should also be monitored for subtherapeutic phenytoin levels if ethosuximide is discontinued.

Summary: Increased serum phenytoin concentrations with concurrent administration of ethosuximide have been reported; however, reports that no interaction occurs with these agents are documented.

Related Drugs: Increased serum phenytoin concentrations have been seen with concurrent methsuximide. A similar interaction is expected to occur between ethosuximide and other hydantoin anticonvulsants and between phenytoin and phensuximide.

Mechanism: Ethosuximide induced inhibition of phenytoin metabolism is a suggested mechanism for this interaction.

Detailed Information: See *EDI,* 5/53.00

Phenytoin-Felbamate

Significance: 2—moderately clinically significant

Potential Effects: Coadministration of felbamate and phenytoin will cause an increase in phenytoin levels and a decrease in felbamate clearance, resulting in phenytoin adverse effects.

Recommendations: As felbamate is added to existing phenytoin therapy, it may be necessary to reduce the dosage of phenytoin (20-33%) in order to control plasma phenytoin concentrations and symptoms of toxicity. Additional reductions of the concomitant phenytoin dosage may also be necessary to minimize side effects and toxicity. Patient serum phenytoin levels and changes in seizure control should be monitored during all phases of therapy.

Summary: Coadministration of phenytoin and felbamate resulted in an increase in plasma phenytoin concentrations and a decrease in felbamate clearance.

Related Drugs: It is not known whether meprobamate would interact similarly with phenytoin. A similar interaction may occur between felbamate and other hydantoin anticonvulsant agents.

Mechanism: Felbamate may act as a competitive inhibitor of phenytoin metabolism.

Detailed Information: See *EDI,* 5/54.50

Phenytoin-Fluconazole

Significance: 1—highly clinically significant

Potential Effects: Fluconazole may decrease the metabolism of phenytoin, leading to increased phenytoin levels and toxicity.

Recommendations: Patients maintained on phenytoin should be closely monitored for increased serum phenytoin levels and phenytoin toxicity if fluconazole is added to, or withdrawn from, therapy. The dose of phenytoin may need to be adjusted.

Summary: The addition of fluconazole to a phenytoin regimen resulted in an increase in serum phenytoin concentration.

Related Drugs: Miconazole has been shown to increase serum phenytoin concentrations. A similar interaction is expected to occur between phenytoin and other imidazole systemic antifungal agents and between fluconazole and other hydantoin anticonvulsants.

Mechanism: Fluconazole may inhibit the hepatic metabolism of phenytoin by interfering with fungal demethylation.

Detailed Information: See *EDI*, 5/54.10

Phenytoin-Fluoxetine

Significance: 2—moderately clinically significant

Potential Effects: The addition of fluoxetine to phenytoin therapy may cause an increase in phenytoin levels and resultant phenytoin toxicity.

Recommendations: Patients receiving concurrent fluoxetine and phenytoin should be monitored for increased phenytoin levels and an increase in phenytoin toxic effects (e.g., nystagmus, gait ataxia, poor muscle tone, lethargy). If phenytoin toxicity occurs, both fluoxetine and phenytoin doses may need to be reduced until toxic signs and symptoms subside.

Summary: Fluoxetine has been shown to increase phenytoin levels, leading to signs and symptoms of phenytoin intoxication.

Related Drugs: An interaction may occur between fluoxetine and other hydantoin anticonvulsants and between phenytoin and other serotonin-selective reuptake inhibitors. Paroxetine may interact with phenytoin.

Mechanism: This interaction may involve the inhibition of the hepatic metabolism of phenytoin by fluoxetine and cause an enhancement of serotonergic neurotransmission, leading to enhanced anticonvulsant effects.

Detailed Information: See *EDI*, 5/54.20

Phenytoin-Folic Acid

Significance: 2—moderately clinically significant

Potential Effects: Folic acid administration (5mg or more per day) to patients stabilized on phenytoin may increase the incidence of seizures. Long-term phenytoin administration may precipitate signs of folic acid deficiency.

Recommendations: If signs of folic acid deficiency are observed in patients receiving phenytoin, folic acid (0.1 to 1mg/day) may be added to therapy. Larger doses of folic acid are not more effective and may cause a loss in seizure control.

Summary: Folic acid administration has been associated with increased seizure frequency and lowered serum phenytoin concentrations. Long-term administration of phenytoin may cause low serum folate concentrations and may precipitate folic acid deficiency.

Related Drugs: The other hydantoin anticonvulsants may also interact with folic acid in a similar manner. There are no drugs related to folic acid.

Mechanism: Phenytoin-induced increases in hepatic metabolizing enzymes may cause a greater demand for folate, and phenytoin may inhibit folate conversion. Folic acid may enhance the parahydroxylation of phenytoin, and higher doses of folate may result in a competitive effect on phenytoin binding sites.

Detailed Information: See *EDI*, 5/55.00

Phenytoin-Ibuprofen

Significance: 2—moderately clinically significant

Potential Effects: Ibuprofen may cause an increase in phenytoin levels.

Recommendations: If these agents are used together, phenytoin levels should be monitored. If increased levels occur, ibuprofen should be discontinued or the dosage of phenytoin decreased.

Summary: The concomitant administration of phenytoin and ibuprofen may increase phenytoin plasma levels, resulting in phenytoin toxicity.

Related Drugs: Phenylbutazone and oxyphenbutazone have been reported to interact with phenytoin (see also Phenytoin-Phenylbutazone, page 126). Other NSAIAs may increase phenytoin plasma levels. A similar interaction is expected to occur between ibuprofen and other hydantoin anticonvulsants.

Mechanism: Ibuprofen may inhibit the hepatic microsomal enzymes responsible for phenytoin metabolism.

Detailed Information: See *EDI,* 5/57.00

Phenytoin-Imipramine

Significance: 3—minimally clinically significant

Potential Effects: Imipramine may cause an increase in phenytoin levels, leading to toxicity. Phenytoin may also cause a decrease in desipramine levels.

Recommendations: Phenytoin levels and signs of toxicity (e.g., nystagmus, gait ataxia, lethargy) should be monitored during cotherapy with imipramine. Since the tricyclics may cause an increase in seizures, the phenytoin dosage may need to be increased. In addition, tricyclic antidepressant levels should be monitored for decreases during concurrent phenytoin therapy.

Summary: Imipramine has been reported to cause an increase in phenytoin levels and phenytoin toxicity.

Related Drugs: The action of other antidepressants on phenytoin levels is varied and conflicting; therefore, it is difficult to determine whether an interaction would occur between phenytoin and the other tricyclic antidepressants and the tetracyclic antidepressants. Amitriptyline, amoxapine, desipramine, imipramine, nortriptyline, and protriptyline have been reported to cause seizures in patients. A similar interaction is expected to occur between imipramine and other hydantoin anticonvulsants.

Mechanism: Imipramine may inhibit the metabolism of phenytoin, which results in increased levels.

Detailed Information: See *EDI,* 5/59.00

Phenytoin-Influenza Virus Vaccine

Significance: 3—minimally clinically significant

Potential Effects: Influenza Virus Vaccine has been shown to increase, decrease, and have no serum phenytoin levels.

Recommendations: Plasma phenytoin levels should be monitored and adjusted if necessary following influenza virus vaccination.

Summary: The administration of influenza virus vaccine was shown to decrease, increase, and have no effect on phenytoin plasma levels.

Related Drugs: It is not known if an interaction would occur between influenza virus vaccine and other hydantoin anticonvulsants.

Mechanism: The influenza virus vaccine is thought to enhance the metabolism of phenytoin. Phenytoin levels may be increased secondary to a decrease in metabolism caused by the influenza virus vaccine.

Detailed Information: See *EDI,* 5/60.10

Phenytoin-Isoniazid

Significance: 2—moderately clinically significant

Recommendations: Patients receiving phenytoin and isoniazid concurrently should have periodic determinations of serum phenytoin concentrations and should be observed closely for signs and symptoms of toxicity (e.g., ataxia, nystagmus). Patients known to be slow acetylators of isoniazid should have the phenytoin dosage reduced when isoniazid is added to the regimen. If phenytoin toxicity occurs, phenytoin should be discontinued or the dosage reduced until toxic signs and symptoms subside. Phenytoin may then be reinstituted and the dosage adjusted until therapeutic concentrations are obtained.

Summary: Isoniazid increases the serum phenytoin concentration, which can result in an increased incidence of phenytoin toxicity.

Related Drugs: Isoniazid may interact with other hydantoin anticonvulsants. Aminosalicylic acid and cycloserine have been shown to interact with phenytoin.

Mechanism: Studies have shown that isoniazid blocks the parahydroxylation of phenytoin and conjugation of the principal metabolite.

Detailed Information: See *EDI*, 5/61.00

Phenytoin-Levodopa

Significance: 3—minimally clinically significant

Recommendations: If the concurrent use of levodopa and phenytoin is necessary, a higher dose of levodopa may be required.

Summary: The therapeutic effects of levodopa were inhibited by the concurrent use of phenytoin, and Parkinson patients showed a worsening of symptoms and a reduction of dyskinesias.

Related Drugs: There are no drugs related to levodopa. A similar interaction may occur between levodopa and other hydantoins; however, documentation is lacking.

Mechanism: The mechanism of this interaction is unknown.

Detailed Information: See *EDI*, 5/63.00

Phenytoin-Levothyroxine

Significance: 3—minimally clinically significant

Recommendations: Since patients may remain euthyroid during concurrent administration of phenytoin and levothyroxine, concomitant use need not be avoided. However, patients should be frequently observed for signs of hypothyroidism. The dose of levothyroxine may need to be increased, since an increase in dose was shown to improve the symptoms of hypothyroidism.

Summary: Data have shown that patients on levothyroxine may develop clinical hypothyroidism after initiation of phenytoin therapy; however, patients remained euthyroid.

Related Drugs: A similar interaction may occur between phenytoin and other thyroid preparations and between levothyroxine and other hydantoin anticonvulsants.

Mechanism: Phenytoin may displace thyroid hormones or it may increase the rate of clearance and catabolism of thyroid hormones.

Detailed Information: See *EDI*, 5/64.10

Phenytoin-Methoxsalen

Significance: 2—moderately clinically significant

Potential Effects: Phenytoin may decrease the serum levels of methoxsalen.

Recommendations: The use of methoxsalen (PUVA therapy) in patients receiving phenytoin may result in treatment failure. However, if phenytoin is discontinued or the dose decreased, methoxsalen serum levels may increase, resulting in serious erythema or blistering reactions. It is not known if adjusting the dose of methoxsalen would be beneficial.

Summary: A patient maintained on phenytoin received PUVA treatment and no beneficial effect was observed. Phenytoin was discontinued, and PUVA therapy had to be stopped secondary to intense PUVA erythema with blisters.

Related Drugs: A similar interaction may occur between methoxsalen and other hydantoin anticonvulsants and between phenytoin and trioxsalen.

Mechanism: Phenytoin may induce the hepatic microsomal enzymes responsible for the metabolism of methoxsalen. There may be a decreased gastrointestinal absorption or altered plasma protein binding of methoxsalen by phenytoin.

Detailed Information: See *EDI*, 5/64.21

Phenytoin-Methylphenidate

Significance: 3—minimally clinically significant

Recommendations: Serum concentrations of phenytoin should be monitored and the dose altered to bring the anticonvulsant level into the therapeutic range.

Summary: Methylphenidate raises serum phenytoin concentration and may cause symptoms of phenytoin toxicity in children; these effects were not seen in adults.

Related Drugs: Primidone has been reported to interact with methylphenidate in a similar manner. A similar interaction is expected to occur with other hydantoin anticonvulsants and methylphenidate.

Mechanism: Methylphenidate is a competitive inhibitor of the hepatic metabolism of phenytoin.

Detailed Information: See *EDI*, 5/65.00

Phenytoin-Metronidazole

Significance: 3—minimally clinically significant

Potential Effects: Concomitant metronidazole therapy may cause an increase in phenytoin levels.

Recommendations: Although these agents may be used together, patients' phenytoin levels should be monitored.

Summary: Metronidazole has been shown to significantly prolong phenytoin's half-life and reduce its clearance; however, in another study, there was no change in the elimination of phenytoin.

Related Drugs: A similar interaction may occur between metronidazole and other hydantoin anticonvulsants. There are no drugs related to metronidazole.

Mechanism: Metronidazole may impair the oxidative metabolism of phenytoin.

Detailed Information: See *EDI*, 5/66.01

Phenytoin-Nifedipine

Significance: 2—moderately clinically significant

Potential Effects: Nifedipine may cause an increase in phenytoin levels, leading to phenytoin toxicity.

Recommendations: Monitor phenytoin levels if nifedipine is added to, or withdrawn from, therapy.

Summary: Nifedipine has been shown to induce signs of phenytoin toxicity revealing nystagmus, dysarthria and cerebellar ataxia.

Related Drugs: A similar interaction may occur between phenytoin and other calcium channel blockers and between nifedipine and other hydantoin anticonvulsants.

Mechanism: Nifedipine may displace phenytoin from plasma proteins or inhibit the parahydroxylation of phenytoin, resulting in increased phenytoin levels.

Detailed Information: See *EDI,* 5/66.30

Phenytoin-Nitrofurantoin

Significance: 3—minimally clinically significant

Recommendations: These agents need not be avoided. However, patients should be monitored for an increase in seizure frequency. If loss of seizure control occurs, the dose of phenytoin may need to be increased or nitrofurantoin may have to be discontinued.

Summary: Phenytoin has been shown to reduce plasma phenytoin levels after the initiation of nitrofurantoin.

Related Drugs: A similar interaction is expected to occur between nitrofurantoin and other hydantoin anticonvulsants. There is a lack of documentation concerning an interaction between phenytoin and furazolidone, and it is not possible to predict whether a similar interaction could occur.

Mechanism: Impaired phenytoin absorption and increased phenytoin metabolism by nitrofurantoin may be responsible.

Detailed Information: See *EDI,* 5/67.00

Phenytoin-Omeprazole

Significance: 2—moderately clinically significant

Potential Effects: Omeprazole may increase the phenytoin area-under-curve.

Recommendations: Caution should be used if omeprazole is added to, or withdrawn from, cotherapy with phenytoin. Phenytoin levels should be monitored, and the dose of phenytoin may need to be adjusted.

Summary: Omeprazole increased the area-under-curve of phenytoin when compared to subjects on phenytoin alone; however, it has been found that omeprazole will not significantly affect the steady-state plasma levels.

Related Drugs: A similar interaction is expected to occur between omeprazole and other hydantoin anticonvulsants. There are no drugs related to omeprazole.

Mechanism: This interaction may result from a decreased elimination or an increased absorption of phenytoin. Omeprazole may inhibit hepatic cytochrome P450 monooxygenase.

Detailed Information: See *EDI,* 5/68.10

Phenytoin-Oral Contraceptive Agents

Significance: 3—minimally clinically significant

Recommendations: Patients may need an alternate form of contraception if phenytoin or other anticonvulsants are required. Also, patients should be monitored for loss of seizure control since an increased phenytoin dose may be necessary.

Summary: The concurrent use of oral contraceptive agents with phenytoin may result in breakthrough bleeding, spotting, and loss of contraceptive effect. Concomitant use of these agents has been reported to lead to loss of seizure control.

Related Drugs: A similar interaction is expected to occur between oral contraceptive agents and other hydantoin anticonvulsants. A similar interaction may occur between phenytoin and other estrogens based on the proposed mechanism.

Mechanism: Phenytoin induces hepatic microsomal enzymes, increasing the rate of metabolism of oral contraceptives. Oral contraceptives cause changes in fluid retention, and this may potentiate a loss of seizure control or may affect the plasma protein binding of phenytoin or inhibit its metabolism.

Detailed Information: See *EDI*, 5/69.00

Phenytoin-Phenobarbital

Significance: 3—minimally clinically significant

Recommendations: Concurrent phenytoin and phenobarbital therapy need not be avoided when indicated. However, the unpredictable clinical outcome of the drug interaction requires that the serum phenytoin concentrations be determined when initiating concurrent therapy, and that phenytoin and phenobarbital concentrations be determined periodically thereafter until the serum drug levels are stabilized. A determination of serum phenytoin and phenobarbital concentrations after three or four weeks of therapy may serve as a good indicator of the quality of the therapeutic regimen. Serum drug concentrations should be determined at the first sign of phenytoin or phenobarbital toxicity. If toxicity occurs, phenytoin or phenobarbital should be discontinued or the dosage should be reduced until toxic signs and symptoms disappear. Then the drug can be reinstituted or the dosages can be adjusted until therapeutic concentrations are attained.

Summary: Phenobarbital may increase, decrease, or cause no change in serum phenytoin concentrations. Other evidence indicates that phenobarbital levels may be increased with concomitant phenytoin.

Related Drugs: Primidone has been shown to interact like phenobarbital with phenytoin (see also Primidone-Phenytoin, page 129). A similar interaction is expected to occur with phenobarbital and other hydantoin anticonvulsants. There is no information regarding possible interactions of other barbiturates with phenytoin.

Mechanism: Phenobarbital induces hepatic microsomal enzyme activity, increasing the rate of metabolism of phenytoin and decreasing its half life. The two drugs may compete for the hepatic microsomal enzyme system.

Detailed Information: See *EDI*, 5/71.00

Phenytoin-Phenylbutazone

Significance: 2—moderately clinically significant

Recommendations: If phenylbutazone, oxyphenbutazone, or sulfin-pyrazone and phenytoin are coadministered, an increase in phenytoin half-life, serum levels, or side effects may occur within the first four weeks of therapy, particularly when phenylbutazone, oxyphenbutazone, or sulfinpyrazone is added to the drug regimen of a patient previously stabilized on phenytoin. If signs and symptoms of phenytoin toxicity develop (e.g., nystagmus, gait ataxia, poor muscle tone, or lethargy), serum phenytoin levels should be determined and doses of phenytoin reduced to establish therapeutic levels.

Summary: Concurrent administration of phenytoin and phenylbutazone may result in a significant increase in the half-life, free fraction, and serum level of phenytoin in some patients.

Related Drugs: Oxyphenbutazone, phenylbutazone, and sulfinpyrazone have been reported to interact with phenytoin in a similar manner. A similar interaction is expected to occur with phenylbutazone, oxyphenbutazone, or sulfinpyrazone and other hydantoin anticonvulsants.

Mechanism: This interaction may be due to the competition for the limited metabolic capacity of hydroxylation enzymes, impaired p-hydroxylation, or phenytoin displacement from its protein binding sites.

Detailed Information: See *EDI,* 5/73.00

Phenytoin-Pyridoxine

Significance: 2—moderately clinically significant

Recommendations: Because not all patients appear to be affected by concurrent pyridoxine and phenytoin, these agents need not be avoided. However, the possibility of an interaction does exist, and patients should be monitored for decreased phenytoin levels or loss of seizure control during concurrent administration.

Summary: Pyridoxine has been shown to cause a marked reduction in phenytoin serum levels.

Related Drugs: A similar interaction is expected to occur between pyridoxine and other hydantoin anticonvulsants, if the mechanism involves induction of hepatic enzymes by pyridoxine. There are no drugs related to pyridoxine.

Mechanism: Pyridoxine may increase the liver enzyme activity responsible for phenytoin metabolism.

Detailed Information: See *EDI,* 5/75.00

Phenytoin-Rifampin

Significance: 2—moderately clinically significant

Recommendations: Patients stabilized on phenytoin should be closely monitored for decreased serum phenytoin concentrations or signs of seizure activity when rifampin is coadministered. Conversely, discontinuation of rifampin in a patient stabilized on phenytoin may necessitate a reduction in the phenytoin dose.

Summary: Rifampin has been shown to decrease serum phenytoin concentrations.

Related Drugs: A similar interaction is expected to occur between rifampin and other hydantoin anticonvulsants. There are no drugs related to rifampin.

Mechanism: Rifampin appears to increase the rate of metabolism of phenytoin, decreasing its half-life and serum concentration.

Detailed Information: See *EDI,* 5/76.10

Phenytoin-Sucralfate

Significance: 2—moderately clinically significant

Potential Effects: Phenytoin levels may be decreased, which may lead to a loss of seizure control.

Recommendations: Monitor phenytoin levels. Phenytoin dosage may need to be increased.

Summary: Sulcralfate was shown to reduce phenytoin's area-under-curve and absorption, risking loss of seizure control.

Related Drugs: Documentation is lacking regarding a similar interaction between sucralfate and other hydantoin anticonvulsants. There are no drugs related to sucralfate.

Mechanism: This mechanism may be related to the physical adsorption of phenytoin by sucralfate.

Detailed Information: See *EDI,* 5/76.30

Phenytoin-Sulfamethizole

Significance: 2—moderately clinically significant

Recommendations: If sulfamethizole and phenytoin are coadministered, an increase in phenytoin half-life, serum levels, or side effects should occur within the first four weeks of therapy, particularly when the sulfonamide is added to the drug regimen of a patient previously stabilized on phenytoin. If signs and symptoms of phenytoin toxicity develop (e.g., nystagmus, gait ataxia, poor muscle tone, or lethargy), serum phenytoin levels should be determined and doses of phenytoin reduced to establish therapeutic levels.

Summary: Sulfamethizole may cause a significant increase in the half-life and serum level of phenytoin.

Related Drugs: Sulfadiazine and sulfamethoxazole, alone and in combination with trimethoprim, have been reported to impair phenytoin metabolism and increase its half-life. Sulfisoxazole does not impair phenytoin metabolism; however, it has been reported to displace phenytoin. It is difficult to predict possible interactions with other sulfonamides and phenytoin. A similar interaction is expected to occur with other hydantoin anticonvulsants and other anticonvulsants metabolized by hepatic microsomal hydroxylation.

Mechanism: Sulfamethizole and phenytoin may compete for the limited metabolic capacity of enzymes. Phenytoin's p-hydroxylation is impaired. Sulfisoxazole displaces phenytoin from its protein binding sites.

Detailed Information: See *EDI,* 5/77.00

Phenytoin-Ticlopidine

Significance: 2—moderately clinically significant

Potential Effects: The addition of ticlopidine to phenytoin therapy may result in increased phenytoin serum levels and toxicity.

Recommendations: The patient should be carefully monitored for changes in phenytoin serum levels and toxicity if ticlopidine is added to or seizures if it is removed from a phenytoin regimen.

Summary: Increased phenytoin serum levels and toxicity resulted when ticlopidine was added to phenytoin therapy.

Related Drugs: Although documentation is lacking regarding an interaction between ticlopidine and the other hydantoin anticonvulsant agents, an interaction may be expected to occur. There are no drugs related to ticlopidine.

Mechanism: It is postulated that this interaction involves ticlopidine's effect on the cytochrome P450$_{2C19}$ isozyme system.

Detailed Information: See *EDI,* 5/78.05

Phenytoin-Trazodone

Significance: 3—minimally clinically significant

Potential Effects: Trazodone may increase phenytoin levels.

Recommendations: Phenytoin levels should be monitored when trazodone is added to, or withdrawn from, therapy.

Summary: The administration of trazodone has been shown to increase phenytoin levels.

Related Drugs: Documentation is lacking regarding an interaction between trazodone and other hydantoin anticonvulsants. There are no drugs related to trazodone.

Mechanism: The mechanism of this interaction is unknown.

Detailed Information: See *EDI,* 5/78.10

Phenytoin-Trimethoprim

Significance: 2—moderately clinically significant

Recommendations: Patients should be monitored for increased phenytoin plasma levels since a lower dosage of phenytoin may be necessary during concurrent use of these agents.

Summary: Trimethoprim has been shown to cause an increased phenytoin elimination half-life and a reduced metabolic clearance rate.

Related Drugs: There are no drugs related to trimethoprim. A similar interaction may occur between trimethoprim and other hydantoin anticonvulsants.

Mechanism: Trimethoprim may inhibit the hepatic metabolism of phenytoin.

Detailed Information: See *EDI,* 5/79.00

Phenytoin-Valproic Acid

Significance: 2—moderately clinically significant

Recommendations: Surveillance of the patient requiring both phenytoin and valproic acid for seizure control should not be limited solely to the serum concentration of total phenytoin, because measurements may grossly underestimate the concentration of free (active) drug. Dosage adjustments should be determined by clinical signs of over- or underdose. Phenytoin serum levels should be determined before valproic acid is administered. After valproic acid is given, a change in serum concentration of phenytoin is used to determine any phenytoin dose adjustments that might be necessary. The measurement of free (active) phenytoin levels should provide a better therapeutic guide than total serum concentrations. The serum concentration of free phenytoin should be determined by ultrafiltration methods or by using saliva samples.

Summary: Valproic acid will decrease phenytoin concentrations and increase the percentage of free phenytoin.

Related Drugs: A similar interaction is expected to occur with valproic acid and other hydantoin anticonvulsants. There are no drugs related to valproic acid; however, sodium valproate and divalproex sodium would be expected to interact in a similar manner.

Mechanism: This interaction will depend on the combination of the displacement of phenytoin from plasma protein binding sites and its reduction in clearance.
Detailed Information: See *EDI,* 5/81.00

Primidone-Acetazolamide
Significance: 3—minimally clinically significant
Recommendations: Patients receiving these agents concomitantly should be monitored for decreases in primidone and/or pheno-barbital serum concentrations or lack of seizure control.
Summary: Concurrent administration of primidone and acetazo-lamide has been reported to decrease or delay the absorption of primidone.
Related Drugs: No documentation exists regarding an interaction between acetazolamide and other barbiturates. No reports exist of barbiturates interacting with other carbonic anhydrase inhibitors.
Mechanism: Acetazolamide may decrease the gastrointestinal absorption of primidone.
Detailed Information: See *EDI,* 5/83.00

Primidone-Phenytoin
Significance: 2—moderately clinically significant
Recommendations: Because these agents are often administered together successfully, their concurrent use need not be avoided. However, patients taking phenytoin and primidone concurrently should be monitored to assure effective anticonvulsant control. Additionally, they may have to be monitored for possible pheno-barbital toxicity.
Summary: Concomitant phenytoin therapy increases the plasma concentrations of phenobarbital, and primidone may increase phenytoin clearance.
Related Drugs: Ethosuximide had no effect on primidone levels, but primidone caused a slight increase in ethosuximide levels. Meth-suximide increased primidone and phenobarbital levels. Pheno-barbital has been shown to interact with phenytoin (see also Phenytoin-Phenobarbital, page 125). An interaction may be expected between primidone and the other hydantoin anticon-vulsants.
Mechanism: Phenytoin may induce the microsomal enzymes responsible for the oxidation of primidone to phenobarbital, or phenytoin may inhibit phenobarbital metabolism or excretion.
Detailed Information: See *EDI,* 5/85.00

Sodium Valproate-Cimetidine
Significance: 3—minimally clinically significant
Recommendations: These agents may be given together; however, valproic acid levels should be monitored. The dose of sodium valproate may need to be decreased.
Summary: Administration of cimetidine has been shown to increase the serum levels of valproic acid.
Related Drugs: Ranitidine did not affect any pharmacokinetic para-meters of sodium valproate. Valproic acid and divalproex sodium would be expected to interact similarly with cimetidine.
Mechanism: Cimetidine may inhibit the hepatic metabolism of sodi-um valproate.
Detailed Information: See *EDI,* 5/86.01

Sodium Valproate-Naproxen

Significance: 3—minimally clinically significant

Recommendations: Patients receiving these agents concurrently should be monitored for valproic acid toxicity. Although the change in free fraction could theoretically alter the relationship between total drug level and clinical response, in practice the magnitude of the interaction does not appear to be sufficiently marked to have clinical relevance for the interpretation of serum drug levels.

Summary: Naproxen was shown to displace valproic acid, increasing the clearance of total drug, but leaving free valproic acid levels unchanged.

Related Drugs: A similar interaction is expected to occur between valproic acid and other NSAIAs. Valproic acid and divalproex sodium would be expected to interact similarly with naproxen.

Mechanism: Naproxen appears to exert a displacing effect on valproic acid, increasing the clearance of total drug, but leaving the clearance of free drug unchanged.

Detailed Information: See *EDI*, 5/86.10

Valproic Acid-Aluminum Hydroxide, Magnesium Hydroxide

Significance: 3—minimally clinically significant

Recommendations: Whether this interaction is clinically significant with steady-state valproic acid therapy or with smaller amounts of antacids is not known. Since antacids are often recommended to relieve gastrointestinal symptoms common to valproic acid administration (indigestion, nausea and vomiting, cramps, diarrhea, etc.), it is important to monitor patients closely for signs of valproic acid toxicity when antacids are used concurrently.

Summary: Aluminum hydroxide-magnesium hydroxide antacid preparations have been shown to significantly increase area-under-curve and steady-state serum levels of valproic acid.

Related Drugs: No drugs are related to valproic acid; however, sodium valproate and divalproex sodium may be expected to interact similarly.

Mechanism: The aluminum/magnesium hydroxide antacid may increase the bioavailability of valproic acid.

Detailed Information: See *EDI*, 5/87.00

Valproic Acid-Amitriptyline

Significance: 3—minimally clinically significant

Potential Effects: Concurrent administration of valproic acid or its derivatives with a tricyclic antidepressant may result in alterations in the pharmacokinetics of either agent.

Recommendations: Monitor for changes in valproic acid levels and tricyclic antidepressant levels when these agents are used together.

Summary: Concurrent administration of valproic acid or its derivatives with a tricyclic antidepressant may result in alterations in the pharmacokinetics of either agent. The clinical significance of this interaction was not determined.

Related Drugs: A similar interaction may occur between valproic acid, divalproex, and valproate with the other tricyclic antidepressants.

Mechanism: The volume of distribution of valproic acid may increase as a result of drug displacement from plasma proteins and/or an enhancement in tissue binding. However, displacement is unlikely since amitriptyline and valproic acid bind predominantly to different classes of plasma proteins. Therefore, an increase in tissue binding of valproic acid by amitriptyline appears more probable. The exact mechanism resulting in increased levels of tricyclic antidepressants is unknown, although it is postulated to involve inhibition of the hydroxylation of the tricyclic agent.

Detailed Information: See *EDI*, 5/88.10

Valproic Acid-Aspirin

Significance: 2—moderately clinically significant

Potential Effects: Aspirin may increase valproic acid half-life, resulting in increased levels of valproic acid and toxicity.

Recommendations: Patients receiving valproic acid should be closely monitored for toxicity if aspirin is added. Especially during a period of febrile illness. Another analgesic/antipyretic may be used as an alternative to aspirin (e.g., acetaminophen).

Summary: Administration of aspirin has been shown to increase valproic acid half-life resulting in increased levels of valproic acid and toxicity.

Related Drugs: A similar interaction is expected to occur between valproic acid and other salicylates. There are no drugs related to valproic acid; however, sodium valproate and divalproex sodium would be expected to interact similarly.

Mechanism: Salicylic acid may compete for active transport sites in the renal tubules or liver. Aspirin may displace valproic acid from plasma proteins and may increase glucuronide excretion, inhibiting the conjugation of valproic acid.

Detailed Information: See *EDI*, 5/89.00

Valproic Acid-Carbamazepine

Significance: 2—moderately clinically significant

Recommendations: Serum valproic acid determinations may be helpful in assessing the need of changing the valproic acid dosage when carbamazepine is added to, or withdrawn from, valproate therapy. There is not enough documentation to substantiate a need to reduce carbamazepine dosage in the presence of valproic acid.

Summary: Concurrent use of carbamazepine and valproic acid results in a decrease in serum valproic acid concentrations. Valproic acid may cause an increase in serum carbamazepine concentrations.

Related Drugs: There are no drugs related to valproic acid; however, sodium valproate and divalproex sodium would be expected to interact similarly.

Mechanism: Carbamazepine is thought to induce hepatic microsomal enzymes, enhancing the metabolism of valproic acid.

Detailed Information: See *EDI*, 5/91.00

Valproic Acid-Chlorpromazine

Significance: 3—minimally clinically significant

Potential Effects: Chlorpromazine may cause an increase in valproic acid levels.

Recommendations: Valproic acid levels should be monitored if these agents are used together. The dose of valproic acid may need to be decreased or haloperidol used instead of chlorpromazine.

Summary: Administration of chlorpromazine was shown to significantly increase the serum levels of valproic acid.

Related Drugs: A similar interaction may occur between valproic acid and other phenothiazines. Haloperidol has been shown to not affect the pharmacokinetic parameters of valproic acid. It is difficult to determine if an interaction would occur between valproic acid and the thioxanthenes, the dihydroindolones and the dibenzoxazepines. There are no drugs related to valproic acid; however, sodium valproate and divalproex sodium would be expected to interact similarly with chlorpromazine.

Mechanism: Chlorpromazine may inhibit the hepatic metabolism of valproic acid.

Detailed Information: See *EDI*, 5/92.10

Valproic Acid-Clonazepam

Significance: 3—minimally clinically significant

Recommendations: The incidence of this interaction is expected to be low. Nevertheless, it should be considered a possibility when these agents are used together. If drowsiness occurs, reduction of the clonazepam dosage may be required.

Summary: Concurrent administration of clonazepam and valproic acid does not appear to cause any alterations in plasma concentrations of either drug; however, some patients have experienced drowsiness.

Related Drugs: Nitrazepam and valproic acid have been reported to cause drowsiness. Valproic acid may increase the free diazepam serum concentration and inhibit diazepam metabolism. A similar interaction is expected to occur between valproic acid and other benzodiazepines. No drugs are related to valproic acid; however, sodium valproate and divalproex sodium would be expected to interact similarly.

Mechanism: Drowsiness may be the result of an increase in benzodiazepine serum levels.

Detailed Information: See *EDI*, 5/93.00

Valproic Acid-Erythromycin

Significance: 2—moderately clinically significant

Potential Effects: The addition of erythromycin to a valproic acid regimen may result in increased valproate levels and toxicity.

Recommendations: Caution should be used in patients maintained on valproic acid if the addition of erythromycin to therapy is contemplated. Possibly an alternative choice of antibiotic therapy should be made.

Summary: Concomitant valproic acid and erythromycin has been shown to result in increased valproic acid serum levels.

Related Drugs: A similar interaction may be expected to occur between valproic acid and other macrolide antibiotics. There are no drugs related to valproic acid; however, sodium valproate and divalproex sodium would be expected to interact similarly.

Mechanism: Erythromycin may inhibit the metabolism of valproate by competitive inhibition of hepatic microsomal enzymes.

Detailed Information: See *EDI*, 5/88.50

Valproic Acid-Felbamate

Significance: 2—moderately clinically significant

Potential Effects: The addition of felbamate to valproic acid results in increased valproic acid plasma drug concentrations.

Recommendations: Patients should be closely monitored for changes in valproic acid serum levels and signs of toxicity with concurrent use of these agents. The dose of one or both agents may need to be adjusted. Initial adverse effects may be minimized by slowly increasing the felbamate dosage or reducing the initial valproic acid dosage during rapid felbamate titration.

Summary: The coadministration of felbamate and valproic acid results in increased steady-state valproate concentrations.

Related Drugs: There are no drugs related to valproic acid. It is not known whether meprobamate would interact similarly with valproic acid. Sodium valproate and divalproex sodium would be expected to interact similarly.

Mechanism: Valproic acid may cause elevations in felbamate concentration through enzyme inhibition.

Detailed Information: See *EDI*, 5/94.50

Valproic Acid-Fluoxetine

Significance: 3—minimally clinically significant

Potential Effects: Serum valproic acid levels may be increased by concurrent fluoxetine.

Recommendations: Patients in whom fluoxetine is added to or discontinued from a valproic acid regimen should be monitored for possible changes in valproic acid serum levels.

Summary: In a single case report, increased serum valproic acid levels resulted when fluoxetine was added.

Related Drugs: Paroxetine has been reported not to interact with valproic acid. No documentation exists regarding an interaction between valproic acid and the other selective serotonin reuptake inhibitors.

Mechanism: It was postulated that fluoxetine may increase valproic acid levels by decreasing the hepatic metabolism of valproic acid.

Detailed Information: See *EDI*, 5/94.70

Valproic Acid-Isoniazid

Significance: 3—minimally clinically significant

Potential Effects: Concurrent use of these agents may result in hepatic and CNS toxicity.

Recommendations: Patients receiving valproic acid and isoniazid concurrently should be monitored for increased liver enzymes and increased central nervous system effects such as vomiting and drowsiness. Valproic acid may need to be discontinued.

Summary: The concurrent use of these agents has been shown to result in hepatic and CNS toxicity.

Related Drugs: There are no drugs related to isoniazid or valproic acid; however, sodium valproate and divalproex sodium would be expected to interact similarly.

Mechanism: Isoniazid may inhibit the metabolism of valproic acid, or valproic acid may increase the risk of isoniazid-induced toxicity.

Detailed Information: See *EDI*, 5/95.00

Chapter Six

Antidepressant Drug Interactions

Amitriptyline-Chlordiazepoxide

Significance: 3—minimally clinically significant

Potential Effects: Concurrent use of these agents may result in impairment of motor function and enhanced anticholinergic effects.

Recommendations: Although a significant interaction is rare, concurrent use of these agents may result in enhanced central nervous system depression. Concurrent use of these agents has not proved to be superior to the tricyclic antidepressant alone. Monitor serum levels of the tricyclic antidepressant.

Summary: The concurrent administration of amitriptyline and chlordiazepoxide may cause impairment of motor function, and chlordiazepoxide may enhance the anticholinergic action of the tricyclic antidepressant.

Related Drugs: Diazepam has been shown to interact with chlordiazepoxide; however, the data are conflicting. Triazolam and tricyclic antidepressants resulted in increased sedation. Alprazolam decreased the clearance of imipramine. Clonazepam has been shown to decrease desipramine serum levels. It is difficult to determine if an interaction would occur with other tricyclic antidepressants and the other benzodiazepines or with the administration of chlordiazepoxide and the other tricyclic antidepressants or the tetracyclic antidepressants.

Mechanism: Amitriptyline and other tricyclic antidepressants may enhance the sedation produced by chlordiazepoxide.

Detailed Information: See *EDI,* 6/1.00

Amitriptyline-Disulfiram

Significance: 3—minimally clinically significant

Potential Effects: Central nervous system changes (organic brain syndrome) may occur if these agents are used together.

Recommendations: Discontinue one or both agents if signs or symptoms of acute organic brain syndrome develop (e.g., impaired consciousness, orientation or memory; hallucinations; illusions).

Summary: Amitriptyline has been shown to exhibit signs of organic brain syndrome when added to disulfiram therapy.

Related Drugs: Disulfiram has been shown to increase imipramine area-under-curve and elimination half-life and increase desipramine area-under-curve. A similar interaction is expected to occur between disulfiram and other tricyclic antidepressants or the tetracyclic antidepressants. There are no drugs related to disulfiram.

Mechanism: Disulfiram and amitriptyline administration may lead to elevated levels of monoamines and dopamine, resulting in organic brain syndromes and psychoses.

Detailed Information: See *EDI,* 6/3.00

Amitriptyline-Fluconazole

Significance: 2—moderately clinically significant

Potential Effects: The addition of fluconazole to the therapy of a patient maintained on amitriptyline may result in increased amitriptyline serum levels and associated toxicity.

Recommendations: Tricyclic antidepressant serum levels should be carefully monitored when fluconazole or other systemic triazole or imidazole antifungal agents are added to or discontinued from concurrent therapy. The dose of the antidepressant may need to be adjusted.

Summary: Concurrent amitriptyline and fluconazole administration resulted in increased amitriptyline levels to as high as 1,464ng/ml (therapeutic range: 150–250ng/ml) and amitriptyline toxicity.

Related Drugs: An interaction may be expected to occur between fluconazole and the other tricyclic antidepressants or between amitriptyline and the other imidazole antifungal agents or triazole antifungal agents. If the interaction occurs by the postulated mechanism, then clomipramine and desipramine would not be expected to interact with fluconazole to the same extent.

Mechanism: The mechanism of this interaction is not known, but it has been suggested that fluconazole and ketoconazole, both known inhibitors of cytochrome $P450_{3A4}$, may interfere with the demethylation of tricyclic antidepressants whose metabolism is mediated by this isoenzyme. It has also been suggested that ketoconazole, which is relatively specific for inhibition of the cytochrome $P450_{3A4}$ isoenzyme, does not significantly affect desipramine metabolism, which is mediated primarily by the cytochrome $P450_{2D6}$ isoenzyme. Also, because the metabolism of clomipramine occurs primarily through cytochrome $P450_{2D6}$, it is possible that clomipramine, like desipramine, may be less likely to interact with fluconazole.

Detailed Information: See *EDI,* 6/4.01

Bupropion-Carbamazepine

Significance: 3—minimally clinically significant

Potential Effects: Concurrent carbamazepine administration may lead to decreased bupropion serum levels and possible decreased pharmacologic effects.

Recommendations: Patients should be carefully monitored for signs of central nervous system toxicity and seizures with concurrent administration of these agents.

Summary: Concurrent carbamazepine and bupropion administration may lead to decreased bupropion serum levels and possible decreased pharmacologic effects. Carbamazepine may decrease bupropion peak plasma concentration and area-under-curve (AUC) values by as much as 87%.

Related Drugs: Bupropion is an antidepressant agent chemically unrelated to the other antidepressant agents; there are no drugs related to carbamazepine. Although unrelated to carbamazepine, valproic acid did not affect the bupropion AUC or peak serum concentration, but it did decrease the time to peak serum concentration. Its sodium salt, sodium valproate, and divalproex sodium would be expected to interact similarly.

Mechanism: It is postulated that the mechanism of this interaction involves the induction by carbamazepine of cytochrome $P450_{3A4}$-mediated hydroxylation of bupropion.

Detailed Information: See *EDI,* 6/4.03

Buspirone-Erythromycin

Significance: 3—minimally clinically significant

Potential Effects: Concurrent administration of buspirone and erythromycin may result in elevated levels of buspirone and a slight increase in buspirone-related adverse effects.

Recommendations: Although the pharmacodynamic changes in a single dose study were small, it would be prudent to reduce the dosage of buspirone during concomitant administration of erythromycin. Buspirone may exhibit nonlinear pharmacokinetics, thus elevations of buspirone during concomitant administration of erythromycin with multiple doses of buspirone may be more dramatic.

Summary: Concurrent administration of buspirone and erythromycin resulted in elevated levels of buspirone and a slight increase in buspirone-related adverse effects. There were interindividual differences in the extent of the interaction.

Related Drugs: Because it is believed that azithromycin does not produce hepatic cytochrome P450 induction or inactivation as erythromycin estolate does, an interaction between buspirone and azithromycin is not likely. Although documentation is lacking, an interaction would be expected to occur between buspirone and the other macrolide antibiotics. Buspirone is an antianxiety agent that is not chemically or pharmacologically related to the benzodiazepines, barbiturates, or other sedative/anxiolytic agents.

Mechanism: Buspirone undergoes extensive first-pass metabolism. It is postulated that erythromycin inhibits the metabolism of buspirone at the cytochrome P450$_{3A4}$ isoenzyme.

Detailed Information: See *EDI,* 6/4.04

Buspirone-Fluoxetine

Significance: 3—minimally clinically significant

Potential Effects: Fluoxetine may decrease the effects of buspirone. Buspirone may augment the effects of fluoxetine.

Recommendations: The concomitant use of buspirone and fluoxetine may be desirable for the treatment of obsessive-compulsive disorder (OCD) or in refractory depression in some patients. However, this combination may decrease the efficacy of buspirone in other conditions.

Summary: The addition of fluoxetine to buspirone therapy may decrease the anxiolytic action of buspirone or may result in adverse effects. The addition of buspirone to fluoxetine therapy in OCD patients may result in augmentation of the effect of fluoxetine.

Related Drugs: A similar effect between buspirone and the other selective serotonin reuptake inhibitors would be expected to occur. Based on the postulated mechanisms, similar effects may result with concurrent buspirone and agents such as venlafaxine or nefazodone that inhibit serotonin reuptake as a part of their mechanism of action. There are no drugs related to buspirone.

Mechanism: The mechanism of this interaction is not known. It has been postulated that efficacy of buspirone in the treatment of OCD is due to its high affinity for the 5-HT1a receptor. The potentiation of fluoxetine by buspirone may cause an effective increase in the amount of synaptic 5-HT. Fluoxetine may impair the oxidative metabolism of buspirone, which may result in increased plasma levels of buspirone.

Detailed Information: See *EDI,* 6/4.05

Desipramine-Quinidine

Significance: 3—minimally clinically significant

Potential Effects: Concurrent quinidine administration may result in a decrease in desipramine clearance.

Recommendations: The interaction between desipramine and quinidine does not occur in all patients, and it appears to be dependent on the metabolic state of the patient. The clinical effects of this interaction have not been clearly established; therefore, patients taking both medications concurrently should be monitored for changes in clinical efficacy and in serum levels early in the course of therapy.

Summary: Concurrent quinidine and desipramine may result in decreased desipramine clearance.

Related Drugs: Nortriptyline and quinidine produced a decrease in nortriptyline metabolism and an increase in the excretion of unchanged nortriptyline. Imipramine oral clearance was decreased when administered concurrently with quinidine sulfate. A similar interaction is expected to occur between quinidine and other tricyclic antidepressant agents.

Mechanism: Inhibition of cytochrome $P450_{DB1}$ metabolism by quinidine is responsible for this interaction.

Detailed Information: See *EDI,* 6/4.06

Desipramine-Thioridazine

Significance: 2—moderately clinically significant

Potential Effects: Thioridazine may inhibit the metabolism of desipramine, resulting in increased levels and toxicity.

Recommendations: Monitor the desipramine level closely during concurrent thioridazine therapy. One or both agents may need to be discontinued or the doses decreased.

Summary: Concomitant use if thioridazine and desipramine has resulted in increased desipramine levels.

Related Drugs: Imipramine and chlorpromazine may result in increased serum levels of either drug. Perphenazine, haloperidol, and thiothixene have been shown to inhibit metabolism of imipramine, and nortriptyline and desipramine have been shown to elevate butaperazine. Fluphenazine has been shown to increase imipramine and desipramine levels. Nortriptyline caused increases in chlorpromazine levels.

Mechanism: This interaction involves an inhibition of desipramine metabolism by thioridazine.

Detailed Information: See *EDI,* 6/4.07

Doxepin-Cholestyramine

Significance: 2—moderately clinically significant

Potential Effects: Concurrent administration of doxepin and cholestyramine may result in decreased serum doxepin levels and an increase in the manifestation of depressive symptoms.

Recommendations: Careful monitoring of antidepressant blood levels and effectiveness should be made in patients receiving concurrent doxepin and cholestyramine.

Summary: A patient maintained on doxepin was administered concurrent cholestyramine, and the serum levels of doxepin and n-desmethyldoxepin, an active metabolite, decreased.

Related Drugs: *In vitro* studies found that amitriptyline, desipramine, imipramine and nortriptyline were significantly adsorbed to cholestyramine in gastric fluid. There are no *in vivo* reports of an interaction between cholestyramine and other tricyclic antidepressants; however, an interaction may be expected to occur. An interaction between tricyclic antidepressants and colestipol may also be expected to occur.

Mechanism: *In vitro,* doxepin has been reported to be 80–83% bound to cholestyramine. One *in vitro* study demonstrated that doxepin adsorption onto cholestyramine decreased with increasing pH of the simulated gastric fluid and with increasing ethanol, suggesting that the true binding effect *in vivo* may be variable.

Detailed Information: See *EDI,* 6/4.10

Doxepin-Propoxyphene

Significance: 3—minimally clinically significant

Recommendations: Further studies are necessary to confirm the interaction; however, patients should be monitored for increased central nervous system side effects. The dose of doxepin may have to be decreased or propoxyphene may need to be discontinued.

Summary: The concurrent use of propoxyphene and doxepin has been shown to result in increased doxepin levels.

Related Drugs: A similar interaction is expected to occur between propoxyphene and other tricyclic antidepressants or maprotiline. No documentation exists regarding a similar interaction between doxepin and other narcotic analgesics.

Mechanism: Propoxyphene may inhibit the hepatic metabolism of doxepin.

Detailed Information: See *EDI,* 6/5.00

Fluoxetine-Aspirin

Significance: 3—minimally clinically significant

Potential Effects: The addition of aspirin following the discontinuation of fluoxetine therapy may result in a display of fluoxetine adverse effects.

Recommendations: The use of concurrent aspirin and fluoxetine should be approached with caution and the patient should be monitored for signs of fluoxetine adverse reactions. It is recommended that fluoxetine be discontinued for longer than 48 hours after the resolution of an allergic reaction before switching to another drug.

Summary: The addition of aspirin following fluoxetine discontinuation because of hives resulted in the reappearance of hives.

Related Drugs: It is not known whether an interaction would occur between fluoxetine and the other salicylates or between aspirin and the other selective serotonin reuptake inhibitors.

Mechanism: A pharmacodynamic interaction may have occurred between aspirin and fluoxetine in which aspirin may have sensitized the patient to develop hives during the falling fluoxetine plasma levels following the discontinuation of fluoxetine. However, the similarities in appearance and distribution of hives with fluoxetine and then with aspirin suggest a pharmacokinetic interaction. Aspirin acetylates serum albumin, which alters the binding of other drugs to this protein. Salicylic acid is strongly bound to serum albumin and can displace other drugs from their protein binding sites. Fluoxetine is approximately 94.5% bound to serum proteins *in vitro.*

Detailed Information: See *EDI,* 6/5.20

Fluoxetine-Clarithromycin

Significance: 3—minimally clinically significant

Potential Effects: The addition of clarithromycin to fluoxetine therapy may result in delirium.

Recommendations: Patients receiving fluoxetine therapy who begin treatment with clarithromycin should be monitored for mental status changes and other signs of fluoxetine toxicity.

Summary: In a case report, the addition of clarithromycin to fluoxetine therapy may have resulted in delirium.

Related Drugs: Although documentation is lacking, based on the proposed mechanism and pharmacologic similarity a similar interaction would be expected to occur between fluoxetine and other macrolide antibiotics except azithromycin. Clarithromycin would be expected to interact with the other selective serotonin reuptake inhibitors and nonselective serotonin reuptake inhibitors.

Mechanism: Clarithromycin may have inhibited the metabolism of fluoxetine at the cytochrome P450 site, resulting in accumulation of fluoxetine.

Detailed Information: See *EDI*, 6/5.50

Fluoxetine-Cyclosporine

Significance: 3—minimally clinically significant

Potential Effects: The addition of fluoxetine to a cyclosporine regimen may result in increased cyclosporine levels and toxicity.

Recommendations: Cyclosporine blood levels should be carefully monitored when fluoxetine is initiated or discontinued in patients maintained on cyclosporine. The dosage of one or both agents may need to be adjusted.

Summary: The addition of fluoxetine to a cyclosporine regimen may result in increased cyclosporine levels and toxicity. However, conflicting data are available.

Related Drugs: A similar interaction would be expected to occur between cyclosporine and the other selective serotonin reuptake inhibitors or the other nonselective serotonin reuptake inhibitor, venlafaxine. There are no drugs related to cyclosporine.

Mechanism: It has been suggested that because cyclosporine is primarily metabolized by the hepatic cytochrome $P450_{3A3/4}$ isoenzyme, drugs that inhibit this isoenzyme may be the most likely to reduce the clearance of cyclosporine and thus produce increases in whole blood levels of cyclosporine. It has also been postulated that inhibition of the cytochrome $P450_{2D6}$ isoenzyme may play a role in the interaction of cyclosporine and fluoxetine.

Detailed Information: See *EDI*, 6/5.70

Fluoxetine-Cyproheptadine

Significance: 2—moderately clinically significant

Potential Effects: The therapeutic effects of fluoxetine may be reversed by the addition of cyproheptadine.

Recommendations: The addition of cyproheptadine to a fluoxetine regimen may result in a decreased effect of fluoxetine. The cyproheptadine may have to be discontinued.

Summary: The therapeutic effects of fluoxetine may be reversed by the addition of cyproheptadine. However, conflicting data are available.

Related Drugs: Paroxetine has interacted with cyproheptadine in a similar fashion. It is not known whether a similar interaction would occur between cyproheptadine and the other selective or nonselective serotonin reuptake inhibitors. It is not known whether a similar interaction would occur between fluoxetine and the other antihistamines.

Mechanism: Fluoxetine's increase of the deficient serotonin activity in bulimia nervosa results in its antibulimic efficacy. Cyprohepta-dine blocks both serotonergic and histaminic function and is effective in reversing sexual dysfunction resulting from antide-pressant use. It is postulated that the effects of fluoxetine, a sero-tonin agonist, are canceled by cyproheptadine, a serotonin antagonist.

Detailed Information: See *EDI*, 6/6.03

Fluoxetine-Marijuana

Significance: 2—moderately clinically significant

Potential Effects: Concurrent use of fluoxetine and marijuana may result in severe mania.

Recommendations: Patients maintained on fluoxetine therapy should be cautioned against the concomitant use of marijuana.

Summary: Marijuana usage by a patient on a fluoxetine regimen resulted in severe mania.

Related Drugs: There are no drugs related to fluoxetine. A similar interaction may occur between fluoxetine and dronabinol.

Mechanism: Marijuana could potentiate the action of fluoxetine at central serotonergic neurons.

Detailed Information: See *EDI*, 6/6.05

Fluoxetine-Tranylcypromine

Significance: 1—highly clinically significant

Potential Effects: Concurrent fluoxetine and tranylcypromine may result in severe toxic and possibly fatal reactions.

Recommendations: The concurrent use of these agents should be avoided. It is recommended that a patient currently maintained on a monoamine oxidase inhibitor have the drug withdrawn for at least 14 days prior to initiating therapy with fluoxetine. A patient currently maintained on fluoxetine should have the drug with-drawn for at least five weeks prior to starting therapy with a monoamine oxidase inhibitor. This five-week period is necessary because of the long half-life (7.6 days) of fluoxetine and its active metabolite, norfluoxetine.

Summary: The administration of tranylcypromine within one to ten days after discontinuation of fluoxetine resulted in adverse effects and death in several patients.

Related Drugs: Phenelzine has produced adverse reactions when combined with or administered shortly after the discontinuation of fluoxetine. Patients being treated with phenelzine or tranyl-cypromine concurrently with sertraline have also experienced adverse reactions. There is a report of three fatal overdoses of concurrent moclobemide and citalopram. Selegiline has also been reported to interact with fluoxetine. Venlafaxine has inter-acted similarly with isocarboxazid and phenelzine. Other selec-tive serotonin reuptake inhibitors may be expected to interact with tranylcypromine, and other monoamine oxidase inhibitors may be expected to interact with the selective serotonin reuptake inhibitors.

Mechanism: The exact mechanism is not known. It has been sug-gested that the combined pharmacologic effects of tranyl-cypromine, which prevents the breakdown of serotonin in the central nervous system (CNS), and fluoxetine, which prevents the reuptake of serotonin into presynaptic neurons, may result in increased serotonin levels in the CNS.

Detailed Information: See *EDI*, 6/6.07

Fluoxetine-Tryptophan

Significance: 3—minimally clinically significant

Potential Effects: Concurrent use of these agents may result in decreased efficacy of fluoxetine. This may result from stimulation of the serotonergic system by a combination of the two agents.

Recommendations: Patients receiving fluoxetine should be monitored for decreased efficacy of fluoxetine when tryptophan is added to their therapy. The tryptophan may need to be discontinued since this has been shown to resolve the adverse effects.

Summary: Administration of tryptophan may decrease the efficacy of fluoxetine.

Related Drugs: There are no drugs related to tryptophan or fluoxetine.

Mechanism: A stimulation of the serotonergic system by the two agents may be the cause of this interaction.

Detailed Information: See *EDI*, 6/6.10

Imipramine-Bupropion

Significance: 3—minimally clinically significant

Potential Effects: Concurrent administration of bupropion and imipramine may result in decreased imipramine and desipramine clearance and increased imipramine and desipramine levels.

Recommendations: Until further studies are performed, patients should be monitored for increased imipramine and desipramine levels and effects during concurrent use of imipramine and bupropion. Other tricyclic antidepressants may also interact in the same way and should be monitored accordingly.

Summary: Concurrent administration of bupropion and imipramine resulted in decreased imipramine and desipramine clearance (by 57% and 82%, respectively) and increased imipramine and desipramine levels.

Related Drugs: A similar interaction may be expected to occur between bupropion and the other tricyclic antidepressants. There are no agents related to bupropion.

Mechanism: Imipramine is converted to desipramine by demethylation via cytochrome P450 isoenzymes 1A2, 2C19, and 3A4. Desipramine and imipramine are also hydroxylated by the 2D6 isoenzyme to 2-hydroxymetabolites. It is possible that bupropion may inhibit the 2D6 isoenzyme and increase levels of both parent and metabolite compounds. It has been postulated that the metabolism of bupropion to hydroxybupropion is mediated by the cytochrome $P450_{3A4}$ isoenzyme which could result in competitive inhibition of imipramine metabolism.

Detailed Information: See *EDI*, 6/7.50

Imipramine-Cimetidine

Significance: 2—moderately clinically significant

Potential Effects: Cimetidine may cause an increase in imipramine levels, leading to increased side effects.

Recommendations: If cimetidine and imipramine are taken together, a decreased dose of imipramine may be necessary. If cimetidine is withdrawn from cotherapy, an increased dose of imipramine may be required. Ranitidine may be used instead of cimetidine.

Summary: Cimetidine may decrease the clearance of imipramine, resulting in increased serum concentrations and consequent anticholinergic adverse effects.

Related Drugs: Cimetidine has been shown to decrease nortriptyline steady-state serum concentration and increase amitriptyline plasma levels, desipramine plasma levels and doxepin's area-under-curve; however, all data do not support these interactions. A similar interaction is expected to occur between cimetidine and other tricyclic antidepressants. Ranitidine has been shown to not alter imipramine, amitriptyline and doxepin's pharmacokinetics. A similar interaction is not expected to occur between imipramine and the other H_2-receptor antagonists, if the mechanism involves hepatic inhibition.

Mechanism: It has been postulated that cimetidine suppresses the conversion of imipramine to desipramine by inhibition of the hepatic metabolism of imipramine.

Detailed Information: See *EDI,* 6/9.00

Imipramine-Epinephrine

Significance: 2—moderately clinically significant

Recommendations: The concurrent use of epinephrine or other direct-acting sympathomimetic amines and tricyclic antidepressants should be avoided. When concurrent therapy is necessary, the initial dose of the sympathomimetic should be lowered, and the patient should be carefully monitored for adverse cardiovascular effects.

Summary: Epinephrine and other direct-acting sympathomimetic amines have shown enhanced cardiovascular effects in those taking imipramine or other tricyclic antidepressants.

Related Drugs: Norepinephrine, phenylephrine, dopamine, and methoxamine have been shown to interact with tricyclic antidepressants. Maprotiline has been shown to reduce tyramine sensitivity. Protriptyline, amitriptyline, and desipramine have been reported to interact with direct-acting sympathomimetics. A similar interaction is expected to occur with other tricyclic antidepressants and imipramine.

Mechanism: There is an enhanced cardiovascular effect because tricyclic antidepressants block the reuptake of norepinephrine, increasing concentrations at receptor sites.

Detailed Information: See *EDI,* 6/11.00

Imipramine-Ethinyl Estradiol

Significance: 3—minimally clinically significant

Recommendations: A patient receiving concurrent ethinyl estradiol and imipramine therapy should be observed for lack of effect or enhanced toxicities of imipramine. Should such effects occur, the dose of one of the agents should be adjusted accordingly. One report suggested reducing the dosage of imipramine by approximately one third when the patient is also taking oral contraceptive agents.

Summary: Patients taking ethinyl estradiol have been reported to be relatively unresponsive to therapy with imipramine.

Related Drugs: Similar reactions have been reported in patients taking conjugated estrogens and imipramine or doxepin. There are no reports with other tricyclic antidepressants or maprotiline. Ethinyl estradiol has been shown to increase elimination half-life, and volume of distribution, and reduce clearance of imipramine. A similar interaction is expected to occur with other estrogenic substances and imipramine.

Mechanism: This interaction may be dose related and dependent on baseline hormonal balance. Imipramine may inhibit oral contraceptive metabolism and enhance the effect of the estrogens.

Detailed Information: See *EDI,* 6/13.00

Imipramine-Levodopa

Significance: 3—minimally clinically significant

Recommendations: Because tricyclic antidepressants have been used successfully and uneventfully for depression in patients with Parkinson's disease, the concurrent use of these agents need not be avoided. However, it is advisable to be aware of a possibility of decreased levodopa levels since a dosage adjustment may be necessary.

Summary: There are data to show that imipramine causes a reduction in the absorption of levodopa.

Related Drugs: A similar interaction is expected to occur between levodopa and other tricyclic antidepressants or tetracyclic antidepressants.

Mechanism: Imipramine may slow gastric emptying time, allowing more time for levodopa to be metabolized and reducing the amount of levodopa available for absorption.

Detailed Information: See *EDI*, 6/15.00

Imipramine-Liothyronine

Significance: 3—minimally clinically significant

Recommendations: Since a patient's thyroid function can affect the response to tricyclic antidepressant agents, patients who fail to respond to such drugs should be examined for hypothyroidism. The addition of liothyronine (25µg/day) to tricyclic antidepressant therapy may be considered in selected patients who do not respond to tricyclic antidepressants alone.

Summary: Liothyronine may enhance and accelerate the onset of the antidepressant effects in euthyroid patients.

Related Drugs: Liothyronine has been shown to potentiate the effect of protriptyline and amitriptyline. A similar interaction is expected to occur with other tricyclic antidepressants and tetracyclic antidepressants. A similar interaction is expected to occur with other thyroid preparations.

Mechanism: The mechanism may involve the thyroid enhancement of antidepressant receptor sensitivity.

Detailed Information: See *EDI*, 6/17.00

Imipramine-Lithium Carbonate

Significance: 3—minimally clinically significant

Potential Effects: Lithium may potentiate the antidepressant effects of imipramine.

Recommendations: Patients maintained on imipramine should be monitored carefully if cotherapy with lithium is instituted. Lithium levels should be monitored, and the dosage of one or both agents may need to be adjusted.

Summary: Concurrent use of imipramine and lithium carbonate may result in increased antidepressant effects.

Related Drugs: A similar interaction is expected to occur with other tricyclic antidepressants and lithium carbonate.

Mechanism: There may be a synergistic effect or a potentiation of the pharmacologic activity of imipramine by lithium. The potentiation of the tricyclic may be due to lithium's enhancement of the serotonin metabolite.

Detailed Information: See *EDI*, 6/18.10

Imipramine-Methyltestosterone

Significance: 3—minimally clinically significant

Recommendations: If paranoid reactions occur during concomitant use of imipramine and methyltestosterone, one or both drugs may have to be discontinued.

Summary: There are data to show that the concurrent use of methyltestosterone and imipramine may cause paranoid reactions.

Related Drugs: A similar interaction is expected to occur between the other tricyclic antidepressants, the tetracyclic antidepressants, and other androgen derivatives.

Mechanism: The mechanism of this interaction is unknown.

Detailed Information: See *EDI,* 6/19.00

Imipramine-Nitroglycerin

Significance: 2—moderately clinically significant

Potential Effects: The occurrence of dry mouth that may be associated with imipramine therapy because of its anticholinergic side effects may prevent the dissolution of sublingual nitroglycerin tablets, resulting in ineffective therapy.

Recommendations: Attempts at increasing salivation (e.g., chewing gum, artificial saliva products) may prove useful in increasing the effectiveness of sublingual nitroglycerin in some patients. If the ineffectiveness of the sublingual nitroglycerin continues, use of the oral, topical, or translingual spray forms of the nitrates or discontinuation of the tricyclic antidepressant may need to be considered.

Summary: There are data to show that imipramine can cause a lack of dissolution of nitroglycerin, secondary to the dry mouth caused by imipramine.

Related Drugs: A similar interaction may occur between sublingual nitroglycerin and other tricyclic antidepressant agents and between imipramine and other nitrates available as a sublingual tablet.

Mechanism: Dry mouth is a common side effect of imipramine therapy because of its anticholinergic effects, making dissolution of the sublingual nitroglycerin difficult.

Detailed Information: See *EDI,* 6/20.10

Imipramine-Reserpine

Significance: 3—minimally clinically significant

Recommendations: These agents should be used concurrently to induce an antidepressant response only in the most recalcitrant patients. Experience with this combination is limited to a few patients, and the risk of adverse effects may outweigh potential therapeutic gains. Also, since reserpine may itself cause depression, this fact should be considered before concurrent administration with imipramine.

Summary: Reserpine used in combination with tricyclic antidepressants has been shown to cause hypotension, flushing, diarrhea, and manic reactions.

Related Drugs: The other tricyclic antidepressants and tetracyclic antidepressants may react similarly. A similar interaction is expected to occur between imipramine and other rauwolfia alkaloids.

Mechanism: When reserpine is added to imipramine therapy, there is a release of norepinephrine into the synapse where imipramine inhibits its reuptake.

Detailed Information: See *EDI,* 6/21.00

Imipramine-Tobacco

Significance: 3—minimally clinically significant

Potential Effects: Tobacco smoking may increase the metabolism of imipramine, leading to decreased levels.

Recommendations: Although no specific adjustments in the imipramine dose need be made in smokers, these patients should be monitored for a decreased response to imipramine.

Summary: There are data to show that tobacco smoking may increase the metabolism of imipramine, leading to decreased levels and response.

Related Drugs: Smoking has been associated with lower plasma amitriptyline and/or nortriptyline levels. Because of conflicting results, it is difficult to determine whether an interaction would occur with tobacco smoking and other tricyclic antidepressants or tetracyclic antidepressants.

Mechanism: The interaction between tobacco and imipramine may result from an increased metabolism of imipramine by tobacco.

Detailed Information: See *EDI,* 6/22.10

Imipramine-Tranylcypromine

Significance: 2—moderately clinically significant

Potential Effects: Concurrent use of these agents may result in hyperpyrexia, excitability, muscular rigidity, fluctuations in blood pressure, convulsions, grand mal seizures, and coma.

Recommendations: Concurrent use of these agents should be avoided. Chlorpromazine has been shown to be useful in treating the effects of this interaction.

Summary: Severe toxic and fatal reactions have been reported when tricyclic antidepressants have been given with a MAOI. However, other studies have described beneficial and uneventful concurrent use. Adverse effects may include hyperpyrexia, excitability, muscular rigidity, fluctuations in blood pressure, convulsions, grand mal seizures, and coma.

Related Drugs: Doxepin, nortriptyline, and protriptyline may interact with MAOIs. Isocarboxazid and amitriptyline have been shown to adversely interact. Tranylcypromine and clomipramine have been shown to cause fatal disseminated intravascular coagulation. Moclobemide with imipramine and clomipramine have been shown to cause serotonin syndrome. A similar interaction may occur with other tricyclic antidepressants. Cyclobenzaprine may react with the MAOIs. Other MAOIs may interact with imipramine.

Mechanism: The MAOIs may enhance the effect of the tricyclic antidepressants through inhibition of microsomal enzymes, or the tricyclic antidepressants may sensitize adrenergic receptors to amines which accumulate extraneuronally.

Detailed Information: See *EDI,* 6/23.00

Nortriptyline-Charcoal

Significance: 3—minimally clinically significant

Recommendations: Activated charcoal may be effective in an acute tricyclic antidepressant overdose, and it may even be useful several hours after the overdose since nortriptyline delays gastric emptying. However, if charcoal is not used for nortriptyline overdose, the administration of these agents should be separated by as much time as possible.

Summary: There are data to show that activated charcoal significantly reduces the absorption of nortriptyline.

Related Drugs: Activated charcoal has been shown to greatly accelerate the elimination of amitriptyline. Other tricyclic and tetracyclic antidepressants may be adsorbed by charcoal. There are no drugs related to charcoal.

Mechanism: Nortriptyline delays gastric emptying, and activated charcoal limits its absorption.

Detailed Information: See *EDI*, 6/24.10

Nortriptyline-Fluoxetine

Significance: 2—moderately clinically significant

Potential Effects: Fluoxetine may inhibit the metabolism of nortriptyline, resulting in increased levels and toxicity.

Recommendations: Patients receiving concurrent fluoxetine and nortriptyline or carbamazepine should be monitored for increased levels of nortriptyline or carbamazepine and toxicity. The dosage of nortriptyline or carbamazepine may need to be decreased.

Summary: The administration of fluoxetine may inhibit the metabolism of nortriptyline, resulting in increased levels.

Related Drugs: Data concerning the coadministration of the tricyclic antidepressant drugs and fluoxetine have been well documented; however, much of the data are conflicting.

Mechanism: Fluoxetine may inhibit the hepatic metabolism of nortriptyline, which may result in elevated plasma levels of nortriptyline.

Detailed Information: See *EDI*, 6/24.30

Nortriptyline-Marijuana

Significance: 2—moderately clinically significant

Potential Effects: The use of marijuana cigarettes while receiving concurrent nortriptyline may result in tachycardia, delirium, and transient cognitive changes.

Recommendations: It was suggested that patients receiving tricyclic antidepressants should be informed of the potential risks of an interaction with marijuana.

Summary: The use of marijuana cigarettes while receiving concurrent nortriptyline resulted in tachycardia, delirium, and transient cognitive changes in a 16-year-old male and a 21-year-old female.

Related Drugs: Another report documents a similar interaction of marijuana and desipramine. A similar interaction may be expected to occur between marijuana and other tricyclic antidepressants. It is not known whether an interaction would occur between nortriptyline and dronabinol, although an interaction would be expected based on the postulated mechanism.

Mechanism: The concurrent use of tricyclic antidepressants may slow the metabolism of tetrahydrocannabinol (THC), thereby increasing levels of THC in the central nervous system. Marijuana, generally in larger doses than were used by these patients, is known to cause symptoms of delirium and tachycardia similar to the ones reported. More data are needed to determine the exact mechanism of this interaction.

Detailed Information: See *EDI*, 6/24.50

Nortriptyline-Phenobarbital

Significance: 3—minimally clinically significant

Recommendations: Although the clinical data are limited, they are sufficient to indicate that phenobarbital will decrease serum nortriptyline levels in patients receiving these drugs concurrently. Because the change in therapeutic effect caused by decreased serum nortriptyline levels is not known, the clinical significance of this drug interaction is difficult to assess. If patients are unresponsive to nortriptyline therapy, concurrent barbiturate therapy should be considered as a possible underlying cause. If additional drugs must be used, the benzodiazepines may be useful in treating anxiety symptoms since they do not affect the metabolism of the tricyclic drugs. Flurazepam, a benzodiazepine, apparently does not affect the metabolism of tricyclic antidepressants; therefore, it maybe an alternative to barbiturate cotherapy.

Summary: Limited data indicate that phenobarbital may decrease the serum concentrations of nortriptyline.

Related Drugs: Amobarbital, pentobarbital, and secobarbital have been suggested to interact similarly with nortriptyline. Desipramine and phenobarbital, and protriptyline and amobarbital undergo a similar interaction. A similar interaction may occur between all other barbiturates, other tricyclic antidepressants, and the tetracyclic antidepressants.

Mechanism: Barbiturates can stimulate the metabolism of the tricyclic antidepressants.

Detailed Information: See *EDI*, 6/25.00

Nortriptyline-Rifampin

Significance: 3—minimally clinically significant

Potential Effects: Concurrent rifampin may induce the metabolism of nortriptyline, resulting in decreased nortriptyline levels.

Recommendations: Nortriptyline serum levels should be closely monitored with the addition or discontinuation of rifampin from concurrent therapy. The dose of nortriptyline may need to be adjusted.

Summary: Nortriptyline serum levels increased following rifampin discontinuation from concurrent nortriptyline therapy.

Related Drugs: Similar interactions between other tricyclic antidepressants and rifampin may be expected to occur. If the interaction occurs based on the proposed mechanism, one would be expected to occur between nortriptyline and rifabutin, which is structurally and pharmacologically related to rifampin.

Mechanism: It is postulated that rifampin, which is known to induce cytochrome P450 enzymatic activity, induces the metabolism of nortriptyline, which undergoes oxidation through this system.

Detailed Information: See *EDI*, 6/26.05

Nortriptyline-Terbinafine

Significance: 2—moderately clinically significant

Potential Effects: The addition of terbinafine to the therapy of a patient maintained on nortriptyline may result in increased nortriptyline serum levels and nortriptyline toxicity.

Recommendations: The addition of terbinafine to the therapy of a patient maintained on nortriptyline should be approached with caution. The patient should be carefully monitored for increased nortriptyline serum levels and toxicity. The dose of nortriptyline may need to be adjusted.

Summary: The addition of terbinafine to the therapy of a patient maintained on nortriptyline resulted in increased nortriptyline levels and nortriptyline toxicity. After discontinuation of terbinafine and normalization of nortriptyline levels, the patient was rechallenged with terbinafine with the same adverse effects.

Related Drugs: It is not known whether an interaction would occur between terbinafine and the other tricyclic antidepressants. It is not known whether a similar interaction would be expected to occur with nortriptyline and butenafine, a benzylamine derivative with a mode of action similar to the allylamine antifungal agent terbinafine.

Mechanism: It has been postulated that the increased nortriptyline concentration was due to a pharmacokinetic interaction because there were no increases in the concentrations of gamma-glutamyl transferase, aspartate aminotransferase, or alanine aminotransferase.

Detailed Information: See *EDI*, 6/26.08

Pargyline-Methyldopa

Significance: 3—minimally clinically significant

Recommendations: Until further clinical studies are performed, the concurrent use of these agents need not be avoided. However, it is prudent to be aware of a possible interaction, and if adverse central nervous system effects develop, it may be advisable to discontinue one or both drugs.

Summary: The concomitant administration of pargyline and methyldopa may result in hallucinations and prolonged nervous system excitement.

Related Drugs: A similar interaction may occur between methyldopa and other monoamine oxidase inhibitors. There are no drugs related to methyldopa.

Mechanism: A combination may be mediated by increased levels of free cerebral catecholamines released from binding sites.

Detailed Information: See *EDI*, 6/26.10

Paroxetine-Cimetidine

Significance: 3—minimally clinically significant

Potential Effects: Serum paroxetine levels may be increased by concurrent cimetidine administration.

Recommendations: The dose of paroxetine may need to be adjusted when cimetidine is added to or removed from concurrent therapy.

Summary: Studies have shown increased serum paroxetine levels may result with cimetidine administration.

Related Drugs: Based on the postulated mechanism, an interaction may be expected to occur between cimetidine and the other serotonin-selective reuptake inhibitors, although documentation is lacking. It cannot be determined whether an interaction would be expected to occur between paroxetine and the other H_2 receptor antagonists.

Mechanism: It is postulated that cimetidine may increase paroxetine levels by inhibiting the hepatic metabolism of paroxetine.

Detailed Information: See *EDI*, 6/26.22

Paroxetine-Dextromethorphan

Significance: 2—moderately clinically significant

Potential Effects: The addition of dextromethorphan to paroxetine may produce serotonin syndrome.

Recommendations: The use of dextromethorphan in patients receiving paroxetine or other agents that inhibit the reuptake of serotonin should be avoided if possible.

Summary: The addition of dextromethorphan to a drug regimen that included paroxetine resulted in serotonin syndrome (mental status changes, restlessness, hypertension, tremor, and myoclonus).

Related Drugs: Fluoxetine has interacted similarly with dextromethorphan and pentazocine; however, in one study, pretreatment with fluoxetine prior to dental surgery had no significant effect on pentazocine analgesia, but significantly attenuated morphine-produced analgesia and shortened morphine's duration of action. When fluvoxamine was added to maintenance methadone therapy, two patients experienced approximately a 20% increase in the methadone plasma level/dose ratio and the remaining three patients had from a 40% to a 100% increase in this ratio. A serotonin-like syndrome has occurred when tramadol was added to a regimen including sertraline. It is likely that a similar effect would occur between dextromethorphan and sertraline and between paroxetine and the narcotic agents related to dextromethorphan. It is also likely that similar effects would occur when dextromethorphan is combined with agents such as nefazodone and venlafaxine that inhibit serotonin reuptake as a part of their mechanism of action.

Mechanism: Dextromethorphan inhibits the reuptake of serotonin at the synapse. The addition of dextromethorphan to a selective serotonin reuptake inhibitor regimen may result in additively or synergistically increased serotonin levels and serotonin syndrome. Concomitant pseudoephedrine and ischemic disease may contribute to the adverse event. The $5-HT_2$ receptors in the brain are responsible for the hallucinogenic effects of lysergic acid diethylamide (LSD), and the synergistic action of fluoxetine and dextromethorphan on serotonin levels may lead to the hallucinations. Because paroxetine is a potent inhibitor of cytochrome $P450_{2D6}$ in *in vitro* studies and has a tenfold greater affinity for this enzyme than does dextromethorphan, it is postulated that the interaction may result from a reduction in the clearance of dextromethorphan and a subsequent increase in dextromethorphan plasma levels.

Detailed Information: See *EDI*, 6/26.24

Paroxetine-Zolpidem

Significance: 3—minimally clinically significant

Potential Effects: Concurrent paroxetine and zolpidem may result in delirium.

Recommendations: The concurrent use of these agents should be approached with caution. The use of an alternative medication for zolpidem may be considered in those patients receiving paroxetine.

Summary: The concomitant administration of zolpidem and paroxetine may have induced delirium in a patient taking paroxetine after receiving her first dose of zolpidem. The delirium resolved spontaneously without treatment within four hours.

Related Drugs: It is not known whether an interaction would occur between zolpidem and the other selective serotonin reuptake inhibitors (SSRIs). It is possible that a similar interaction may occur between zolpidem and the SSRIs that are highly protein bound, fluoxetine and sertraline.

Mechanism: It has been proposed that since both paroxetine and zolpidem are highly protein bound, this interaction may occur through competition for binding sites. Both of these agents are known to only infrequently cause hallucinations without the presence of other drugs. Further studies are needed.

Detailed Information: See *EDI*, 6/26.27

Phenelzine-Buspirone

Significance: 3—minimally clinically significant

Potential Effects: Concurrent administration of buspirone and a monoamine oxidase inhibitor (MAOI) may result in blood pressure elevation.

Recommendations: Concurrent therapy with a MAOI and buspirone is not recommended. However, if these agents are administered together, the patient's blood pressure should be carefully monitored.

Summary: There are data to show that the concurrent administration of buspirone and a MAOI may result in blood pressure elevation.

Related Drugs: Tranylcypromine was shown to exhibit a similar interaction. A similar interaction is expected to occur between buspirone and other MAOIs. Furazolidone and procarbazine may interact similarly with buspirone.

Mechanism: The affinity of buspirone for serotonin receptors may explain the observed change in blood pressure.

Detailed Information: See *EDI*, 6/26.30

Phenelzine-Clonazepam

Significance: 3—minimally clinically significant

Potential Effects: Concurrent use of these agents may result in a tyramine-type reaction.

Recommendations: The concomitant use of phenelzine and clonazepam should be approached with caution. The patient should be monitored for signs of a tyramine-type reaction (e.g., headache, flushing, hypertension). The dose of one or both agents may need to be decreased, or one may need to he discontinued.

Summary: Concurrent administration of phenelzine and clonazepam resulted in a tyramine-type reaction.

Related Drugs: A similar interaction is expected to occur between clonazepam and other MAOIs, and between clonazepam and furazolidone, procarbazine, or selegiline. An interaction may occur between phenelzine and other benzodiazepines.

Mechanism: Clonazepam and other benzodiazepines may elevate serotonin levels.

Detailed Information: See *EDI*, 6/26.31

Phenelzine-Levodopa

Significance: 1—highly clinically significant

Recommendations: Levodopa and monoamine oxidase inhibitors should not be administered concurrently. If an antidepressant must be used in a patient receiving levodopa, a tricyclic antidepressant should be considered. If a monoamine oxidase inhibitor must be used concurrently with levodopa, a carbidopa-levodopa combination product should be considered instead of levodopa alone. The effects of monoamine oxidase inhibition usually last two weeks after the drug is discontinued; therefore, levodopa should not be given until at least four weeks after the monoamine oxidase inhibitor is discontinued.

Summary: Levodopa has been documented to cause a significant rise in blood pressure as well as flushing and palpitations when used in combination with phenelzine.

Related Drugs: Isocarboxazid, pargyline and tranylcypromine have been shown to exhibit a similar interaction. This interaction would be expected to occur with agents that possess MAOI activity. There are no drugs related to levodopa.

Mechanism: The concurrent administration of carbidopa, a peripheral decarboxylase inhibitor, with levodopa may suppress the hypertensive reaction caused by monoamine oxidase inhibitors.

Detailed Information: See *EDI,* 6/27.00

Phenelzine-Sulfisoxazole

Significance: 3—minimally clinically significant

Recommendations: If an increased incidence of adverse effects occurs following concurrent administration of these agents, one or both drugs may need to be discontinued. In a case report, symptoms subsided upon discontinuation of sulfisoxazole.

Summary: There are data to show that coadministration of these agents may cause an increased incidence of adverse effects.

Related Drugs: A similar interaction is expected to occur between sulfisoxazole and other MAOIs or between phenelzine and other sulfonamides.

Mechanism: The concurrent use of these agents may saturate the acetylation mechanism, resulting in higher plasma levels and increased side effects.

Detailed Information: See *EDI,* 6/28.10

Pimozide-Sulfamethoxazole, Trimethoprim

Significance: 3—minimally clinically significant

Potential Effects: Combination sulfamethoxazole-trimethoprim may alter a patient's response to pimozide.

Recommendations: Patients receiving these agents together should be closely monitored for changes in their response to pimozide.

Summary: There are data to show that administration of sulfamethoxazole-trimethoprim may alter a patient's response to pimozide.

Related Drugs: It is not known if a similar interaction would occur between pimozide and other sulfonamides. There are no drugs related to pimozide.

Mechanism: This interaction may have occurred at pimozide's receptor site.

Detailed Information: See *EDI,* 6/28.30

Tranylcypromine-Atracurium

Significance: 3—minimally clinically significant

Potential Effects: Concurrent use of these agents may result in hypertension.

Recommendations: Patients should be monitored for hypotension during co-therapy with these agents. If necessary, phentolamine may be useful in reversing the hypertension.

Summary: There are data to show that administration of tranylcypromine when patients are induced with atracurium may result in hypertension.

Related Drugs: It is difficult to determine if a similar interaction would occur between atracurium and other MAOIs or between tranylcypromine and other nondepolarizing neuromuscular blocking agents.

Mechanism: The mechanism of this interaction is not known.

Detailed Information: See *EDI,* 6/28.50

Tranylcypromine-Phenylpropanolamine

Significance: 1—highly clinically significant

Recommendations: Patients receiving monoamine oxidase inhibitors should be instructed to avoid indirect-acting sympathomimetic agents, foods containing tyramine, and nonprescription items with the potential to interact (e.g., cough and cold preparations). Symptoms such as headache, gastrointestinal upset, fever, and visual disturbances should be pointed out as indicators of hypertension caused by such combinations. Marked elevation of blood pressure under these circumstances may be treated by alpha-adrenergic blocking agents like phentolamine (5mg intramuscularly or intravenously).

Summary: Indirect acting sympathomimetic amines may cause an abrupt elevation of blood pressure when administered with tranylcypromine or other MAOIs, resulting in hypertensive crisis.

Related Drugs: Other MAOIs have been reported to interact with other indirect-acting sympathomimetics. Pseudoephedrine may interact similarly. Mixed acting sympathomimetics have been shown to interact with monoamine oxidase inhibitors. Procarbazine and dopamine administered with indirect and mixed acting sympathomimetics may cause hypertensive reactions. Furazolidone has been shown to interact with indirect acting sympathomimetics (see also Furazolidone-Amphetamine, page 185).

Mechanism: The stimulation of norepinephrine released by the indirect-acting adrenergic agents results in an increase of neurotransmitters. The enhancement results from an inhibition of the hepatic microsomal enzymes.

Detailed Information: See *EDI,* 6/29.00

Tranylcypromine-Propranolol

Significance: 4—not clinically significant

Recommendations: One study suggests that monamine oxidase inhibitors should be discontinued at least two weeks before the institution of propranolol therapy, but this is a theoretical consideration only and no clinical interaction has been documented. Therefore, this combination need not be avoided at this time.

Summary: The concomitant administration of tranylcypromine and propranolol does not result in an increase in pressor activity or tachycardia.

Related Drugs: Documentation is lacking regarding an interaction between other MAOIs and other beta-blocking agents and with

furazolidone and procarbazine.
Mechanism: The mechanism of this interaction is unknown.
Detailed Information: See *EDI,* 6/31.00

Tranylcypromine-Tryptophan

Significance: 3—minimally clinically significant
Potential Effects: Use of these agents together may cause sudden changes in mental status.
Recommendations: Use these agents together with caution. Monitor patients for mental status changes. Tryptophan may need to be discontinued.
Summary: There are data to show that coadministration of these agents may cause sudden changes in mental status, exhibiting symptoms such as hyperreflexia, ankle clonus, nystagmus, incoordination, tremor, myoclonic jerks, and nausea.
Related Drugs: Phenelzine was shown to have a similar interaction. A similar interaction may occur between tryptophan and other MAOIs. There are no drugs related to tryptophan.
Mechanism: This interaction may result from a stimulation of the serotonergic system by the combination of the two agents.
Detailed Information: See *EDI,* 6/33.00

Trazodone-Fluoxetine

Significance: 3—minimally clinically significant
Potential Effects: Fluoxetine may decrease the metabolism of trazodone, resulting in increased levels.
Recommendations: Monitor patients for increased trazodone levels and side effects when fluoxetine is added to trazodone therapy.
Summary: There are data to show that the ratio of trazodone plasma level to dose increases when fluoxetine is added to therapy, decreasing trazodone levels.
Related Drugs: There are no drugs related to fluoxetine or trazodone.
Mechanism: Fluoxetine may decrease the hepatic metabolism of trazodone, resulting in an increase in plasma levels and adverse reactions.
Detailed Information: See *EDI,* 6/35.00

Venlafaxine-Cimetidine

Significance: 3—minimally clinically significant
Potential Effects: Concurrent use of venlafaxine and cimetidine may result in an inhibition of venlafaxine first-pass metabolism.
Recommendations: The concomitant use of these agents may result in a more pronounced interaction in the elderly and in patients with hepatic impairment or pre-existing hypertension. Therefore, caution is advised with such patients, and dosage adjustments may be necessary.
Summary: Cimetidine may inhibit the first-pass metabolism of venlafaxine.
Related Drugs: It is not known whether an interaction would occur between venlafaxine and other H_2-receptor antagonists. There are no drugs related to venlafaxine.
Mechanism: Cimetidine may inhibit venlafaxine metabolism to its active metabolite, increase the plasma concentrations of venlafaxine and lower the concentrations of the active metabolite.
Detailed Information: See *EDI,* 6/37.00

Chapter Seven

Antihypertensive Drug Interactions

Bethanidine-Mazindol

Significance: 2—moderately clinically significant

Recommendations: The concomitant use of these agents may need to be avoided. If concurrent use is required, blood pressure should be monitored frequently.

Summary: A report has shown that mazindol reversed the antihypertensive effect of bethanidine and caused a loss of bethanidine-induced side effects.

Related Drugs: Other antihypertensives related to bethanidine may interact with mazindol. Other anorexiants that possess indirect-acting sympathomimetic activity may interact with bethanidine (see Guanethidine-Dextroamphetamine, page 163). Phenylpropanolamine has been shown to antagonize the antihypertensive effects of bethanidine.

Mechanism: Anorexiants with indirect-acting sympathomimetic activity may compete with bethanidine for uptake or displace bethanidine from adrenergic neurons.

Detailed Information: See *EDI,* 7/1.00

Captopril-Allopurinol

Significance: 3—minimally clinically significant

Recommendations: Until further clinical studies are done, the concurrent use of these agents need not be avoided. However, these drugs should be prescribed with caution, especially in patients with chronic renal failure. One or both drugs may need to be discontinued.

Summary: The coadministration of allopurinol and captopril have been shown to result in Stevens-Johnson syndrome, pyrexia, arthralgia, and myalgia.

Related Drugs: There are no drugs related to captopril or allopurinol.

Mechanism: Allopurinol and captopril have been associated with skin eruptions of the erythema multiforme type and, in some cases, have led to toxic epidermal necrolysis and Stevens-Johnson syndrome.

Detailed Information: See *EDI,* 7/2.10

Captopril-Aluminum Hydroxide, Magnesium Carbonate, Magnesium Hydroxide

Significance: 3—minimally clinically significant

Potential Effects: The antacid combination may decrease the bioavailability of captopril.

Recommendations: If these agents are used together, their administration should be separated by as much time as possible.

Summary: There are data to show that coadministration of these agents will cause a decrease in captopril concentration and in the bioavailability of captopril.

Related Drugs: A similar interaction may occur between captopril and other antacids because of pharmacologic similarity. It is not known if a similar interaction would occur between the antacid combinations and other ACE inhibitors.

Mechanism: A transient rise in gastric pH caused by the antacid preparation may have increased the ionization of captopril, decreasing membrane penetration.

Detailed Information: See *EDI,* 7/2.30

Captopril-Aspirin

Significance: 2—moderately clinically significant

Recommendations: Patients should be closely monitored for blood pressure changes during concurrent use of these agents. If blood pressure control decreases, discontinuation of the aspirin may be necessary.

Summary: Coadministration of captopril and aspirin showed a decreased antihypertensive.

Related Drugs: There are no drugs related to captopril. A similar interaction is expected to occur between captopril and other salicylates.

Mechanism: Aspirin may interfere with the release of vasodilating prostaglandins enhanced by long-term captopril therapy.

Detailed Information: See *EDI*, 7/3.00

Captopril-Chlorpromazine

Significance: 3—minimally clinically significant

Potential Effects: Concurrent use of these agents may result in hypotension.

Recommendations: If these agents are used together, blood pressure should be closely monitored. One or both agents may need to be discontinued.

Summary: Data have shown that the coadministration of these agents may cause hypotension.

Related Drugs: An interaction may occur between chlorpromazine and other ACE inhibitors and between captopril and other phenothiazines, thioxanthenes, butyrophenones, dihydroindolones, and dibenzoxazepines.

Mechanism: A synergistic effect may have occurred when chlorpromazine and captopril were used concurrently.

Detailed Information: See *EDI*, 7/4.10

Captopril-Furosemide

Significance: 2—moderately clinically significant

Potential Effects: Furosemide may induce severe postural hypotension in patients receiving captopril.

Recommendations: The hypotension is transient. If it occurs, place the patient in a supine position and, if needed, start an IV with normal saline.

Summary: There are data to show that coadministration of these agents may induce severe postural hypotension; however, this hypotensive response is transient.

Related Drugs: Enalapril and furosemide have been shown to potentiate renal problems; however, conflicting data are available. A similar interaction is expected to occur between captopril and other loop diuretics, thiazide diuretics, mercurial diuretics, and thiazide-related diuretics.

Mechanism: Furosemide, as well as other diuretics that cause sodium and water loss, may exaggerate the hypotensive state.

Detailed Information: See *EDI*, 7/5.00

Captopril-Indomethacin

Significance: 2—moderately clinically significant

Potential Effects: Indomethacin may decrease or abolish the antihypertensive effect of captopril.

Recommendations: Blood pressure should be monitored if indomethacin is added to, or withdrawn from, captopril therapy. Indomethacin may need to be discontinued.

Summary: There are data to show that coadministration of indomethacin and captopril has led to a decreased or a total invalidation of the antihypertensive effect of captopril.

Related Drugs: Enalapril was not affected by indomethacin or sulindac; however, conflicting data are available. A similar interaction is expected to occur between captopril and other NSAIAs. An interaction may also be expected to occur between indomethacin and other ACE inhibitors.

Mechanism: Indomethacin, which inhibits endogenous prostaglandin synthesis, may interfere with the release of vasodilating prostaglandins.

Detailed Information: See *EDI*, 7/7.00

Captopril-Naloxone

Significance: 3—minimally clinically significant

Potential Effects: Naloxone may decrease the hypotensive effect of captopril.

Recommendations: Monitor the patient's blood pressure if these agents are used together.

Summary: There are data to show that coadministration of these agents may lead to a decrease in the hypotensive effect of captopril.

Related Drugs: A similar interaction may occur between captopril and naltrexone.

Mechanism: Administration of the opiate antagonist naloxone with captopril would prevent a decrease in baroreflex sensitivity, attenuating the hypotensive response to the captopril.

Detailed Information: See *EDI*, 7/8.10

Captopril-Potassium Chloride

Significance: 3—minimally clinically significant

Potential Effects: The concurrent use of these agents may cause an increase in potassium levels.

Recommendations: Monitor potassium levels when using these agents together. The dose of either agent may need to be reversed or discontinued.

Summary: There are data to show that coadministration of these agents may increase serum potassium; however, no clinical signs or symptoms associated with hyperkalemia were present. There are data indicating that coadministration of these agents caused no change in serum potassium.

Related Drugs: The other ACE inhibitors would also be expected to interact with potassium chloride. Captopril may also be expected to interact with other potassium salts.

Mechanism: Concurrent administration of captopril and a potassium supplement may result in an additive pharmacologic effect, increasing serum potassium concentrations.

Detailed Information: See *EDI*, 7/8.30

Captopril-Probenecid

Significance: 3—minimally clinically significant

Recommendations: Because it is not clear whether a moderate increase in captopril levels will have any significant effect on the antihypertensive action of captopril, the concurrent use of these agents need not be avoided. However, it is prudent to monitor the patient's blood pressure regularly, and a decrease in the dose of captopril may be necessary.

Summary: There are data to show that probenecid reduces the total body clearance and renal clearance of captopril, increasing captopril levels.

Related Drugs: There are no drugs related to captopril. A similar interaction is expected to occur between captopril and sulfinpyrazone.

Mechanism: Probenecid may interfere with tubular secretion of drugs and this may interfere with captopril excretion.

Detailed Information: See *EDI*, 7/9.00

Clonidine-Cyclosporine

Significance: 2–moderately clinically significant

Potential Effects: Concurrent administration of clonidine and cyclosporine may result in elevated levels of cyclosporine. Clonidine may help prevent cyclosporine-induced renal toxicity.

Recommendations: Cyclosporine levels should be monitored in patients maintained on cyclosporine in whom clonidine is initiated or discontinued. Dosage adjustments of cyclosporine may be necessary or clonidine may need to be discontinued.

Summary: Concurrent administration of clonidine and cyclosporine resulted in elevated levels of cyclosporine from 300–927µg/L (therapeutic range: 150–300µg/L) within five days, despite a reduction in cyclosporine dosage. Following the discontinuation of clonidine, cyclosporine levels decreased rapidly to below 200µg/L within two days. In other studies, bone marrow transplant patients and renal allograft recipients also had elevated levels of cyclosporine, but mean serum creatinine levels were significantly lower than in patients who did not receive clonidine.

Related Drugs: There are no agents related to cyclosporine or clonidine.

Mechanism: It is postulated that clonidine inhibits the metabolism of cyclosporine by the cytochrome P450 enzyme system. It is also postulated that clonidine's beneficial effects on kidney function may be the result of a combination of clonidine's inhibition of renin release, reduction in the responsiveness of the kidneys to vasopressin, and reduction of preglomerular vasoconstriction.

Detailed Information: See *EDI*, 7/9.80

Clonidine-Naloxone

Significance: 3—minimally clinically significant

Potential Effects: Patients taking clonidine who are given naloxone may have a diminished antihypertensive effect.

Recommendations: If a loss of antihypertensive control occurs, naloxone may need to be discontinued or another antihypertensive chosen.

Summary: Several studies have shown that the concurrent administration of clonidine and naloxone decreases the antihypertensive effect of clonidine; however, there are conflicting data available.

Related Drugs: Naltrexone has been shown to inhibit the hypotension and bradycardia produced by clonidine. There are no drugs related to clonidine.

Mechanism: This interaction may result from the similarities that may exist between central alpha adrenergic receptors and opiate receptors.

Detailed Information: See *EDI*, 7/10.10

Clonidine-Propranolol

Significance: 1—highly clinically significant

Potential Effects: Abrupt discontinuation of clonidine from cotherapy with propranolol results in severe hypertension and tachycardia.

Recommendations: Propranolol should be discontinued well in advance of clonidine withdrawal. Labetalol may be substituted for propranolol, or it may be used to reverse the resulting hypertension after clonidine withdrawal.

Summary: The rapid discontinuation of clonidine from combined therapy with propranolol may produce severe symptoms of sympathetic activity, rapid blood pressure elevations and a paradoxic hypertension.

Related Drugs: Timolol and metoprolol have been documented to exhibit a similar interaction. It is not known if other beta cardioselective beta blocking agents would interact similarly. Other noncardioselective beta-blocking agents may interact similarly to propranolol.

Mechanism: Propranolol neutralizes the vasodilatory effect of beta$_2$-adrenergic receptors. When clonidine is stopped, neurotransmitters are released and manifest vasoconstriction.

Detailed Information: See *EDI*, 7/11.00

Clonidine-Rifampin

Significance: 4—not clinically significant

Recommendations: Rifampin has not been shown to alter the elimination of clonidine, and no special precautions need to be taken when these two agents are used concomitantly.

Summary: The results of a study involving six normal volunteers indicates that no change occurred in the elimination kinetics of clonidine during rifampin administration.

Related Drugs: There are no drugs related to rifampin or clonidine.

Mechanism: Clonidine is biotransformed by the liver and eliminated unchanged by the kidney. Rifampin does not appear to induce the metabolism of clonidine.

Detailed Information: See *EDI*, 7/13.00

Enalapril-Azathioprine

Significance: 3—minimally clinically significant

Potential Effects: Concurrent use of azathioprine and an ACE inhibitor may result in hematological changes such as anemia, neutropenia, or granulocytopenia.

Recommendations: Patients receiving concurrent azathioprine and an ACE inhibitor should be closely monitored for hematological changes.

Summary: Concurrent use of azathioprine and enalapril resulted in significantly reduced hematocrit and hemoglobin.

Related Drugs: Captopril has been reported to reduce white blood cell counts when combined with azathioprine. Based on the postulated mechanism and pharmacologic similarity, an interaction would be expected to occur between azathioprine and the other ACE inhibitors and between enalapril and the other nitrosourea alkylating agents, although documentation is lacking.

Mechanism: The exact mechanism of this interaction is unknown. The impairment of hematopoiesis by azathioprine may have made any inherent ability of ACE inhibitors to trigger anemia, possibly through decreased or low erythropoietin or hemolysis, clinically significant.

Detailed Information: See *EDI*, 7/14.00

Enalapril-Rifampin

Significance: 3—minimally clinically significant

Potential Effects: Rifampin may increase the clearance of enalapril leading to hypertensive control.

Recommendations: Patients maintained on enalapril should be closely monitored for changes in blood pressure if rifampin cotherapy is instituted. The rifampin may need to be discontinued or the enalapril dose may need to be adjusted.

Summary: Concurrent administration of enalapril and rifampin may result in a decrease in the effects of enalapril.

Related Drugs: It is not known whether an interaction would occur between rifampin and other ACE inhibitors. There are no drugs related to rifampin.

Mechanism: Rifampin may enhance the renal clearance of enalaprilat.

Detailed Information: See *EDI*, 7/14.50

Guanethidine-Alcohol, Ethyl

Significance: 2—moderately clinically significant

Recommendations: Patients prescribed guanethidine should be informed of the following: (1) concurrent alcohol ingestion may increase the incidence of guanethidine-induced orthostatic hypotension, dizziness, and syncope, thus alcohol intake should be limited, if possible; (2) these adverse reactions are most likely to occur during hot weather or while standing for long periods, rising rapidly from a sitting or prone position, or exercising; (3) if such symptoms occur, one should lie, sit, or squat immediately.

Summary: Alcohol may enhance the orthostatic hypotension and syncope caused by guanethidine.

Related Drugs: Other drugs pharmacologically related to guanethidine may interact with alcohol.

Mechanism: Alcohol may inhibit the ability of a patient taking guanethidine to respond to orthostatic changes.

Detailed Information: See *EDI*, 7/15.00

Guanethidine-Chlorpromazine

Significance: 1—highly clinically significant

Recommendations: Because this interaction is clinically significant, patients should not receive chlorpromazine and guanethidine concomitantly, if possible. If concurrent administration is required, patients should be closely monitored for a reversal of the hypotensive effect of guanethidine. The dose of guanethidine may have to be increased to maintain the hypotensive effect. Antihypertensive drugs, such as methyldopa, which do not interact with chlorpromazine may be considered as alternatives to guanethidine. Also, molindone, which does not appear to alter the antihypertensive effect of guanethidine, may be a suitable alternative to chlorpromazine.

Summary: Chlorpromazine may reverse the antihypertensive effects of guanethidine.

Related Drugs: Chlorpromazine may interact with guanethidine to a greater degree than other phenothiazines, thioxanthenes, and dibenzoxazepines. Administration of haloperidol and thiothixene has been shown to cause a significant increase in blood pressure. Molindone does not alter the antihypertensive effects of guanethidine. Bethanidine, debrisoquin, and guanadrel may be expected to interact with chlorpromazine.

Mechanism: Guanethidine exerts its antihypertensive effects by competing with norepinephrine. Chlorpromazine apparently blocks the transport of guanethidine into the neuron.

Detailed Information: See *EDI*, 7/17.00

Guanethidine-Desipramine

Significance: 1—highly clinically significant

Recommendations: The concurrent administration of guanethidine and desipramine or other tricyclic antidepressants should be avoided. If cotherapy is selected, the patient should be closely monitored for one to two weeks, with the expectation that the guanethidine dose may have to be increased. High doses (300mg) of guanethidine have been successful in overcoming the antidepressant antagonism. Antihypertensive agents such as prazosin, atenolol, or other beta blockers may be considered as guanethidine substitutes since they do not interact with desipramine. The antidepressant doxepin (in doses less than 150mg daily) may be substituted for desipramine. However, doxepin in this dosage rarely produces an adequate antidepressant effect.

Summary: The antihypertensive effect of guanethidine has been shown to be antagonized within three to seven days of initiating desipramine therapy.

Related Drugs: Amitriptyline, imipramine, protriptyline, nortriptyline, and doxepin have been shown to inhibit the antihypertensive effects of guanethidine. Cyclobenzaprine may antagonize the antihypertensive effect of guanethidine. Bethanidine and debrisoquin have shown a loss of antihypertensive effect when administered with tricyclic antidepressants. An interaction may occur between desipramine and guanadrel.

Mechanism: Desipramine antagonizes guanethidine's antihypertensive and neuronal blocking effects, and this is dependent upon the concentration of guanethidine.

Detailed Information: See *EDI*, 7/19.00

Guanethidine-Dextroamphetamine

Significance: 2—moderately clinically significant

Recommendations: The reversal of guanethidine's effect by dextroamphetamine, and its resultant effect on blood pressure, suggests that the two drugs should not be administered concurrently. If dextroamphetamine and antihypertensive therapy are indicated for the treatment of a given patient, clonidine, methyldopa, or a beta blocking agent whose effect has not been reported to be antagonized by dextroamphetamine should be considered. In addition, since the effect of guanethidine on blood pressure is known to last for several days after discontinuation, the effects of amphetamines on blood pressure must be monitored even after guanethidine discontinuation because these patients may quickly revert to pretreatment levels of blood pressure. One should also note that this prolonged antihypertensive effect of guanethidine may also enhance the effect of alternative forms of blood pressure control, even after drug therapy has been altered.

Summary: The concurrent use of guanethidine and dextroamphetamine may result in a decrease in the antihypertensive effect of guanethidine.

Related Drugs: Bethanidine, debrisoquin, and guanadrel have shown to decrease antihypertensive effects. Methamphetamine, ephedrine, methylphenidate, and mephentermine have shown a similar effect. Phenylpropanolamine has antagonized the effects of bethanidine. The interaction of other direct and mixed acting sympathomimetics with guanethidine are discussed in another monograph (see Guanethidine-Phenylephrine, page 164).

Mechanism: The antihypertensive effect of guanethidine is the result of its ability to block the release of norepinephrine.

Detailed Information: See *EDI*, 7/21.00

Guanethidine-Hydrochlorothiazide

Significance: 2—moderately clinically significant

Recommendations: The addition of hydrochlorothiazide to long-term guanethidine therapy may result in the need to reduce the dose of guanethidine. The thiazide diuretic will enhance the antihypertensive effect of guanethidine. Patients should be informed of the possible occurrence of dizziness or syncope from the enhanced antihypertensive effect of the combination therapy.

Summary: Concurrent hydrochlorothiazide and guanethidine therapy reduces sodium and water retention and increases blood volume, necessitating a decrease in guanethidine.

Related Drugs: Other diuretics that possess antihypertensive properties may be expected to undergo a similar interaction with guanethidine. Bethanidine, debrisoquin, and guanadrel may be expected to interact with hydrochlorothiazide.

Mechanism: The thiazides appear to cause fluid and sodium depletion, and long-term use of guanethidine results in a progressive resistance to its antihypertensive effect because of increasing sodium retention and edema formation.

Detailed Information: See *EDI*, 7/23.00

Guanethidine-Minoxidil

Significance: 2—moderately clinically significant

Recommendations: It is recommended that guanethidine be discontinued at least one week before initiation of minoxidil, if possible. If not possible, it is suggested that minoxidil therapy be started in a hospital setting and that the patient remain in the hospital until the severe orthostatic effects dissipate or until the patient learns how to avoid activities that produce these effects.

Summary: The coadministration of guanethidine and minoxidil may result in profound orthostatic hypotension.

Related Drugs: Bethanidine, debrisoquin, and guanadrel may be expected to produce a similar hypotensive episode with minoxidil. There are no drugs related to minoxidil.

Mechanism: Guanethidine is known to cause orthostatic hypotension, and minoxidil may accentuate this effect.

Detailed Information: See *EDI,* 7/25.00

Guanethidine-Phenelzine

Significance: 2—moderately clinically significant

Recommendations: To avoid any risk in compromise of blood pressure control, MAO inhibitors should not be added to any antihypertensive regimen including guanethidine. Careful monitoring of blood pressure is required if this combination cannot be avoided.

Summary: Addition of a MAOI to guanethidine may result in a compromise in the antihypertensive effectiveness of guanethidine.

Related Drugs: Other MAOIs may be expected to interact similarly with guanethidine. Bethanidine, debrisoquin, and guanadrel may interact in the same manner.

Mechanism: MAOIs antagonize guanethidine's hypotensive effect by interfering with catecholamine depletion.

Detailed Information: See *EDI,* 7/27.00

Guanethidine-Phenylephrine

Significance: 2—moderately clinically significant

Recommendations: A compromise in blood pressure control may occur when direct or mixed-acting sympathomimetic agents are used by patients who are receiving or have recently received guanethidine. The concurrent use of these agents should be avoided.

Summary: Direct and mixed acting sympathomimetics may antagonize the hypotensive effects of patients pretreated with guanethidine, resulting in hypertension.

Related Drugs: Bethanidine, debrisoquin, and guanadrel may show potential to interact in the same manner. Other sympathomimetics may show an effect similar to phenylephrine's. Interactions between indirect-acting sympathomimetics and guanethidine are discussed in another monograph (see Guanethidine-Dextroamphetamine, page 163).

Mechanism: Guanethidine blocks the release of norepinephrine, causing a supersensitivity, and this may be related to guanethidine indirectly interfering with neuron amine uptake and/or a sensitizing action of the drug.

Detailed Information: See *EDI,* 7/29.00

Guanfacine-Phenobarbital

Significance: 3—minimally clinically significant

Potential Effects: Phenobarbital induces the metabolism of guanfacine leading to decreased blood pressure control.

Recommendations: Monitor blood pressure closely if phenobarbital is added to, or discontinued from, a guanfacine regimen. The guanfacine dose may need to be adjusted.

Summary: The antihypertensive effect of guanfacine may be decreased by the addition of phenobarbital.

Related Drugs: A similar interaction is expected to occur between guanfacine and other barbiturates. There are no drugs related to guanfacine.

Mechanism: Enzyme induction of guanfacine metabolism by phenobarbital may be the cause of this interaction.

Detailed Information: See *EDI*, 7/30.05

Hydralazine-Indomethacin

Significance: 3—minimally clinically significant

Potential Effects: The hypotensive effect of hydralazine may be blocked or decreased by indomethacin.

Recommendations: Monitor the patient's blood pressure when using these agents together.

Summary: There are data to show that administration of indomethacin may block or decrease the hypotensive effect of hydralazine; however, conflicting data are available.

Related Drugs: Diclofenac was shown to diminish the antihypertensive effect of hydralazine. It is not known if a similar interaction would occur between hydralazine and other NSAIAs. There are no drugs related to hydralazine.

Mechanism: Indomethacin, by inhibiting prostaglandin synthesis, may attenuate the hypotensive response to hydralazine.

Detailed Information: See *EDI*, 7/30.10

Methyldopa-Amitriptyline

Significance: 3—minimally clinically significant

Recommendations: Based on the information available, it would seem that an interaction between methyldopa and amitriptyline is unlikely to occur in most patients; however, it is prudent to monitor blood pressure if tricyclic antidepressants are added to methyldopa therapy. An interaction between clonidine and desipramine is more firmly established and appears to occur regularly, although it can be overcome by increasing the dose of clonidine. Patients who receive tricyclic antidepressants in combination with clonidine should have their blood pressure closely monitored during the first several days of combined therapy. Alternatively, the tetracyclic antidepressant maprotiline may be substituted for the tricyclic antidepressant if clonidine therapy is chosen.

Summary: Loss of blood pressure control occurred when amitriptyline was added to a methyldopa regimen.

Related Drugs: Methyldopa was reported not to interact with desipramine. Clonidine has been reported to interact with tricyclic antidepressants. Imipramine has been reported to antagonize the antihypertensive effects of clonidine. Guanabenz may interact similarly with other tricyclic antidepressants. Mianserin was shown to have no interaction with the antihypertensive action of clonidine or methyldopa.

Mechanism: Methyldopa and clonidine depend on central alpha-adrenergic stimulation, and the tricyclic antidepressants could directly antagonize their effect.

Detailed Information: See *EDI*, 7/31.00

Methyldopa-Ferrous Sulfate

Significance: 2—moderately clinically significant

Potential Effects: Concurrent use of these agents may decrease the hypertensive effects of methyldopa.

Recommendations: Patients should be monitored closely if ferrous sulfate is added to, or withdrawn from, concomitant therapy with methyldopa. The dose of methyldopa may need to be adjusted.

Summary: Ferrous sulfate may decrease the absorption of methyldopa, decreasing its hypertensive effects.

Related Drugs: Ferrous gluconate has been shown to decrease excretion and absorption of methyldopa. Ferrous fumarate would be expected to interact in a similar manner. There are no drugs related to methyldopa.

Mechanism: The decrease in excretion of methyldopa is due to a reduction in methyldopa absorption and an increase in methyldopa sulfation, and the decrease in absorption may result from chelation of methyldopa.

Detailed Information: See *EDI,* 7/32.50

Methyldopa-Haloperidol

Significance: 3—minimally clinically significant

Recommendations: Reports suggest that the concurrent use of these agents can lead to abnormal central nervous system symptoms. Although the incidence may be low, it is important to be aware of this possible interaction. Should central nervous system symptoms occur, discontinuation of haloperidol should resolve the reaction.

Summary: Data have shown that dementia has occurred after haloperidol was added to an existing methyldopa regimen.

Related Drugs: A similar interaction is expected to occur with the phenothiazines, thioxanthenes, dihydroindolones and dibenzoxazepines. There are no drugs related to methyldopa.

Mechanism: This interaction results from an additive inhibition of dopamine in the central nervous system.

Detailed Information: See *EDI,* 7/33.00

Methyldopa-Levodopa

Significance: 3—minimally clinically significant

Recommendations: Although several reports indicate that concurrent use of levodopa and methyldopa may produce a beneficial effect on the symptoms of parkinsonism without increasing the risk of adverse drug reactions, the possibility that this combination influences the therapeutic response to levodopa in certain patients should be considered. The occurrence of side effects such as vomiting and drowsiness induced by either drug may require a dose reduction or discontinuation of methyldopa.

Summary: Coadministration of levodopa and methyldopa can result in increased therapeutic effectiveness of either drug or adverse effects, depending on dose of either drug used.

Related Drugs: There are no drugs related to levodopa or methyldopa.

Mechanism: This interaction may be due to additive or synergistic hypotensive effects.

Detailed Information: See *EDI,* 7/35.00

Methyldopa-Norepinephrine

Significance: 2—moderately clinically significant

Recommendations: It is important to be aware of a possible inter-action between methyldopa and norepinephrine or other sympa-thomimetics (direct, indirect, and mixed acting), which may lead to hypertension. Phentolamine or another alpha-adrenergic blocking agent may be useful if hypertension does occur. It may also be necessary to discontinue the sympathomimetic amine. The norepinephrine dose should initially be reduced when used concurrently with methyldopa, and one study suggests beginning with one-tenth the usual dose.

Summary: The pressor effect of norepinephrine was found to increase and to be prolonged with the concurrent administration of methyldopa. A possible hypertensive episode may result.

Related Drugs: Other direct-acting sympathomimetics may interact similarly with methyldopa. The pressor effect of tyramine was found to be increased when coadministered with methyldopa. Phenylpropanolamine was reported to cause a severe hyperten-sive reaction. A similar interaction is expected to occur between methyldopa and other mixed and indirect-acting sympath-omimetics.

Mechanism: There may be an additive effect between the false transmitter and normal transmitter at the same alpha receptor sites, or methyldopa's metabolites may facilitate the access to alpha-adrenergic receptor sites.

Detailed Information: See *EDI*, 7/37.00

Methyldopa-Phenobarbital

Significance: 4—not clinically significant

Recommendations: The clinical significance of the potential inter-action between methyldopa and phenobarbital has not been substantiated. Therefore, it appears that no dosage adjustments or additional precautions are necessary when these two agents are administered concurrently.

Summary: Barbiturate therapy could result in lowered methyldopa blood levels.

Related Drugs: Other barbiturates may act in a similar manner with phenobarbital. There are no drugs related to methyldopa.

Mechanism: Phenobarbital may increase methyldopa metabolism, resulting in decreased serum methyldopa levels.

Detailed Information: See *EDI*, 7/39.00

Methyldopa-Phenoxybenzamine

Significance: 3—minimally clinically significant

Potential Effects: Use of these agents together may cause urinary incontinence, especially in patients who undergo a bilateral lum-bar sympathectomy.

Recommendations: If urinary incontinence occurs, phenoxybenza-mine may need to be discontinued.

Summary: There are data to show that coadministration of these agents may cause urinary incontinence.

Related Drugs: A similar interaction is expected to occur with the other nonspecific alpha-adrenergic blocking agents. Phen-tolamine may produce a similar interaction with methyldopa. There are no drugs related to methyldopa.

Mechanism: Methyldopa and phenoxybenzamine may decrease alpha-adrenergic stimulation of the bladder, increasing cholinergic activity and leading to the relaxation of the trigone and contraction of the detrusor.

Detailed Information: See *EDI*, 7/40.10

Methyldopa-Propranolol

Significance: 2—moderately clinically significant

Recommendations: These interactions are potentially serious. It would seem prudent to consider the possibility of this interaction in patients taking methyldopa and beta-adrenergic blocking agents, especially when a drug or clinical situation may cause an increased release of the neurotransmitter.

Summary: There are data to show that coadministration of methyldopa and propranolol leads to increased blood pressure.

Related Drugs: Other nonselective beta blocking agents may interact in a similar manner with methyldopa.

Mechanism: Beta-blocking agents, when administered concurrently, would block the beta receptor activity, allowing the alpha receptor activity to occur unopposed, resulting in hypertension.

Detailed Information: See *EDI*, 7/41.00

Nitroprusside-Captopril

Significance: 3—minimally clinically significant

Recommendations: Patients who are receiving captopril for control of hypertension and who require nitroprusside for acute lowering of blood pressure should be closely monitored to prevent extreme hypotension.

Summary: The concurrent administration of captopril with nitroprusside can reduce the dosage requirement for nitroprusside while maintaining adequate hypotensive control.

Related Drugs: A similar interaction may occur between nitroprusside and other ACE inhibitors. There are no drugs related to nitroprusside.

Mechanism: The concurrent use of these two drugs can diminish the body's compensatory mechanism to nitroprusside-induced hypotension and reduce the dose of nitroprusside required.

Detailed Information: See *EDI*, 7/42.10

Prazosin-Indomethacin

Significance: 2—moderately clinically significant

Recommendations: Patients' blood pressure should be closely monitored during concurrent use of these agents. An increased prazosin dose may be necessary.

Summary: The concurrent use of prazosin and indomethacin may reduce the hypotensive effect of prazosin.

Related Drugs: There are no drugs related to prazosin. A similar interaction is expected to occur with other NSAIAs and prazosin, if the mechanism involves prostaglandin inhibition.

Mechanism: Indomethacin prevents the rise in plasma renin activity that is seen following the administration of prazosin.

Detailed Information: See *EDI*, 7/43.00

Prazosin-Propranolol

Significance: 2—moderately clinically significant

Recommendations: Patients should be advised of the increased risk involved with the first dose of prazosin, especially when it is added to a beta-blocking agent. Initiation of prazosin treatment with a dose of 0.5mg or less has been suggested.

Summary: The concurrent use of prazosin and propranolol may enhance the acute postural hypotensive reaction.

Related Drugs: Prazosin and alprenolol exhibited a similar interaction. A similar interaction is expected to occur between prazosin and other beta-blocking agents. There are no drugs related to prazosin.

Mechanism: The compensatory responses of the heart, after the first dose of prazosin, is blocked by the beta-blockade produced by propranolol.

Detailed Information: See *EDI,* 7/45.00

Prazosin-Verapamil

Significance: 3—minimally clinically significant

Recommendations: Patients should be monitored for a rapid decrease in blood pressure if the agents are used concurrently. A decreased prazosin dose may be necessary.

Summary: The concurrent administration of verapamil and prazosin have been shown to decrease systolic and diastolic blood pressures.

Related Drugs: Prazosin and nifedipine resulted in an acute hypotensive response; however, conflicting data are available. A similar interaction may occur between prazosin and other calcium channel blockers. There are no drugs related to prazosin.

Mechanism: This greater hypotensive activity may be due in part to a pharmacokinetic interaction that enhances the bioavailability of prazosin. A pharmacodynamic interaction at the level of vascular smooth muscle or compensatory cardiac activity may also play a role.

Detailed Information: See *EDI,* 7/46.10

Reserpine-Ephedrine

Significance: 2—moderately clinically significant

Recommendations: Patients receiving reserpine who are not responsive to therapeutic doses of ephedrine should be switched to a direct acting sympathomimetic agent such as norepinephrine or phenylephrine. The direct acting adrenergic agents will bypass the vesicle depletion action of reserpine and initiate the desired hypertensive action. Should norepinephrine be used, the added reuptake action of this agent will partially restore normal catecholamine activity. Smaller doses of direct acting sympathomimetics may be sufficient since the vasculature in reserpine treated patients is often more sensitive to these drugs.

Summary: The indirect sympathomimetic action of ephedrine may be antagonized as a result of depletion of norepinephrine from adrenergic vesicles by reserpine.

Related Drugs: Amphetamine, methylphenidate, tyramine, and phenylpropanolamine may interact with reserpine. Other rauwolfia alkaloids may interact with ephedrine.

Mechanism: When reserpine is given before ephedrine, it may antagonize the indirect action of ephedrine, resulting in a decreased cardiovascular response to this sympathomimetic.

Detailed Information: See *EDI,* 7/47.00

Reserpine-Halothane

Significance: 3—minimally clinically significant

Recommendations: Clinical evidence indicates that long-term reserpine therapy is not a contraindication to anesthesia and surgery. However, patients on reserpine therapy should be observed for any unexpected hypotensive episodes during administration of halothane, particularly when there is associated blood loss, excessive speed of induction of anesthesia, surgical manipulation, position change, or excessive amount of anesthetic agents used. If reserpine is not withdrawn before surgery and if hypotension does occur, an exacerbated effect may be noticed since the endogenous catecholamines have already been chronically depleted by reserpine. Therefore, the use of an indirect-acting sympathomimetic agent would be ineffective, and a direct-acting sympathomimetic agent would be required to treat the hypotension.

Summary: Several studies have suggested that administration of halothane in patients receiving reserpine may be tolerated without increased risk of hypotension; however, conflicting data are available.

Related Drugs: Other anesthetic agents may interact similarly with reserpine. Other rauwolfia alkaloids may interact with halothane and other general anesthetics.

Mechanism: Halothane adds to the catecholamine depleting action of reserpine, causing enhanced depressant effects on the heart and resulting in decreased cardiac output and hypotension.

Detailed Information: See *EDI,* 7/49.00

Sodium Nitroprusside-Esmolol

Significance: 3—minimally clinically significant

Potential Effects: Esmolol may potentiate sodium nitroprusside hypotension.

Recommendations: Monitor patients for excessive hypotension during concurrent use of these agents.

Summary: The hypotensive action of sodium nitroprusside is potentiated when esmolol is given concurrently.

Related Drugs: No documentation exists regarding an interaction between sodium nitroprusside and other cardioselective beta-blocking agents or the noncardioselective beta-blocking agents. There are no drugs related to sodium nitroprusside.

Mechanism: The activation of the renin-angiotensin system and the production of angiotensin II is thought to be the cause of resistance to the effects of sodium nitroprusside.

Detailed Information: See *EDI,* 7/51.00

Spironolactone-Cholestyramine

Significance: 2—moderately clinically significant

Potential Effects: Concurrent spironolactone and cholestyramine may result in metabolic acidosis and hyperkalemia.

Recommendations: Concurrent cholestyramine and spironolactone should be approached with caution. Patients receiving concurrent therapy should be monitored for potential acidosis and hyperkalemia. Either cholestyramine or spironolactone may need to be discontinued.

Summary: Concurrent spironolactone and cholestyramine may have resulted in metabolic acidosis and hyperkalemia in patients with pre-existing hepatic dysfunction.

Related Drugs: Although documentation is lacking, based on the proposed mechanism a similar reaction would be expected to occur between spironolactone and the other anion exchange resin and between cholestyramine and the other potassium sparing diuretics.

Mechanism: Bicarbonate has been shown to bind to cholestyramine, an anionic exchange resin. It is postulated that cholestyramine may have exchanged chloride for bicarbonate and concurrent spironolactone may have prevented the kidneys from adequately acidifying the urine and correcting the excess chloride and loss of bicarbonate.

Detailed Information: See *EDI,* 7/52.00

Chapter Eight

Anti-infective
Drug Interactions

Acyclovir-Probenecid

Significance: 3—minimally clinically significant

Recommendations: Until further information concerning this inter-action is available, the clinical significance is difficult to assess. However, when acyclovir is used parenterally with probenecid, the resulting reduced elimination of acyclovir should be consid-ered and any necessary dosage adjustments made.

Summary: The administration of probenecid caused a decrease in the elimination rate of acyclovir.

Related Drugs: A similar interaction may occur between acyclovir and sulfinpyrazone. There are no drugs related to acyclovir.

Mechanism: Acyclovir is eliminated by urinary excretion, by glomerular filtration and tubular secretion. Probenecid blocks the tubular secretion of acyclovir.

Detailed Information: See *EDI*, 8/1.00

Ampicillin-Allopurinol

Significance: 3—minimally clinically significant

Recommendations: The concurrent use of these agents need not be avoided; however, one or both drugs may have to be discon-tinued if a rash develops.

Summary: The concurrent use of allopurinol and ampicillin may result in an increased incidence of drug-induced skin rash.

Related Drugs: Similar results were reported in patients receiving both allopurinol and amoxicillin. A similar interaction may occur between bacampicillin and hetacillin. There are no drugs related to allopurinol.

Mechanism: It is not known if the increased rash incidence is the result of a drug-drug interaction or an ampicillin-hyperuricemia interaction.

Detailed Information: See *EDI*, 8/3.00

Ampicillin-Oral Contraceptive Agents

Significance: 2—moderately clinically significant

Potential Effects: Ampicillin may decrease the effect of the oral con-traceptive agents.

Recommendations: The concomitant use of oral contraceptive agents and ampicillin need not be avoided. However, the poten-tial for reduced efficacy of the oral contraceptive should be a consideration in patients receiving both drugs.

Summary: Ampicillin may cause a loss of contraceptive protection.

Related Drugs: Oral contraceptive failures have been further report-ed for amoxicillin, penicillin G, and oxacillin. A similar interaction is expected to occur with other penicillins.

Mechanism: Antibiotics destroy gut flora and prevent steroid reab-sorption, resulting in lower than normal concentrations.

Detailed Information: See *EDI*, 8/5.00

Bacampicillin–N-Acetylcysteine

Significance: 3—minimally clinically significant

Potential Effects: Bacampicillin may decrease the absorption of N-acetylcysteine (NAC), resulting in decreased levels.

Recommendations: Patients being administered oral NAC should be monitored for decreased plasma levels of NAC if bacampicillin is added to the regimen, and the dosage should be adjusted as necessary. Erythromycin has been shown not to interact significantly with NAC.

Summary: Administration of bacampicillin resulted in a decrease in the NAC peak concentration.

Related Drugs: A similar interaction may occur between NAC and other penicillins. There are no drugs related to NAC.

Mechanism: Absorption of bacampicillin is dose-dependent. A capacity-limited transport system exists in the intestine for the aminopenicillins and NAC may be expected to utilize the same transport system.

Detailed Information: See *EDI,* 8/6.50

Cefoperazone-Alcohol, Ethyl

Significance: 2—moderately clinically significant

Potential Effects: A disulfiram-like reaction may occur when alcohol is ingested while a patient is receiving cefoperazone.

Recommendations: Patients receiving cefoperazone or other cephalosporins with a methyltetrazolethiol side chain should avoid ingesting products containing alcohol.

Summary: A disulfiram-like reaction including symptoms like flushing, tachycardia, bronchospasm, sweating, nausea, and vomiting may occur in patients ingesting alcohol and receiving cefoperazone.

Related Drugs: Moxalactam, cefamandole and cefotetan have exhibited this reaction. Cefoperazone, cefonicid and ceforanide may exhibit an interaction with alcohol. An interaction would not be expected to occur between alcohol and other cephalosporins that do not have the methyltetrazolethiol side chain.

Mechanism: Disulfiram-like reactions are caused when there is interference with acetaldehyde dehydrogenase activity and acetaldehyde subsequently accumulates.

Detailed Information: See *EDI,* 8/7.00

Cefotaxime-Cimetidine

Significance: 3—minimally clinically significant

Potential Effects: Concurrent bolus administration of cimetidine and cefotaxime has been reported to result in tachycardia.

Recommendations: If a bolus of cimetidine is given with cefotaxime, the patient should be monitored for tachycardia. The use of continuous infusion of cimetidine may circumvent the tachycardia.

Summary: There are data to show that coadministration of cimetidine and cefotaxime results in tachycardia.

Related Drugs: It is not known if a similar interaction would occur between cimetidine and other cephalosporins or between cefotaxime and other H_2-receptor antagonists.

Mechanism: The mechanism of this interaction is not known.

Detailed Information: See *EDI,* 8/8.10

Cephaloridine-Furosemide

Significance: 2—moderately clinically significant

Recommendations: Concurrent use of furosemide and cephaloridine should be avoided in patients with even mild pre-existing renal disease or impaired renal function, the elderly, and those receiving other nephrotoxic drugs. Use of a less nephrotoxic cephalosporin may be preferable if this combination is required, and renal function should be monitored regularly.

Summary: Cephaloridine nephrotoxicity may be enhanced by concurrent furosemide administration, but reports are complicated.

Related Drugs: Cephacetrile and cephalothin have exhibited a similar interaction. There is no documentation regarding a similar interaction with bumetanide. No other reports have appeared involving an interaction between cephaloridine and the thiazide diuretics or the thiazide-related diuretics.

Mechanism: An additive stimulation of renin release by both agents may lead to acute renal failure. Furosemide inhibits water reabsorption, leading to a higher concentration of cephaloridine. Natriuresis may lead to higher concentrations of cephaloridine.

Detailed Information: See *EDI,* 8/9.00

Cephalothin-Colistimethate

Significance: 2—moderately clinically significant

Recommendations: Renal function should be closely monitored if these drugs are used together or sequentially. It has been recommended that the colistimethate dosage be determined according to kidney function rather than body weight.

Summary: Concurrent use of cephalothin and colistimethate have been associated with an increased risk of nephrotoxicity.

Related Drugs: Other cephalosporins may interact in a similar manner with colistimethate or other polypeptide antibiotics.

Mechanism: Cephalothin may interfere with the renal excretion of colistimethate.

Detailed Information: See *EDI,* 8/11.00

Cephalothin-Probenecid

Significance: 2—moderately clinically significant

Potential Effects: Administration of probenecid and a cephalosporin may result in higher and prolonged serum cephalosporin concentrations with a resultant increase in potential nephrotoxicity.

Recommendations: Concurrent use of a cephalosporin and probenecid will increase and prolong the serum levels of the cephalosporin. Conversely, probenecid has been shown to decrease the half-life of ceftriaxone. These elevated serum levels may increase the potential nephrotoxicity of the cephalosporin, and the dosage may need to be reduced.

Summary: Concurrent administration of probenecid and a cephalosporin results in higher and prolonged serum cephalosporin concentrations.

Related Drugs: There are many cephalasporins that have been documented to interact similarly with probenecid.

Mechanism: Probenecid may compete with the antibiotic for active renal secretion by the proximal tubule. The volume of distribution of the cephalosporin may be restricted by probenecid.

Detailed Information: See *EDI,* 8/13.00

Chloramphenicol-Acetaminophen

Significance: 3—minimally clinically significant

Potential Effects: Acetaminophen may increase the clearance of chloramphenicol. In the presence of malnutrition, the net effect may be a decrease in chloramphenicol.

Recommendations: Because of conflicting results, it is not possible to recommend avoiding the concurrent administration of acetaminophen and chloramphenicol. However, it is prudent to be aware of a possible interaction between these agents. Patients should be closely monitored since a dosage adjustment of either agent may be necessary.

Summary: Acetaminophen may increase the clearance of chloramphenicol; however, there are conflicting data available.

Related Drugs: There are no drugs related to chloramphenicol or acetaminophen.

Mechanism: Acetaminophen and chloramphenicol may compete for metabolism, resulting in a decreased clearance of chloramphenicol. The increased clearance of chloramphenicol may be a result of increased glucuronidation of chloramphenicol.

Detailed Information: See *EDI,* 8/14.10

Chloramphenicol-Phenobarbital

Significance: 3—minimally clinically significant

Recommendations: It will be necessary to carefully monitor patients who receive these agents concomitantly. Chloramphenicol dosage may need to be significantly increased within a few days of initiating combined therapy. The possible rise in phenobarbital concentrations may cause sedation or other toxic symptoms, thereby necessitating a decreased phenobarbital dosage.

Summary: Concurrent administration of these agents has resulted in decreased chloramphenicol serum concentrations in infants and children.

Related Drugs: A similar interaction is expected to occur between chloramphenicol and other barbiturates.

Mechanism: Chloramphenicol may inhibit phenobarbital metabolism.

Detailed Information: See *EDI,* 8/15.00

Chloramphenicol-Rifampin

Significance: 2—moderately clinically significant

Recommendations: Since there is a risk that serum concentrations of chloramphenicol will be reduced to subtherapeutic levels when rifampin is administered concomitantly, it appears prudent to monitor these concentrations when rifampin is added to chloramphenicol therapy, and consideration may be given to increasing the dose of chloramphenicol.

Summary: This interaction may lead to a decrease in the effectiveness of chloramphenicol.

Related Drugs: There are no drugs related to chloramphenicol or rifampin.

Mechanism: Rifampin can increase the rate of glucuronide, and chloramphenicol is metabolized by glucuronide conjugation.

Detailed Information: See *EDI,* 8/16.01

Chloroquine-Cimetidine

Significance: 3—minimally clinically significant

Potential Effects: Cimetidine may inhibit the metabolism of chloroquine, resulting in increased levels.

Recommendations: Concurrent use of these agents should be done with caution. Ranitidine, or possibly famotidine, may be an alternative to cimetidine.

Summary: There are data to show that administration of cimetidine may inhibit the metabolism of chloroquine, resulting in increased levels.

Related Drugs: Ranitidine did not significantly alter chloroquine pharmacokinetics. An interaction may occur between cimetidine and other aminoquinolines.

Mechanism: Cimetidine may inhibit the hepatic mixed-function oxidases responsible for chloroquine's metabolism.

Detailed Information: See *EDI,* 8/16.03

Chloroquine-Cyclosporine

Significance: 2—moderately clinically significant

Potential Effects: Concurrent administration of cyclosporine and chloroquine may result in an increase in cyclosporine levels and serum creatinine.

Recommendations: Cyclosporine levels and serum creatinine should be monitored in patients receiving cyclosporine when chloroquine is initiated or discontinued. The dose of cyclosporine may need to be significantly lowered.

Summary: In two case reports, concurrent administration of cyclosporine and chloroquine resulted in an increase in cyclosporine levels and serum creatinine.

Related Drugs: It is not known if there is an interaction between chloroquine and tacrolimus. Although documentation is lacking, based on the proposed mechanism a similar interaction would be expected to occur between cyclosporine and hydroxychloroquine or primaquine.

Mechanism: One set of authors proposed that chloroquine may have increased cyclosporine levels by interfering with cyclosporine metabolism either by direct action at the cytochrome P450 site or by decreasing enzyme release from lysosomes.

Detailed Information: See *EDI,* 8/16.07

Chloroquine-Kaolin

Significance: 3—minimally clinically significant

Recommendations: Simultaneous administration of these agents should be avoided. It may be best to separate the administration of these drugs by at least four hours to reduce the possibility of an interaction. The dose of chloroquine may need to be increased.

Summary: There are data to show that administration of kaolin can result in a decrease in the chloroquine area-under-curve and in chloroquine plasma level and absorption.

Related Drugs: It is not known if a similar interaction would occur between kaolin and other aminoquinolines. There are no drugs related to kaolin; however, it is possible that other aluminum salts may interact similarly with chloroquine.

Mechanism: The gastrointestinal absorption of chloroquine may decrease because of the adsorption of chloroquine onto the surface of kaolin.

Detailed Information: See *EDI*, 8/16.10

Chloroquine-Levothyroxine

Significance: 3—minimally clinically significant

Potential Effects: The addition of chloroquine to a stable levothyroxine regimen may result in an increase in the thyroid stimulating hormone (TSH) concentration.

Recommendations: TSH levels should be monitored if chloroquine is added to or discontinued from the therapy of a patient maintained on levothyroxine. The dose of levothyroxine may need to be adjusted.

Summary: The addition of chloroquine to a stable levothyroxine regimen may have resulted in an increase in the TSH, which returned to normal one week after discontinuation of the chloroquine. Upon rechallenge, TSH levels increased from 3.2 to 26mU/L and, after two months, reached 54.7mU/L. Free tri-iodothyronine concentrations also increased. Four weeks after completing therapy, levels of TSH and free tri-iodothyronine returned to normal ranges.

Related Drugs: It is not known whether a similar interaction would occur between chloroquine and dextrothyroxine or between levothyroxine and hydroxychloroquine or primaquine.

Mechanism: The mechanism of this interaction is not known. However, it is postulated that chloroquine increases the catabolism of thyroid hormones by enzymatic induction.

Detailed Information: See *EDI*, 8/16.20

Ciprofloxacin-Aluminum Hydroxide, Magnesium Hydroxide

Significance: 2—moderately clinically significant

Potential Effects: Concurrent use of ciprofloxacin and aluminum hydroxide/magnesium hydroxide may result in decreased absorption of ciprofloxacin, leading to a decrease in serum levels.

Recommendations: Patients receiving these agents concomitantly should be monitored for decreased ciprofloxacin levels and/or efficacy. The dose of ciprofloxacin may need to be increased or an alternative antacid may need to be considered.

Summary: The concurrent administration of ciprofloxacin and a combination antacid containing aluminum hydroxide and magnesium hydroxide resulted in a decrease in plasma ciprofloxacin levels by as much as 94%.

Related Drugs: Calcium carbonate antacid has shown both no effect and a decrease in ciprofloxacin area-under-curve and bioavailability. Dairy products also may cause a significant decrease in ciprofloxacin bioavailability. A similar interaction was noted with lomefloxacin and aluminum/magnesium hydroxide. Single doses of bismuth subsalicylate did not significantly alter ciprofloxacin absorption. Because of conflicting results, it is difficult to determine if an interaction would occur between ciprofloxacin and the other antacids; however, a similar interaction may be expected to occur with those antacids that contain aluminum or magnesium ions. A decrease of 73% in serum ofloxacin levels has been seen with aluminum hydroxide/magnesium hydroxide use, and the antacid combination has reportedly decreased the antibiotic efficacy of norfloxacin. Enoxacin bioavailability was decreased by 49–73% when magnesium/aluminum hydroxide was given 0.5–2 hours prior to administration of the antibiotic. The bioavailability of enoxacin was not affected when the antacid was given eight hours before or two hours after enoxacin administration. A similar interaction has been described with pefloxacin. The concurrent administration of levofloxacin and aluminum hydroxide, rufloxacin and magnesium/aluminum hydroxides, and fleroxacin with calcium-rich foods have all demonstrated similar interactions. Since the fluoroquinolones have been modified chemically to a great extent compared to the other quinolones, cinoxacin and nalidixic acid, it is difficult to determine if an interaction would occur with these two agents.

Mechanism: Reduced levels of ciprofloxacin may result from reduced gastrointestinal absorption probably related to the formation of inactive chelate complexes between ciprofloxacin and the aluminum and magnesium ions. In one report, supplementation of agar media for testing quinolone sensitivities with magnesium sulfate results in the production of smaller inhibition zone diameters as compared to agar that has not been supplemented with magnesium sulfate. Fewer effects or no effects were noted with agar supplemented with zinc sulfate or calcium nitrate.

Detailed Information: See *EDI,* 8/16.30

Ciprofloxacin-Cyclosporine

Significance: 2—moderately clinically significant

Potential Effects: Ciprofloxacin may increase cyclosporine levels, resulting in nephrotoxicity.

Recommendations: Patients maintained on cyclosporine should be monitored for increased cyclosporine levels and for signs of nephrotoxicity when ciprofloxacin is added to therapy.

Summary: There are data to show that administration of ciprofloxacin may increase cyclosporine levels resulting in nephrotoxicity.

Related Drugs: Norfloxacin was shown to exhibit a similar interaction. It is not known if an interaction would occur between cyclosporine and other quinolone antibacterials. There are no drugs related to cyclosporine.

Mechanism: There may be a synergistic nephrotoxicity between ciprofloxacin and cyclosporine.

Detailed Information: See *EDI,* 8/16.45

Ciprofloxacin-Ferrous Sulfate

Significance: 2—moderately clinically significant

Potential Effects: Ferrous sulfate has been shown to decrease ciprofloxacin peak concentrations and area under curve.

Recommendations: The concurrent use of ciprofloxacin and ferrous sulfate should be avoided. This is prudent since decreased ciprofloxacin absorption occurs even with separation of administration of these agents.

Summary: Concurrent ciprofloxacin and ferrous sulfate resulted in a decrease in the ciprofloxacin peak serum concentration.

Related Drugs: Multiple vitamin and/or mineral preparations have shown similar changes in ciprofloxacin concentrations. Ferrous sulfate and zinc sulfate have been shown to reduce excretion of norfloxacin. A similar interaction may occur between the ferrous salts and other fluoroquinolone anti-infective agents. It is difficult to determine if an interaction would occur with cinoxacin or nalidixic acid.

Mechanism: A ciprofloxacin-Fe+3 complex formation has been demonstrated *in vitro* in pH conditions similar to the small bowel.

Detailed Information: See *EDI*, 8/16.48

Ciprofloxacin-Nutritional Supplements

Significance: 3—minimally clinically significant

Potential Effects: Concurrent administration of ciprofloxacin and nutritional supplement products may result in changes in ciprofloxacin pharmacokinetics.

Recommendations: Further studies are needed to determine the potential for clinical significance of this interaction. Until that time, it is recommended that patients receiving concurrent therapy with fluoroquinolones and nutritional supplements be closely monitored for efficacy of their anti-infective therapy.

Summary: Studies of ciprofloxacin administered concurrently with three different nutritional supplements have documented varying effects of these products on ciprofloxacin pharmacokinetics. Conflicting results have been seen with ciprofloxacin and Osmolite®, with one study reporting a reduction of 26% in the maximum concentration (C_{max}) and of 33% in the area-under-curve (AUC) of the antibiotic. The second study did not report any significant reduction in absorption of ciprofloxacin. Results with Pulmocare® have also shown significant decreases in C_{max} and AUC. When ciprofloxacin was administered in conjunction with Resource®, no significant differences were noted in either C_{max} or time to C_{max} (T_{max}); however, the AUC for ciprofloxacin was reduced by 25%. The combination of ciprofloxacin and Ensure revealed significant lowering of the C_{max} by 53% and lengthening of the T_{max}. The AUC for ciprofloxacin was substantially reduced, with a resultant 72% reduction in the bioavailability of the antibiotic.

Related Drugs: Ofloxacin has also been studied when used in combination with Ensure®. The nutritional product's coadministration resulted in a decrease in the C_{max} of 64% and lengthened the T_{max} of ofloxacin. The AUC for ofloxacin was also increased, resulting in an 88% reduction in ofloxacin's bioavailability. Similar interactions may occur between other enteral nutritional supplements and these or other fluoroquinolones. Since the fluoroquinolones have been modified chemically to a great extent compared to the other quinolones, cinoxacin and nalidixic acid, it is difficult to determine if an interaction would also occur with these agents.

Mechanism: Many nutritional supplements contain divalent cations that may be involved in a chelation reaction with ciprofloxacin. This type of interaction has been reported in the past with concurrent administration of ciprofloxacin with antacids, sucralfate, and ferrous sulfate.

Detailed Information: See *EDI*, 8/16.49

Cyclosporine-Amphotericin B

Significance: 2—moderately clinically significant

Potential Effects: Concurrent use of these agents may result in nephrotoxicity.

Recommendations: Monitor serum creatinine levels carefully. The dose of cyclosporine may need to be decreased or an alternative therapy used.

Summary: There are data to show that concurrent use of these agents may result in nephrotoxicity. There are data available indicating that amphotericin B increases cyclosporine concentrations.

Related Drugs: There are no drugs related to cyclosporine or amphotericin B.

Mechanism: Cyclosporine alone is potentially nephrotoxic, and the addition of amphotericin B may increase cyclosporine concentrations and the occurrence of nephrotoxicity.

Detailed Information: See *EDI*, 8/2.50

Dapsone-Rifampin

Significance: 3—minimally clinically significant

Potential Effects: Rifampin may induce the metabolism of dapsone, leading to decreased levels.

Recommendations: If rifampin is used on a regular basis with dapsone, the patient should be monitored for decreased dapsone efficacy or levels. The dosage of dapsone may need to be increased.

Summary: There are data to show that coadministration of rifampin may induce the metabolism of dapsone, leading to decreased levels.

Related Drugs: There are no drugs related to dapsone or rifampin.

Mechanism: Rifampin may induce the hepatic microsomal enzymes responsible for the metabolism of dapsone.

Detailed Information: See *EDI*, 8/16.50

Dapsone-Trimethoprim

Significance: 3—minimally clinically significant

Potential Effects: Concurrent use of these agents may result in increased serum levels of both drugs.

Recommendations: The concurrent administration of dapsone and trimethoprim results in increased serum concentration of both drugs. This may result in an increased cure rate for AIDS-associated *Pneumocystis carinii* pneumonia. Patients receiving this therapy should be observed for a greater risk of developing methemoglobinemia.

Summary: Concurrent administration of dapsone and trimethoprim resulted in an increase in the serum concentration of both agents.

Related Drugs: There are no drugs related to either dapsone or trimethoprim.

Mechanism: A competitive inhibition may occur between dapsone and/or monoacetyldapsone and trimethoprim for renal secretion.

Detailed Information: See *EDI*, 8/16.70

Doxycycline-Carbamazepine

Significance: 2—moderately clinically significant

Recommendations: To maintain adequate serum levels of doxycycline, the antibiotic should be given every 12 hours to patients on long-term therapy with carbamazepine, or another noninteracting tetracycline product may be used.

Summary: The administration of doxycycline to patients receiving carbamazepine therapy will result in a reduction of antimicrobial effectiveness.

Related Drugs: For tetracycline, methacycline, oxytetracycline, demeclocycline, and chlortetracycline, half-lives and quantity excreted have not been shown to be affected by carbamazepine. There is a lack of data concerning whether this interaction occurs with minocycline.

Mechanism: Carbamazepine is known to induce liver enzymes and possibly accelerate the metabolism of doxycycline.

Detailed Information: See *EDI,* 8/17.00

Doxycycline-Phenobarbital

Significance: 2—moderately clinically significant

Recommendations: A higher dosage of doxycycline or a normal dosage of a noninteracting tetracycline derivative should be used during concurrent administration with phenobarbital.

Summary: Doxycycline serum levels, half-life, and urinary excretion may be reduced by concurrent administration of phenobarbital.

Related Drugs: Amobarbital and pentobarbital have been reported to decrease the half-life of doxycycline, and other barbiturates may be expected to interact similarly. A similar interaction is expected to occur with minocycline.

Mechanism: Phenobarbital induces hepatic microsomal enzymes, resulting in enhanced doxycycline elimination.

Detailed Information: See *EDI,* 8/19.00

Doxycycline-Phenytoin

Significance: 2—moderately clinically significant

Recommendations: The clinical response to doxycycline in patients receiving concurrent anticonvulsants should be monitored closely. It has been suggested that doxycycline's daily dose be doubled.

Summary: The concurrent use of doxycycline and phenytoin may result in a decreased half-life of doxycycline, lower serum levels and an inadequate antibacterial effect.

Related Drugs: Other tetracycline derivatives were shown to be unaffected by these anticonvulsants. A similar interaction is expected to occur with minocycline and with the other hydantoin anticonvulsants.

Mechanism: The decrease in half-life of doxycycline has been attributed to the induction of microsomal enzymes by phenytoin.

Detailed Information: See *EDI,* 8/21.00

Erythromycin-Cimetidine

Significance: 3—minimally clinically significant

Potential Effects: Concurrent erythromycin and cimetidine may result in increased erythromycin levels with possible erythromycin-induced reversible hearing loss.

Recommendations: Patients receiving concurrent cimetidine and erythromycin (especially high dose erythromycin) in the presence of renal insufficiency should be monitored for hearing loss.

Summary: Concurrent erythromycin and cimetidine resulted in increased erythromycin levels and one report of erythromycin-induced deafness.

Related Drugs: Although documentation is lacking, based on the postulated mechanism and pharmacologic and structural similarity a similar interaction would be expected to occur between cimetidine and the other macrolide antibiotics (except azithromycin) and between erythromycin and the other H_2 receptor antagonists.

Mechanism: It is thought that cimetidine may have increased erythromycin levels by inhibiting the metabolism of erythromycin at the cytochrome P450 site or by increasing erythromycin absorption from the gastrointestinal tract.

Detailed Information: See *EDI*, 8/21.50

Erythromycin-Cyclosporine

Significance: 1—highly clinically significant

Potential Effects: Erythromycin causes an increase in cyclosporine levels, which can lead to nephrotoxicity and neurotoxicity.

Recommendations: Concurrent used of these agents should be avoided. Monitor cyclosporine levels and renal function if these agents must be used together.

Summary: There are data to show that erythromycin causes an increase in cyclosporine levels, and this interaction may lead to nephrotoxicity and neurotoxicity.

Related Drugs: A similar interaction may occur between cyclosporine and other macrolide antibiotics. There are no drugs related to cyclosporine.

Mechanism: Erythromycin may inhibit the hepatic metabolism of cyclosporine.

Detailed Information: See *EDI*, 8/22.01

Erythromycin-Ergotamine

Significance: 2—moderately clinically significant

Potential Effects: The concurrent use of these agents may result in the development of the clinical signs of ergotism.

Recommendations: If clinical signs of ergotism develop during concurrent administration of these agents, one or both drugs may need to be discontinued and the patient treated symptomatically. It has been shown that nitroprusside reduces the duration of vasospasm.

Summary: The concurrent administration of erythromycin and ergotamine may result in the development of the clinical signs of ergotism as evidenced by peripheral vasospasm, dysesthesia, and renal ischemia. This effect occurred with small doses of ergotamine (1.2–2mg). Concurrent erythromycin and ergotamine may also result in lower extremity ischemia.

Related Drugs: Concurrent use of ergotamine and troleandomycin has been reported to cause peripheral vasospasm. A similar interaction occurred between ergotamine and oleandomycin. Dihydroergotamine, administered concurrently with erythromycin, troleandomycin, or ponsinomycin has shown similar results. The concurrent administration of erythromycin and bromocriptine resulted in a 268% increase in bromocriptine area-under-curve and a 4.6-fold increase in bromocriptine maximum concentration. An interaction between erythromycin and the other ergot alkaloids may be expected to occur.

Mechanism: The mechanism is unknown. Erythromycin may interfere with the hepatic metabolism of ergotamine. It has been shown in animal models that the cytochrome $P450_{3A1}$ isozyme induced by macrolides is similar to the metabolite-cytochrome P-450 complex formed by macrolides that impairs the metabolism of dihydroergotamine.

Detailed Information: See *EDI,* 8/22.03

Erythromycin-Terfenadine

Significance: 1—highly clinically significant

Potential Effects: Concurrent use of these agents may result in increased terfenadine levels with cardiotoxicity.

Recommendations: The concurrent use of these agents is contraindicated according to the manufacturer's package insert for terfenadine. Loratadine or cetirizine may be alternatives to terfenadine; azithromycin may be an alternative to erythromycin.

Summary: Concurrent erythromycin and terfenadine may result in increased terfenadine levels and possible cardiotoxicity, studies have shown.

Related Drugs: There have been reports of serious cardiac events with concomitant troleandomycin and terfenadine. Similar cardiac events have been reported with concomitant terfenadine and josamycin. Clarithromycin may interact with terfenadine in a manner similar to erythromycin, but azithromycin does not interact with terfenadine. Though erythromycin caused a significant increase in loratidine concentration, there were no statistically significant changes in any electrocardiogram parameter, including QT_c interval. Although documentation is lacking, based on the proposed mechanism and structural and pharmacologic similarity a similar interaction would be expected to occur between terfenadine or astemizole and other macrolide antibiotics.

Mechanism: It is postulated that erythromycin and clarithromycin inhibit the cytochrome P450 metabolism of terfenadine and astemizole, thus allowing an increase in plasma levels. The cardiac changes produced by elevated levels of terfenadine and astemizole may be due to the ability of terfenadine and astemizole to inhibit the delayed rectifier potassium channel.

Detailed Information: See *EDI,* 8/22.07

Ethambutol-Aluminum Hydroxide

Significance: 3—minimally clinically significant

Recommendations: The results of a study do not indicate that the concomitant administration of aluminum hydroxide and ethambutol should be avoided. Should a patient receiving these agents exhibit a reduced antitubercular effectiveness, the possibility of this interaction should be considered.

Summary: Aluminum hydroxide may delay or reduce the absorption of ethambutol.

Related Drugs: Other antacids containing aluminum salts may delay the absorption of ethambutol.

Mechanism: Aluminum hydroxide is thought to reduce ethambutol absorption by delaying gastric emptying.

Detailed Information: See *EDI*, 8/22.10

Furazolidone-Amphetamine

Significance: 1—highly clinically significant

Recommendations: Tyramine containing foods, amphetamines, other indirect acting sympathomimetic agents, and mixed acting sympathomimetics are contraindicated in patients receiving furazolidone.

Summary: Furazolidone has a progressive and generalized monoamine oxidase inhibition, and concurrent administration of amphetamine could result in a hypertensive crisis.

Related Drugs: Tyramine has been reported to interact with furazolidone. Other sympathomimetics may have the potential for interacting with furazolidone. Other monoamine oxidase inhibitors have been shown to interact with indirect-acting sympathomimetics (see also Tranylcypromine-Phenylpropanolamine, page 153). Procarbazine may be expected to interact similarly.

Mechanism: Inhibition of monoamine oxidase by furazolidone causes a supersensitivity to amphetamine because of an increased amount of norepinephrine released.

Detailed Information: See *EDI*, 8/23.00

Gentamicin-Carbenicillin

Significance: 1—highly clinically significant

Recommendations: To prevent *in vitro* inactivation, the antibiotics should not be mixed in infusion fluids. There apparently is no contraindication for using these agents together in patients with normal renal function. For patients with renal failure, the dosage of the aminoglycoside and the penicillin must be adjusted for renal impairment and the serum levels of both agents should be monitored. Concurrent use of neomycin and orally administered penicillins should be avoided.

Summary: Concurrent gentamicin and carbenicillin are more effective against certain susceptible organisms than either drug alone; however, gentamicin can be significantly diminished if mixed with carbenicillin *in vitro*.

Related Drugs: Carbenicillin and ticarcillin have been reported to cause the *in vitro* inactivation of sisomicin, netilmicin, tobramycin, amikacin and gentamicin. Ampicillin and penicillin G decrease gentamicin activity when mixed *in vitro*.

Mechanism: Semisynthetic penicillins chemically interact with aminoglycosides forming biologically inactive amides.

Detailed Information: See *EDI*, 8/25.00

Gentamicin-Cephalothin

Significance: 1—highly clinically significant

Recommendations: Patients receiving these drugs concurrently should be observed and monitored closely for signs of nephrotoxicity. High doses of either antibiotic given over an extended period should be avoided. If the concurrent use of these drugs is chosen, the dosage should be based on renal function.

Summary: Concurrent use of gentamicin and cephalothin have been associated with an increased risk of nephrotoxicity, acute renal failure and the development of an acquired Fanconi syndrome.

Related Drugs: Tobramycin and cephalothin have increased risks of nephrotoxicity. Tobramycin and moxalactam have resulted in a increase in tobramycin clearance. Gentamicin and cephalexin were shown to cause hypokalemia. Other aminoglycosides may interact similarly with cephalothin and other cephalosporins.

Mechanism: Gentamicin appears to affect the proximal tubule, and cephalothin may cause acute tubular necrosis. These actions may be additive or there may be a mutual enhancement of toxicity.

Detailed Information: See *EDI,* 8/27.00

Gentamicin-Indomethacin

Significance: 2—moderately clinically significant

Potential Effects: Indomethacin may decrease the glomerular filtration rate, which may increase gentamicin levels and the risk of nephrotoxicity.

Recommendations: Aminoglycoside levels should be closely monitored during concomitant indomethacin therapy and the aminoglycoside dose decreased if necessary. It was suggested that the aminoglycoside dose be decreased prior to indomethacin administration.

Summary: There are data to show that administration of indomethacin may decrease the glomerular filtration rate, increasing gentamicin levels and the risk of nephrotoxicity.

Related Drugs: Amikacin and indomethacin were shown to exhibit a similar interaction. A similar interaction may occur between indomethacin and other aminoglycosides and between gentamicin and other NSAIAs.

Mechanism: Aminoglycoside elimination is dependent on glomerular filtration rate, and indomethacin has been shown to reduce this.

Detailed Information: See *EDI,* 8/28.10

Gentamicin-Polymyxin B

Significance: 2—moderately clinically significant

Recommendations: With rare exception, the combination of these two drugs can, and should, be avoided because of the availability of safer, less toxic combinations. If the interaction does occur, the patient should be supported, as necessary, until the effects dissipate.

Summary: Both gentamicin and polymyxin B may cause nephrotoxicity and neuromuscular blockade; the combination of the two drugs may increase the risk of these side effects.

Related Drugs: Kanamycin and polymyxin resulted in an apneic episode. Neomycin, streptomycin, and kanamycin appear to have the greatest potential for causing neuromuscular blockade; gentamicin and tobramycin are less likely. The potential for other aminoglycosides to cause neuromuscular blockade and nephrotoxicity exists. The polypeptide antibiotics are nephrotoxic.

Mechanism: The toxicities of these two groups of drugs are additive.

Detailed Information: See *EDI,* 8/29.00

Gentamicin-Vancomycin

Significance: 3—minimally clinically significant

Potential Effects: The concomitant use of these agents may result in increased nephrotoxicity. However, two studies found no increase in nephrotoxicity with concomitant administration.

Recommendations: Monitor drug levels and renal function closely during concurrent therapy with these agents. By proper dosing, it may be possible to avert, minimize or reverse nephrotoxicity. Further study of this interaction is needed.

Summary: Concurrent vancomycin and gentamicin have been shown to cause nephrotoxicity; however, not all data support this.

Related Drugs: Vancomycin with tobramycin or amikacin have shown a similar interaction. A similar interaction may occur between vancomycin and other parenteral aminoglycosides. There are no drugs related to vancomycin.

Mechanism: Nephrotoxicity is an additive or synergistic effect of vancomycin and the aminoglycoside.

Detailed Information: See *EDI*, 8/30.01

Griseofulvin-Cyclosporine

Significance: 3—minimally clinically significant

Potential Effects: The addition of griseofulvin to a cyclosporine regimen may result in decreased cyclosporine blood levels.

Recommendations: Patients maintained on cyclosporine should be carefully monitored for changes in cyclosporine blood levels and possible precipitation of rejection events or toxicity if griseofulvin is added to therapy or discontinued. The dose of cyclosporine may need to be adjusted.

Summary: The addition of griseofulvin to a cyclosporine regimen resulted in decreased cyclosporine blood levels.

Related Drugs: There are no drugs related to cyclosporine or griseofulvin.

Mechanism: The mechanism of this interaction is not known.

Detailed Information: See *EDI*, 8/30.05

Griseofulvin-Oral Contraceptive Agents

Significance: 2—moderately clinically significant

Potential Effects: Griseofulvin may increase the metabolism of oral contraceptive agents, leading to breakthrough bleeding and loss of contraceptive effectiveness.

Recommendations: The concomitant use of these agents need not be avoided. However, the potential for reduced contraceptive efficacy should be a consideration when these drugs are used concurrently.

Summary: Griseofulvin may increase the metabolism of oral contraceptive agents, leading to breakthrough bleeding and loss of contraceptive effectiveness.

Related Drugs: There are no drugs related to griseofulvin.

Mechanism: Griseofulvin may induce the metabolism of the oral contraceptive agents, with a corresponding decrease in estrogen concentration.

Detailed Information: See *EDI*, 8/30.10

Griseofulvin-Phenobarbital

Significance: 3—minimally clinically significant

Recommendations: The clinical course of patients taking griseofulvin and phenobarbital concurrently should be closely followed. If the clinical response is inadequate, the dose of griseofulvin may need to be increased.

Summary: Administration of phenobarbital may decrease serum levels of griseofulvin.

Related Drugs: The effect of concurrent administration of other barbiturates on serum griseofulvin levels has not been studied.

Mechanism: Phenobarbital may induce enzymes, increasing the metabolism of the griseofulvin.

Detailed Information: See *EDI,* 8/31.00

Imipenem, Cilastatin-Cyclosporine

Significance: 2—moderately clinically significant

Potential Effects: The concomitant administration of imipenem-cilastatin and cyclosporine may result in mental disturbances as well as changes in cyclosporine serum levels.

Recommendations: Patients receiving concomitant therapy with these agents should be monitored for disturbances of the central nervous system (CNS) and changes in cyclosporine levels. The dosage of cyclosporine may need to be adjusted, or imipenem-cilastatin may need to be discontinued.

Summary: The concomitant administration of imipenem-cilastatin and cyclosporine resulted in mental disturbances (including confused states, agitation, intensive tremor, seizures, myoclonus, and jacksonian fits) as well as increases in cyclosporine blood levels, although conflicting data in animals indicate concurrent administration results in decreasing cyclosporine levels. Another study showed that the administration of the imipenem-cilastatin with cyclosporine may result in a decrease in cyclosporine-related nephrotoxicity.

Related Drugs: There are no drugs related to imipenem-cilastatin or cyclosporine.

Mechanism: The mechanism is unknown. However, both imipenem and cyclosporine alone are known to produce CNS disturbances, and it is possible the metabolism of cyclosporine is inhibited by imipenem, resulting in increased cyclosporine levels and side effects. The mechanism of decreased cyclosporine-related nephrotoxicity may be the result of a decrease in cyclosporine levels caused by imipenem-cilastatin or a decrease in tubular uptake of cyclosporine caused by cilastatin.

Detailed Information: See *EDI,* 8/32.10

Isoniazid-Aluminum Hydroxide

Significance: 3—minimally clinically significant

Recommendations: Single high doses of isoniazid are more effective in arresting tuberculosis than the same amount of drug in divided doses. Although the clinical significance of this interaction is not known, high peak serum concentrations of isoniazid appear to be important in antitubercular therapy. Therefore, isoniazid should be administered at least one hour before antacid administration.

Summary: Administration of aluminum hydroxide may decrease the peak serum levels and delay or decrease the absorption of isoniazid.

Related Drugs: It is difficult to determine whether an interaction would occur between isoniazid and other antacids. There are no drugs related to isoniazid.

Mechanism: Aluminum hydroxide delays gastric emptying and causes retention of isoniazid in the stomach, causing lower peak serum concentrations.

Detailed Information: See *EDI*, 8/33.00

Isoniazid-Disulfiram

Significance: 3—minimally clinically significant

Recommendations: Until further documentation is provided, patients receiving isoniazid and disulfiram concurrently should be monitored for the occurrence of central nervous system (CNS) effects such as dizziness, irritability, lethargy, and uncoordination. If these signs or symptoms occur, dosage reduction or discontinuation of disulfiram should be considered.

Summary: The concurrent use of isoniazid and disulfiram has been reported to result in adverse CNS effects.

Related Drugs: There are no drugs related to isoniazid or disulfiram.

Mechanism: The combination of isoniazid and disulfiram results in altered dopamine metabolism in the brain, resulting in an accumulation of methylated byproducts.

Detailed Information: See *EDI*, 8/35.00

Isoniazid-Meperidine

Significance: 3—minimally clinically significant

Recommendations: Patients should be monitored for adverse reactions during concurrent use of these agents. If lethargy or hypotension occurs, meperidine may need to be discontinued. Also, since morphine was shown not to interact in a particular patient, it may be considered as a suitable alternative to meperidine.

Summary: There are data to show that coadministration of these agents has caused lethargy and hypotension.

Related Drugs: There are no drugs related to isoniazid. Documentation is lacking regarding a similar interaction between isoniazid and other narcotic analgesics.

Mechanism: The mechanism of this interaction is unknown.

Detailed Information: See *EDI*, 8/37.00

Isoniazid-Prednisolone

Significance: 3—minimally clinically significant

Recommendations: If concurrent administration of isoniazid and prednisolone is necessary, the dose of isoniazid may need to be increased.

Summary: There are data to show that administration of prednisolone lowered isoniazid plasma levels.

Related Drugs: A similar interaction may occur between isoniazid and other corticosteroids. There are no drugs related to isoniazid.

Mechanism: Prednisolone may increase the hepatic metabolism and/or renal clearance of isoniazid.

Detailed Information: See *EDI*, 8/39.00

Isoniazid-Propranolol

Significance: 3—minimally clinically significant

Potential Effects: Propranolol may decrease the clearance of isoniazid.

Recommendations: Until further clinical studies are done, the concurrent administration of propranolol and isoniazid need not be avoided. However, patients should be monitored since a decreased dose of isoniazid may be necessary.

Summary: There are data to show that administration of propranolol may decrease the clearance of isoniazid.

Related Drugs: A similar interaction is expected to occur with the beta-blocking agents that are not extensively hepatically metabolized, if the mechanism involves inhibition of the metabolism of isoniazid by propranolol. It is not known if the other beta-blocking agents that are extensively metabolized in the liver would interact with isoniazid. There are no drugs related to isoniazid.

Mechanism: Propranolol may inhibit the acetylation of isoniazid in the liver.

Detailed Information: See *EDI,* 8/40.10

Isoniazid-Pyridoxine

Significance: 3—minimally clinically significant

Potential Effects: Pyridoxine may reduce the antitubercular effects of isoniazid. Peripheral neuropathy may be increased.

Recommendations: Concurrent administration of pyridoxine and isoniazid does not reduce the effectiveness of isoniazid in eradicating tubercle bacilli. The use of concurrent pyridoxine-isoniazid therapy is currently advocated; however, caution should be observed for possible paradoxical vitamin B_6 deficiency.

Summary: There are data to show that pyridoxine may reduce the antitubercular effects of isoniazid. Peripheral neuropathy may be increased.

Related Drugs: There are no drugs related to isoniazid or pyridoxine.

Mechanism: An excess of the pyridoxine moiety may saturate the activating enzymes, resulting in paradoxical vitamin B_6 deficiency.

Detailed Information: See *EDI,* 8/41.00

Isoniazid-Rifampin

Significance: 2—moderately clinically significant

Potential Effects: Incidence of hepatotoxicity may be increased when taking these agents together.

Recommendations: Patients should be aware of the signs and symptoms of hepatotoxicity when taking these agents concurrently. In children, limiting the isoniazid dose to 10mg/Kg and the rifampin dose to 15mg/Kg may help to minimize the toxicity.

Summary: Rifampin is frequently combined with isoniazid to treat tuberculosis; however, hepatotoxicity has been reported to occur more frequently.

Related Drugs: There are no drugs related to rifampin or isoniazid.

Mechanism: Liver damage caused by isoniazid is related to formation of hepatotoxic metabolites and is enhanced by enzyme-inducing drugs such as rifampin.

Detailed Information: See *EDI,* 8/43.00

Itraconazole-Buspirone

Significance: 3—minimally clinically significant

Potential Effects: Concurrent administration of buspirone and itraconazole may result in elevated levels of buspirone and a slight increase in buspirone-related adverse effects.

Recommendations: Although the pharmacodynamic changes in a single dose study were small, it would be prudent to reduce the dosage of buspirone during concomitant administration of itraconazole. Buspirone may exhibit nonlinear pharmacokinetics, thus elevations of buspirone during concomitant administration of itraconazole with multiple doses of buspirone may be more dramatic.

Summary: Concurrent administration of buspirone with itraconazole resulted in elevated buspirone maximum concentration by thirteenfold and a slight increase in buspirone-related adverse effects.

Related Drugs: Based on the proposed mechanism, an interaction would be expected to occur between buspirone and the other systemic azole antifungal agents.

Mechanism: Buspirone undergoes extensive first-pass metabolism. It is postulated that itraconazole inhibits the metabolism of buspirone at the cytochrome P450$_{3A4}$ isoenzyme.

Detailed Information: See *EDI*, 8/44.15

Itraconazole-Didanosine

Significance: 2—moderately clinically significant

Potential Effects: Concurrent didanosine and itraconazole may result in decreased absorption of itraconazole.

Recommendations: It would be prudent to administer these two agents at least two hours apart. Itraconazole serum levels should be monitored to insure that levels remain within a range that will not lead to treatment failure.

Summary: Decreased itraconazole absorption occurred when coadministered with didanosine, resulting in decreased itraconazole levels and clinical effect.

Related Drugs: Ketoconazole has been reported to decrease the absorption of didanosine, but the reverse has not been shown. Based on structural and pharmacologic similarity and the postulated mechanism, an interaction would be expected to occur between didanosine and the other imidazole antifungal agents. It is unknown whether other antiretroviral agents will interact with itraconazole or the other imidazole antifungals.

Mechanism: Ketoconazole and itraconazole require an acidic media for predictable dissolution to occur, and solubility decreases as pH increases. Didanosine is formulated to prevent destruction by gastric acid. This formulation can cause an increase in gastric pH; thus a decrease in solubility and absorption of itraconazole may be expected.

Detailed Information: See *EDI*, 8/44.30

Kanamycin-Ethacrynic Acid

Significance: 1—highly clinically significant

Recommendations: The concurrent use of these agents should be avoided whenever possible. Extreme caution as well as dose reduction and continuous monitoring of eighth cranial nerve function should be followed if concurrent administration is necessary.

Summary: Concurrent administration of kanamycin and ethacrynic acid may result in an increased incidence of ototoxic effects.

Related Drugs: Ethacrynic acid and other aminoglycoside antibiotics have been reported to interact in a similar manner. Bumetanide and furosemide have been reported to interact with the aminoglycosides, causing transient to permanent hearing problems.

Mechanism: A possible synergistic ototoxic effect may be involved with these two agents, or there may be a reduced antibiotic clearance.

Detailed Information: See *EDI*, 8/45.00

Ketoconazole-Aluminum Hydroxide, Magnesium Hydroxide

Significance: 2—moderately clinically significant

Potential Effects: Concurrent administration of ketoconazole with an antacid may decrease ketoconazole absorption.

Recommendations: A prudent regimen would be to administer the two agents as far apart as possible. Since there is no information on how long antacids affect intragastric pH, antacids should be administered after ketoconazole dosages.

Summary: Concurrent administration of ketoconazole with an antacid decreased ketoconazole absorption. In one study, ketoconazole area-under-curve was decreased by 41% when given with the antacid combination compared with ketoconazole administration in the fasting state.

Related Drugs: The administration of sodium bicarbonate, alone and with aluminum hydroxide, has resulted in subtherapeutic concentrations of ketoconazole and treatment failure. Administration of a single dose of fluconazole with an antacid containing aluminum hydroxide and magnesium hydroxide resulted in no statistically significant changes in fluconazole pharmacokinetics when compared to fluconazole administration alone. Although other antacids may also interfere with the absorption of ketoconazole and fluconazole, documentation is lacking. It is not known if the other azole antifungal agents would interact with antacids.

Mechanism: Ketoconazole requires acidic media for predictable dissolution to occur, and solubility decreases as pH increases. The antacid presumably increases the intragastric pH, thereby decreasing dissolution and subsequent absorption.

Detailed Information: See *EDI*, 8/47.00

Ketoconazole-Cimetidine

Significance: 2—moderately clinically significant

Potential Effects: Concurrent administration of ketoconazole with cimetidine may result in decreased absorption of ketoconazole.

Recommendations: In patients receiving concurrent therapy with ketoconazole and an H_2 receptor antagonist, consider monitoring ketoconazole levels. The dosage of ketoconazole may need to be increased or the H_2 receptor antagonist may need to be discontinued.

Summary: Concurrent administration of ketoconazole and cimetidine resulted in decreased absorption of ketoconazole. Administration of ketoconazole in an acidified solution two hours after cimetidine increased ketoconazole levels when compared to ketoconazole administration alone and with cimetidine.

Related Drugs: Ranitidine has shown a similar interaction with ketoconazole. An interaction between ketoconazole and the other H_2
receptor antagonists would be expected to occur. It is not known
whether an interaction would occur between cimetidine and the
other imidazole antifungal agents. The administration of fluconazole with cimetidine resulted in no significant interactions. It is not
known whether an interaction would occur between the parenterally administered H_2 receptor antagonists and the imidazole antifungal agents.

Mechanism: Ketoconazole requires acidic media for predictable
dissolution to occur, and solubility decreases as pH increases.
The H_2 receptor antagonist increases the intragastric pH, thereby
decreasing dissolution and subsequent absorption of ketoconazole.

Detailed Information: See *EDI*, 8/48.50

Ketoconazole-Cyclosporine

Significance: 1—highly clinically significant

Potential Effects: Ketoconazole may cause an increase in
cyclosporine levels.

Recommendations: Avoid using these agents together. If they are
used together, monitor cyclosporine levels and renal function.

Summary: There are data to show that administration of ketoconazole may cause an increase in cyclosporine levels. Because
cyclosporine alone is nephrotoxic, the combination of these
agents may lead to an increased risk of nephrotoxicity.

Related Drugs: Similar interactions have been reported with itraconazole and fluconazole. A similar interaction may occur
between other systemic imidazole antifungal agents and
cyclosporine. There are no drugs related to cyclosporine.

Mechanism: This interaction may be due to an increase in
cyclosporine absorption, competition for hepatic biotransformation, competition for cell-binding sites, ketoconazole-induced
inhibition of hepatic metabolism, or competition for an excretion
pathway.

Detailed Information: See *EDI*, 8/49.00

Ketoconazole-Methylprednisolone

Significance: 2—moderately clinically significant

Potential Effects: Ketoconazole inhibits the metabolism of methylprednisolone, which may result in enhanced methylprednisolone
side effects. Ketoconazole may also enhance the cortisol sup-
pressive effects of methylprednisolone.

Recommendations: Patients should be monitored for enhanced
adverse effects of methylprednisolone when receiving concurrent
ketoconazole. The dose of methylprednisolone may need to be
decreased. One report recommends reducing the methylprednisolone dose by 50% when used with ketoconazole.

Summary: There are data to show that administration of ketoconazole may inhibit the metabolism of methylprednisolone, resulting
in enhanced methylprednisolone side effects.

Related Drugs: Ketoconazole was reported to increase plasma
prednisolone. A similar interaction may occur with methylprednisolone and ketoconazole and other corticosteroids. There are
no drugs related to ketoconazole.

Mechanism: Ketoconazole may inhibit the hepatic metabolism of methylprednisolone.

Detailed Information: See *EDI,* 8/50.01

Ketoconazole-Omeprazole

Significance: 2—moderately clinically significant

Potential Effects: The concurrent administration of ketoconazole and omeprazole may result in decreased ketoconazole absorption.

Recommendations: Ketoconazole serum levels should be monitored in patients receiving concurrent ketoconazole and omeprazole. The dosage of ketoconazole may need to be increased or omeprazole may need to be discontinued. Administration of an acidic beverage with ketoconazole may improve ketoconazole absorption in some patients.

Summary: The concurrent administration of ketoconazole and a single dose of omeprazole resulted in decreased ketoconazole absorption. Area-under-curve and maximum concentration decreased by 98.9% and 99%, respectively, when compared to ketoconazole administration alone.

Related Drugs: The administration of a single dose of fluconazole on day seven of omeprazole treatment resulted in no significant changes in fluconazole. It is not known whether an interaction would be expected to occur between omeprazole and the other imidazole antifungal agents. An interaction between ketoconazole and the other proton pump inhibitors would be expected to occur.

Mechanism: Ketoconazole requires acidic media for predictable dissolution to occur, and solubility decreases as pH increases. Omeprazole increases the intragastric pH, thereby decreasing dissolution and subsequent absorption.

Detailed Information: See *EDI,* 8/50.06

Ketoconazole-Rifampin

Significance: 2—moderately clinically significant

Potential Effects: Concurrent administration of ketoconazole and rifampin may result in decreased ketoconazole serum levels and efficacy.

Recommendations: It is important to monitor the patient for a decrease in ketoconazole efficacy when rifampin is added. Administering the two agents at separate times (at least 12 hours apart) appears to prevent the decrease in rifampin but not ketoconazole serum levels. Concurrent fluconazole and rifabutin may offer an alternative.

Summary: Concurrent rifampin and ketoconazole has been shown to result in a decrease in ketoconazole serum levels.

Related Drugs: Rifampin has been shown to cause a significant decrease in itraconazole serum levels with concurrent therapy. In spite of decreased itraconazole concentrations with rifabutin, this combination has been reported to be potentially synergistic when used to treat cryptococcoses. A similar interaction resulting in decreased fluconazole concentrations has been reported with concomitant rifampin. Patients receiving concurrent rifabutin and fluconazole showed a decrease in the incidence of *Mycobacterium avium* bacteremia. There was an increase in the incidence of leukopenia with combination therapy compared to rifabutin alone. Although no documentation exists, because of structural and pharmacological similarities an interaction may be expected to occur between rifampin or rifabutin and the other imidazole antifungal agents.

Mechanism: It has been suggested that rifampin increased the metabolism of ketoconazole. It is possible that ketoconazole interfered with the absorption of rifampin. Fluconazole is a potent inhibitor of cytochrome P450 hepatic enzyme systems. It has been noted to increase both the maximum concentration and area-under-curve of rifabutin and its D-acetyl metabolite.

Detailed Information: See *EDI,* 8/50.10

Ketoconazole-Sucralfate

Significance: 3—minimally clinically significant

Potential Effects: Concurrent sucralfate and ketoconazole may decrease ketoconazole bioavailability.

Recommendations: It has been suggested that, in some patients, clinical failure of therapy may be associated with the concomitant administration of sucralfate and ketoconazole. It is recommended that the administration of sucralfate and ketoconazole be separated by as much time as possible to decrease the potential effect of sucralfate on ketoconazole bioavailability.

Summary: Concurrent sucralfate and ketoconazole resulted in decreased ketoconazole bioavailability.

Related drugs: It is not known whether an interaction would occur between sucralfate and other imidazole antifungal agents or between ketoconazole and other aluminum salts.

Mechanism: The mechanism of this interaction is not known, but it is not pH related.

Detailed Information: See *EDI,* 8/50.40

Ketoconazole-Terfenadine

Significance: 1—highly clinically significant

Potential Effects: Concurrent use of ketoconazole (or itraconazole) and terfenadine will result in a decrease in the metabolism and clearance of terfenadine, resulting in increased levels and cardiotoxicity.

Recommendations: The concurrent use of terfenadine or astemizole with either ketoconazole or itraconazole is contraindicated according to the manufacturers' product information for these agents. Loratadine or cetirizine may be alternatives to terfenadine or astemizole.

Summary: The addition of ketoconazole to terfenadine therapy has resulted in elevations in levels of terfenadine. The resulting increase in terfenadine serum levels has been associated with occurrence of Torsades de Pointes arrhythmia and a risk of sudden cardiac death.

Related Drugs: Itraconazole and terfenadine have been reported to cause a similar arrhythmia. Ketoconazole was shown to be an inhibitor of *in vitro* astemizole metabolism. Based on the postulated mechanism, concurrent ketoconazole and loratadine may be expected to result in elevated levels of loratadine; however, no electrocardiographic changes have been reported. Fluconazole may not cause arrhythmias when combined with terfenadine. Although documentation is lacking regarding an interaction between the piperidine H_1 receptor antagonists and the other imidazole antifungal agents, an interaction may be expected to occur based on the postulated mechanism and structural similarity.

Mechanism: Ketoconazole has been shown to inhibit drug metabolism possibly by inhibition of the cytochrome P450 enzyme system. Terfenadine is metabolized to a great degree by the liver, presumably by cytochrome P450 oxidative metabolism. It is thought that the arrhythmia experienced by patients was due to an increase in serum concentration of either terfenadine or its acid metabolite.

Detailed Information: See *EDI,* 8/50.60

Lincomycin-Erythromycin

Significance: 3—minimally clinically significant

Recommendations: Although there are insufficient data to conclude that an interaction occurs between lincomycin and erythromycin, the clinician should be aware of the possibility of the development of cross interference. This may offset any therapeutic advantage of combining these agents. If possible, concurrent use of lincomycin and erythromycin should be avoided.

Summary: Erythromycin can theoretically antagonize the activity of lincomycin by blocking access to ribosomal binding sites.

Related Drugs: Other macrolide antibiotics and chloramphenicol may also interfere with the activity of lincomycin.

Mechanism: Erythromycin has a greater affinity for the 50S ribosomal unit; therefore, erythromycin could block the effects of lincomycin by displacing it from the binding site or by preventing binding.

Detailed Information: See *EDI,* 8/51.00

Lincomycin-Kaolin

Significance: 1—highly clinically significant

Recommendations: In patients receiving lincomycin who require antidiarrheal therapy, products that do not contain kaolin should be considered. When a kaolin-containing product must be used, it should be given at least two hours before lincomycin.

Summary: Kaolin reduces the gastrointestinal absorption of lincomycin.

Related Drugs: Kaolin had no effect on the extent of clindamycin absorption.

Mechanism: The physical coating action of kaolin on the intestinal mucosa and kaolin's adsorbent property may be responsible for this interaction.

Detailed Information: See *EDI,* 8/53.00

Metronidazole-Chloroquine

Significance: 2—moderately clinically significant

Potential Effects: Concurrent use of these agents may result in acute dystonic reactions.

Recommendations: Concurrent used of these agents should be avoided. Sulfadoxine and pyrimethamine may be used in place of chloroquine for malaria if concurrent metronidazole is to be used.

Summary: There are data to show that coadministration of these agents has led to acute dystonic reactions—restlessness, facial grimacing, and coarse tremors.

Related Drugs: A similar interaction may occur between metronidazole and hydroxychloroquine or primaquine. There are no drugs related to metronidazole.

Mechanism: Chloroquine and metronidazole decrease neuronal calcium uptake/availability, which may decrease dopamine levels, resulting in dystonic reactions.

Detailed Information: See *EDI,* 8/54.05

Metronidazole-Cimetidine

Significance: 3—minimally clinically significant

Potential Effects: Cimetidine may inhibit the metabolism of metronidazole.

Recommendations: The concurrent administration of metronidazole and cimetidine need not be avoided. However, monitor for metronidazole side effects (e.g., convulsive seizures, peripheral neuropathy). The dose of metronidazole may need to be adjusted.

Summary: There are data to show that administration of cimetidine may inhibit the metabolism of metronidazole; however, all data do not support the existence of this interaction.

Related Drugs: There are no drugs related to metronidazole. A similar interaction may occur between metronidazole and other H_2-receptor antagonists.

Mechanism: Cimetidine may inhibit the hepatic metabolism of metronidazole by interfering with the microsomal cytochrome P450 mono-oxygenase system.

Detailed Information: See *EDI,* 8/54.10

Metronidazole-Disulfiram

Significance: 2—moderately clinically significant

Potential Effects: Concomitant metronidazole and disulfiram may result in an alternation of the effects of disulfiram, which may include acute psychosis, confusion, or visual and auditory hallucinations.

Recommendations: Concurrent administration of these agents should be avoided if possible. If concomitant use is necessary, one or both drugs may need to be discontinued if symptoms occur.

Summary: There are data to show that administration of metronidazole may result in an alternation of the effects of disulfiram, which may include acute psychosis, confusion, or visual and auditory hallucinations.

Related Drugs: A similar interaction may occur between metronidazole and calcium carbamide and monosulfiram and between disulfiram and anti-infective agents related to metronidazole.

Mechanism: Metronidazole may have an attenuated disulfiram effect.

Detailed Information: See *EDI,* 8/55.00

Metronidazole-Phenobarbital

Significance: 2—moderately clinically significant

Potential Effects: Phenobarbital may increase the hepatic metabolism of metronidazole, resulting in decreased levels of metronidazole.

Recommendations: Patients receiving metronidazole therapy should be observed for a lack of, or a decrease in, antimicrobial response during the concurrent administration of phenobarbital. An increased dose of metronidazole may be necessary.

Summary: There are data to show that administration of phenobarbital may increase the hepatic metabolism of metronidazole, resulting in decreased levels of metronidazole.

Related Drugs: A similar interaction may occur between metronidazole and other barbiturates. There are no drugs related to metronidazole.

Mechanism: Phenobarbital, a known hepatic enzyme inducer, increases the hepatic metabolism of metronidazole.

Detailed Information: See *EDI*, 8/57.00

Nitrofurantoin-Magnesium Trisilicate

Significance: 3—minimally clinically significant

Recommendations: Although concurrent use of these agents need not be avoided, it may be best to separate their administration by as much time as possible. The dose of nitrofurantoin may need to be increased.

Summary: Administration of magnesium trisilicate was shown to result in a decrease in both the rate and extent of nitrofurantoin absorption, and this may result in a decrease in antimicrobial effectiveness.

Related Drugs: Aluminum hydroxide, magnesium carbonate, and magnesium hydroxide decreased nitrofurantoin absorption. Because of variable results, it is difficult to determine whether an interaction would occur between nitrofurantoin and other antacids. There are no drugs related to nitrofurantoin.

Mechanism: The decreased gastrointestinal absorption of nitrofurantoin may be due to its subsequent slow and incomplete release from the antacid surface.

Detailed Information: See *EDI*, 8/58.10

Nitrofurantoin-Probenecid

Significance: 3—minimally clinically significant

Recommendations: The significance of this interaction is difficult to determine for several reasons. Reports of a nitrofurantoin-probenecid interaction in clinical practice have been sparse. Second, the lower doses of probenecid frequently used in clinical practice would not exert as great an effect on nitrofurantoin excretion and systemic accumulation as the doses of 500 to 1000mg every two hours used experimentally. An additional factor for consideration involves renal dysfunction. Systemic accumulation and decreased urinary excretion of nitrofurantoin occurred in patients in whom serum creatinine levels were greater than about 2.5 to 3mg% (normal, 0.6 to 1.2mg%). Thus, patients with decreased renal efficiency may not be good candidates for nitrofurantoin therapy. An increase in nitrofurantoin dosage in an attempt to enhance urine levels would only serve to increase the likelihood of systemic accumulation and the adverse effects associated with increased serum levels. Thus, concurrent administration of these drugs should be avoided whenever possible.

Summary: Concurrent administration of probenecid decreases the renal clearance of nitrofurantoin and increases the serum levels of the nitrofurantoin, and this has been associated with the onset of polyneuropathies.

Related Drugs: Sulfinpyrazone may have an effect on nitrofurantoin excretion similar to that of probenecid.

Mechanism: Probenecid is known to inhibit the tubular secretion of many compounds and presumably exerts the same effect with nitrofurantoin.

Detailed Information: See *EDI*, 8/59.00

Nitrofurantoin-Propantheline

Significance: 3—minimally clinically significant

Recommendations: The concurrent use of these agents need not be avoided. However, it is prudent to separate the administration of these drugs by as much time as possible.

Summary: The concurrent use of nitrofurantoin and propantheline causes an increase in nitrofurantoin absorption and excretion.

Related Drugs: There are no drugs related to nitrofurantoin. A similar interaction may occur with other anticholinergics.

Mechanism: It has been suggested that propantheline decreases gastric emptying time because of its ability to reduce gastric motility, increasing nitrofurantoin bioavailability.

Detailed Information: See *EDI*, 8/61.00

Norfloxacin-Sucralfate

Significance: 2—moderately clinically significant

Potential Effects: Sucralfate may decrease norfloxacin absorption, resulting in decreased levels and efficacy.

Recommendations: Concurrent use of these agents should be avoided.

Summary: The bioavailability of norfloxacin is reduced in the presence of sucralfate.

Related Drugs: Sulcralfate was shown to decrease the bioavailability of ciprofloxacin. It is difficult to determine if an interaction would occur with cinoxacin or nalidixic acid. There are no drugs related to sucralfate.

Mechanism: Reduced levels of norfloxacin may occur because of reduced gastrointestinal absorption, possibly related to the formation of inactive norfloxacin aluminum chelates.

Detailed Information: See *EDI*, 8/62.10

Penicillin-Aspirin

Significance: 3—minimally clinically significant

Recommendations: The limited clinical data prevent definite assessment of the clinical significance of this drug interaction. Concurrent use of high doses of aspirin has been suggested to increase the clinical benefits of penicillin, but the possible toxicities resulting discourage such therapy.

Summary: Aspirin significantly increases penicillin serum concentrations and half-life.

Related Drugs: Aspirin has reduced the serum protein binding of cloxacillin, dicloxacillin, nafcillin, and oxacillin. There appear to be no reports that the other salicylates affect the disposition of penicillin.

Mechanism: Aspirin may displace penicillin from its protein binding sites, or there may be competition of the two drugs for the same renal secretory sites in the proximal tubule.

Detailed Information: See *EDI*, 8/63.00

Penicillin-Chloramphenicol

Significance: 4—not clinically significant

Recommendations: There is no unequivocal clinical evidence that chloramphenicol causes any significant antagonism of the bactericidal effect of penicillin. Therefore, concurrent use of these antibiotics need not be avoided in the limited circumstances where such therapy is indicated.

Summary: The bacteriostatic action of chloramphenicol may antagonize the bactericidal action of penicillin; however, several variables such as the organisms involved and the doses used can affect the potential interaction.

Related Drugs: Administration of chloramphenicol and ampicillin and chlor-amphenicol and procaine penicillin were found to be superior treatments to chloramphenicol alone. A similar interaction may occur between chloramphenicol and other penicillins. There are no drugs related to chloramphenicol.

Mechanism: Chloramphenicol inhibits protein synthesis, which may mask the bactericidal action of penicillin.

Detailed Information: See *EDI*, 8/65.00

Penicillin-Chlortetracycline

Significance: 2—moderately clinically significant

Recommendations: Tetracycline may cause a clinically significant antagonism of penicillin in situations where rapid bactericidal activity is necessary (e.g., pneumococcal meningitis). There is no clinical evidence supporting a penicillin-tetracycline interaction with infections where rapid bacterial kill is not critical. Even in those cases where no antagonism occurs, there is no justification for concurrent use of penicillin and tetracycline.

Summary: Tetracycline derivatives may antagonize the bactericidal action of penicillin G under conditions where rapid bacterial kill is desired. Increased incidence of mortality and reinfection have been reported in patients receiving chlortetracycline and penicillin G.

Related Drugs: Antagonism of the action of all other penicillins may be expected based on their common mechanism of action. All tetracyclines may be expected to interact in a similar manner with penicillin.

Mechanism: Spheroplast formation, a preceding step in the lysis of bacteria exposed to penicillin, is inhibited by tetracyclines.

Detailed Information: See *EDI*, 8/67.00

Penicillin-Erythromycin

Significance: 3—minimally clinically significant

Recommendations: Penicillins should not be used routinely in combination with erythromycin. Although concurrent administration has revealed synergism, indifference and antagonism have also been reported and are most likely the result of differences in microorganisms studied and their related susceptibilities to these antibiotics. If these drugs are used concurrently, both the minimum inhibitory concentration and the minimum bactericidal concentration should be checked to ensure a synergistic bactericidal effect.

Summary: Concomitant usage of penicillin and erythromycin may result in synergism, antagonism, or no alteration of the combined antibacterial effect.

Related Drugs: Penicillin G, penicillin V, ampicillin, and methicillin have been documented to interact with erythromycin. Cephalosporins may interact with erythromycin in a similar manner.

Mechanism: Erythromycin exerts a bacteriostatic effect resulting in decreased bacterial cytoplasmic growth and a decreased susceptibility to cellular lysis induced by bactericidal drugs such as penicillin.

Detailed Information: See *EDI*, 8/69.00

Penicillin-Probenecid

Significance: 3—minimally clinically significant

Recommendations: Complications during concurrent administration of these drugs result from increased antibiotic levels and are encountered most frequently during long-term treatment. It may be advisable to reduce the dosage of penicillin when probenecid is combined with the antibiotic and to monitor the penicillin serum levels.

Summary: Concurrent administration of penicillin and probenecid results in higher and more sustained serum penicillin levels.

Related Drugs: All penicillins may interact in a similar manner with probenecid. There are many penicillin analogs that have been reported to interact with probenecid.

Mechanism: Probenecid may compete with other weak organic acids and diminish tubular secretion of such compounds, or it may decrease the apparent volume of distribution, resulting in a larger penicillin fraction in the central compartment.

Detailed Information: See *EDI*, 8/71.00

Polymyxin B-Prochlorperazine

Significance: 2—moderately clinically significant

Recommendations: Caution should be used when concurrently administering polymyxin B and prochlorperazine or other polypeptide antibiotics and phenothiazines. Ventilatory assistance should be made available.

Summary: In one case report, a patient who received intravenous polymyxin B experienced severe apnea after the administration of prochlorperazine.

Related Drugs: A similar interaction was documented after the concurrent administration of colistin and promethazine. A similar interaction may occur with other polypeptide antibiotics and other phenothiazines.

Mechanism: The development of apnea in these patients may result from a synergistic neuromuscular blockade.

Detailed Information: See *EDI*, 8/73.00

Rifampin-Aminosalicylic Acid

Significance: 4—not clinically significant

Recommendations: It may not be possible to know if a granule formulation contains bentonite. However, it was demonstrated that separating the administration of these two agents by 8 to 12 hours prevented the interaction.

Summary: Aminosalicylic acid granules have been reported to decrease the bioavailability and pharmacologic activity of rifampin. Another study found that the reduction was caused by bentonite, an excipient in the aminosalicylic acid granules.

Related Drugs: There are no drugs related to rifampin or aminosalicylic acid.

Mechanism: Physical adsorption of rifampin is the likely mechanism in this interaction.

Detailed Information: See *EDI*, 8/75.00

Rifampin-Clofibrate

Significance: 3—minimally clinically significant

Recommendations: In order to achieve therapeutic plasma concentrations of clofibrate, it may be necessary to increase the dose of clofibrate when it is administered concomitantly with rifampin.

Summary: There are data to show that administration of rifampin significantly reduces the plasma levels of clofibric acid.

Related Drugs: There are no drugs related to clofibrate or rifampin.

Mechanism: Rifampin may enhance the hepatic metabolism of clofibrate and the renal excretion of its metabolite.

Detailed Information: See *EDI,* 8/76.10

Rifampin-Cyclosporine

Significance: 1—highly clinically significant

Potential Effects: Rifampin causes a decrease in cyclosporine levels which may lead to graft rejections. Avoid using these agents together.

Recommendations: If they must be given together, cyclosporine levels should be monitored frequently.

Summary: There are data to show that administration of rifampin causes a decrease in cyclosporine levels, which may lead to graft rejections. When rifampin was discontinued, cyclosporine levels were shown to increase dramatically.

Related Drugs: There are no drugs related to cyclosporine or rifampin.

Mechanism: Rifampin, a known inducer of hepatic microsomal enzymes, increases the metabolism and clearance of cyclosporine.

Detailed Information: See *EDI,* 8/76.30

Rifampin-Oral Contraceptive Agents

Significance: 1—highly clinically significant

Potential Effects: Concurrent rifampin may increase the metabolism of oral contraceptive agents, leading to breakthrough bleeding and loss of contraceptive effectiveness.

Recommendations: Although some women may take these agents concomitantly without risk, there is no way to predict who will be affected. Some prescribers may choose to warn patients that spotting and breakthrough bleeding are signs of diminished contraceptive effectiveness, and alternative forms of contraception should be used. Others may choose to recommend an alternative contraception method.

Summary: Concurrent administration of rifampin and oral contraceptive agents have been shown to result in an increased incidence of menstrual disorders and pregnancies.

Related Drugs: A similar interaction may occur between oral contraceptive agents and rifabutin.

Mechanism: Antibiotics destroy gut flora and may prevent steroid reabsorption, resulting in lower than normal concentrations of the contraceptive. Rifampin is a microsomal enzyme inducer, increasing the hydroxylation of estrogens.

Detailed Information: See *EDI,* 8/77.00

Rifampin-Prednisolone

Significance: 2—moderately clinically significant

Recommendations: A reduced corticosteroid activity may be expected when rifampin is coadministered, necessitating an increased steroid dose. One approximation is to double the daily steroid dose when rifampin therapy is initiated. Patients stabilized on both agents may require a steroid dosage decrease when rifampin is discontinued.

Summary: Prednisolone disposition is altered by rifampin, resulting in a decreased corticosteroid activity. Rifampin was further implicated in the decreased serum area-under-curve and increased clearance of prednisolone.

Related Drugs: Similar changes in corticosteroid disposition have been reported for cortisone acetate, fludrocortisone, cortisol (hydrocortisone), and methylprednisolone. A similar interaction may occur with other corticosteroids. There are no drugs related to rifampin.

Mechanism: Rifampin induces hepatic metabolizing enzymes, leading to an increased metabolism of the steroid.

Detailed Information: See *EDI,* 8/79.00

Rifampin-Probenecid

Significance: 4—not clinically significant

Recommendations: At this point, there appears to be no advantage of adding probenecid to rifampin therapy with the goal of increasing rifampin's plasma levels or decreasing its rate of metabolism.

Summary: Rifampin and probenecid have been the subject of conflicting data designed to evaluate whether the addition of probenecid to rifampin therapy would add any therapeutic benefit.

Related Drugs: There are no drugs related to rifampin. It is not known if an interaction occurs between rifampin and sulfinpyrazone.

Mechanism: Both agents may compete at the plasma membrane, increasing peak serum rifampin levels, or individual patient variations could cause the serum levels of rifampin to increase.

Detailed Information: See *EDI,* 8/81.00

Sulfadiazine-Cyclosporine

Significance: 2—moderately clinically significant

Potential Effects: The addition of sulfadiazine to cyclosporine therapy may result in decreased cyclosporine levels.

Recommendations: The addition of sulfadiazine to the therapy of a patient maintained on cyclosporine requires close monitoring of cyclosporine levels. The dose of cyclosporine may need to be adjusted, especially when high daily sulfonamide doses are required.

Summary: Sulfadiazine therapy may result in a decreased cyclosporine concentration.

Related Drugs: Sulfamethoxydiazine was shown to decrease cyclosporine. It is not known whether an interaction would occur between cyclosporine and other sulfonamides, but one may occur.

Mechanism: The different effects of the related sulfonamides on cyclosporine levels are dependent on the absolute dosage used.

Detailed Information: See *EDI,* 8/82.50

Sulfamethazine/Trimethoprim-Cyclosporine

Significance: 3—minimally clinically significant

Recommendations: Patients should be observed for a decrease in cyclosporine serum levels. Until further studies are done, an increase in the cyclosporine dose, use of an alternative antibiotic, or use of the oral rather than the intravenous route of administration for the antibiotics may be necessary.

Summary: Administration of trimethoprim and sulfamethazine may result in undetectable cyclosporine serum levels, potentiating graft rejection.

Related Drugs: There are no drugs related to cyclosporine. It is not known whether other sulfonamides would interact similarly with cyclosporine.

Mechanism: The mechanism of this interaction is unknown.

Detailed Information: See *EDI*, 8/83.00

Sulfamethoxazole/Trimethoprim-Oral Contraceptive Agents

Significance: 3—minimally clinically significant

Potential Effects: The estrogenic effects of oral contraceptives may be increased in women receiving sulfamethoxazole-trimethoprim.

Recommendations: It is unlikely that clinical problems will arise in women taking long-term oral contraceptive agents who are given short courses of sulfamethoxazole-trimethoprim.

Summary: There are data to show that administration of sulfamethoxazole-trimethoprim may increase the estrogenic effects of oral contraceptives; however, all data do not support this interaction.

Related Drugs: Documentation is lacking regarding an interaction between oral contraceptive agents and other sulfonamides.

Mechanism: The enhanced effects of ethinylestradiol may be due to the inhibition of steroid microsomal hydroxylation enzymes in the liver by sulfamethoxazole.

Detailed Information: See *EDI*, 8/84.10

Sulfasalazine-Ampicillin

Significance: 3—minimally clinically significant

Recommendations: Sulfasalazine is often used in the management of inflammatory bowel disease. Patients receiving this drug should be monitored for loss of therapeutic efficacy when ampicillin is added to their therapy.

Summary: Ampicillin was shown to affect the extent of absorption, reducing the availability of sulfasalazine.

Related Drugs: There is no documentation regarding an interaction between sulfasalazine and the other penicillins. It is difficult to determine whether an interaction would occur between ampicillin and the other sulfonamides.

Mechanism: The mechanism of this interaction is unknown.

Detailed Information: See *EDI*, 8/85.00

Terbinafine-Cyclosporine

Significance: 2—moderately clinically significant

Potential Effects: Concurrent terbinafine and cyclosporine administration may result in a decrease in cyclosporine trough blood levels.

Recommendations: Cyclosporine blood levels should be monitored whenever terbinafine is added to or discontinued from concurrent therapy. Cyclosporine levels should be closely monitored in patients whose levels are at the lower end of the therapeutic range.

Summary: The addition of terbinafine to the therapy of several patients maintained on cyclosporine resulted in a decrease in mean cyclosporine trough blood levels. However, conflicting data are available.

Related Drugs: There are no drugs related to terbinafine or cyclosporine.

Mechanism: Terbinafine may induce cyclosporine metabolism even though studies have shown that terbinafine is not a significant enzyme inducer *in vitro*.

Detailed Information: See *EDI,* 8/86.00

Tetracycline-Aluminum Hydroxide

Significance: 1—highly clinically significant

Potential Effects: Concurrent used may decrease absorption of tetracycline because of chelation.

Recommendations: If these agents must be used together, separate the administration by at least two hours.

Summary: Concurrent administration of aluminum hydroxide containing antacids or products containing divalent ions and tetracycline significantly decreases the gastrointestinal absorption of tetracycline.

Related Drugs: Most tetracycline analogs may interact in a similar manner with aluminum hydroxide and/or dairy products. Minocycline absorption is not notably influenced by food and dairy products, but aluminum, calcium, and magnesium ions may impair absorption. Sucralfate may prevent absorption of tetracycline. Bismuth subsalicylate has been shown to decrease tetracycline absorption and decrease the bioavailability of doxycycline.

Mechanism: Tetracycline forms relatively insoluble chelates with divalent and trivalent metallic ions.

Detailed Information: See *EDI,* 8/87.00

Tetracycline-Cimetidine

Significance: 3—minimally clinically significant

Recommendations: Further studies are needed to elucidate this interaction; however, patients should be monitored for a decrease in the efficacy of tetracycline. The dose of tetracycline may need to be increased. Alternatively, the use of the oral solution of tetracycline, which was shown not to interact, might be considered.

Summary: The concurrent use of tetracycline and cimetidine resulted in a reduction in the tetracycline plasma concentration, a decrease in the area-under-curve, and a reduction in excretion.

Related Drugs: A similar interaction may occur between cimetidine and other tetracyclines or between tetracycline and other H_2-receptor antagonists, if the mechanism involves an increased gastric pH.

Mechanism: Dissolution of the capsule form of tetracycline depends on gastric acidity, and cimetidine raises gastric pH.

Detailed Information: See *EDI,* 8/89.00

Tetracycline-Ferrous Sulfate

Significance: 1—highly clinically significant

Recommendations: Ferrous sulfate should not be given simultaneously with tetracycline or tetracycline analogs. When it is necessary for patients to receive both agents orally, this interaction may be avoided by administering the ferrous sulfate not less than three hours before or two hours after the tetracycline.

Summary: The concurrent oral administration of ferrous sulfate and tetracycline causes an interference with the absorption of tetracycline and the ferrous ion.

Related Drugs: The absorption of most tetracycline analogs will be decreased with concurrent administration of ferrous salts. Ferrous gluconate and fumarate have been shown to interact with the tetracyclines, and ferrous lactate may also interact in a similar manner.

Mechanism: Ferric and ferrous ions have been shown to form chelates with tetracyclines.

Detailed Information: See *EDI,* 8/91.00

Tetracycline-Oral Contraceptive Agents

Significance: 2—moderately clinically significant

Potential Effects: The concurrent use of these agents may result in loss of contraceptive efficacy.

Recommendations: The majority of women may take these agents concomitantly without risk, but there seems no way to predict who will be affected. Some prescribers may choose to warn patients that spotting and breakthrough bleeding are signs of diminished contraceptive effectiveness, and alternative forms of contraception should be used. Others may choose to recommend an alternative contraceptive method.

Summary: The concurrent use of tetracycline and oral contraceptive agents has led to contraceptive failure.

Related Drugs: Oxytetracycline has been reported to exhibit a similar interaction. The other tetracycline derivatives may interact with oral contraceptive agents.

Mechanism: Antibiotics destroy the gut flora and prevent steroid reabsorption, resulting in lower than normal concentrations of the contraceptive.

Detailed Information: See *EDI,* 8/93.00

Tetracycline-Sodium Bicarbonate

Significance: 4—not clinically significant

Recommendations: The incidence of the tetracycline-sodium bicarbonate interaction is not known, and there is conflicting evidence regarding the occurrence of adverse effects. A cautious regimen would be to administer the drugs as far apart as possible. There is no documentation whether this interaction will occur when tetracycline is administered in a liquid dosage form.

Summary: There are data to show that administration of sodium bicarbonate will reduce tetracycline absorption; however, all data do not support this.

Related Drugs: There appear to be no reports on the effect of sodium bicarbonate on any other tetracycline analog.

Mechanism: Tetracycline dissolves slower at a higher intragastric pH.

Detailed Information: See *EDI,* 8/95.00

Tetracycline-Thimerosal

Significance: 3—minimally clinically significant

Recommendations: Reactions to thimerosal-containing contact lens solution are common. Delayed hypersensitivity reactions have also been reported. However, when patients develop a reaction after long-term use, another explanation for the reaction is necessary. Until additional cases are reported in the literature, the concurrent use of these agents need not be avoided. Should an ocular reaction occur, one or both drugs may have to be withdrawn.

Summary: Tetracycline appears to potentiate ocular reactions when thimerosal-containing contact lens solution is being used.

Related Drugs: Other tetracyclines may interact similarly with thimerosal.

Mechanism: Tetracyclines are known to penetrate into ocular fluid and may chelate the mercury in thimerosal.

Detailed Information: See *EDI*, 8/96.10

Tobramycin-Miconazole

Significance: 3—minimally clinically significant

Potential Effects: Intravenously administered miconazole may cause a decrease in tobramycin levels.

Recommendations: Closely monitor tobramycin levels when these agents are used together.

Summary: There are data to show that administration of miconazole may cause a decrease in tobramycin levels.

Related Drugs: It is not known if miconazole would interact similarly with other aminoglycosides. There are no drugs related to miconazole.

Mechanism: The miconazole vehicle may cause an increased cellular uptake of tobramycin, leading to an increased volume of distribution.

Detailed Information: See *EDI*, 8/96.21

Troleandomycin-Methylprednisolone

Significance: 2—moderately clinically significant

Potential Effects: Troleandomycin may inhibit the metabolism of methylprednisolone, leading to increased levels and possible adverse steroid effects.

Recommendations: Patients should be monitored for corticosteroid toxicity during concomitant use. Erythromycin may be an alternate to troleandomycin because it interacts to a lesser extent. The concurrent use of these agents may be beneficial for some patients.

Summary: There are data to show that administration of troleandomycin may inhibit the metabolism of methylprednisolone, leading to increased levels and increased adverse effects.

Related Drugs: Erythromycin and oleandomycin alter methylprednisolone disposition. Prednisolone is unaffected by troleandomycin. A similar interaction may occur with other corticosteroids and troleandomycin.

Mechanism: The interaction may result from a macrolide antibiotic inhibition of methylprednisolone metabolism.

Detailed Information: See *EDI*, 8/96.30

Troleandomycin-Oral Contraceptive Agents

Significance: 2—moderately clinically significant

Recommendations: The large number of cases of cholestasis in women taking both troleandomycin and oral contraceptives strongly suggests a marked cholestatic effect from this association; therefore, women taking oral contraceptives should avoid taking troleandomycin.

Summary: The use of troleandomycin in women taking oral contraceptive agents has caused jaundice.

Related Drugs: Documentation is lacking describing a similar interaction with the other macrolide antibiotics.

Mechanism: The explanation for jaundice associated with troleandomycin is not known.

Detailed Information: See *EDI,* 8/97.00

Vidarabine-Allopurinol

Significance: 2—moderately clinically significant

Recommendations: Until further information concerning this interaction is available, caution is warranted when these two drugs are used simultaneously.

Summary: There are data to show that coadministration of allopurinol and vidarabine may cause severe neurotoxicity.

Related Drugs: There are no drugs related to allopurinol or vidarabine.

Mechanism: Inhibition of xanthine oxidase by allopurinol could increase the drug levels of vidarabine, producing adverse effects.

Detailed Information: See *EDI,* 8/99.00

Zidovudine-Acetaminophen

Significance: 3—minimally clinically significant

Potential Effects: Concomitant use of these agents may result in neutropenia and/or changes in zidovudine serum levels.

Recommendations: Patients on zidovudine therapy should be closely monitored for symptoms of toxicity when acetaminophen is added to the regimen. The dosage of zidovudine may have to be adjusted.

Summary: There are data to show that concomitant use of these agents may result in neutropenia and changes in zidovudine serum levels. There are no significant changes in acetaminophen serum levels.

Related Drugs: There are no drugs related to zidovudine or acetaminophen.

Mechanism: Acetaminophen and zidovudine are both metabolized by hepatic glucuronidation, and this could explain the decreased zidovudine plasma levels after acetaminophen administration.

Detailed Information: See *EDI,* 8/100.10

Zidovudine-Acyclovir

Significance: 3—minimally clinically significant

Potential Effects: The concurrent use of zidovudine and acyclovir may result in increased lethargy and decreased alertness.

Recommendations: Since it is likely these two agents will be administered concurrently because herpes simplex infections are common in AIDS patients, patients should be observed for increased lethargy and decreased alertness. If this effect occurs, acyclovir may need to be discontinued.

Summary: There are data to show that coadministration of these agents can produce dramatic lethargy and fatigue.

Related Drugs: There are no drugs related to zidovudine or acyclovir.

Mechanism: The mechanism of this interaction is not known.

Detailed Information: See *EDI,* 8/101.00

Zidovudine-Probenecid

Significance: 2—moderately clinically significant

Potential Effects: Probenecid will decrease the metabolism of zidovudine, resulting in increased zidovudine levels.

Recommendations: The use of concomitant zidovudine and probenecid should be approached with caution. The patient should be monitored for increased levels of zidovudine and its active metabolite. The dose of zidovudine may need to be reduced.

Summary: Probenecid may inhibit the metabolism of zidovudine, causing increased zidovudine levels.

Related Drugs: It is not known whether a similar interaction would occur between zidovudine and sulfinpyrazone. There are no drugs related to zidovudine.

Mechanism: The mechanism may be due to inhibition of zidovudine glucuronidation by probenecid.

Detailed Information: See *EDI*, 8/105.00

Chapter Nine

Antineoplastic
Drug Interactions

Bleomycin-Cisplatin

Significance: 3—minimally clinically significant

Potential Effects: Bleomycin total clearance may decrease during successive cycles of concurrent administration with cisplatin as cumulative doses of cisplatin increase.

Recommendations: Patients receiving concurrent therapy with bleomycin and cisplatin should be monitored closely for cisplatin-induced changes in renal function, which may alter the clearance of bleomycin. The bleomycin dosage may need to be adjusted.

Summary: Bleomycin total clearance decreased during successive cycles of concurrent administration with cisplatin as cumulative doses of cisplatin increased. Greater effects appeared to occur at cisplatin doses greater than 300mg/m, although this relationship was not proven to be statistically significant. Bleomycin toxicity was not observed.

Related Drugs: It is not known if a similar interaction would be expected to occur between bleomycin and carboplatin. There are no drugs related to bleomycin.

Mechanism: It is postulated that cisplatin administration results in changes in renal function that alter the elimination of bleomycin, although nonrenal mechanisms for the decrease are not ruled out. It has been shown that cisplatin-induced renal damage persists even when serum creatinine values return to normal. Also, serious renal dysfunction has reportedly occurred in children who receive long-term therapy with cisplatin.

Detailed Information: See *EDI*, 9/0.50

Carmustine-Cimetidine

Significance: 2—moderately clinically significant

Recommendations: Patients receiving these agents concurrently should be monitored for the appearance of bone marrow suppression. If suppression is detected, cimetidine should be discontinued.

Summary: There are data to show that concomitant cimetidine and carmustine have an additive bone marrow depressant effect.

Related Drugs: There are no published reports of an additive effect between other antineoplastic nitrosoureas and cimetidine. It is unknown whether ranitidine would interact similarly.

Mechanism: Both drugs have bone marrow suppressant properties which would appear to be additive during cotherapy.

Detailed Information: See *EDI*, 9/1.00

Cyclophosphamide-Allopurinol

Significance: 2—moderately clinically significant

Recommendations: The routine prophylactic use of allopurinol to prevent hyperuricemia may not be advisable during chemotherapy with alkylating agents. Patients who receive these drugs concurrently should be monitored for signs of bone marrow depression (leukopenia, thrombocytopenia, and pancytopenia).

Summary: The concurrent administration of cyclophosphamide and allopurinol may enhance the bone marrow depression induced by cyclophosphamide; however, all data do not support this.

Related Drugs: No specific interactions have been reported with other alkylating agents. There are no drugs related to allopurinol.

Mechanism: The mechanism is unknown; however, allopurinol does affect liver enzyme systems, and cyclophosphamide undergoes hepatic oxidation.

Detailed Information: See *EDI*, 9/3.00

Cyclophosphamide-Chloramphenicol

Significance: 2—moderately clinically significant

Recommendations: Cyclophosphamide must be converted to active metabolites to produce its antineoplastic activity. Therefore, concomitant administration with chloramphenicol may delay or partially inhibit cyclophosphamide's antineoplastic activity. This interaction is clinically significant and should be avoided.

Summary: Chloramphenicol has been shown to inhibit the metabolism of cyclophosphamide.

Related Drugs: There are no drugs related to cyclophosphamide or chloramphenicol.

Mechanism: Chloramphenicol is thought to inhibit the hepatic biotransformation of cyclophosphamide.

Detailed Information: See *EDI*, 9/4.10

Cyclophosphamide-Indomethacin

Significance: 3—minimally clinically significant

Potential Effects: Concurrent use of these agents may result in water intoxication.

Recommendations: Concurrent indomethacin and low-dose cyclophosphamide therapy should be approached with caution because of the possibility of acute water intoxication. Appropriate supportive measures should be employed if water intoxication occurs.

Summary: Concurrent administration of indomethacin and cyclophosphamide induced acute water intoxication.

Related Drugs: An interaction may occur between cyclophosphamide and other NSAIAs. It is not known whether an interaction may occur between indomethacin and other antineoplastic alkylating agents.

Mechanism: Inhibition of prostaglandins may result in an increase in anti-diuretic hormone, which may have precipitated the water intoxication.

Detailed Information: See *EDI*, 9/5.10

Cyclophosphamide Fluorouracil-Hydrochlorothiazide Methotrexate

Significance: 3—minimally clinically significant

Recommendations: Patients' neutrophil counts should be monitored closely during concurrent use of these agents. If neutropenia develops, the dose of the thiazide diuretic may need to be lowered or the drug discontinued.

Summary: The concurrent use of hydrochlorothiazide and cancer chemotherapy combinations have resulted in granulocytopenia.

Related Drugs: The same interaction was shown to occur with chlorothiazide and trichlormethiazide. A similar interaction may occur with all thiazide diuretics and thiazide-related diuretics.

Mechanism: The mechanism is unknown.

Detailed Information: See *EDI*, 9/5.00

Cyclophosphamide-Methotrexate

Significance: 3—minimally clinically significant

Recommendations: Although further clinical studies are necessary, clinicians should be aware of the possibility of decreased levels of the active metabolites of cyclophosphamide.

Summary: The concurrent administration of methotrexate and cyclophosphamide may result in the inhibition of the metabolism of cyclophosphamide.

Related Drugs: There are no drugs related to cyclophosphamide or methotrexate.

Mechanism: Methotrexate may inhibit the metabolism of cyclophosphamide, decreasing the formation of the active metabolites of cyclophosphamide.

Detailed Information: See *EDI*, 9/6.01

Cyclophosphamide-Prednisone

Significance: 3—minimally clinically significant

Recommendations: Administration of concomitant prednisolone and cyclophosphamide appears not to significantly alter the metabolism of cyclophosphamide. Although the concurrent administration of these agents is often utilized as therapy for various malignancies, concomitant prednisone use may necessitate an increase in cyclophosphamide dosage.

Summary: The concurrent administration of oral cyclophosphamide and prednisone resulted in no difference in cyclophosphamide half-life.

Related Drugs: The metabolism of cyclophosphamide was not altered by the concomitant administration of prednisolone; however, it has also been shown to immediately prolong cyclophosphamide half-life. It is difficult to determine the influence of other corticosteroids on cyclophosphamide disposition.

Mechanism: The increased metabolism of cyclophosphamide is thought to result from the induction of hepatic enzymes by prednisone.

Detailed Information: See *EDI*, 9/6.10

Doxorubicin-Phenobarbital

Significance: 3—minimally clinically significant

Recommendations: Although it was not determined if the efficacy of doxorubicin was decreased with concurrent phenobarbital, patients should be monitored, as the dose of doxorubicin may need to be increased to obtain optimal drug efficacy.

Summary: There are data to show that coadministration of these agents may potentially result in a decrease in the therapeutic effect of doxorubicin.

Related Drugs: It may be expected that all barbiturates would interact similarly with doxorubicin. Daunorubicin may be expected to interact also.

Mechanism: Phenobarbital, because of hepatic microsomal enzyme induction, may affect the metabolism of doxorubicin.

Detailed Information: See *EDI*, 9/6.21

Etoposide-Cyclosporine

Significance: 2—moderately clinically significant

Potential Effects: Concurrent administration of cyclosporine and etoposide may result in a decrease in etoposide clearance and an increase in etoposide levels. Cyclosporine may also increase the sensitivity of certain multidrug-resistant cell lines to etoposide.

Recommendations: In patients receiving concurrent therapy with etoposide and high-dose cyclosporine, etoposide dosages should be reduced 50%. Dosages may need further adjustment in patients with renal or hepatic impairment.

Summary: Concurrent administration of cyclosporine resulted in a decrease in etoposide clearance and an increase in etoposide levels. Cyclosporine may increase the etoposide sensitivity of certain multidrug-resistant cell lines.

Related Drugs: A similar interaction has occurred with the concomitant administration of cyclosporine and teniposide; however, there was significant interpatient variation. There are no drugs related to cyclosporine.

Mechanism: It is postulated that cyclosporine decreases etoposide P-gp-mediated excretion in the brush border of the proximal renal tubule and luminal surface of the biliary tract in the liver, thus explaining the decrease in both renal and nonrenal clearance of etoposide. Cyclosporine may also inhibit etoposide metabolism at the P-450 isoenzyme system.

Detailed Information: See *EDI*, 9/6.26

Fluorouracil-Cimetidine

Significance: 3—minimally clinically significant

Recommendations: Until further clinical studies are done, the concurrent administration of these two agents should be used with caution. If signs of 5-fluorouracil toxicity develop (e.g., stomatitis or esophagopharyngitis, rapidly falling white blood cell count, leukopenia, gastrointestinal effects), the dose of 5-fluorouracil may need to be decreased.

Summary: There are data to show that coadministration of these agents did not exhibit any significant pharmacokinetic alterations; however, use of these agents concomitantly should be done with caution.

Related Drugs: A similar interaction may occur with floxuridine. A similar interaction is not expected to occur between 5-fluorouracil and other H_2-receptor antagonists, if the mechanism involves hepatic enzyme inhibition by cimetidine.

Mechanism: The interaction between 5-fluorouracil and cimetidine may result from a reduction in liver blood flow caused by cimetidine or from cimetidine's inhibition of the hepatic metabolism of 5-fluorouracil.

Detailed Information: See *EDI*, 9/6.30

Interleukin-2–Dexamethasone

Significance: 2—moderately clinically significant

Potential Effects: Concurrent use of these agents may result in a decrease in the antitumor effectiveness of interleukin-2.

Recommendations: Because concurrent use of dexamethasone with interleukin-2 may reduce the antitumor effectiveness of interleukin-2, the concurrent use of these agents should be avoided.

Summary: Concurrent interleukin-2 and dexamethasone may result in a decreased interleukin-2 antineoplastic effect.

Related Drugs: A similar interaction may occur between interleukin-2 and other corticosteroids. There are no drugs related to interleukin-2.

Mechanism: The mechanism of this interaction is not known, but it may be related to the immunosuppressive effects of dexamethasone on interleukin-2-induced tumor necrosis factor synthesis.

Detailed Information: See *EDI*, 9/6.60

Lomustine-Theophylline

Significance: 3—minimally clinically significant

Recommendations: Evidence is insufficient to indicate that theophylline should not be used concurrently with lomustine, although one should be aware that thrombocytopenia and myelotoxicity are possible during combined therapy with these agents.

Summary: A patient receiving theophylline and lomustine for medulloblastoma developed epistaxis and thrombocytopenia.

Related Drugs: There have been no reports of similar interactions with theophylline and other alkylating agents. A synergistic effect was seen with theophylline and carmustine in mice. A similar interaction is expected to occur with other theophylline derivatives. Dyphylline may also be expected to interact with lomustine.

Mechanism: The mechanism is unknown, but it has been suggested that theophylline may disrupt normal platelet function.

Detailed Information: See *EDI*, 9/7.00

Melphalan-Cyclosporine

Significance: 2—moderately clinically significant

Recommendations: Since renal impairment may occur with the concomitant use of cyclosporine and melphalan, patients' renal function should be closely monitored when these agents are administered concurrently.

Summary: There are data to show that coadministration of cyclosporine and melphalan may lead to the development of severe renal failure; however, some patients experienced mild, or no, renal failure.

Related Drugs: There are no drugs related to melphalan or cyclosporine.

Mechanism: The mechanism of this interaction is unknown; however, it may involve a direct effect on the kidney rather than an effect on the absorption or metabolism of cyclosporine. Both of these agents have been documented to cause renal impairment alone.

Detailed Information: See *EDI*, 9/8.10

Mercaptopurine-Allopurinol

Significance: 1—highly clinically significant

Potential Effects: Allopurinol decreases the first-pass metabolism of mercaptopurine, resulting in an increase in mercaptopurine serum levels and toxic effects.

Recommendations: The initial dose of oral mercaptopurine should be reduced to one-third or one-fourth of the presently recommended dosage level when allopurinol is administered concurrently. Subsequent adjustments of mercaptopurine dosages should be made on the basis of clinical response and/or toxicity.

Summary: The concurrent administration of mercaptopurine and allopurinol has been shown to result in a clinically significant increase in the pharmacologic and toxic effects of mercaptopurine.

Related Drugs: Azathioprine has been shown to interact with allopurinol. There are no drugs related to allopurinol.

Mechanism: Mercaptopurine metabolite is catalyzed by the enzyme xanthine oxidase, and allopurinol inhibits the action of xanthine oxidase, reducing the rate of mercaptopurine inactivation and resulting in higher blood levels.

Detailed Information: See *EDI*, 9/9.00

Methotrexate-Alcohol, Ethyl

Significance: 3—minimally clinically significant

Recommendations: Because of the possibility that ethyl alcohol may increase the hepatotoxic potential of methotrexate, patients receiving this drug should be advised to minimize consumption of products containing ethyl alcohol.

Summary: Concurrent methotrexate therapy and ethyl alcohol consumption may lead to greater incidence of hepatotoxicity.

Related Drugs: Benzyl alcohol, a preservative in some methotrexate preparations, has been implicated as a contributor to neurologic side effects when methotrexate is administered intrathecally. Preservative-free parenteral preparations should be used for the intrathecal route of administration.

Mechanism: A specific mechanism for a methotrexate and ethyl alcohol interaction is not known. It has been observed that high concentrations of ethyl alcohol weakly inhibit transport and may lead to higher intrahepatic concentrations of methotrexate.

Detailed Information: See *EDI*, 9/11.00

Methotrexate-Aspirin

Significance: 1—highly clinically significant

Recommendations: Administration of aspirin should be avoided in patients receiving methotrexate when an acceptable alternative drug is available. Acetaminophen has been used concurrently with methotrexate without causing an increase in methotrexate toxicity. If concurrent administration is necessary, the patient should be observed closely for methotrexate toxicity.

Summary: The concurrent administration of methotrexate and aspirin may result in elevated or prolonged serum concentrations of methotrexate, increasing toxicity.

Related Drugs: All salicylates and their combination products may interact with methotrexate. There are no drugs related to methotrexate.

Mechanism: Aspirin is capable of displacing methotrexate from plasma proteins *in vitro*, and methotrexate and aspirin have a common elimination pathway. Aspirin may compete with, and inhibit, methotrexate elimination.

Detailed Information: See *EDI*, 9/13.00

Methotrexate-Cisplatin

Significance: 2—moderately clinically significant

Potential Effects: Pretreatment with cisplatin may increase the incidence of methotrexate toxicity.

Recommendations: Because of the possible serious nature of this interaction, extreme caution should be exercised when using these agents concurrently. Methotrexate levels and blood counts should be carefully monitored.

Summary: Administration of methotrexate following pretreatment with cisplatin resulted in methotrexate toxicity and death. Severe stomatitis, myelosuppression and renal failure were observed.

Related Drugs: It is not known if cisplatin would interact with the other antineoplastic antimetabolites. There are no drugs related to cisplatin.

Mechanism: The mechanism is not known.

Detailed Information: See *EDI*, 9/14.10

Methotrexate-Cytarabine

Significance: 3—minimally clinically significant

Potential Effects: Concurrent use of these agents may result in enhanced cell-kill. Methotrexate may also increase mercaptopurine levels.

Recommendations: Although there are inconclusive reports regarding this interaction, patients receiving concurrent methotrexate and cytarabine should be closely monitored. Concurrent methotrexate and topical fluorouracil should be avoided.

Summary: Administration of cytarabine before initiation of methotrexate therapy enhances methotrexate. Conversely, the cytarabine can be enhanced when methotrexate is administered before the initiation of cytarabine therapy.

Related Drugs: Methotrexate was found to increase mercaptopurine's area-under-curve and levels. Fluorouracil 2% cream was shown to cause erythema, blisters and necrosis when administered with methotrexate. It is not known if methotrexate would enhance the cell-kill of the other antineoplastic antimetabolites.

Mechanism: Many factors are involved in the mechanism of the interaction of these two chemotherapeutic agents. These include the order of administration of the agents, the time interval between administration and the complexities of the enzyme-substrate system within a given patient. Thus the exact outcome of the interaction can be variable from patient to patient.

Detailed Information: See *EDI,* 9/15.00

Methotrexate-Etretinate

Significance: 2—moderately clinically significant

Potential Effects: Concurrent use of these agents may result in hepatotoxicity.

Recommendations: Monitor drug levels and hepatic function when these agents are coadministered. The dosage of one or both agents may need to be changed.

Summary: There are data to show that coadministration of these agents results in hepatotoxicity; however, not all data support this. An absence of significant side effects and no evidence of hepatotoxicity have been documented.

Related Drugs: A similar interaction may occur between methotrexate and isotretinoin.

Mechanism: Increased hepatotoxicity may be due to an additive effect of these two potentially hepatotoxic agents. Etretinate may also interfere with the metabolism or excretion of methotrexate.

Detailed Information: See *EDI,* 9/16.05

Methotrexate-Ketoprofen

Significance: 2—moderately clinically significant

Potential Effects: Ketoprofen may increase methotrexate levels, leading to serious methotrexate toxicity.

Recommendations: Avoid using these agents together. If ketoprofen is to be administered, it should not be given for at least 24 hours after the last methotrexate dose.

Summary: Simultaneous administration of ketoprofen was associated with prolonged and striking enhancement of serum methotrexate levels.

Related Drugs: Indomethacin, ibuprofen and diclofenac were shown to increase methotrexate levels, potentiating toxicity. Phenylbutazone therapy has been shown to cause fever, oral ulcerations, severe bone marrow suppression, and septicemia when given with methotrexate. A similar interaction may occur between methotrexate and the other NSAIAs. There are no drugs related to methotrexate.

Mechanism: This interaction may be explained by the inhibition of renal prostaglandin synthesis by ketoprofen, which decreases renal perfusion rate and inhibits methotrexate clearance. Competitive renal secretion of these two drugs may be another explanation.

Detailed Information: See *EDI,* 9/16.10

Methotrexate-Leucovorin

Significance: 1—highly clinically significant

Recommendations: The evidence shows that leucovorin reverses methotrexate-induced inhibition of folic acid antagonism. Beneficial results in some diseases are obtained by intramuscular or intravenous methotrexate administration followed by intramuscular leucovorin. The optimal interval between the administration of the two drugs is six hours or less. Effective leucovorin doses have ranged from 4 to 12mg. Methotrexate dosage can be greater than usual (up to 600mg/Kg) when consecutive leucovorin administration is used.

Summary: Methotrexate toxicity can be greatly reduced by consecutive administration of leucovorin within six hours. "Leucovorin rescue" can be accomplished while maintaining the therapeutic effectiveness of methotrexate against tumors.

Related Drugs: There are no drugs related to methotrexate or leucovorin.

Mechanism: Methotrexate is a folic acid antagonist. Leucovorin is an active metabolite of folic acid.

Detailed Information: See *EDI,* 9/17.00

Methotrexate-Neomycin

Significance: 2—moderately clinically significant

Recommendations: Patients should be monitored during concurrent use of these agents. An increased dose of methotrexate may be necessary, or, in the case of kanamycin, the dose of methotrexate may need to be reduced.

Summary: The concurrent use of oral neomycin and methotrexate has resulted in a reduced methotrexate absorption, necessitating an increased methotrexate dose.

Related Drugs: Paromomycin also reduced the absorption of methotrexate. Kanamycin has been reported to increase methotrexate plasma levels. There are no drugs related to methotrexate.

Mechanism: Neomycin is known to produce malabsorption of many drugs, and this may be the mechanism here; however, further study is needed.

Detailed Information: See *EDI,* 9/19.00

Methotrexate-Omeprazole

Significance: 2—moderately clinically significant

Potential Effects: Increased methotrexate levels may result with concurrent administration of omeprazole.

Recommendations: Omeprazole should be withdrawn in patients several days prior to methotrexate therapy to avoid methotrexate toxicity.

Summary: Increased methotrexate levels may result with concurrent administration of omeprazole, a case report suggested.

Related Drugs: Although documentation is lacking, based on the proposed mechanism a similar interaction may be expected to occur between methotrexate and lansoprazole. It is not known whether a similar interaction would occur between omeprazole and other folic acid antagonists related to methotrexate (trimetrexate and aminopterin).

Mechanism: It is postulated that omeprazole may inhibit the active secretion of methotrexate from the kidney.

Detailed Information: See *EDI*, 9/20.00

Methotrexate-Probenecid

Significance: 1—highly clinically significant

Recommendations: Although the concurrent use of these agents need not be avoided, it is important to monitor methotrexate plasma levels and lower the dose of methotrexate when necessary.

Summary: The concurrent use of methotrexate and probenecid leads to a marked increase in serum methotrexate levels.

Related Drugs: There are no drugs related to methotrexate. A similar interaction may occur between methotrexate and sulfinpyrazone if the mechanism involves inhibition of renal tubular transport.

Mechanism: Probenecid may inhibit the excretion of methotrexate by the renal and biliary routes, and displacement of methotrexate from plasma albumin binding sites by probenecid may also contribute.

Detailed Information: See *EDI*, 9/21.00

Methotrexate-Procarbazine

Significance: 2—moderately clinically significant

Potential Effects: Procarbazine may predispose patients to nephrotoxicity with concurrent methotrexate.

Recommendations: Consideration should be given to allowing an interval of at least 72 hours between the administration of the final dose of procarbazine and the initiation of high-dose methotrexate therapy. Renal function should be closely monitored, and methotrexate therapy may need to be modified or discontinued.

Summary: Concurrent therapy with high-dose methotrexate and procarbazine may increase the nephrotoxicity of methotrexate.

Related Drugs: It is not known if an interaction would occur between metho-trexate and other MAOIs. There are no drugs related to methotrexate.

Mechanism: Procarbazine may have a transient effect on the kidneys and alter the renal excretion of methotrexate. If the excretion of methotrexate is delayed, there will be further impairment of renal function.

Detailed Information: See *EDI*, 9/22.10

Methotrexate-Sodium Bicarbonate

Significance: 3—minimally clinically significant

Recommendations: Although urinary alkalinization with an agent such as sodium bicarbonate is used in high-dose methotrexate therapy, it is important to monitor the patient for decreased methotrexate levels.

Summary: Sodium bicarbonate has been shown to increase the renal elimination of methotrexate.

Related Drugs: There are no drugs related to methotrexate. If the mechanism deals with urinary alkalinization, then other agents capable of alkalinizing the urine may be expected to interact similarly.

Mechanism: A urinary pH greater than 8.0 may result in a significant increase in the urinary elimination rate of methotrexate.

Detailed Information: See *EDI,* 9/23.00

Methotrexate-Sulfamethoxazole, Trimethoprim

Significance: 1—highly clinically significant

Potential Effects: The use of these agents together can induce folate deficiency, leading to megaloblastic anemia.

Recommendations: If these agents are used together, the patient's hematologic status should be monitored closely for signs of folate deficiency anemia. The administration of folic acid may be considered.

Summary: There are data to show that coadministration of these agents can induce folate deficiency, leading to megaloblastic anemia. Sulfamethoxazole and trimethoprim have been shown to alter the pharmacokinetics of methotrexate; however, all data do not support this.

Related Drugs: Methotrexate plasma protein binding and renal clearance have been shown to be decreased by sulfisoxazole. A similar interaction may occur between methotrexate and other sulfonamides. There are no drugs related to methotrexate.

Mechanism: Methotrexate and cotrimoxazole act synergistically to produce significant folate deficiency, leading to megaloblastic changes.

Detailed Information: See *EDI,* 9/25.00

Mitomycin-Etoposide

Significance: 3—minimally clinically significant

Potential Effects: The concurrent use of these agents may result in dyspnea, tachycardia, and diaphoresis.

Recommendations: Until further studies are done to confirm the occurrence of this interaction, no specific recommendations can be made with regard to this therapy. However, it is prudent to be aware of the possible sudden dyspnea that may occur with concurrent mitomycin and etoposide.

Summary: There are data to show that coadministration of these agents may lead to dyspnea, tachycardia, diaphoresis, and the absence of bronchospasm or rales.

Related Drugs: There are no drugs related to mitomycin or etoposide.

Mechanism: The mechanism of this interaction is not known.

Detailed Information: See *EDI,* 9/26.01

Mitomycin-Vinblastine

Significance: 2—moderately clinically significant

Potential Effects: The concomitant use of these agents may result in pulmonary toxicity. It has been stated that the incidence of abrupt pulmonary toxicity with this combination is 3% to 6%.

Recommendations: Patients receiving these agents should be closely monitored for pulmonary toxicity. If this occurs, bronchodilators or mechanical support may be required. Continuing concomitant therapy in these patients should be avoided.

Summary: Several case studies have reported the occurrence of pulmonary toxicity in patients receiving combination therapy with mitomycin and vinblastine for lung cancer.

Related Drugs: A similar interaction may occur between mitomycin and vincristine. There are no drugs related to mitomycin.

Mechanism: Pulmonary edema resulting from the administration of mitomycin and vinblastine may be the underlying mechanism.

Detailed Information: See *EDI*, 9/27.00

Mitotane-Spironolactone

Significance: 2—moderately clinically significant

Potential Effects: Concurrent mitotane and spironolactone administration may result in antagonism of the therapeutic effectiveness of mitotane.

Recommendations: The therapeutic effectiveness of mitotane should be closely monitored in patients receiving these agents concurrently. Alternative therapy may need to be considered.

Summary: Concurrent mitotane and spironolactone administration resulted in antagonism of the therapeutic effectiveness of mitotane.

Related Drugs: An interaction may be expected to occur between mitotane and the other potassium-sparing diuretics.

Mechanism: The mechanism is not known, but it has been postulated that spironolactone may reverse patients' hypokalemia with probable adrenocortical hyperplasia.

Detailed Information: See *EDI*, 9/28.30

Paclitaxel-Cisplatin

Significance: 2—moderately clinically significant

Potential Effects: The sequence of administration of paclitaxel and cisplatin may affect efficacy and the severity of neutropenic side effects.

Recommendations: In chemotherapy regimens that include both paclitaxel and cisplatin, paclitaxel should be administered prior to cisplatin. Consideration should be given to administering paclitaxel prior to the concurrent administration of paclitaxel and cisplatin.

Summary: The sequence of administration of paclitaxel and cisplatin may affect efficacy and the severity of neutropenic side effects. Additive cytotoxic effects were seen *in vitro* when paclitaxel was administered prior to cisplatin. Antagonistic effects were seen when cisplatin was administered prior to paclitaxel. Synergistic cell kills may occur when paclitaxel is administered before concurrent administration of paclitaxel and cisplatin. In one *in vitro* study, the administration of combination paclitaxel and cisplatin significantly increased cell kills over those produced by cisplatin alone only when cisplatin followed paclitaxel, not when paclitaxel followed cisplatin. In an *in vivo* dose escalating study, the administration of cisplatin prior to paclitaxel resulted in more profound neutropenia than when the order was reversed. Paclitaxel clearance was 20% lower when paclitaxel was administered following cisplatin than prior to cisplatin.

Related Drugs: Concurrent administration of carboplatin and paclitaxel or the administration of paclitaxel followed by carboplatin
has been shown to be more effective than the administration of
carboplatin followed by paclitaxel. However, conflicting data are
available. Based on the proposed mechanism and pharmacologic similarity, a similar interaction may be expected to occur
between docetaxol and cisplatin.

Mechanism: Paclitaxel's cytotoxic effects are thought to result from
its effects on the microtubules that are present during mitosis.
Administration of cisplatin prior to paclitaxel is thought to
decrease the number of cells entering mitosis, thereby decreasing the cytotoxic effects of paclitaxel. Administration of paclitaxel
following cisplatin has been shown to result in a decrease in
paclitaxel clearance, which may be responsible for the increase
in severity of neutropenia.

Detailed Information: See *EDI,* 9/28.50

Vinblastine-Erythromycin

Significance: 3—minimally clinically significant

Potential Effects: The concurrent administration of these agents
may lead to increased vinblastine toxicity.

Recommendations: It is recommended that patients receiving vinblastine therapy should not be administered concurrent erythromycin. If these agents are given together, the toxicity
observed may be typical of much higher doses of vinblastine.

Summary: Concurrent vinblastine and erythromycin resulted in
severe neutropenia and myalgia.

Related Drugs: It is not known whether an interaction would occur
between vinblastine and the other macrolide antibiotic agents. A
similar interaction may be expected to occur between erythromycin and the other vinca alkaloids.

Mechanism: Erythromycin has been reported to potentiate a number
of drugs by interference with cytochrome P450-mediated metabolism, and vinblastine or vindesine metabolism has been shown
to be mediated by cytochrome P450 isozymes. Inhibition of the
cytochrome P450-mediated metabolism of vinblastine by erythromycin is likely the mechanism for the observed interaction.

Detailed Information: See *EDI,* 9/30.00

Chapter Ten

Antipsychotic and Antianxiety Drug Interactions

Alprazolam-Fluoxetine

Significance: 2—moderately clinically significant

Potential Effects: Fluoxetine may decrease the metabolism of alprazolam, resulting in increased effects of alprazolam.

Recommendations: The dose of benzodiazepines which undergo extensive phase I hepatic metabolism may need to be lowered in patients receiving therapy with selective serotonin reuptake inhibitors or nefazodone.

Summary: Concurrent administration of alprazolam and fluoxetine resulted in decreased clearance and increased effects of alprazolam.

Related Drugs: Fluoxetine has been reported to interact with diazepam and clonazepam. Fluvoxamine significantly interacted with diazepam and alprazolam. A study with triazolam and fluoxetine could not be evaluated for an interaction. Paroxetine has been reported to not significantly interact with oxazepam. Sertraline decreased diazepam clearance in one report by 13%. Nefazodone interacted with both alprazolam and triazolam, while venlafaxine did not interact with diazepam. If the mechanism involves inhibition of benzodiazepine metabolism, then the benzodiazepines metabolized by phase I reactions would be expected to interact similarly. An interaction with the benzodiazepines metabolized by phase II reactions is not likely to occur.

Mechanism: It is thought that fluoxetine decreased the hepatic metabolism of diazepam, decreasing the clearance and increasing the half-life. The selective-serotonin reuptake inhibitors and nefazodone may decrease the metabolism of phase I hepatically metabolized benzodiazepines through competitive inhibition at the cytochrome P450 site.

Detailed Information: See *EDI,* 10/0.04

Buspirone-Cimetidine

Significance: 4—not clinically significant

Potential Effects: Cimetidine does not markedly alter any pharmacokinetic parameters of buspirone.

Recommendations: Since a clinically significant interaction between buspirone and cimetidine is unlikely, buspirone may be considered as an alternative antianxiety agent.

Summary: In one study, concurrent administration of cimetidine and buspirone did not alter the pharmacokinetic profile of buspirone.

Related Drugs: Although documentation is lacking, buspirone would also not be expected to interact with the other H_2 receptor antagonists.

Mechanism: The administration of cimetidine did not markedly alter any pharmacokinetic parameters of buspirone.

Detailed Information: See *EDI,* 10/0.07

Chlordiazepoxide-Ketoconazole

Significance: 3—minimally clinically significant

Potential Effects: Concurrent administration of imidazole antimycotics with phase I metabolized benzodiazepines may result in decreased clearance of benzodiazepines and increased levels and clinical effects of benzodiazepines.

Recommendations: Patients should be observed for an increase in the effects of chlordiazepoxide or other phase I metabolized benzodiazepines. The dose of these benzodiazepines may need to be decreased.

Summary: Concurrent ketoconazole administration resulted in a decrease of chlordiazepoxide clearance and volume of distribution.

Related Drugs: Both ketoconazole and itraconazole have been reported to interact with triazolam and midazolam. Based on the postulated mechanism, the other benzodiazepines that are metabolized by phase I reactions may also be expected to interact with ketoconazole and itraconazole, although documentation is lacking. Due to structural and pharmacologic similarity, chlordiazepoxide, triazolam, and midazolam may be expected to interact with the other imidazole antifungal agents.

Mechanism: Ketoconazole has been shown to be a potent inhibitor of the cytochrome P450$_{3A4}$ enzyme system, thus blocking the metabolism of chlodiazepoxide. Before this induction occurs, the ketoconazole may compete with the chlordiazepoxide for transport, thereby increasing the volume of distribution and decreasing clearance.

Detailed Information: See *EDI*, 10/0.10

Chlorpromazine-Alcohol, Ethyl

Significance: 2—moderately clinically significant

Recommendations: Patients receiving chlorpromazine should be warned that alcohol ingestion may produce enhanced CNS depression. Concurrent use may impair their ability to drive an automobile and operate hazardous machinery. Oral prescription and nonprescription products containing alcohol, as well as alcoholic beverages, should be used with caution.

Summary: Concurrent use of chlorpromazine and alcohol may cause an intensification of the CNS depression of each drug. Alcohol may precipitate extrapyramidal reactions.

Related Drugs: Thioridazine may produce less CNS depression in combination with alcohol. Other phenothiazines, thioxanthenes, butyrophenones, dihydroindolones and dibenzoxazepines may interact in a similar manner.

Mechanism: Alcohol may precipitate extrapyramidal reactions in patients on phenothiazines by inducing a temporary brain dysfunction.

Detailed Information: See *EDI*, 10/1.00

Chlorpromazine-Aluminum Hydroxide, Magnesium Hydroxide

Significance: 3—minimally clinically significant

Recommendations: It is not known whether magnesium hydroxide and aluminum hydroxide alone have an effect on chlorpromazine absorption, but documentation indicates the combination of ingredients did alter chlorpromazine absorption. Therefore, until further clinical evidence is available, antacid products containing aluminum hydroxide and magnesium hydroxide, or those containing magnesium trisilicate, should be administered one hour before or two hours after chlorpromazine administration.

Summary: Chlorpromazine absorption from the gastrointestinal tract may be altered by the simultaneous administration of antacids.

Related Drugs: Other phenothiazines, thioxanthenes, butyrophenones, dihydroindolones and dibenzoxazepines may interact. Trisilicate gel antacids have been shown to decrease chlorpromazine levels, whereas calcium carbonate-glycine antacids do not.

Mechanism: Administration of aluminum and magnesium containing antacids decreases the gastrointestinal absorption and serum levels of chlorpromazine.

Detailed Information: See *EDI*, 10/3.00

Chlorpromazine-Amphetamine

Significance: 2—moderately clinically significant

Potential Effects: These agents may exert opposing effects on monoaminergic function in the central and peripheral nervous system if used concurrently.

Recommendations: Simultaneous use of chlorpromazine and amphetamine should be restricted to treating amphetamine overdose cases. A chlorpromazine dose of 1mg/Kg intramuscularly has been recommended. This may be followed by 0.5mg/Kg intramuscularly after 30 minutes if necessary to control recurrence of excitement. Conversely, overdosage with chlorpromazine generally is best managed with supportive measures alone.

Summary: Chlorpromazine and amphetamine are pharmacologic antagonists. These two drugs exert opposing effects on monoaminergic function in the central and peripheral nervous system. This antagonistic relationship has been utilized clinically in the management of amphetamine overdosage. Inclusion of either agent in a therapeutic regimen of the other could prove counterproductive. The amphetamines may antagonize the antipsychotic effect of the phenothiazine.

Related Drugs: Chlorpromazine is a multifunctional antagonist to several neurotransmitters. Other phenothiazines exhibit somewhat different potencies in their ability to interfere with the actions of norepinephrine or dopamine, the neurotransmitters generally believed involved in the stimulatory actions of amphetamine. Thus one would presume that other phenothiazine derivatives such as the thioxanthenes as well as the dihydroindolone and dibenzoxazepine would also exhibit antagonism of amphetamine actions with varying degrees of potency. Other antipsychotic agents such as haloperidol, a butyrophenone that possesses dopamine blocking activity and significant alpha-adrenergic blocking activity, may also effectively antagonize the actions of amphetamine. Other indirect-acting sympathomimetics as well as direct and mixed-acting sympathomimetics, which characteristically produce central and peripheral stimulation, would logically be expected to undergo antagonism by chlorpromazine.

Mechanism: The precise mechanism involved in the antagonism of amphet-amine by chlorpromazine is not known, but it appears to involve quite complex pharmacodynamic interplay with monoaminergic effector and control. Thioridazine has been associated with electrocardiogram repolarization abnormalities more frequently than other neuroleptics, and it has been reported to have induced ventricular arrhythmias and fatalities in some cases.

Detailed Information: See *EDI*, 10/5.00

Chlorpromazine-Benztropine

Significance: 2—moderately clinically significant

Recommendations: Use of benztropine should probably be reserved to treat those responsive aspects of extrapyramidal syndrome (EPS) that can arise during chlorpromazine therapy. Clinical evidence suggests that relatively short-term treatment (three to four months) with benztropine may suffice to effectively deal with drug-induced parkinsonism. Refractory EPS cases may be a result of suboptimal serum concentrations of anticholinergic medication. Additive anticholinergic actions of benztropine and chlorpromazine may be hazardous in angle closure glaucoma or in individuals hyperresponsive to parasympathetic blockade.

Summary: The interaction between chlorpromazine and benztropine is used in managing certain movement disorders resulting from the antipsychotic-induced extrapyramidal syndrome (EPS).

Related Drugs: Virtually all antipsychotic drugs are able to induce EPS to varying extents. Other phenothiazines, thioxanthenes, dihydroindolones and dibenzoxazepines are expected to interact in a similar manner with benztropine. Other anticholinergic drugs commonly used in the treatment of parkinsonism may be effective in treating chlorpromazine-induced parkinsonism.

Mechanism: Chlorpromazine-induced parkinsonism appears to arise from a functional increase of cholinergic activity secondary to dopamine receptor blockade.

Detailed Information: See *EDI*, 10/7.00

Chlorpromazine-Diazoxide

Significance: 2—moderately clinically significant

Recommendations: Patients' blood glucose should be closely monitored if chlorpromazine and diazoxide are to be used concurrently. The dose of diazoxide may need to be decreased.

Summary: A child on long-term diazoxide and bendroflumethiazide treatment developed severe hyperglycemia after administration of chlorpromazine.

Related Drugs: There are no drugs related to diazoxide. The phenothiazines, thioxanthenes, butyrophenones, dihydroindolones and dibenzoxazepines may interact in a similar manner with diazoxide.

Mechanism: The mechanism of this interaction is unknown; however, chlorpromazine has been reported to result in hyperglycemia.

Detailed Information: See *EDI*, 10/9.00

Chlorpromazine-Levodopa

Significance: 3—minimally clinically significant

Recommendations: The effect of levodopa and chlorpromazine on each other is unpredictable. In instances where no alternative drugs are available and both drugs must be used, the patient should be observed closely for a deterioration in levodopa's growth hormone stimulating or antiparkinsonian effects, or a decrease in the therapeutic effect of chlorpromazine.

Summary: Levodopa and chlorpromazine may antagonize each other when these drugs are administered together.

Related Drugs: Other phenothiazines, thioxanthenes, butyrophenones, dihydroindolones and dibenzoxazepines may interact in a similar manner with levodopa. There are no drugs related to levodopa.

Mechanism: Chlorpromazine and levodopa have opposing actions at central dopaminergic receptor sites.

Detailed Information: See *EDI*, 10/11.00

Chlorpromazine-Lithium Carbonate

Significance: 2—moderately clinically significant

Potential Effects: Lithium carbonate may cause a decrease in chlorpromazine levels. Neurotoxicity may also occur when these agents are used together.

Recommendations: Monitor patients for decreased chlorpromazine levels or neurotoxicity when these agents are used together. Dosage adjustments or discontinuation of one or both agents may be necessary.

Summary: Concurrent administration of chlorpromazine and lithium carbonate has been shown to decrease plasma chlorpromazine levels, and neurotoxic and/or somnambulistic episodes have been reported.

Related Drugs: There are no drugs related to lithium carbonate. Interactions between lithium carbonate and other antipsychotics are discussed in other monographs (see Lithium Carbonate-Haloperidol, page 241, and Lithium Carbonate-Thioridazine, page 245).

Mechanism: The decreased chlorpromazine levels may be due to a lithium-induced delay in gastric emptying, decreasing bioavailability of chlorpromazine, or to a decreased chlorpromazine absorption.

Detailed Information: See *EDI*, 10/13.00

Chlorpromazine-Phenobarbital

Significance: 3—minimally clinically significant

Recommendations: Since long-term administration of barbiturates might decrease the effectiveness of chlorpromazine by decreasing serum levels, the dosage of chlorpromazine may need to be increased. However, if the barbiturate is discontinued, chlorpromazine toxicity might result, and the dose would have to be readjusted.

Summary: The long-term administration of phenobarbital may decrease serum chlorpromazine levels, but no change in therapeutic response is documented.

Related Drugs: Chlorpromazine may enhance the action of some barbiturates. Other phenothiazines, thioxanthenes, butyrophenones, dihydroindolones and dibenzoxazepines may interact in a similar manner with phenobarbital.

Mechanism: Phenobarbital may increase the induction of hepatic microsomal enzymes, decreasing serum chlorpromazine levels. The sedative action of barbiturates is primarily the result of depression on the arousal system.

Detailed Information: See *EDI*, 10/15.00

Chlorpromazine-Piperazine

Significance: 3—minimally clinically significant

Recommendations: From analysis of the data available regarding the potential interaction between chlorpromazine and piperazine, this combination appears devoid of serious risk. Individuals receiving this combined therapy should be carefully monitored for any manifestations of seizure disorders. Renal dysfunction may impair elimination of piperazine and potentially enhance the ability of this drug to elicit toxicity or interact with chlorpromazine.

Summary: There has been a report of the concurrent use of chlorpromazine and piperazine leading to convulsions.

Related Drugs: There is a lack of documentation concerning a similar interaction with other phenothiazines, thioxanthenes, butyrophenones, dihydroindolones and dibenzoxazepines. There are no drugs related to piperazine.

Mechanism: Chlorpromazine alone lowers the seizure threshold and, given in combination with piperazine, it may cause convulsions.

Detailed Information: See *EDI*, 10/17.00

Chlorpromazine-Tobacco

Significance: 3—minimally clinically significant

Recommendations: Patients stabilized on chlorpromazine may exhibit altered responses to the drug if they change their smoking habits. Cessation of smoking may require decreased drug dosage to minimize sedation.

Summary: Smoking causes a decrease in chlorpromazine-induced drowsiness, sedation and hypotension.

Related Drugs: A similar interaction may occur with other phenothiazines, thioxanthenes, butyrophenones, dihydroindolones and dibenzoxazepines.

Mechanism: An increased dosage requirement in smokers could result from induction of chlorpromazine metabolism.

Detailed Information: See *EDI,* 10/18.01

Clorazepate-Aluminum Hydroxide, Magnesium Hydroxide

Significance: 3—minimally clinically significant

Recommendations: Although concurrent use of these agents need not be avoided, it may be best to separate their administration by as much time as possible to avoid any possible interaction.

Summary: These agents have been shown to reduce the rate and extent of desmethyldiazepam, the metabolite of clorazepate; however, all data do not support this interaction.

Related Drugs: It is difficult to determine whether clorazepate would interact with other antacids or if an interaction would occur between aluminum hydroxide-magnesium hydroxide antacids and other benzodiazepines due to conflicting results.

Mechanism: The rate of clorazepate conversion to desmethyldiazepam depends on the presence of strong acid and may be decreased by the presence of the antacid.

Detailed Information: See *EDI,* 10/18.10

Clorazepate-Influenza Virus Vaccine

Significance: 3—minimally clinically significant

Potential Effects: Influenza virus vaccine may inhibit the metabolism of clorazepate, leading to increased side effects.

Recommendations: The concurrent use of these agents need not be avoided; however, patients should be monitored for disorientation. The dose of clorazepate may need to be decreased or the clorazepate discontinued.

Summary: There are data to show that coadministration of these agents may lead to disorientation and lethargy.

Related Drugs: It is not known if an interaction would occur between influenza virus vaccine and other benzodiazepines due to conflicting results.

Mechanism: Influenza virus vaccine may inhibit the hepatic metabolism of clorazepate.

Detailed Information: See *EDI,* 10/18.30

Clozapine-Caffeine

Significance: 3—minimally clinically significant

Potential Effects: Concurrent clozapine and caffeinated beverages may result in exacerbation of psychotic episodes, increased clozapine levels, and tachycardia.

Recommendations: Patients receiving therapy with clozapine who ingest caffeine should be monitored for exacerbation of psychotic symptoms and increased clozapine levels and adverse effects. Although the manufacturer states that the use of caffeine may help decrease the sedative effects of clozapine, some patients may need to be instructed to avoid caffeine-containing beverages and medications.

Summary: The concurrent use of clozapine with caffeinated beverages may result in exacerbation of psychotic episodes, increased clozapine levels, or tachycardia.

Related Drugs: There are no drugs related to clozapine. Documentation is lacking regarding a similar interaction between clozapine and the other xanthine derivatives.

Mechanism: Although the exact mechanism of this interaction is unknown, it is speculated that adenosine A2a receptor antagonism by caffeine results in increased dopamine activation at the D_2 receptor site. It has been postulated that the combination of clozapine, caffeine, and electroconvulsive therapy (ECT) may result in supraventricular tachycardia, although there are reports of caffeine-associated cardiac rhythm disturbances during ECT and tachycardia has been reported during clozapine use alone.

Detailed Information: See *EDI*, 10/18.45

Clozapine-Carbamazepine

Significance: 1—highly clinically significant

Potential Effects: The concurrent use of carbamazepine and clozapine may result in decreased levels of clozapine, which may result in decreased antipsychotic control. Concurrent use may also result in ataxia. Additionally, both agents may increase the risk of agranulocytosis.

Recommendations: The potential for severe bone marrow depression by either clozapine or carbamazepine alone indicates that this combination should only be used with appropriate monitoring and when absolutely necessary. A clozapine dosage adjustment may be necessary to avoid subtherapeutic or toxic levels when carbamazepine is added to or discontinued from concurrent therapy.

Summary: The concurrent use of carbamazepine and clozapine resulted in decreased levels of clozapine by as much as 75%, which may have resulted in decreased antipsychotic control. Concurrent use may have also resulted in ataxia. Additionally, both agents have been shown to increase the risk of agranulocytosis.

Related Drugs: There are no drugs related to clozapine or carbamazepine.

Mechanism: Carbamazepine is known to be an inducer of liver microsomal enzyme systems regulating the inactivation of a variety of drugs, and it has been shown to substantially decrease the plasma levels of other neuroleptics. Similarly, the abrupt discontinuation of carbamazepine can markedly increase the plasma levels of concomitantly used neuroleptics. Carbamazepine has been reported to cause neutropenia, agranulocytosis, and aplastic anemia. Clozapine may also cause neutropenia, leukopenia, and granulocytopenia. It is not known if the bone marrow toxicity is an additive or synergistic effect due to the interaction between clozapine and carbamazepine.

Detailed Information: See *EDI*, 10/18.47

Clozapine-Cimetidine

Significance: 2—moderately clinically significant

Potential Effects: Cimetidine may decrease the metabolism of clozapine, resulting in increased levels and toxicity.

Recommendations: Concurrent use of clozapine and cimetidine should be approached with caution. The patient should be monitored for symptoms of clozapine toxicity, and the clozapine dose may need to be reduced. Ranitidine may be an alternative to cimetidine.

Summary: Increased clozapine serum levels may result if cimetidine is added to therapy, thereby increasing adverse reactions to clozapine.

Related Drugs: Although ranitidine binds readily to clozapine P450 *in vitro*, doses of 300mg/day have shown no similar effect on clozapine levels. The addition of cimetidine has resulted in excessive sedation, necessitating a reduction in chlorpromazine dosage in schizophrenic patients. Chronic administration of cimetidine may produce a fall in steady-state plasma chlorpromazine percent ratios. Conflicting studies with concurrent cimetidine and haloperidol in animal models have reported that cimetidine does not affect haloperidol--induced catalepsy and that cimetidine blocks the cataleptogenic effect of chlorpromazine. It is difficult to determine whether the other phenothiazines as well as molindone, loxapine, or pimozide would interact with cimetidine. It is also not known if an interaction would be expected to occur between clozapine and the other H_2-receptor antagonists.

Mechanism: It has been postulated that cimetidine may decrease the metabolism of clozapine due to cimetidine's cytochrome P450 inhibitory effect.

Detailed Information: See *EDI,* 10/18.50

Clozapine-Erythromycin

Significance: 2—moderately clinically significant

Potential Effects: The addition of erythromycin to clozapine therapy may result in increased clozapine levels and tonic-clonic seizure.

Recommendations: Patients receiving clozapine and erythromycin concurrently should be monitored for signs of clozapine toxicity. Alternative antibiotic therapy may need to be instituted or the dose of clozapine may need to be reduced.

Summary: The addition of erythromycin to clozapine therapy may have resulted in increased clozapine levels and tonic-clonic seizure activity in a patient.

Related Drugs: It is expected that if the mechanism of the interaction is secondary to hepatic microsomal inhibition, clarithromycin and troleandomycin would interact and azithromycin, dirithromycin, and spiramycin would not. Documentation of this is lacking.

Mechanism: The mechanism of this interaction is unknown. Both clozapine and erythromycin are metabolized by the hepatic microsomal enzyme system. Erythromycin may have inhibited the metabolism of clozapine, resulting in increased clozapine levels.

Detailed Information: See *EDI,* 10/18.60

Clozapine-Fluvoxamine

Significance: 2—moderately clinically significant

Potential Effects: Concurrent therapy with clozapine and fluvoxamine may result in increased clozapine levels and clozapine-related side effects.

Recommendations: Concurrent therapy with clozapine and a selective serotonin reuptake inhibitor (SSRI) need not be avoided. However, clozapine levels should be monitored and the patient should be monitored for signs of clozapine toxicity. The dosage of either clozapine or the SSRI may need to be adjusted or one or both agents may need to be discontinued.

Summary: Concurrent therapy with clozapine and fluvoxamine resulted in increased clozapine levels by as much as 269% and, in some reports, clozapine-related side effects.

Related Drugs: Paroxetine and sertraline have also been shown to increase clozapine levels. There are no drugs related to clozapine.

Mechanism: It is postulated that the metabolism of clozapine is inhibited by fluoxetine, fluvoxamine, paroxetine, and sertraline. Clozapine is metabolized at multiple cytochrome P450 isoenzymes, including $P450_{1A2}$.

Detailed Information: See *EDI*, 10/18.80

Diazepam-Alcohol, Ethyl

Significance: 2—moderately clinically significant

Potential Effects: Concurrent use of diazepam with alcohol causes increased central nervous system (CNS) depression.

Recommendations: Patients receiving diazepam should be informed of the potentially serious effects of concomitant use of alcohol.

Summary: Diazepam and ethyl alcohol will lead to enhanced disruption of psychomotor performance and increased CNS depression.

Related Drugs: Temazepam and the other short-acting or intermediate-acting benzodiazepines tend to result in fewer alcohol interactions. Midazolam with alcohol results in impairment of immediate recall. Reports have been conflicting regarding the actions of chlordiazepoxide. An interaction may occur between alcohol and other benzodiazepines, although the extent of the interaction is difficult to determine.

Mechanism: There appears to be an unknown pharmacodynamic mechanism causing additive CNS depressant effect.

Detailed Information: See *EDI*, 10/19.00

Diazepam-Aminophylline

Significance: 3—minimally clinically significant

Potential Effects: Aminophylline may decrease the sedative effects of diazepam.

Recommendations: If diazepam is being used for its sedative effects, the dose may need to be increased during concomitant aminophylline therapy.

Summary: Aminophylline has been shown to antagonize diazepam-induced anesthesia, sedation, somnolence, and impairment in thinking and psychomotor performance.

Related Drugs: A similar interaction may occur between diazepam and other theophylline derivatives. Caffeine has also been shown to antagonize the effects of diazepam and lorazepam.

Mechanism: Aminophylline and other xanthines may compete with diazepam at receptor sites, may depress GABA transmission or may interfere with adenosine receptors.

Detailed Information: See *EDI*, 10/20.10

Diazepam-Cimetidine

Significance: 2—moderately clinically significant

Potential Effects: Cimetidine may decrease the metabolism of diazepam, leading to increased side effects such as sedation, fatigue, or drowsiness.

Recommendations: If these agents are given together, the patient should be monitored for increased side effects. A noninteracting benzodiazepine or famotidine or ranitidine may be considered.

Summary: Cimetidine has been found to increase the absorption and to significantly impair the elimination of diazepam, resulting in a potentiation of the sedative effects of diazepam.

Related Drugs: Chlordiazepoxide, alprazolam, triazolam, nitrazepam and midazolam have all been shown to interact with cimetidine in varying degrees. Other benzodiazepines dependent on phase I reactions would be expected to interact with cimetidine. Cimetidine does not alter the elimination of oxazepam, lorazepam or temazepam; lorazepam absorption is enhanced with concomitant cimetidine. Ranitidine has been shown to reduce diazepam's steady-state plasma levels and increase plasma clearance. Famotidine has been shown to have no effect on any pharmacokinetic parameters of diazepam.

Mechanism: Cimetidine may inhibit hepatic microsomal drug metabolism, causing a reduction in the hepatic elimination of diazepam.

Detailed Information: See *EDI,* 10/21.00

Diazepam-Disulfiram

Significance: 3—minimally clinically significant

Potential Effects: Concurrent use of diazepam in patients receiving disulfiram may lead to enhanced sedation.

Recommendations: Present documentation suggests that the benzodiazepines that undergo N-demethylation, including diazepam, will be affected by disulfiram. It may be necessary to reduce the dosage of these particular benzodiazepines if concurrent use with disulfiram is required. An alternative may be to use oxazepam, lorazepam, or any other benzodiazepine that does not undergo N-demethylation. It is also important to realize that drowsiness is one of the most common side effects of disulfiram, and this may lead to an additive effect with use of benzodiazepines.

Summary: Concurrent use of diazepam in patients receiving disulfiram may lead to enhanced sedation.

Related Drugs: Chlordiazepoxide, oxazepam and lorazepam have been shown to interact with disulfiram in varying degrees. A similar interaction may occur between diazepam and other antialcoholic agents. A similar interaction is expected to occur with those benzodiazepines whose metabolic pathway is dependent on phase I reactions.

Mechanism: Disulfiram inhibits N-demethylation and C-hydroxylation of diazepam and the glucuronidation of the metabolites so formed.

Detailed Information: See *EDI,* 10/25.00

Diazepam-Fluoxetine

Significance: 3—minimally clinically significant

Potential Effects: Fluoxetine may decrease the metabolism of diazepam.

Recommendations: Further studies are necessary to determine clinical significance. No changes were reported in psychomotor response, so dosage modification of either drug is unnecessary.

Summary: Fluoxetine was found to not affect the psychomotor responses of diazepam.

Related Drugs: A similar interaction is expected to occur with other benzodiazepines metabolized by phase I reactions.

Mechanism: Fluoxetine may decrease the hepatic metabolism of diazepam.

Detailed Information: See *EDI*, 10/26.50

Diazepam-Isoniazid

Significance: 3—minimally clinically significant

Recommendations: The reduction in diazepam clearance is small but may necessitate a decreased diazepam dosage in some patients.

Summary: Isoniazid has been shown to prolong diazepam half-life and decrease diazepam clearance.

Related Drugs: There are no drugs related to isoniazid. A similar interaction is expected to occur with other benzodiazepines metabolized by phase I reactions, if the mechanism involves inhibition of hepatic enzymes by isoniazid.

Mechanism: Isoniazid inhibits hepatic microsomal drug metabolism, and this may cause a decrease in diazepam clearance.

Detailed Information: See *EDI*, 10/27.00

Diazepam-Levodopa

Significance: 3—minimally clinically significant

Recommendations: Clinical data about this drug interaction are insufficient to recommend avoiding the concurrent use of levodopa and benzodiazepines. However, one should be alert for evidence of worsening parkinsonism in patients previously stabilized on levodopa who are receiving this drug combination.

Summary: Concurrent administration of diazepam and levodopa may result in a diminished antiparkinson effect of levodopa.

Related Drugs: Chlordiazepoxide, nitrazepam, flurazepam and oxazepam have been used with levodopa without any significant loss in antiparkinson activity. It is difficult to predict possible interactions of other benzodiazepines with levodopa. Levodopa-carbidopa may interact with benzodiazepines in a similar manner.

Mechanism: Benzodiazepines are known to increase the brain's acetylcholine content, possibly antagonizing the beneficial dopamine-mediated response to levodopa.

Detailed Information: See *EDI*, 10/29.00

Diazepam-Omeprazole

Significance: 3—minimally clinically significant

Potential Effects: Concurrent administration of diazepam and omeprazole may result in a decrease in the mean clearance of diazepam.

Recommendations: Patients maintained on omeprazole should be monitored for enhanced diazepam response with concurrent administration of these agents.

Summary: Concurrent administration of diazepam and omeprazole resulted in a decrease in the mean clearance of diazepam by up to 54% and an increase in diazepam half-life by as much as 130%.

Related Drugs: When added to triazolam and lorazepam therapy, omeprazole has caused gait disturbance. Dizziness and difficulty walking have also been reported when omeprazole was added to flurazepam therapy. *In vitro,* omeprazole has inhibited the metabolism of midazolam. The other benzodiazepines metabolized by N-demethylation or hydroxylation may be expected to interact similarly; however, it is not known if those dependent on glucuronidation would interact. Lansoprazole and pantoprazole have shown no significant effects on diazepam pharmacokinetics.

Mechanism: It is postulated that the decrease in diazepam clearance is an effect of omeprazole's inhibition of the cytochrome P450 enzyme system. Diazepam is metabolized by the $P450_{2C19}$ and $P450_{3A}$ isozymes. Lansoprazole, pantoprazole, and omeprazole are also metabolized by the $P450_{2C19}$ and $P450_{3A}$ isozymes and inhibit these isozymes. Pantoprazole is also metabolized by a cytosolic sulfotransferase, a conjugating enzyme.

Detailed Information: See *EDI,* 10/30.10

Diazepam-Oral Contraceptive Agents

Significance: 3—minimally clinically significant

Potential Effects: Oral contraceptive agents may alter the metabolism of diazepam, resulting in increased diazepam levels.

Recommendations: Although a direct relationship between the plasma concentration of diazepam and its clinical effect is not clearly established, patients who are taking oral contraceptives should be closely monitored for increased diazepam effects. A dosage adjustment may be necessary in some patients.

Summary: There are data to show that coadministration of these agents may lead to an increased diazepam effect.

Related Drugs: The data regarding the coadministration of oral contraceptives and benzodiazepines are very conflicting.

Mechanism: Estrogens may bind to cytochrome P450 and decrease the amount of the hepatic oxidative drug-metabolizing enzyme system necessary in diazepam oxidation.

Detailed Information: See *EDI,* 10/31.00

Diazepam-Propranolol

Significance: 3—minimally clinically significant

Potential Effects: Propranolol may inhibit the metabolism of diazepam.

Recommendations: If increased effects of diazepam are observed during concurrent administration with propranolol, the dose of diazepam may need to be decreased.

Summary: There are data to show that coadministration of these agents may lead to the increased effects of diazepam, and it has been documented that these agents did impair measures of subjective arousal and mood.

Related Drugs: The data regarding the use of the benzodiazepines and beta-blockers are conflicting, and it is suggested that the use of these agents be monitored closely and dosage adjustments made when required.

Mechanism: Propranolol may inhibit the metabolism of diazepam, and the inhibition of diazepam's metabolism has been found to be proportional to the degree of lipid solubility of the beta-blocking agent.

Detailed Information: See *EDI,* 10/32.10

Diazepam-Rifampin

Significance: 3—minimally clinically significant

Potential Effects: Rifampin may induce the metabolism of diazepam, resulting in decreased levels.

Recommendations: Patients receiving rifampin, either alone or in combination therapy, may have markedly enhanced diazepam clearance, and may therefore require higher doses of diazepam.

Summary: There are data to show that administration of rifampin may lead to an enhanced diazepam clearance and a reduced half-life, maximum concentration and area-under-curve, and this may necessitate higher doses of diazepam.

Related Drugs: A similar interaction is expected to occur with the other benzodiazepines metabolized by phase I and rifampin, if the mechanism involves induction of hepatic enzymes by rifampin. There are no drugs related to rifampin.

Mechanism: Rifampin, a known enzyme inducer, may be the primary cause of this interaction.

Detailed Information: See *EDI,* 10/33.00

Diazepam-Tobacco

Significance: 3—minimally clinically significant

Potential Effects: Tobacco may decrease the sedative effect of diazepam. The dose of diazepam, in most cases, need not be changed in patients who use tobacco.

Recommendations: However, in some patients, the dose of diazepam may need to be increased.

Summary: There are data to show that smokers who were administered diazepam experienced less sedation.

Related Drugs: The data regarding smokers who use benzodiazepines are conflicting, and it is suggested that the use of these agents be monitored closely and dosage adjustments made when required.

Mechanism: The constituents of cigarette smoke may stimulate a more rapid metabolism of diazepam and other benzodiazepines.

Detailed Information: See *EDI,* 10/34.10

Fluphenazine-Clonidine

Significance: 3—minimally clinically significant

Recommendations: Since the discontinuation of clonidine causes neurologic symptoms to disappear, this is the course of action suggested in patients developing such symptoms. Hydralazine has been substituted for clonidine with no similar interaction.

Summary: In one patient receiving clonidine and chlorthalidone, administration of fluphenazine led to acute organic brain syndrome.

Related Drugs: There are no drugs related to clonidine. Other phenothiazines, thioxanthenes, butyrophenones, dihydroindolones and dibenzoxazepines may interact in a similar manner.

Mechanism: Clonidine, a potent alpha-adrenergic agonist, when combined with fluphenazine, a potent dopamine blocker, may result in a relative adrenergic dominance.

Detailed Information: See *EDI,* 10/35.00

Haloperidol-Carbamazepine

Significance: 2—moderately clinically significant

Potential Effects: Carbamazepine may cause a decrease in haloperidol levels.

Recommendations: Monitor the patient's mental status and haloperidol levels if carbamazepine is added to, or withdrawn from, therapy.

Summary: There are data to show that administration of carbamazepine may cause a decrease in haloperidol levels; however, all data do not support this interaction.

Related Drugs: Because the mechanism of this interaction is unclear, it is not known if the phenothiazines, thioxanthenes, butyrophenones, dihydroindolones and dibenzoxazepines would interact with carbamazepine. There are no drugs related to carbamazepine.

Mechanism: Carbamazepine may increase haloperidol's metabolism, or haloperidol may facilitate intracellular transport of carbamazepine; however, this is not documented.

Detailed Information: See *EDI,* 10/36.10

Haloperidol-Fluoxetine

Significance: 3—minimally clinically significant

Potential Effects: Addition of fluoxetine to haloperidol therapy may cause extrapyramidal symptoms.

Recommendations: Patients maintained on haloperidol should be carefully monitored for extrapyramidal symptoms if fluoxetine is added to therapy. One or both agents may need to be discontinued.

Summary: There are data to show that a patient maintained on haloperidol developed extrapyramidal symptoms when administered fluoxetine.

Related Drugs: It is not known if an interaction would occur between fluoxetine and other antipsychotic agents such as the phenothiazines, thioxanthenes, butyrophenones, dihydroindolones and dibenzoxazepines. There are no drugs related to fluoxetine.

Mechanism: The mechanism of this interaction is not known.

Detailed Information: See *EDI,* 10/36.30

Haloperidol-Rifampin

Significance: 2—moderately clinically significant

Potential Effects: Concurrent administration of haloperidol and rifampin may result in decreased levels of haloperidol.

Recommendations: Patients receiving haloperidol who are started on rifampin should be monitored for decreased haloperidol levels and decreased effectiveness of haloperidol. Patients maintained on haloperidol in whom rifampin is discontinued should be monitored for increased haloperidol levels and possible adverse effects. The dose of haloperidol may need to be adjusted.

Summary: Concurrent administration of haloperidol and rifampin resulted in decreased levels of haloperidol. Discontinuation of rifampin from concurrent therapy with haloperidol resulted in increased haloperidol levels.

Related Drugs: An interaction would be expected to occur between the other butyrophenones and rifampin as well as between haloperidol and rifabutin.

Mechanism: Rifampin has been shown to induce the cytochromes $P450_{3A}$, $P450_{2C}$, and $P450_{2D6}$. Haloperidol is metabolized by several cytochrome P450 isozymes, including $P450_{2D6}$ and $P450_{1A2}$. Rifampin may induce the metabolism of haloperidol at the $P450_{2D6}$ isozyme site.

Detailed Information: See *EDI*, 10/36.45

Haloperidol-Tacrine

Significance: 2—moderately clinically significant

Potential Effects: Concurrent administration of haloperidol and tacrine may result in parkinsonian symptoms.

Recommendations: Patients receiving concurrent therapy with haloperidol and tacrine should be monitored for parkinsonian symptoms. One or both agents may need to be discontinued.

Summary: Concurrent administration of haloperidol and tacrine resulted in parkinsonian symptoms. After discontinuation and resolution of symptoms, rechallenge with the two drugs produced the same adverse effects.

Related Drugs: It is not known if the other antipsychotic agents such as the phenothiazines, thioxanthenes, as well as molindone, loxapine, clozapine, risperidone, and pimozide would interact with tacrine. There are no drugs related to tacrine.

Mechanism: It is postulated that a tacrine-induced increase in cholinergic activity enhances basal ganglia sensitivity to haloperidol's dopamine-blocking ability. Concurrent administration may result in increased striatal acetylcholine activity, resulting in parkinsonian symptoms.

Detailed Information: See *EDI*, 10/36.60

Lithium Carbonate-Acetazolamide

Significance: 1—highly clinically significant

Recommendations: It is important to measure lithium serum levels during concurrent use of these agents. A higher dose of lithium carbonate may be necessary.

Summary: There are data to show that the administration of acetazolamide causes an increase in the excretion of lithium, necessitating an increase in lithium dosages.

Related Drugs: A similar interaction is expected to occur between lithium carbonate and other carbonic anhydrase inhibitors.

Mechanism: Acetazolamide may increase the renal excretion of lithium by alkalinization of the urine or by impairing the proximal tubular reabsorption of lithium.

Detailed Information: See *EDI*, 10/37.00

Lithium Carbonate-Acyclovir

Significance: 3—minimally clinically significant

Potential Effects: The addition of acyclovir to a lithium carbonate regimen may result in increased lithium levels and toxicity.

Recommendations: Patients should be carefully monitored for increased serum lithium levels and toxicity with concurrent administration of lithium carbonate and high-dose intravenous acyclovir. Further studies are needed.

Summary: The addition of intravenous acyclovir to a lithium carbonate regimen resulted in increased serum lithium levels from 0.8meq/L to 3.4meq/L (normal range: 0.6–1.2meq/L) and lithium toxicity.

Related Drugs: It is not known whether an interaction would be expected to occur between lithium and the other nucleoside analogues. There are no drugs related to lithium.

Mechanism: Since both of these agents are primarily eliminated unchanged in the kidneys and the percentage of acyclovir excreted increases with increasing dose, acyclovir serum concentrations attained following intravenous acyclovir doses of 10mg/Kg may impair the clearance of lithium. Further studies are needed to validate this hypothesis. The bioavailability of oral acyclovir ranges from 15–30%; it has been postulated that it may be unlikely that increased serum lithium levels will occur with concurrent lithium carbonate and oral acyclovir.

Detailed Information: See *EDI,* 10/37.50

Lithium Carbonate-Alcohol, Ethyl

Significance: 3—minimally clinically significant

Potential Effects: Alcohol may cause an increase in lithium levels.

Recommendations: The use of these agents together need not be avoided; however, lithium levels should be closely monitored in patients who use alcohol.

Summary: There are data to show that alcohol may cause an increase in lithium levels; however, all data do not support this, and there are conflicting reports.

Related Drugs: There are no drugs related to lithium carbonate.

Mechanism: The mechanism of this interaction is not known.

Detailed Information: See *EDI,* 10/38.10

Lithium Carbonate-Carbamazepine

Significance: 2—moderately clinically significant

Potential Effects: Neurotoxicity may occur when these agents are used together.

Recommendations: Monitor patients for neurotoxicity when these agents are used concurrently. One or both agents may need to be discontinued.

Summary: There are data to show that coadministration of these agents may cause neurotoxicity; however, data have shown that use of these agents does not potentiate neurotoxicity.

Related Drugs: There are no drugs related to lithium carbonate or carbamazepine.

Mechanism: This interaction may be related to the combined, mutual effects of lithium carbonate and carbamazepine on sodium metabolism or on nerve conduction velocity.

Detailed Information: See *EDI,* 10/39.00

Lithium Carbonate-Chlorothiazide

Significance: 1—highly clinically significant

Recommendations: Although several studies have pointed out specific instances in which lithium and chlorothiazide are useful (e.g., lithium polyuria and lithium-induced nephrogenic diabetes insipidus) when given concurrently, in general they should not be used together. If these drugs must be given simultaneously, the patient should be observed closely for signs and symptoms of lithium-induced neurotoxicity or cardiotoxicity, and a lower dose of lithium may be required. The potassium-sparing diuretics, spironolactone and triamterene, did not affect serum lithium concentrations in a small group of patients and may be safer diuretics to use concurrently with lithium. Amiloride, another potassium-sparing diuretic, may also be considered.

Summary: Concurrent administration of chlorothiazide may result in enhanced cardiotoxicity and neurotoxicity secondary to lithium.

Related Drugs: Any thiazide diuretic that promotes or enhances the excretion of both sodium and potassium may interact with lithium. The loop diuretics, the mercurial diuretics, other thiazides and other thiazide-related diuretics may interact with lithium.

Mechanism: Long-term thiazide administration may lead to an increase in the reabsorption of lithium and a subsequent decrease in lithium clearance.

Detailed Information: See *EDI*, 10/41.00

Lithium Carbonate-Cisplatin

Significance: 3—minimally clinically significant

Potential Effects: Cisplatin therapy may temporarily decrease lithium levels.

Recommendations: Monitor lithium levels when cisplatin therapy (cisplatin and fluid load) are added to lithium therapy. The decrease in lithium levels should return to baseline shortly after completion of therapy.

Summary: There are data to show that cisplatin therapy may temporarily decrease lithium levels; however, fluid load, which is part of cisplatin therapy, may be responsible for the decreased lithium levels.

Related Drugs: There are no drugs related to lithium or cisplatin.

Mechanism: The decreased lithium levels occurred because of enhanced renal elimination of lithium.

Detailed Information: See *EDI*, 10/42.10

Lithium Carbonate-Diazepam

Significance: 3—minimally clinically significant

Potential Effects: The use of these agents together may result in hypothermia associated with coma, reduced pulse rates, and lowering of systolic blood pressure.

Recommendations: The use of these agents together need not to be avoided. If hypothermia occurs, one or both drugs may need to be discontinued.

Summary: The concurrent use of lithium carbonate and diazepam has been shown to result in hypothermia associated with coma, reduced reflexes, decreased pulse and a low systolic blood pressure.

Related Drugs: There is no documentation regarding a similar interaction between lithium carbonate and the other benzodiazepines. There are no drugs related to lithium carbonate.

Mechanism: The mechanism of this interaction is unknown.

Detailed Information: See *EDI*, 10/43.00

Lithium Carbonate-Enalapril

Significance: 2—moderately clinically significant

Potential Effects: Enalapril may increase lithium levels, leading to toxicity.

Recommendations: Patients should be monitored for signs of lithium toxicity, increased lithium levels, and a decrease in renal function when concurrent enalapril is administered. The dose of lithium may need to be decreased or enalapril may need to be discontinued.

Summary: The addition of lithium carbonate to the therapy of a patient maintained on enalapril resulted in increased serum lithium levels.

Related Drugs: Lisinopril has been shown to potentiate lithium carbonate toxicity. A similar interaction may occur between lithium carbonate and other ACE inhibitors. A similar interaction would be expected to occur between enalapril and lithium citrate.

Mechanism: The increase in lithium serum concentration may be because of the loss of sodium ions and decreased fluid volume.

Detailed Information: See *EDI*, 10/44.10

Lithium Carbonate-Fluoxetine

Significance: 2—moderately clinically significant

Potential Effects: Fluoxetine may increase lithium levels, resulting in toxicity.

Recommendations: Patients on lithium therapy should be closely monitored for increased lithium levels if fluoxetine is administered. The dose of lithium may need to be decreased or fluoxetine may need to be discontinued. Paroxetine may be a potential agent for alternative therapy.

Summary: Increased lithium levels may occur when coadministered with fluoxetine.

Related Drugs: Sertraline and lithium carbonate exhibited a similar interaction. Fluvoxamine and lithium therapy resulted in somnolence.

Mechanism: Fluoxetine has been reported to cause mania, and manic patients have a greater vulnerability to neurotoxicity associated with lithium. There may be a possible synergistic antidepressant effect between lithium and fluoxetine.

Detailed Information: See *EDI*, 10/44.30

Lithium Carbonate-Haloperidol

Significance: 2—moderately clinically significant

Recommendations: Lithium's onset of action occurs several days after therapy is begun. Therefore, haloperidol is usually added during the acute manic phase and then its dose is tapered and finally discontinued. It is preferable to avoid using these agents together during the acute manic phase since there is a higher risk of combined toxicity at that time. If this combination of drugs is to be used during the acute manic symptoms, a conservative lithium dosage is recommended.

Summary: Concomitant administration of lithium carbonate and haloperidol has been reported to cause confusion, extrapyramidal and cerebellar dysfunction, and, in some cases, permanent brain damage and irreversible dyskinesias.

Related Drugs: There are no drugs related to lithium carbonate. The interactions between lithium carbonate and other antipsychotics are discussed in other monographs (see Chlorpromazine-Lithium Carbonate, page 227, and Lithium Carbonate-Thioridazine, page 245).

Mechanism: The mechanism is not known. It has been suggested that this interaction may be dose related.

Detailed Information: See *EDI*, 10/45.00

Lithium Carbonate-Indomethacin

Significance: 2—moderately clinically significant

Potential Effects: Indomethacin may cause an increase in lithium levels, possibly resulting in lithium toxicity.

Recommendations: Monitor patients and lithium levels carefully if these agents are used together. The dose of lithium may need to be decreased or sulindac may possibly be used instead of indomethacin.

Summary: The addition of indomethacin to a stable lithium carbonate regimen resulted in increased lithium plasma levels and toxicity (e.g., polyuria, delirium, lethargy).

Related Drugs: Other nonsteroidal anti-inflammatory drugs (NSAIDs) that have been reported to interact with lithium carbonate resulting in increased lithium levels include ibuprofen, diclofenac, piroxicam, phenylbutazone, mefenamic acid, tiaprofenic acid, naproxen, and ketorolac. Although the interaction with sulindac is conflicting (causing both increased and decreased serum lithium levels), an interaction between lithium and other NSAIDs would be expected to occur. There are no drugs related to lithium.

Mechanism: Prostaglandins may play an important role in renal lithium clearance. Concurrent administration of NSAIDs (prostaglandin synthesis inhibitors) with lithium reduces renal lithium clearance, causing an increase in plasma lithium concentrations. Enhanced renal reabsorption of lithium induced by indomethacin is another possible explanation. The mechanism of action of sulindac's paradoxical effect on lithium is not known. However, it has been suggested that sulindac has a sparing effect on renal prostaglandin synthesis. A possible mechanism may be a sparing effect on intrarenal cyclooxygenase since sulindac is broken down into inactive metabolites (sulindac sulfoxide and sulindac sulfone) in the kidney. Since lithium is approximately 80% reabsorbed in the proximal tubule, the addition of tiaprofenic acid may result in enhanced tubular lithium reabsorption.

Detailed Information: See *EDI,* 10/47.00

Lithium Carbonate-Mazindol

Significance: 2—moderately clinically significant

Recommendations: When an anorexic agent such as mazindol is used concurrently with lithium therapy, care should be taken to assure that sodium intake remains adequate so that increased serum lithium concentrations and possible toxicity are avoided. It may be necessary to lower the dose of lithium during concurrent administration of mazindol.

Summary: Lithium intoxication has been observed in a case where lithium carbonate and mazindol were administered simultaneously.

Related Drugs: Other anorexic agents should be used cautiously. There are no drugs related to lithium carbonate.

Mechanism: A compensatory increase in lithium reabsorption may occur, resulting in a decreased lithium clearance. Dieting and a decrease in sodium intake may induce lithium intoxications.

Detailed Information: See *EDI,* 10/49.00

Lithium Carbonate-Methyldopa

Significance: 2—moderately clinically significant

Potential Effects: The use of these agents together may result in lithium toxicity despite normal lithium levels.

Recommendations: If toxicity occurs, the dose of lithium should be decreased or another antihypertensive used.

Summary: Several case reports have shown that the concurrent administration of lithium carbonate and methyldopa may result in signs of lithium toxicity despite the presence of therapeutic serum lithium levels.
Related Drugs: There are no drugs related to lithium carbonate or methyldopa.
Mechanism: Methyldopa may exacerbate the CNS response to lithium or may increase the brain uptake of lithium.
Detailed Information: See *EDI,* 10/51.00

Lithium Carbonate-Metoprolol

Significance: 2—moderately clinically significant
Recommendations: Because all beta-blocking agents can improve lithium-induced tremors, it is advisable to use a cardioselective agent such as metoprolol in patients with bronchospastic problems.
Summary: In two patients with a history of bronchospastic disease, the use of metoprolol produced objective and subjective improvement of lithium carbonate-induced tremors.
Related Drugs: Propranolol, pindolol and nadolol have been shown to act like metoprolol, but these are contraindicated in bronchospastic disease. A similar interaction may occur with other noncardioselective beta-blocking agents. The other cardioselective beta-blocking agents would act like metoprolol.
Mechanism: The mechanism of this interaction is not fully known; however, both beta₁ and beta₂ receptors have been implicated in essential tremor.
Detailed Information: See *EDI,* 10/53.00

Lithium Carbonate-Metronidazole

Significance: 2—moderately clinically significant
Potential Effects: Metronidazole may increase the incidence of lithium nephrotoxicity.
Recommendations: Patients should be closely monitored for the development of renal complications during concurrent use of these agents. Also, lithium, creatinine, and electrolyte levels should be monitored. Lithium may need to be discontinued or the dosage tapered.
Summary: The administration of metronidazole and lithium carbonate has resulted in toxic reactions to lithium.
Related Drugs: There are no drugs related to lithium carbonate or metronidazole.
Mechanism: The mechanism of this interaction is not known.
Detailed Information: See *EDI,* 10/54.10

Lithium Carbonate-Norepinephrine

Significance: 3—minimally clinically significant
Recommendations: If a patient on lithium carbonate is to receive norepinephrine, a higher dose of norepinephrine may be necessary to achieve the desired pressor response.
Summary: Lithium carbonate has been shown to decrease the pressor response to norepinephrine.
Related Drugs: A similar interaction may be expected between lithium carbonate and other direct acting sympathomimetics. Documentation is lacking regarding a similar interaction with other mixed acting sympathomimetics. Tyramine has been shown to not alter lithium carbonate. The indirect acting sympathomimetics

have been reported to increase lithium levels (see also Lithium Carbonate-Mazindol, page 242). There is no documentation regarding a similar interaction between lithium carbonate and other indirect acting sympathomimetics. There are no drugs related to lithium carbonate.

Mechanism: The mechanism of this interaction is unknown.

Detailed Information: See *EDI*, 10/55.00

Lithium Carbonate-Phenytoin

Significance: 3—minimally clinically significant

Recommendations: Until further documentation is available, patients receiving concurrent therapy of lithium and phenytoin should be observed for clinical signs of lithium toxicity. Since toxicity has been reported in the presence of normal therapeutic levels, therapy should be closely supervised. Dosing adjustments of lithium may be required.

Summary: There are data to show that administration of phenytoin may potentiate clinical signs of lithium toxicity, and toxicity has been reported in the presence of normal therapeutic levels.

Related Drugs: There is a lack of documentation regarding an interaction between lithium and other hydantoin derivatives. There are no drugs related to lithium carbonate.

Mechanism: The mechanism of this interaction is unknown.

Detailed Information: See *EDI*, 10/57.00

Lithium Carbonate-Potassium Iodide

Significance: 2—moderately clinically significant

Recommendations: Patients receiving lithium carbonate should avoid taking nonprescription or prescription iodine-containing preparations. The appearance of goiter or detection of abnormal chemical thyroid tests is not an indication to discontinue lithium therapy. However, it is appropriate to discontinue any iodine-containing drugs and to stabilize thyroid status with appropriate drugs.

Summary: The concurrent administration of lithium carbonate and potassium iodide or other iodine-containing compounds may enhance the hypothyroid and goitrogenic effects of either drug.

Related Drugs: An interaction between lithium carbonate and iso-propamide iodide has been reported. All prescription, nonprescription and radiographic products containing iodine may enhance lithium's antithyroid effects. There are no drugs related to lithium carbonate.

Mechanism: Concurrent use of these compounds could have additive or synergistic hypothyroid effects.

Detailed Information: See *EDI*, 10/59.00

Lithium Carbonate-Tetracycline

Significance: 2—moderately clinically significant

Potential Effects: Concurrent use of these agents may lead to lithium toxicity or a decrease in lithium levels.

Recommendations: Caution should be used when concurrently administering lithium and tetracycline, since lithium levels may be increased or decreased by tetracycline. Serum lithium concentrations should be determined routinely, and the dose of lithium adjusted accordingly.

Summary: The concurrent administration of lithium carbonate and tetracycline may cause serum concentrations of lithium to increase and may lead to lithium toxicity; however, there are conflicting data.

Related Drugs: Documentation is lacking regarding an interaction between lithium carbonate and other tetracyclines.

Mechanism: The mechanism of this interaction is unknown.

Detailed Information: See *EDI*, 10/61.00

Lithium Carbonate-Theophylline

Significance: 2—moderately clinically significant

Potential Effects: Theophylline and caffeine may increase lithium clearance, resulting in decreased lithium levels.

Recommendations: Monitor lithium levels closely if theophylline or caffeine is added to or withdrawn from cotherapy. The dosage of lithium may need to be changed.

Summary: Theophylline and caffeine may increase lithium clearance, resulting in decreased lithium clearances by 51%. It has been suggested that theophylline infusions might be an alternative to hemodialysis in lithium intoxications requiring an immediate reduction in lithium concentration.

Related Drugs: It has been shown that aminophylline increases the lithium/creatinine clearance ratio, which may result in decreased serum lithium below the therapeutic level. Lithium levels increased 23.9% from baseline following caffeine withdrawal and returned to baseline following resumption of caffeine. A similar interaction may be expected between lithium carbonate and the other theophylline derivatives. There are no drugs related to lithium carbonate.

Mechanism: The mechanism of this interaction is related to an increase in the renal excretion of lithium by the theophylline derivative aminophylline.

Detailed Information: See *EDI*, 10/63.00

Lithium Carbonate-Thioridazine

Significance: 2—moderately clinically significant

Recommendations: Plasma level monitoring of either agent is of questionable value in preventing the occurrence of neurotoxic symptoms, since many patients experienced neurotoxic symptoms with plasma concentrations within the therapeutic range. Routine electroencephalogram monitoring may aid in the detection or prevention of neurotoxicity; however, it is recommended that therapy be based on the total clinical picture. Conservative use of both agents is warranted, and dosage adjustments of one or both agents may be necessary. If possible, it would be preferable to use only one agent.

Summary: Neurotoxic symptoms and somnambulistic episodes have been observed in patients simultaneously receiving lithium carbonate and thioridazine.

Related Drugs: Neurotoxic or somnambulistic episodes have also been reported when lithium was coadministered with thiothixene, fluphenazine, perphenazine, and chlorpromazine (see Chlorpromazine-Lithium Carbonate, page 227). Other phenothiazines, thioxanthenes, dihydroindolones and dibenzoxazepines may interact similarly with lithium. Haloperidol may also interact with lithium carbonate (see Lithium Carbonate-Haloperidol, page 241). There are no drugs related to lithium carbonate.

Mechanism: The neurotoxicity-type symptoms may be a potentiation or a pharmacologic summation of the antipsychotic agents and lithium.

Detailed Information: See *EDI*, 10/65.00

Lithium Carbonate-Verapamil

Significance: 2—moderately clinically significant

Potential Effects: Concurrent lithium and calcium channel blockers may result in signs of neurotoxicity or decreased lithium levels with or without manic symptoms.

Recommendations: Patients receiving concurrent therapy with lithium and calcium channel blockers should be monitored for development of manic symptoms or neurotoxicity. Lithium levels should be monitored if calcium channel blockers are added to or withdrawn from therapy; however, neurotoxicity may develop at therapeutic or subtherapeutic lithium levels.

Summary: In case reports, concurrent lithium and verapamil resulted in symptoms of neurotoxicity or decreased lithium levels with or without manic symptoms.

Related Drugs: Patients receiving diltiazem and lithium have been reported to have similar reactions. Nifedipine was reported not to interact with lithium in one case report. Documentation is lacking regarding a similar interaction between lithium carbonate and the other calcium channel blockers; however, based on the proposed mechanism an interaction may be expected to occur.

Mechanism: It has been postulated that the decrease in serum lithium concentration by verapamil results from (1) enhancement of lithium excretion from improved cardiac output due to correction of arrhythmias or (2) a shift of extracellular lithium to an intracellular compartment because of calcium slow channel blocker inhibition of the sodium-potassium ATPase pump. The neurotoxicity that was induced by concurrent lithium and calcium channel blockers may result from similar effects of both agents on neurosecretory processes. Concurrent use may also result in an acute increase in dopamine availability secondary to an increase in dopamine synthesis triggered by lithium and verapamil-induced blockade of dopamine autoreceptors.

Detailed Information: See *EDI*, 10/66.10

Lorazepam-Probenecid

Significance: 3—minimally clinically significant

Potential Effects: Probenecid may decrease the metabolism of lorazepam, leading to increased lorazepam plasma concentrations and potentiated side effects.

Recommendations: If these agents are used together, the patient should be monitored for an increase in lorazepam side effects (e.g., sedation).

Summary: There are data to show that administration of probenecid decreases clearance and prolongs the mean elimination half-life, creating a potential for increased adverse effects.

Related Drugs: The other benzodiazepines with primary metabolic pathways dependent on phase II reactions may interact similarly with probenecid. It is not known if other benzodiazepines metabolized by phase I reactions would interact with probenecid. It is not known if an interaction would occur between lorazepam and sulfinpyrazone.

Mechanism: Probenecid may reduce lorazepam clearance by inhibiting glucuronyl transferase activity, decreasing the formation of lorazepam glucuronide.

Detailed Information: See *EDI*, 10/66.30

Loxapine-Sumatriptan

Significance: 3-minimally clinically significant

Potential Effects: Concurrent administration of loxapine and suma-triptan may result in a dystonic reaction or other extrapyramidal side effects.

Recommendations: Concurrent use of sumatriptan and antipsy-chotics should be approached with caution. Patients receiving antipsychotics should be monitored for extrapyramidal side effects following sumatriptan administration.

Summary: In a single case report, a patient being treated with loxap-ine developed a dystonic reaction within 15 minutes of sumatrip-tan administration.

Related Drugs: Although documentation is lacking, based on the postulated mechanism a similar interaction may be expected to occur between sumatriptan and the phenothiazines, the thioxan-thines, as well as haloperidol and molindone.

Mechanism: Concurrent administration of loxapine and sumatriptan may predispose the patient to a dystonic reaction because of an additive pharmacologic effect.

Detailed Information: See EDI, 10/66.35

Midazolam-Erythromycin

Significance: 2—moderately clinically significant

Potential Effects: Erythromycin may inhibit the metabolism of mida-zolam, possibly leading to increased effects of midazolam.

Recommendations: Patients should be observed for increased midazolam effect, especially drowsiness, when erythromycin is administered concurrently. The dose of midazolam may need to be lowered.

Summary: Concurrent midazolam and erythromycin resulted in increased midazolam levels.

Related Drugs: Erythromycin, roximthromycin, and troleandomyin have been shown to interact with triazolam, while azithromycin has been shown not to interact. If the mechanism involves inhibi-tion of the metabolism of triazolam by erythromycin, then a simi-lar interaction may be expected to occur between erythromycin and the other benzodiazepines metabolized by phase I reac-tions; however, documentation is lacking. Although there is no documentation, erythromycin would not be expected to interact with the other benzodiazepines metabolized by phase II reac-tions.

Mechanism: The proposed mechanism is one of hepatic microso-mal inhibition, causing elevated midazolam concentrations.

Detailed Information: See *EDI,* 10/66.42

Midazolam-Thiopental

Significance: 3—minimally clinically significant

Potential Effects: Concurrent use of these agents may result in a synergistic anesthetic effect.

Recommendations: Patients receiving concurrent midazolam and thiopental should be monitored for a possible synergistic effect. The dose of one or both agents may need to be reduced.

Summary: There are data to show that coadministration of the agents may cause a supra-additive anesthesia effect.

Related Drugs: A similar reaction may occur between thiopental and other benzodiazepines and between midazolam and other barbi-turates.

Mechanism: This interaction involves the GABA receptor and the barbiturate binding sites. Binding to these sites can allosterically modify the benzodiazepine receptor. Barbiturates may enhance the binding of benzodiazepines.

Detailed Information: See *EDI*, 10/66.45

Olanzapine-Fluvoxamine

Significance: 3—minimally clinically significant

Potential Effects: Concurrent administration of fluvoxamine and olanzapine may result in a decrease in olanzapine clearance and increased olanzapine levels.

Recommendations: Patients receiving concurrent therapy with olanzapine and fluvoxamine should be monitored for increased olanzapine effects. The dosage of olanzapine may need to be adjusted, or fluvoxamine may need to be discontinued.

Summary: Concurrent administration of fluvoxamine and olanzapine resulted in a decrease in olanzapine clearance and increased olanzapine levels. In one study, olanzapine maximum concentration and area-under-curve increased by 84% and 119%, respectively.

Related Drugs: A similar interaction would be expected to occur between olanzapine and the other selective serotonin reuptake inhibitors and the nonselective serotonin reuptake inhibitors. It is not known whether fluvoxamine would interact with the other antipsychotic agents chemically unrelated to olanzapine.

Mechanism: It is postulated that olanzapine's metabolism is mediated by the cytochrome $P450_{1A2}$ isozyme system and that fluvoxamine inhibits this same system. It is thus speculated that fluvoxamine inhibits the metabolism of olanzapine.

Detailed Information: See *EDI*, 10/66.47

Oxazepam-Diflunisal

Significance: 3—minimally clinically significant

Potential Effects: Diflunisal may decrease oxazepam levels.

Recommendations: The dose of oxazepam may need to be increased if these agents are used together.

Summary: In one study, concurrent administration of diflunisal and oxazepam resulted in decreased oxazepam concentrations.

Related Drugs: Aspirin has been reported to increase the activity of midazolam. Midazolam has been reported to have no interaction with diflunisal. The other benzodiazepines with primary metabolic pathways dependent on phase II reactions may interact similarly with diflunisal based on the proposed mechanism; however, documentation is lacking. It is not known if a similar interaction would occur between oxazepam and the other salicylates; however, they may also interact because salicylates compete for protein binding with oxazepam.

Mechanism: It has been suggested that this interaction results from a presystemic displacement of oxazepam from its plasma protein binding sites by diflunisal. Also, inhibition of the tubular secretion of oxazepam glucuronide by the glucuronides of diflunisal may be involved.

Detailed Information: See *EDI*, 10/66.50

Perphenazine-Disulfiram

Significance: 3—minimally clinically significant

Potential Effects: Disulfiram may decrease perphenazine plasma concentration levels along with its sulfoxide metabolite.

Recommendations: Patients receiving oral perphenazine and disulfiram concurrently should be observed for exacerbated psychotic symptoms. The dosage of disulfiram and the oral form of perphenazine may need to be adjusted.

Summary: There are data to show that administration of disulfiram may decrease perphenazine plasma concentration levels along with its sulfoxide metabolite.

Related Drugs: A similar interaction may occur between disulfiram and other phenothiazines, thioxanthenes, butyrophenones, dihydroindolones, and dibenzoxazepines. A similar interaction is not expected to occur between perphenazine and other antialcoholic agents.

Mechanism: Disulfiram may activate the liver enzymes inactivating perphenazine.

Detailed Information: See *EDI,* 10/67.00

Pimozide-Fluoxetine

Significance: 3—minimally clinically significant

Potential Effects: The addition of fluoxetine to the therapy of a patient maintained on pimozide may result in an increase in pimozide adverse effects.

Recommendations: Patients should be monitored for bradycardia, changes in sensorium, or other signs of pimozide side effects when fluoxetine or pimozide is added to a regimen including the other. The dosage of one or both drugs may need to be adjusted.

Summary: Increased pimozide adverse effects were seen when fluoxetine was added to the therapy of patients maintained on pimozide. Effects included bradycardia, galactorrhea, and a change in sensorium.

Related Drugs: An oculogyric crisis occurred in a nine-year-old after paroxetine was added to pimozide therapy and reoccurred upon rechallenge with the two drugs. It is not known if a similar interaction would occur between pimozide and the other selective serotonin reuptake inhibitors, though this may be possible based on the proposed mechanism of action.

Mechanism: It is hypothesized that fluoxetine may decrease the plasma clearance of pimozide, increasing plasma levels of pimozide, possibly because of impaired hepatic microsomal activity. It is also possible that the two drugs, which both can cause bradycardia, exert additive effects in the patient.

Detailed Information: See *EDI,* 10/68.50

Promazine-Charcoal

Significance: 3—minimally clinically significant

Recommendations: Activated charcoal may be an effective treatment in an acute promazine overdose. It should be administered as soon as possible, and subsequent doses should be given to increase promazine elimination. However, if charcoal is not used for promazine overdose, the administration of these agents should be separated by as much time as possible.

Summary: The concomitant administration of activated charcoal and promazine decreases the rate and extent of promazine absorption.

Related Drugs: It is expected that the other phenothiazines will also be adsorbed to charcoal. There are no drugs related to charcoal.

Mechanism: It has been suggested that activated charcoal adsorbs promazine.

Detailed Information: See *EDI*, 10/69.00

Temazepam-Diphenhydramine

Significance: 2—moderately clinically significant

Potential Effects: In one case report, the concurrent use of these agents in a pregnant patient resulted in the delivery of a stillborn infant.

Recommendations: These agents should not be used together in pregnant patients because of the potentially serious consequences.

Summary: There are data to show that coadministration of diphenhydramine and temazepam resulted in violent intrauterine fetal movements leading to the delivery of a stillborn infant.

Related Drugs: It is difficult to determine if a similar interaction would occur between temazepam and other antihistamines or between diphenhydramine and other benzodiazepines.

Mechanism: Both drugs cross the placenta. Antihistamines cause vasoconstriction of the placenta, increasing the maternal-fetal exchange, and antihistamines also have an embryotoxic effect. Diphenhydramine may affect the metabolism of temazepam.

Detailed Information: See *EDI*, 10/70.10

Thioridazine-Bromocriptine

Significance: 2—moderately clinically significant

Recommendations: The concurrent use of thioridazine and bromocriptine should be used with caution, and patients should be monitored for increased prolactin levels. Thioridazine may need to be discontinued, as this interaction appears to be reversible.

Summary: There are data to show that coadministration of these agents will increase prolactin levels. A temporary loss of vision was documented to occur with coadministration of these therapies.

Related Drugs: A similar interaction may occur between bromocriptine and other phenothiazines, thioxanthenes, butyrophenones, dihydroindolones, and dibenzoxazepines. There are no drugs related to bromocriptine.

Mechanism: It has been suggested that thioridazine diminishes the prolactin-lowering ability of bromocriptine.

Detailed Information: See *EDI*, 10/71.00

Triazolam-Ketoconazole

Significance: 1—highly clinically significant

Potential Effects: Concurrent administration of imidazole antimycotics with phase I metabolized benzodiazepines may result in decreased clearance of benzodiazepines and increased levels and clinical effects of benzodiazepines.

Recommendations: The concurrent administration of either alprazolam or triazolam with either itraconazole or ketoconazole is contraindicated according to the manufacturer's product labeling. The concurrent administration of other combinations of imidazole antifungals and phase I metabolized benzodiazepines need not be avoided. However, patients should be observed for an increase in the effects of the benzodiazepines. The dose of the benzodiazepine may need to be decreased.

Summary: Concurrent administration of imidazole antimycotics with phase I metabolized benzodiazepines may result in decreased clearance of benzodiazepines and increased levels, clinical effects, and adverse effects of benzodiazepines including increased sedation and amnesiac effects.

Related Drugs: Based on the postulated mechanism, benzodiazepines that are metabolized by phase I (N-dealkylation or hydroxylation) may be expected to interact with fluconazole, itraconazole, and ketoconazole. It is not known if these imidazole antifungal agents would interact with the benzodiazepines. Alprazolam, chlordiazepoxide, midazolam, and triazolam may be expected to interact with the other imidazole antifungals.

Mechanism: It is believed that the imidazole antifungals inhibit the metabolism of the benzodiazepines by inhibition of the cytochrome $P450_{3A4}$ enzyme system.

Detailed Information: See *EDI*, 10/73.00

Chapter Eleven

Beta-Adrenergic Blocking Agents' Drug Interactions

Atenolol-Ampicillin

Significance: 3—minimally clinically significant

Potential Effects: Ampicillin may decrease the effects of atenolol. Also, beta-blockers may increase the risk of anaphylactic reactions to the penicillins.

Recommendations: Monitor patients for lack of atenolol's effects when administered with ampicillin. Observe patients for signs of anaphylactic reactions when taking beta-blocking agents and penicillins together.

Summary: There are data to show that ampicillin administration may decrease the effects of atenolol.

Related Drugs: It is not known if a similar interaction would occur between atenolol and other penicillins or between ampicillin and other beta-blocking agents. There is an increased risk of penicillin anaphylactic reactions with beta-blocking agents (see also Propranolol-Allergenic Extracts, page 256).

Mechanism: The mechanism of this interaction is unknown.

Detailed Information: See *EDI*, 11/1.00

Atenolol-Calcium Carbonate

Significance: 3—minimally clinically significant

Recommendations: The patient's response to atenolol should be monitored during administration of concurrent calcium salts, and the atenolol dose may need to be adjusted.

Summary: The administration of calcium carbonate was shown to reduce the peak plasma concentration and decrease the area-under-curve of atenolol. A reduction in beta-blockade was demonstrated, but blood pressure response did not significantly change.

Related Drugs: A similar interaction would be expected to occur with the other calcium salts. There is no documentation regarding a similar interaction with the other beta-blocking agents.

Mechanism: The gastrointestinal absorption of atenolol is impaired by calcium salts, although other mechanisms may exist.

Detailed Information: See *EDI*, 11/3.00

Atenolol-Propantheline

Significance: 3—minimally clinically significant

Recommendations: Although the concurrent use of these agents need not be avoided, it may be necessary to decrease the dose of atenolol or separate the administration of the drugs by as much time as possible.

Summary: Propantheline was shown to prolong the absorption and the time to peak, and to increase the area-under-curve, of atenolol.

Related Drugs: Metoprolol and propranolol exhibited similar interactions with propantheline. A similar interaction is expected to occur between propantheline and other beta-blocking agents and between atenolol and other anticholinergics.

Mechanism: Propantheline, by decreasing gastrointestinal motility, increases the absorption of atenolol.

Detailed Information: See *EDI*, 11/4.01

Labetalol-Glutethimide

Significance: 3—minimally clinically significant

Recommendations: If a decreased response to labetalol occurs during concurrent administration of glutethimide, the dose of labetalol may need to be increased or the glutethimide discontinued.

Summary: The administration of glutethimide resulted in a significant reduction in labetalol area-under-curve and systemic bioavailability, necessitating a possible increase in labetalol dosage.

Related Drugs: A similar interaction is expected to occur between glutethimide and other hepatically metabolized beta-blocking agents if the mechanism involves enzyme induction by glutethimide. The agents that are not extensively metabolized by the liver would not be expected to interact with glutethimide. There are no drugs related to glutethimide.

Mechanism: Glutethimide, a known hepatic microsomal oxidative enzyme inducer, increases the metabolism of labetalol.

Detailed Information: See *EDI,EDI,* 11/4.10

Labetalol-Halothane

Significance: 2—moderately clinically significant

Recommendations: The interaction may be of benefit in some patients since hypotension may be induced, causing a decrease in arterial pressure unaccompanied by tachycardia, thereby reducing blood loss during surgery. However, if this effect is not desired, the concentration of halothane may need to be decreased or the use of another anesthetic considered. It was reported that dopamine, a beta agonist acting on different receptors in the myocardium than either epinephrine or isoproterenol, may be useful as an inotropic agent in patients experiencing this interaction.

Summary: The administration of halothane and labetalol has been shown to result in myocardial depression, a decrease in arterial blood pressure, cardiac output, peripheral resistance, a fall in heart rate and an increase in central venous pressure.

Related Drugs: A similar interaction may occur between halothane and other beta-blocking agents; however, it is difficult to determine the extent of the interaction. The other halogenated inhalation anesthetics may interact with labetalol.

Mechanism: A synergism between labetalol's alpha and beta receptor blockade and halothane's myocardial depressant activity has been revealed.

Detailed Information: See *EDI,* 11/4.30

Metoprolol-Amiodarone

Significance: 2—moderately clinically significant

Potential Effects: Concurrent use of the agents results in severe bradycardia.

Recommendations: Monitor patients closely for bradycardia during concurrent use. If this occurs, metoprolol should be discontinued, and a sympathomimetic agent may be required. Atenolol might be an alternative to metoprolol.

Summary: Metoprolol may interact with amiodarone by producing severe bradycardia.

Related Drugs: There has been documentation of an interaction between amiodarone and propranolol. Because of conflicting results, it is not known whether an interaction would occur between amiodarone and other beta-adrenergic blocking agents.

Mechanism: The mechanism by which metoprolol and amiodarone produce severe bradycardia and hypotension has not been established.

Detailed Information: See *EDI,* 11/4.50

Metoprolol-Oral Contraceptive Agents

Significance: 3—minimally clinically significant

Potential Effects: Oral contraceptives may decrease the metabolism of metoprolol.

Recommendations: Although concurrent use of these agents need not be avoided, patients should be monitored for a possible increase in the effects of metoprolol.

Summary: There are data to show that oral contraceptive agents may decrease the metabolism and increase the effects of metoprolol.

Related Drugs: Propranolol and acebutolol have been shown to interact with oral contraceptive agents. Because of conflicting results, it is not known if an interaction would occur between oral contraceptive agents and other hepatically metabolized beta-blocking agents. A similar interaction is not expected to occur with beta-blocking agents that do not undergo significant hepatic metabolism.

Mechanism: Oral contraceptive agents inhibit hepatic microsomal enzymes, leading to a reduction in first-pass hepatic metabolism of metoprolol and propranolol.

Detailed Information: See *EDI*, 11/5.00

Metoprolol-Pentobarbital

Significance: 2—moderately clinically significant

Recommendations: The dosage regimen of orally administered metoprolol may have to be increased if prescribed concomitantly with long-term (longer than ten days) pentobarbital therapy. The barbiturates do not seem to change the bioavailability of beta-blockers administered intravenously. Patients should be observed for a less than optimal therapeutic effect. Alternatively, timolol or one of the beta-blockers not dependent on hepatic first-pass metabolism (atenolol, nadolol, and pindolol) may be substituted.

Summary: Pentobarbital has been reported to reduce the plasma concentration and bioavailability of metoprolol.

Related Drugs: Phenobarbital has been shown to increase the clearance of propranolol. Pentobarbital has reduced the plasma concentrations and bioavailability of alprenolol. Timolol or the beta-blocking agents not dependent on first-pass hepatic metabolism have been shown not to interact. A similar interaction may occur between metoprolol and other barbiturates.

Mechanism: Pentobarbital and phenobarbital have been reported to induce liver enzymes, reducing the plasma concentrations of the beta-blocking agents dependent on hepatic metabolism.

Detailed Information: See *EDI*, 11/7.00

Metoprolol-Rifampin

Significance: 2—moderately clinically significant

Recommendations: During concurrent use of these agents, blood pressure changes should be carefully monitored as the dose of metoprolol may need to be increased.

Summary: Rifampin, when administered concurrently with metoprolol, reduced the area-under-curve of metoprolol.

Related Drugs: There are no drugs related to rifampin. Propranolol has been shown to interact with rifampin. A similar interaction is not expected to occur with other beta-blocking agents that are not extensively metabolized by first-pass hepatic metabolism.

Mechanism: Rifampin, a known inducer of hepatic microsomal enzymes, is probably responsible for this interaction.

Detailed Information: See *EDI*, 11/9.00

Nadolol-Phenelzine

Significance: 3—minimally clinically significant

Potential Effects: Bradycardia and a decrease in the pulse rate may occur with concurrent administration of nadolol and phenelzine.

Recommendations: A careful observation should be made of the pulse rates with coadministration of nadolol and phenelzine. One review suggests that monoamine oxidase inhibitor therapy should be discontinued at least two weeks prior to the institution of propranolol therapy.

Summary: A patient on nadolol therapy experienced bradycardia when phenelzine was added to the regimen.

Related Drugs: Metoprolol with phenelzine has been shown to cause changes in pulse. Documentation is lacking regarding an interaction between other monoamine oxidase inhibitors and other beta-blocking agents and with furazolidone and procarbazine.

Mechanism: The mechanism of this interaction is unknown.

Detailed Information: See *EDI*, 11/10.50

Propranolol-Alcohol, Ethyl

Significance: 3—minimally clinically significant

Recommendations: Alcohol alone may lead to incidences of angina and tachycardia. It is possible that the concomitant use of these agents potentiates these adverse reactions as well as other side effects involving neurologic functions. It is prudent to caution patients regarding the concurrent use of propranolol and alcohol.

Summary: The elimination of propranolol is increased by concomitant administration of alcohol, and the blood pressure reducing effect of propranolol may be diminished.

Related Drugs: The beta-blocking agents that undergo extensive hepatic metabolism may be affected by concurrent alcohol ingestion. The beta-blocking agents that are not extensively metabolized by the liver are expected to interact similarly with alcohol.

Mechanism: Blood flow to the liver is increased by alcohol through vascular dilation, resulting in an increased amount of propranolol presented to the liver for metabolism.

Detailed Information: See *EDI*, 11/11.00

Propranolol-Allergenic Extracts

Significance: 3—minimally clinically significant

Recommendations: Although anaphylaxis may occur with the use of the allergenic extract alone, patients receiving a beta-blocking agent who are given immunotherapy may experience an exaggerated anaphylactic reaction. Aggressive therapy may be required if such an interaction occurs. Further documentation of the extent of such an interaction is necessary.

Summary: A patient experienced an anaphylactic reaction to a monthly allergenic extract injection after being started on propranolol therapy. Severe hypertension was also reported in this patient.

Related Drugs: Other beta-blocking agents may have the same ability to potentiate anaphylactic reactions as propranolol.

Mechanism: Beta receptor blockade may potentiate anaphylactic reactions by decreasing intracellular cyclic AMP, lowering the threshold for mediator release by mast cells.

Detailed Information: See *EDI*, 11/12.10

Propranolol-Aluminum Hydroxide

Significance: 3—minimally clinically significant

Recommendations: The clinical significance of the changes in bioavailability have not been determined for any of the beta-blocking agents. Until such data are available, it would seem prudent to separate the dosages of the antacid and beta-blockers by as much time as possible.

Summary: Concomitant administration of propranolol and aluminum hydroxide gel resulted in a decrease in propranolol bioavailability.

Related Drugs: Because of conflicting results, it is difficult to determine whether an interaction would occur between aluminum hydroxide and other beta-blockers.

Mechanism: The proposed mechanisms involve propranolol being adsorbed to, or complexing with, the antacid compound, inhibiting gastrointestinal absorption.

Detailed Information: See *EDI,* 11/13.00

Propranolol-Aminoglutethimide

Significance: 3—minimally clinically significant

Recommendations: Although no special precautions are necessary at this time, the patient's blood pressure should still be periodically monitored following the concomitant use of propranolol and aminoglutethimide.

Summary: A case of lethargy, skin rash, and hypotension was reported in a patient with metastatic cancer taking propranolol following the addition of aminoglutethimide.

Related Drugs: An interaction may occur between aminoglutethimide and other beta-blocking agents. Glutethimide has been shown to interact in a different manner with labetalol (see Labetalol-Glutethimide, page 253).

Mechanism: Aminoglutethimide may exert an antithyroid-like effect, and propranolol may enhance this effect. Propranolol may cause vasodilation and hypotension.

Detailed Information: See *EDI,* 11/14.01

Propranolol-Aspirin

Significance: 3—minimally clinically significant

Recommendations: Patients' blood pressure should be monitored closely during concurrent use of these agents. If a loss of blood pressure control is noted, the dose of propranolol may need to be increased or aspirin may need to be discontinued. Further studies are needed.

Summary: Administration of aspirin with propranolol has been shown to increase diastolic blood pressure.

Related Drugs: A similar interaction may occur between aspirin and other beta-blocking agents. An interaction may occur between propranolol and other salicylates; however, documentation is lacking.

Mechanism: Aspirin may inhibit the prostaglandins responsible for vasodilation, resulting in an increase in blood pressure.

Detailed Information: See *EDI,* 11/14.10

Propranolol-Chlorpheniramine

Significance: 4—not clinically significant

Recommendations: The possibility of an interaction between these agents, though remote, should be considered when they are coadministered.

Summary: Chlorpheniramine could theoretically inhibit the beta-adrenergic blocking effect of propranolol and enhance its quinidine-like effect.

Related Drugs: Other beta-adrenergic blocking agents could also be affected by the antihistamines.

Mechanism: Chlorpheniramine has been shown to prevent the uptake of catecholamines at the adrenergic nerve terminal, raising the concentration at the adrenergic receptor sites.

Detailed Information: See *EDI,* 11/15.00

Propranolol-Chlorpromazine

Significance: 2—moderately clinically significant

Potential Effects: The concomitant administration of these agents may result in increased levels of either agent.

Recommendations: Patients receiving chlorpromazine and propranolol concurrently should be monitored for increased levels of both agents, as well as for symptoms of chlorpromazine toxicity (e.g., delirium, grand mal seizure). The dose of either agent may need to be decreased.

Summary: The concurrent administration of propranolol and chlorpromazine has been shown to increase levels of each other.

Related Drugs: A similar interaction is expected to occur between phenothiazines, thioxanthenes, butyrophenones, dihydroindolones and dibenzoxazepines and propranolol. A similar interaction is expected to occur with other beta-blocking agents extensively metabolized by the liver, if the mechanism involves a decreased first-pass hepatic metabolism. It is not known if the beta-blocking agents that do not exhibit an extensive first-pass metabolism would be expected to interact with chlorpromazine.

Mechanism: The bioavailability of propranolol is increased as a result of a decrease in the first-pass hepatic metabolism by chlorpromazine.

Detailed Information: See *EDI,* 11/17.00

Propranolol-Cholestyramine

Significance: 3—minimally clinically significant

Recommendations: Concomitant administration of cholestyramine and propranolol need not be avoided; however, patients receiving long-term propranolol therapy who have cholestyramine added to, or withdrawn from, their therapy may require an adjustment in the propranolol dosage.

Summary: Cholestyramine administration may necessitate an adjustment in propranolol dosage in some patients.

Related Drugs: Other beta-blocking agents may interact similarly with cholestyramine.

Mechanism: This interaction may result from the formation of a nonabsorbable complex by propranolol and cholestyramine.

Detailed Information: See *EDI,* 11/18.10

Propranolol-Cimetidine

Significance: 1—highly clinically significant

Potential Effects: Cimetidine inhibits the metabolism of propranolol, resulting in increased propranolol levels and effects.

Recommendations: Patients receiving these agents concurrently should be monitored for increased beta-blocking activity. The dose of either agent may need to be reduced, or alternative agents to cimetidine (famotidine, ranitidine) or propranolol (atenolol, pindolol) that do not interact may be considered.

Summary: Concurrent administration of cimetidine and propranolol have resulted in an increase in propranolol plasma concentrations. Resting pulse rates may be significantly lower when cimetidine is administered with propranolol.

Related Drugs: Cimetidine interacted similarly with metoprolol and labetalol. Because of conflicting results, it is difficult to determine whether an interaction would occur between cimetidine and other beta-blocking agents. Ranitidine has been shown to interact similarly to cimetidine; however, all data do not support this. Propranolol would not be expected to interact with famotidine.

Mechanism: Cimetidine reduces hepatic blood flow, decreasing the extraction rate of propranolol, and it may inhibit propranolol metabolism.

Detailed Information: See *EDI,* 11/19.00

Propranolol-Cocaine

Significance: 2—moderately clinically significant

Potential Effects: Cocaine-associated coronary vasoconstriction may be potentiated by propranolol.

Recommendations: Concurrent use of propranolol and cocaine should probably be avoided.

Summary: Cocaine-induced coronary vasoconstriction is potentiated by propranolol.

Related Drugs: A similar interaction may occur between cocaine and other beta-adrenergic blocking agents.

Mechanism: Propranolol potentiates the effects of cocaine.

Detailed Information: See *EDI,* 11/20.50

Propranolol-Desipramine

Significance: 3—minimally clinically significant

Recommendations: Since substantial clinical evidence is lacking with respect to specific interactions of desipramine with propranolol, no additional precautions are necessary when these drugs are given concurrently. However, precautions appropriate to the individual use of these drugs should be observed.

Summary: The use of propranolol in patients receiving desipramine requires caution until reports are fully substantiated.

Related Drugs: Other beta-blocking agents may interact with desipramine in a similar manner to propranolol.

Mechanism: Desipramine may antagonize propranolol in myocardial tissue and may counteract the bradycardia and decrease the inotropic effects produced by propranolol.

Detailed Information: See *EDI,* 11/21.00

Propranolol-Diatrizoate

Significance: 3—minimally clinically significant

Potential Effects: Administration of these agents together may result in hypotension.

Recommendations: Further documentation of the incidence of adverse reactions to radiocontrast agents with concurrent beta-blocking drug therapy is necessary before the extent of such an interaction can be determined. In order to minimize the likelihood of such an interaction, one study recommended withdrawing the beta-blocking agent for two to three days before radiologic examination and administering an antihistamine two hours before examination. However, abruptly withdrawing beta-blocker therapy can be associated with the development of other adverse reactions. Until further information is available, practitioners should be aware of the possibility of hypotension development with concurrent radiocontrast agent and beta-blocker use.

Summary: A patient taking propranolol received sodium meglumine diatrizoate and experienced severe reactions characterized by progressive erythema of the upper extremities, hypotension, and tachycardia.

Related Drugs: Nadolol was documented to cause a similar interaction. The other beta-blocking agents may have the same ability to potentiate hypotensive reactions of diatrizoate. It is not known if other radiopaque agents would interact similarly with propranolol.

Mechanism: Iodinated contrast agents may cause histamine release and the development of hypotension or an anaphylactic reaction.

Detailed Information: See *EDI,* 11/22.10

Propranolol-Epinephrine

Significance: 1—highly clinically significant

Recommendations: Sympathomimetic drugs with alpha agonist activity should be avoided if possible or used very cautiously in patients taking nonselective beta antagonists. This includes the use of local anesthetics with epinephrine. It has been recommended that the epinephrine dose not exceed 3mg/Kg every 30 minutes in these patients, with continuous blood pressure and pulse monitoring. If possible, a cardioselective beta$_1$-blocking agent (acebutolol, atenolol, and metoprolol) may be cautiously used in place of propranolol, beginning a few days before the patient is scheduled to receive the sympathomimetic drug.

Summary: Administration of epinephrine with propranolol may result in a considerable increase in systolic and diastolic blood pressure and a marked decrease in heart rate, potentiating a stroke.

Related Drugs: There are ample data indicating that epinephrine may interact with other beta-blockers; however, the data are conflicting. Epinephrine has been documented to interact with beta-blocking ophthalmic preparations as well.

Mechanism: Concurrent administration of propranolol and epinephrine results in blocking of the beta agonist activity of epinephrine while the alpha adrenergic effects are unopposed.

Detailed Information: See *EDI,* 11/23.00

Propranolol-Ergotamine

Significance: 3—minimally clinically significant

Recommendations: In certain patients receiving concomitant propranolol and ergot alkaloids, the dose of the ergot alkaloid may need to be adjusted downward.

Summary: There are data to show that administration of propranolol may necessitate an adjustment downward of the ergot alkaloids. Peripheral vasoconstriction and migraine headache have been reported when propranolol was added to the regimen.

Related Drugs: A similar interaction is not expected to occur between the beta$_1$ cardioselective beta-blocking agents, if the mechanism involves the blocking of the vasodilatory effect of beta$_2$-adrenergic receptors in the vessels. The other noncardioselective beta-blocking agents may interact similarly with ergotamine. The other ergot alkaloids may interact with propranolol.

Mechanism: Vasodilation is blocked by the noncardioselective beta-adrenergic blocking agents, allowing the ergot alkaloid to produce a maximum vasoconstriction.

Detailed Information: See *EDI*, 11/25.00

Propranolol-Flecainide

Significance: 3—minimally clinically significant

Potential Effects: Use of these agents together may result in an increase in plasma levels of both drugs and an additive effect on cardiac function.

Recommendations: Use of these agents together need not routinely be avoided. However, the patient's cardiac status should be monitored.

Summary: There are data to show that coadministration of these agents may result in an increase in plasma levels of both drugs and an additive effect on cardiac function.

Related Drugs: A similar interaction may occur between flecainide and other beta-blocking agents. It is not known whether an interaction would occur between propranolol and the other class IC antiarrhythmic agents.

Mechanism: The mechanism of this interaction is unknown.

Detailed Information: See *EDI*, 11/26.10

Propranolol-Fluoxetine

Significance: 2—moderately clinically significant

Potential Effects: Increased cardiac effects of propranolol may be seen following the addition of fluoxetine.

Recommendations: Patients receiving concurrent selective serotonin reuptake inhibitors and beta-blockers should be monitored closely for increased pharmacologic action of beta-blockers. The beta-blocker dosage may need to be decreased.

Summary: Increased cardiac effects of propranolol have been seen following the addition of fluoxetine.

Related Drugs: Similar interactions have been reported between fluoxetine and metoprolol, sertraline and propranolol, and fluvoxamine and both metoprolol and propranolol. Although documentation is lacking, based on the proposed mechanism fluoxetine would be expected to interact with the other beta-adrenergic blockers which undergo hepatic metabolism and a similar reaction would be expected to occur between paroxetine and the hepatically metabolized beta-blockers.

Mechanism: It was postulated that fluoxetine may increase the duration of action of 5-HT in the atrium, thus impairing atrioventricular conduction, and that fluoxetine may inhibit the metabolism of metoprolol and other lipophilic beta-blockers which undergo extensive first-pass metabolism by the cytochrome P450 enzyme. Sertraline and the other selective serotonin reuptake inhibitors may worsen coronary artery disease by causing vasoconstriction in affected coronary arteries.

Detailed Information: See *EDI*, 11/26.50

Propranolol-Furosemide

Significance: 2—moderately clinically significant

Recommendations: The concurrent use of these agents need not be avoided. However, patients should be closely monitored, and a corresponding dosage adjustment of either agent should be made if necessary.

Summary: The concurrent administration of furosemide and propranolol results in higher blood levels of propranolol, and this increase can be accompanied by a simultaneous increase in beta-adrenergic blockade.

Related Drugs: Documentation is lacking regarding an interaction between furosemide and other beta-blocking agents. A similar interaction is expected to occur between propranolol and the other loop diuretics.

Mechanism: A furosemide-induced reduction in extracellular fluid volume may be responsible for this mechanism.

Detailed Information: See *EDI,* 11/27.00

Propranolol-Hydralazine

Significance: 3—minimally clinically significant

Recommendations: The clinical significance of the increased propranolol bioavailability has not been determined in long-term administration studies. Some patients may develop symptoms of propranolol toxicity (e.g., bradycardia, bronchospasm). If such symptoms appear, plasma propranolol should be monitored, and decreasing the propranolol dosage may be indicated.

Summary: Concurrent administration of hydralazine and propranolol significantly increases the bioavailability of propranolol and may enhance the antihypertensive effect of hydralazine.

Related Drugs: Hydralazine resulted in similar plasma concentration increases with metoprolol, but not with nadolol or acebutolol. Labetalol may interact with hydralazine similarly to propranolol. Beta-blocking agents that do not undergo significant first-pass metabolism would not interact with hydralazine. There are no drugs related to hydralazine.

Mechanism: Hydralazine may enhance the systemic availability of propranolol by alteration of first-pass clearance.

Detailed Information: See *EDI,* 11/29.00

Propranolol-Indomethacin

Significance: 2—moderately clinically significant

Potential Effects: Indomethacin may reduce the hypotensive effects of propranolol.

Recommendations: Patients' blood pressure should be closely monitored when these agents are used together. The dose of propranolol may need to be increased or the indomethacin discontinued.

Summary: Indomethacin therapy may reduce the hypotensive effects of propranolol.

Related Drugs: A similar interaction is expected to occur between indomethacin and other beta-blocking agents. Oral and ophthalmic indomethacin did not affect the ability of ophthalmic timolol to lower intraocular pressure. Since NSAIAs inhibit prostaglandin synthesis to some extent, a similar interaction is expected to occur with propranolol.

Mechanism: Indomethacin inhibits the prostaglandin responsible for vasodilation, resulting in an increase in blood pressure.

Detailed Information: See *EDI,* 11/31.00

Propranolol-Misoprostol

Significance: 3—minimally clinically significant

Potential Effects: Misoprostol may increase propranolol levels.

Recommendations: No special precautions appear necessary at the present time, since the existence and clinical significance of a misoprostol-propranolol interaction has not been established.

Summary: The addition of misoprostol to propranolol therapy may result in an increase in the maximum plasma propranolol concentration.

Related Drugs: No additional information is available concerning an interaction between misoprostol and other beta adrenergic blocking agents; therefore, it is not known whether a reaction would be expected to occur. There are no drugs related to misoprostol.

Mechanism: This interaction may result from changes in hepatic blood flow or reduced gastric acid secretion.

Detailed Information: See *EDI*, 11/32.05

Propranolol-Pravastatin

Significance: 3—minimally clinically significant

Potential Effects: Propranolol may decrease the bioavailability of pravastatin.

Recommendations: Although the patient should be monitored during concurrent propranolol and pravastatin administration, the clinical significance of the decrease in pravastatin concentration is likely to be small.

Summary: The coadministration of propranolol with pravastatin has been shown to decrease the pravastatin total mean serum concentration-time curve.

Related Drugs: A similar interaction is expected to occur between propranolol and other HMG-CoA reductase inhibitors. The other beta-adrenergic blocking agents that are primarily hepatically metabolized may interact. It is not known whether an interaction would occur between pravastatin and other beta-adrenergic blocking agents that are not hepatically metabolized or between propranolol and other HMG-CoA reductase inhibitors.

Mechanism: Beta-adrenergic blocking agents decrease hepatic blood flow, increasing first-pass clearance of drugs having high extraction ratios.

Detailed Information: See *EDI*, 11/32.50

Propranolol-Quinidine

Significance: 3—minimally clinically significant

Potential Effects: Propranolol may reduce the clearance of quinidine. Concurrent therapy may possibly result in orthostatic hypotension. However, these agents may have a beneficial effect when used together for arrhythmias.

Recommendations: Concurrent administration of these agents may be therapeutically beneficial in certain patients. However, patients should be monitored for quinidine levels and orthostatic hypotension.

Summary: There are data to show that administration of propranolol may reduce the clearance of quinidine and result in orthostatic hypotension.

Related Drugs: It would be expected that other beta-adrenergic blockers would exert the same beneficial effect with quinidine. It is not known if propranolol would interact with the quinine.

Mechanism: The mechanism of the decreased clearance of quinidine by propranolol is not known.

Detailed Information: See *EDI,* 11/33.00

Propranolol-Thyroid

Significance: 2—moderately clinically significant

Recommendations: Although a specific drug interaction has not been determined, it is prudent to be aware of a possible interaction while treating a patient with a thyroid abnormality. Therefore, when using a thyroid drug concurrently with propranolol or metoprolol, the dose of the beta-blocking agent may need to be increased. Alternatively, a noninteracting beta-blocking agent may be used.

Summary: Several studies indicate that patients taking a thyroid drug may show a decreased bioavailability of propranolol; however, other studies show conflicting results.

Related Drugs: Metoprolol undergoes extensive first-pass metabolism and is altered in the hyperthyroid state. Those beta-blocking agents that do not undergo significant first-pass metabolism do not appear to be affected by hyperthyroidism. A similar interaction may be expected between propranolol and other thyroid drugs.

Mechanism: The decreased bioavailability of propranolol and metoprolol results from an increase in presystemic clearance related to the extent of first-pass metabolism. In the hypothyroid state, the interaction may be produced by a decrease in presystemic clearance.

Detailed Information: See *EDI,* 11/35.00

Propranolol-Tobacco

Significance: 2—moderately clinically significant

Potential Effects: Smoking decreased the levels of propranolol.

Recommendations: If a patient stabilized on propranolol changes smoking habits, the dose of propranolol may need to be adjusted.

Summary: Smoking has resulted in reduced steady-state serum propranolol concentrations and increased propranolol clearance.

Related Drugs: The other beta-blocking agents dependent on hepatic metabolism may interact similarly with tobacco. The beta-blocking agents that are not dependent on hepatic metabolism may not interact with tobacco.

Mechanism: Tobacco is known to induce hepatic microsomal enzymes, and propranolol is eliminated by hepatic clearance.

Detailed Information: See *EDI,* 11/37.00

Timolol, Ophthalmic-Acetazolamide

Significance: 3—minimally clinically significant

Potential Effects: The use of the agents together in patients with chronic obstructive pulmonary disease (COPD) may result in acidosis.

Recommendations: The concurrent administration of acetazolamide and ophthalmic timolol, especially in patients with COPD, should be done with caution. If acidosis occurs, one or both agents may need to be discontinued. The use of ophthalmic betaxolol, a cardioselective agent, may be considered as an alternative to ophthalmic timolol.

Summary: There are data to show that coadministration of these agents in patients with COPD may result in acidosis.

Related Drugs: A similar interaction may occur between acetazolamide and other oral and ophthalmic noncardioselective beta blocking agents. A similar interaction may occur between ophthalmic timolol and other carbonic anhydrase inhibitors.

Mechanism: Acetazolamide produces metabolic acidosis by blocking the renal excretion of hydrogen ions.

Detailed Information: See *EDI*, 11/38.10

Timolol, Ophthalmic-Prednisone

Significance: 2—moderately clinically significant

Potential Effects: The use of these agents together may cause an increase in the serum potassium level.

Recommendations: Monitor the patient's serum potassium level when these agents are used together. The ophthalmic timolol may need to be discontinued.

Summary: There are data to show that coadministration of these agents may cause an increase in serum potassium levels.

Related Drugs: A similar interaction may occur between prednisone and other beta blocking agents as well as the other ophthalmic beta blocking agents. A similar interaction is expected to occur between ophthalmic timolol and other corticosteroids.

Mechanism: Therapy with beta-blocking agents can cause small increases in potassium levels by suppression of renin and aldosterone release and by preventing $beta_2$-receptor mediated hepatic and skeletal muscle potassium uptake.

Detailed Information: See *EDI*, 11/39.00

Chapter Twelve

Cardiac Glycoside
Drug Interactions

Digitalis-Calcium Chloride (intravenous)

Significance: 2—moderately clinically significant

Recommendations: If intravenous administration of calcium is necessary in patients receiving digitalis therapy, it is recommended that this procedure be accomplished slowly and with caution. If cardiac toxicity does develop from intravenous calcium administration to a digitalized patient, supportive measures without additional antiarrhythmics may be sufficient, based on studies of massive digitalis intoxication. Calcium chelation with ethylenediaminetetraacetic acid (EDTA) may produce only transient improvement while adding its own toxicity; therefore, it has been considered unsatisfactory in treating digitalis toxicity in general.

Summary: Effects of digitalis glycosides on the heart are increased by extracellular concentrations of ionic calcium. Intravenous administration of calcium salts during digitalis therapy may result in altered cardiac electrophysiologic activity.

Related Drugs: The other digitalis glycosides may interact in a similar manner. Multiple forms of calcium compounds are available for parenteral administration and may interact in a similar manner with the digitalis glycosides.

Mechanism: Elevated extracellular concentrations of Ca^{+2} facilitate inward calcium fluxes and modify transmembrane potentials and stronger contractions of cardiac muscle.

Detailed Information: See *EDI*, 12/1.00

Digitalis-Phenytoin

Significance: 2—moderately clinically significant

Recommendations: With appropriate safeguards, phenytoin appears to be a useful adjunct to management of digitalis-induced supraventricular arrhythmias. It must be borne in mind that certain individuals may not respond, or may experience a worsening in cardiac function, after therapeutic doses of phenytoin. Long-term antiarrhythmic treatment with phenytoin may increase the elimination of digitalis, so use of an alternate antiarrhythmic drug may be advantageous. If phenytoin is deleted from combination therapy with digitalis, appropriate adjustment of the cardiac glycoside dosage may be necessary.

Summary: The administration of phenytoin to a patient experiencing supraventricular cardiotoxicity from digitalis has been utilized as a positive interaction with beneficial results.

Related Drugs: The other digitalis glycosides may interact in a similar manner with phenytoin. A similar interaction is expected to occur with other hydantoin anticonvulsants and digitalis.

Mechanism: Phenytoin antagonizes supraventricular arrhythmias induced by digitalis overdosage through a pharmacodynamic interaction on the membranes of myocardial pacemaker cells.

Detailed Information: See *EDI*, 12/3.00

Digitalis-Reserpine

Significance: 3—minimally clinically significant

Recommendations: It may be wise to consider the many alternatives to reserpine for controlling hypertension in patients using digitalis glycosides. If reserpine is necessary in a digitalized individual, it can be successfully used, but careful observation of the patient is in order. If atrial fibrillation pre-exists, the potential for this adverse drug interaction appears to be greatly enhanced.

Summary: The clinical literature documents an interaction between cardiac glycosides and reserpine characterized by enhanced cardiotoxicity.

Related Drugs: A similar interaction is expected to occur with other digitalis glycosides and reserpine. Other rauwolfia alkaloids may interact with digitalis.

Mechanism: Direct or indirect effects of these two drugs may actually underlie this interaction.

Detailed Information: See *EDI*, 12/5.00

Digitoxin-Aminoglutethimide

Significance: 3—minimally clinically significant

Potential Effects: Aminoglutethimide may increase the clearance of digitoxin, leading to decreased digitoxin levels.

Recommendations: Although concurrent use of these agents need not be avoided, digitoxin levels should be monitored and the dosage increased if necessary.

Summary: There are data to show that administration of aminoglutethimide may increase the clearance of digitoxin, leading to decreased digitoxin levels.

Related Drugs: Digitalis may interact in a similar manner with aminoglutethimide. The other digitalis glycosides would not be expected to interact with aminoglutethimide. A similar interaction may occur between glutethimide and digitoxin.

Mechanism: Aminoglutethimide increases the metabolism of digitoxin.

Detailed Information: See *EDI*, 12/6.10

Digitoxin-Cholestyramine

Significance: 2—moderately clinically significant

Potential Effects: Cholestyramine may bind to digitoxin in the gastrointestinal tract, decreasing absorption and increasing elimination.

Recommendations: Monitor digitalis levels when these agents are used together. Separating administration by 1.5 hours or using digoxin capsules may avoid this interaction. Cholestyramine may be useful in treating digoxin toxicity.

Summary: Concurrent administration of cholestyramine and digitoxin can decrease the gastrointestinal absorption of digitoxin and result in reduced bioavailability.

Related Drugs: Administration of cholestyramine and digoxin resulted in reduced digoxin bioavailability. Based on the proposed mechanism, cholestyramine may interact with other digitalis glycosides. A similar interaction is expected to occur between colestipol and other digitalis glycosides.

Mechanism: Cholestyramine has been reported to bind digitoxin in the gastrointestinal tract, inhibiting absorption and enterohepatic circulation and resulting in reduced reabsorption and increased fecal excretion of digitoxin.

Detailed Information: See *EDI*, 12/7.00

Digitoxin-Phenobarbital

Significance: 2—moderately clinically significant

Recommendations: When phenobarbital or another barbiturate is added to the regimen of a patient receiving digitoxin, careful monitoring for underdigitalization should be performed. It may be necessary to increase the digitoxin dose in some patients. Conversely, patients receiving combined therapy should be monitored carefully for digitalis toxicity if the barbiturate is withdrawn from the regimen.

Summary: Phenobarbital may decrease plasma digitoxin levels and shorten the digitoxin half-life.

Related Drugs: Digitalis leaf may interact in a similar manner with phenobarbital. Other barbiturates would interact with cardiac glycosides in a similar manner.

Mechanism: Phenobarbital may increase the metabolism of digitoxin to digoxin through hepatic microsomal enzymes.

Detailed Information: See *EDI*, 12/9.00

Digitoxin-Phenylbutazone

Significance: 3—minimally clinically significant

Recommendations: Patients should be closely monitored during concurrent therapy, and the dose of digitoxin may need to be increased.

Summary: Phenylbutazone reduced serum digitoxin levels.

Related Drugs: A similar interaction is expected to occur between digitoxin and oxyphenbutazone and between phenylbutazone and other digitalis glycosides.

Mechanism: Phenylbutazone may increase the hepatic metabolism of digitoxin.

Detailed Information: See *EDI*, 12/11.00

Digitoxin-Rifampin

Significance: 1—highly clinically significant

Recommendations: Patients should be monitored for underdigitalization during concurrent therapy with rifampin. It would be expected that the dosage of the glycoside will need to be increased within the first week of cotherapy.

Summary: Serum digitoxin concentrations can be significantly reduced with concurrent use of rifampin.

Related Drugs: Rifampin has caused subtherapeutic digoxin serum concentrations. A similar interaction is expected to occur with rifampin and other digitalis glycosides. There are no drugs related to rifampin.

Mechanism: Rifampin increases the metabolism of digitoxin.

Detailed Information: See *EDI*, 12/13.00

Digoxin-Acarbose

Significance: 3—minimally clinically significant

Potential Effects: Concurrent administration of digoxin and acarbose may result in subtherapeutic levels of digoxin.

Recommendations: Serum digoxin levels should be monitored in patients receiving concurrent therapy with digoxin and acarbose. The dosage of digoxin may need to be adjusted or acarbose may need to be discontinued.

Summary: Concurrent administration of digoxin and acarbose resulted in subtherapeutic levels of digoxin as low as 0.48ng/ml (therapeutic range: 0.8–2.1ng/ml).

Related Drugs: A similar reaction would be expected to occur between acarbose and the other digitalis glycosides. There are no drugs related to acarbose.

Mechanism: The exact mechanism is unknown. An acarbose-induced change in gastrointestinal transit may alter the absorption of digoxin or acarbose may adsorb digoxin molecules. Alternatively, acarbose may inhibit the hydrolysis of digoxin prior to absorption, resulting in alterations in the digoxin laboratory analysis, since less genin, a digoxin hydrolysate, would be available to cross-react in the assay.

Detailed Information: See *EDI,* 12/15.00

Digoxin-Aluminum Hydroxide, Magnesium Hydroxide, Magnesium Trisilicate

Significance: 2—moderately clinically significant

Potential Effects: Simultaneous administration of aluminum- or magnesium-containing antacids may decrease the gastrointestinal absorption of digoxin.

Recommendations: Oral digoxin tablets should not be given simultaneously with certain antacids (e.g., aluminum/magnesium hydroxide and magnesium trisilicate). When both digoxin and antacids are indicated, antacid preparations containing magnesium trisilicate, magnesium hydroxide, and aluminum hydroxide should be administered at least one to two hours before or after the digoxin. Serum digoxin levels and the clinical status of the patient should be monitored carefully for signs of underdigitalization. The use of digoxin with concurrent sucralfate should be monitored for decreased effects of digoxin. The sucralfate may have to be discontinued.

Summary: Administration of antacids containing magnesium trisilicate, magnesium hydroxide, and aluminum hydroxide may significantly decrease the gastrointestinal absorption of digoxin.

Related Drugs: The other digitalis glycosides may interact with antacids to a variable degree. The extent to which other magnesium- or aluminum-containing antacids affect digoxin absorption is not known. Sucralfate was shown to decrease digoxin area-under-curve.

Mechanism: The adsorptive capacity of antacids may be responsible for decreased digoxin absorption. Liquid antacids coat digoxin tablets and may interfere with dissolution or disintegration. Digoxin may bind to sucralfate, decreasing the extent of absorption.

Detailed Information: See *EDI,* 12/17.00

Digoxin-Aminosalicylic Acid

Significance: 3—minimally clinically significant

Recommendations: Patients' digoxin serum levels should be monitored during concomitant use of these agents. An increased digoxin dose may be necessary, or separating the administration of the two drugs by as much time as possible may be beneficial.

Summary: Concurrent administration of digoxin and aminosalicylic acid resulted in a reduced digoxin area-under-curve.

Related Drugs: A similar interaction may occur between aminosalicylic acid and other digitalis glycosides. There are no drugs related to aminosalicylic acid.

Mechanism: Decreased gastrointestinal absorption of digoxin is believed to be the mechanism in this interaction.

Detailed Information: See *EDI,* 12/19.00

Digoxin-Amiodarone

Significance: 1—highly clinically significant

Potential Effects: Amiodarone causes an increase in digoxin levels, which may result in digoxin toxicity.

Recommendations: Monitor patients for signs of digoxin toxicity and increased digoxin levels. The dose of digoxin may need to be decreased.

Summary: Several studies and case reports have shown that the concurrent administration of digoxin and amiodarone results in significant increases in digoxin serum levels, digoxin toxicity and side effects.

Related Drugs: A similar interaction may occur between amiodarone and other digitalis glycosides. There are no drugs related to amiodarone.

Mechanism: Amiodarone decreases renal and nonrenal clearance of digoxin, probably by a decrease in renal tubular secretion, or amiodarone may displace digoxin from its tissue binding sites.

Detailed Information: See *EDI,* 12/20.01

Digoxin-Captopril

Significance: 2—moderately clinically significant

Potential Effects: Captopril may cause an increase in digoxin levels.

Recommendations: Monitor patients for increased digoxin levels when these agents are used together.

Summary: There are data to show that administration of captopril may cause an increase in digoxin levels; however, studies have also shown that digoxin levels may slightly decrease.

Related Drugs: A similar interaction may occur between deslanoside and captopril, if the mechanism involves a reduced renal clearance of digoxin. A similar interaction may occur between digoxin and other ACE inhibitors.

Mechanism: Captopril increases digoxin levels by reducing digoxin's renal clearance.

Detailed Information: See *EDI,* 12/20.03

Digoxin-Charcoal

Significance: 3—minimally clinically significant

Recommendations: Activated charcoal appears to be effective in the treatment of an acute digoxin overdose, especially in doses of 50 to 100G, and one report suggests that it may also be effective in some cases of more chronic intoxications. However, if charcoal is not being used in this situation, it may be advisable to separate the administration of these agents by as much time as possible.

Summary: Activated charcoal has been shown to reduce the absorption and lower serum levels of digoxin.

Related Drugs: It may be expected that charcoal will reduce the absorption of the other digitalis glycosides.

Mechanism: Activated charcoal adsorbs digoxin, limiting its gastrointestinal absorption.

Detailed Information: See *EDI,* 12/20.10

Digoxin-Cimetidine

Significance: 3—minimally clinically significant

Recommendations: Until further studies are done, the concurrent use of these agents need not be avoided. However, because of digoxin's low therapeutic index, serum digoxin levels should be monitored. An increased digoxin dose may be necessary.

Summary: There are data to show that cimetidine administration may decrease digoxin levels; however, all data do not support this interaction.

Related Drugs: The other digitalis glycosides may interact similarly with cimetidine. Documentation is lacking regarding a similar interaction between digoxin and other H_2-receptor antagonists.

Mechanism: Cimetidine may increase gastric pH, resulting in a decrease in digoxin absorption.

Detailed Information: See *EDI,* 12/20.30

Digoxin-Cyclophosphamide, Prednisone, Procarbazine, Vincristine

Significance: 2—moderately clinically significant

Potential Effects: Use of these agents together may result in a decrease in digoxin levels.

Recommendations: Monitor digoxin levels in patients taking these agents together. Digitoxin or digoxin capsules may be an alternative to digoxin tablets.

Summary: There are data to show that administration of these agents with digoxin may lead to a decrease in digoxin levels.

Related Drugs: Digoxin has been shown to interact with other combination cytotoxic therapies; however, the data are conflicting. Because of conflicting results, it is difficult to determine if an interaction would occur with other digitalis glycosides.

Mechanism: Combination cytotoxic agents may reduce gastrointestinal absorption of digoxin, possibly resulting from impairment of the intestinal mucosal membrane by the cytotoxic drugs.

Detailed Information: See *EDI,* 12/21.00

Digoxin-Cyclosporine

Significance: 2—moderately clinically significant

Potential Effects: Cyclosporine may increase digoxin levels, resulting in toxicity.

Recommendations: Monitor digoxin levels and cardiac status closely during concomitant therapy with cyclosporine.

Summary: There are data to show that administration of cyclosporine can increase digoxin levels, potentiating toxicity; however, the data are conflicting.

Related Drugs: It is not known if an interaction would occur between cyclosporine and other digitalis glycosides. There are no drugs related to cyclosporine.

Mechanism: Decreased digoxin clearance may be a result of a cyclosporine-induced reduction in renal blood flow.

Detailed Information: See *EDI,* 12/22.10

Digoxin-Diazepam

Significance: 2—moderately clinically significant

Potential Effects: Concurrent digoxin and diazepam may result in an increase in digoxin half-life and a decrease in digoxin urinary excretion.

Recommendations: Patients should be monitored for an increase in digoxin levels, and a lower dose of digoxin may be necessary.

Summary: There are data to show that administration of diazepam may increase digoxin levels.

Related Drugs: A similar interaction is expected to occur between digoxin and deslanoside if the interaction results from a renal mechanism. Other benzodiazepines have been documented to interact with digoxin; however, the data are conflicting.

Mechanism: The mechanism of this interaction is unknown.

Detailed Information: See *EDI*, 12/23.00

Digoxin-Disopyramide

Significance: 3—minimally clinically significant

Recommendations: Until further studies are done, the concurrent use of these agents need not be avoided, and no special precautions appear necessary.

Summary: The concurrent use of disopyramide does not significantly affect serum digoxin levels.

Related Drugs: It is not known whether an interaction would occur between disopyramide and other digitalis glycosides. There are no drugs related to disopyramide.

Mechanism: The mechanism of this interaction is unknown.

Detailed Information: See *EDI*, 12/25.00

Digoxin-Erythromycin Base

Significance: 1—highly clinically significant

Potential Effects: The addition of erythromycin to a stable digoxin regimen may result in increased digoxin serum levels and toxicity.

Recommendations: Digoxin serum concentrations should be monitored when initiating or discontinuing concurrent erythromycin therapy. Patients who are receiving erythromycin and being digitalized should be closely monitored for overdigitalization.

Summary: The addition of erythromycin to the therapy of patients maintained on digoxin resulted in increased serum digoxin levels by as much as 104% and digoxin toxicity.

Related Drugs: One patient with a stable digoxin regimen experienced a 270% increase in digoxin serum levels after starting clarithromycin. Other erythromycin salts and macrolide antibiotics would be expected to undergo a similar interaction with digoxin. It is not known if an interaction would occur between erythromycin and the other digitalis glycosides.

Mechanism: Approximately 10% of the patients who receive digoxin convert a substantial portion of it to digoxin reduction products. These metabolites are not taken up as well by cardiac muscle and have less cardiac activity and some are more rapidly excreted in the urine. These products are formed predominantly by the bacteria in the gastrointestinal tract. The antibiotic, by destroying the bacteria, decreases digoxin metabolism, which would account for the increased digoxin serum concentrations.

Detailed Information: See *EDI*, 12/27.00

Digoxin-Esmolol

Significance: 3—minimally clinically significant

Potential Effects: Concurrent administration of oral digoxin and a beta-blocking agent may result in an increase in the mean digoxin area-under-curve (AUC).

Recommendations: Concurrent use of these agents need not be avoided. However, digoxin levels should be monitored closely during concomitant beta-blocker therapy, especially at the initiation or discontinuation of beta-blocker therapy.

Summary: Concurrent administration of oral digoxin and esmolol resulted in an increase in the mean digoxin AUC. Other pharmacologic parameters were not affected. The clinical significance was not determined.

Related Drugs: Studies have shown conflicting results with carvedilol, nadolol, atenolol, propranolol, and sotalol; therefore it would be difficult to determine if an interaction would occur between digoxin and other beta-blocking agents. It is also not known if an interaction would occur between esmolol and the other digitalis glycosides.

Mechanism: The mechanism whereby esmolol increased the digoxin AUC is not known; however, it is unlikely that esmolol altered the clearance of digoxin. It has been suggested that the oral bioavailability of digoxin may have been increased as a result of intestinal vasodilation.

Detailed Information: See *EDI,* 12/28.01

Digoxin-Flecainide

Significance: 3—minimally clinically significant

Potential Effects: Flecainide may cause an increase in digoxin levels.

Recommendations: Until further clinical studies are available, the concurrent administration of digoxin and flecainide need not be avoided. However, digoxin levels should be routinely monitored since the dose of digoxin may need to be decreased.

Summary: There are data to show that flecainide administration may cause an increase in digoxin levels. Adverse effects reported were mild and included tiredness, dizziness, nausea, and weakness.

Related Drugs: Encainide showed no significant change in digoxin levels. It is not known if flecainide would interact with other digitalis glycosides.

Mechanism: The mechanism of this interaction is unknown.

Detailed Information: See *EDI,* 12/28.10

Digoxin-Fluoxetine

Significance: 2—moderately clinically significant

Potential Effects: The addition of fluoxetine to the therapy of a patient stabilized on digoxin may result in increased digoxin levels and digoxin toxic effects.

Recommendations: If fluoxetine is added to or discontinued from the therapy of a patient maintained on digoxin, the patient should be carefully monitored for serum digoxin level changes and toxicity. The digoxin dosage may need to be adjusted or an alternative to fluoxetine may need to be contemplated.

Summary: The addition of fluoxetine to the therapy of a patient stabilized on digoxin resulted in increased digoxin levels (from 1.4nmol/L to 4.2nmol/L) and digoxin toxic effects.

Related Drugs: In separate studies, sertraline, paroxetine, and flu-voxamine had no significant effects on digoxin pharmacokinetics. Based on structural and pharmacologic similarity, an interaction may be expected to occur between digoxin and citalopram, although this interaction is not expected to be of clinical significance. It is not known whether a similar interaction would be expected to occur between fluoxetine and the other digitalis glycosides.

Mechanism: The mechanism of this interaction is not known.

Detailed Information: See *EDI,* 12/28.50

Digoxin-Furosemide

Significance: 2—moderately clinically significant

Potential Effects: Concurrent administration of these agents may result in increased digoxin effect and toxicity resulting from hypokalemia.

Recommendations: Monitor the patient's potassium level and cardiac status with concurrent administration of these agents.

Summary: Concurrent administration of digoxin and furosemide resulted in cardiac arrhythmias.

Related Drugs: Digitalis and digitoxin have also been reported to interact with diuretics. Deslanoside may be expected to interact similarly based on pharmacologic similarity. All potassium-depleting diuretics, including thiazides, other loop diuretics, the mercurial diuretic mersalyl, and thiazide-related diuretics may be expected to interact with digoxin similarly. Amphotericin B, although structurally and pharmacologically unrelated to the potassium-sparing diuretics, has caused hypokalemia, which can predispose patients to digoxin toxicity.

Mechanism: Digoxin acts on excitable tissues of the myocardium to inhibit sodium/potassium dependent ATPase. In hypokalemia there is less extracellular potassium available to exchange for intracellular sodium through remaining sodium pump activity, and membranes become even more depolarized. Thus, furosemide and other diuretics enhance the electrophysiologic effects of digoxin primarily by disturbing the normal potassium gradient across cell membranes.

Detailed Information: See *EDI,* 12/29.00

Digoxin-Ginseng

Significance: 3—minimally clinically significant

Potential Effects: Concomitant ginseng and digoxin administration may lead to increased digoxin serum levels.

Recommendations: Patients should be carefully monitored for apparent changes in digoxin serum levels and possible toxicity with concurrent use of these agents. The dose of digoxin may need to be adjusted.

Summary: Elevated digoxin serum levels have occurred with concomitant digoxin and Siberian ginseng administration. No digoxin or digitoxin contamination was found in the ginseng capsules.

Related Drugs: It is not known whether a similar interaction would be expected to occur between ginseng and the other digitalis glycosides.

Mechanism: Siberian ginseng contains eleutherosides, which are chemically related to cardiac glycosides such as digoxin. Since no digoxin toxicity has been reported, it is unlikely that these compounds are converted to digoxin *in vivo* or that the elimination of digoxin is impaired. It is possible that the serum assay may have measured another compound, perhaps an eleutheroside or its derivative. Further studies are needed.

Detailed Information: See *EDI*, 12/30.05

Digoxin-Heparin

Significance: 3—minimally clinically significant

Recommendations: Until further clinical studies are done, the concurrent use of these agents need not be avoided. However, caution should be used in patients receiving high dose heparin therapy, and digoxin levels should be monitored frequently.

Summary: The concomitant use of these agents should be used with caution.

Related Drugs: It is not known if heparin would interact with other digitalis glycosides.

Mechanism: Heparin releases free fatty acids, and these strongly bind to serum albumin and may remove digoxin from the albumin sites.

Detailed Information: See *EDI*, 12/30.10

Digoxin-Hydroxychloroquine

Significance: 2—moderately clinically significant

Recommendations: Patients should be closely monitored for signs of digoxin toxicity during concurrent use of these agents, and the dose of digoxin may need to be reduced.

Summary: There are data to show that administration of hydroxychloroquine may increase serum digoxin levels.

Related Drugs: A similar interaction is expected to occur between the other digitalis glycosides and other aminoquinolines.

Mechanism: The mechanism of this interaction is unknown; however, hydroxychloroquine is related to quinidine, and the interaction between digoxin and quinidine is well documented (see Digoxin-Quinidine, page 280).

Detailed Information: See *EDI*, 12/31.00

Digoxin-Ibuprofen

Significance: 2—moderately clinically significant

Potential Effects: Ibuprofen may increase digoxin levels when added to therapy. One study reported an initial change in digoxin levels, but no change in digoxin levels after 28 days of cotherapy.

Recommendations: Monitor digoxin levels during concurrent therapy. The dose of digoxin may need to be decreased.

Summary: Ibuprofen may increase serum digoxin levels; however, there was no significant difference in digoxin levels after 28 days of concomitant therapy.

Related Drugs: A similar interaction is expected to occur between deslanoside and digitalis or digitoxin, if the mechanism involves a decreased renal excretion. Because of conflicting reports, it is difficult to determine if an interaction would occur between digoxin and the other NSAIAs.

Mechanism: NSAIAs are known to depress kidney function, and there may be a decreased digoxin renal excretion.

Detailed Information: See *EDI*, 12/33.00

Digoxin-Itraconazole

Significance: 2—moderately clinically significant

Potential Effects: The addition of itraconazole to the therapy of a patient maintained on digoxin may result in increased digoxin serum levels.

Recommendations: Digoxin serum levels should be carefully monitored if itraconazole is added to, or withdrawn from, concurrent therapy. The dose of digoxin may need to be adjusted, and as much as a 75% decrease in digoxin dose may be needed with concurrent itraconazole. Ketoconazole may be a suitable alternative, but further controlled clinical studies are needed.

Summary: There are data to show that itraconazole may increase digoxin serum levels in digoxin maintained patients.

Related Drugs: An interaction may occur between itraconazole and other digitalis glycosides. Because of conflicting data, it is not known if an interaction would occur between digoxin and other imidazole antifungal agents.

Mechanism: The mechanism of the interaction is unknown.

Detailed Information: See *EDI*, 12/34.50

Digoxin-Kaolin

Significance: 2—moderately clinically significant

Recommendations: A steady-state study indicates that the interaction is not of major clinical significance, although other studies report a significant decrease in digoxin bioavailability. Administering the kaolin-pectin suspension at least two hours after digoxin appears to avoid the interaction. If the agents must be administered simultaneously, then digoxin as the soft gelatin capsule or the elixir is recommended. The patient receiving both digoxin and kaolin-pectin suspension concurrently should be observed for signs and symptoms of underdigitalization.

Summary: Concurrent administration of kaolin-pectin suspension and digoxin tablets resulted in a significant reduction in digoxin bioavailability.

Related Drugs: A similar interaction is expected to occur between kaolin-pectin and other digitalis glycosides. Digoxin has been shown to be decreased by concurrent diphenoxylate and atropine.

Mechanism: Kaolin may prevent the gastrointestinal absorption of digoxin by adsorption of digoxin, or kaolin may alter the gastrointestinal motility.

Detailed Information: See *EDI*, 12/35.00

Digoxin-Methyldopa

Significance: 3—minimally clinically significant

Recommendations: Patients receiving methyldopa and digoxin concurrently should be observed carefully for symptomatic bradycardia. If sinus bradycardia occurs during concomitant therapy, hydralazine has been shown to be a beneficial alternative to methyldopa.

Summary: There are data to show that methyldopa administration may sometimes cause symptomatic bradycardia in patients on digoxin.

Related Drugs: A similar interaction is expected to occur between methyldopa and other digitalis glycosides. There are no drugs related to methyldopa.

Mechanism: Digoxin could augment the sympatholytic action of methyldopa.

Detailed Information: See *EDI,* 12/36.10

Digoxin-Metoclopramide

Significance: 2—moderately clinically significant

Recommendations: Metoclopramide will influence digoxin absorption less from fast-dissolving digoxin tablets, digoxin capsules, or liquid preparations than from slow-dissolving tablets. Thus, slow-dissolving preparations may underdigitalize patients currently receiving metoclopramide. Digoxin serum concentrations should therefore be monitored when these agents are used concomitantly.

Summary: Metoclopramide was shown to increase serum digoxin concentrations; however, the pharmacokinetic changes will depend on the formulation of digoxin used.

Related Drugs: A similar interaction is expected to occur with other digitalis glycosides and metoclopramide. There are no drugs related to metoclopramide.

Mechanism: Peristalsis caused by metoclopramide may reduce the time digoxin is at the absorption site, causing less drug to be absorbed.

Detailed Information: See *EDI,* 12/37.00

Digoxin-Mexiletine

Significance: 4—not clinically significant

Potential Effects: Mexiletine does not affect digoxin levels.

Recommendations: The concurrent administration of digoxin and mexiletine need not be avoided. Because of the lack of interaction, mexiletine may be considered as an alternative antiarrhythmic agent to other agents that have been shown to interact with digoxin (e.g., quinidine), although further study is needed to support this statement.

Summary: Mexiletine was shown to have no significant effect on serum digoxin levels.

Related Drugs: It is not known if an interaction would occur between digoxin and lidocaine or tocainide, or between mexiletine and the other digitalis glycosides.

Mechanism: Mexiletine does not appear to affect the serum levels of digoxin.

Detailed Information: See *EDI,* 12/38.10

Digoxin-Moricizine

Significance: 4—not clinically significant

Potential Effects: Moricizine does not appear to alter digoxin levels.

Recommendations: Concurrent administration need not be avoided. Moricizine may be an alternative agent to those antiarrhythmics that interact with digoxin during concurrent digoxin therapy.

Summary: An interaction does not appear to occur between digoxin and moricizine.

Related Drugs: There are no reports demonstrating an interaction between moricizine and other digitalis glycosides. There are no drugs related to moricizine.

Mechanism: Moricizine does not appear to affect the serum levels of digoxin.

Detailed Information: See *EDI,* 12/38.30

Digoxin-Neomycin

Significance: 2—moderately clinically significant

Recommendations: The interaction was seen with neomycin dosages from 1.0G to 3.0G with tablets or solutions of both digoxin and neomycin, or when neomycin was given three or six hours before digoxin. Therefore, if neomycin is added to, or withdrawn from, concurrent digoxin therapy, patients must be monitored for changing digoxin serum concentrations and dosage adjustments should be made. Patients receiving neomycin who are being digitalized should be closely monitored for underdigitalization.

Summary: Concurrent administration of neomycin sulfate has been shown to depress serum digoxin concentrations.

Related Drugs: A similar interaction is expected to occur between neomycin and other digitalis glycosides or between digoxin and other available oral aminoglycosides.

Mechanism: Neomycin may cause a precipitation of digoxin, or neomycin may change the intestinal membrane permeability.

Detailed Information: See *EDI,* 12/39.00

Digoxin-Penicillamine

Significance: 2—moderately clinically significant

Recommendations: Patients should be monitored for decreased digoxin levels. The dose of digoxin may need to be increased.

Summary: Concurrent use of digoxin and penicillamine results in significantly reduced serum digoxin levels.

Related Drugs: There is no documentation regarding a similar interaction between penicillamine and other digitalis glycosides. There are no drugs related to penicillamine.

Mechanism: The exact mechanism is not known.

Detailed Information: See *EDI,* 12/41.00

Digoxin-Prazosin

Significance: 2—moderately clinically significant

Potential Effects: Prazosin may increase digoxin levels.

Recommendations: Patients maintained on digoxin should be monitored closely if prazosin is added to, or withdrawn from, cotherapy. The dose of digoxin may need to be adjusted.

Summary: There are data to show that prazosin administration may increase digoxin levels.

Related Drugs: It is not known if a similar interaction would occur between prazosin and other digitalis glycosides or between digoxin and other alpha-1-adrenergic blocking agents.

Mechanism: Prazosin may cause an increase in oral absorption, reduce tubular secretion, reduce hepatic clearance or alter the protein binding of digoxin.

Detailed Information: See *EDI,* 12/42.10

Digoxin-Propafenone

Significance: 2—moderately clinically significant

Potential Effects: Propafenone may cause an increase in digoxin levels.

Recommendations: Concurrent use of digoxin and propafenone should be approached with caution. Digoxin levels should be monitored and the dose of digoxin may need to be adjusted.

Summary: Concurrent use of propafenone may increase digoxin serum levels.

Related Drugs: Flecainide has been shown to interact with digoxin; however, the data are conflicting. It is not known if propafenone would interact with other digitalis glycosides or if an interaction would occur between digoxin and indecainide.

Mechanism: Reduced renal elimination of digoxin may partially explain the serum digoxin concentration increase during concurrent propafenone administration.

Detailed Information: See *EDI*, 12/42.30

Digoxin-Propantheline

Significance: 1—highly clinically significant

Recommendations: The problem presented by a patient who requires propantheline and digoxin can be circumvented by the selection of quickly absorbed digoxin preparations—either rapidly solubilized tablets or liquid digoxin. The soft gelatin capsule form of digoxin might also be considered because of its rapid dissolution. Should digitalized patients experience symptoms indicative of digitalis glycoside intoxication with the use of propantheline or similar drug, it may be from excessive absorption of digoxin from a slowly disintegrating tablet. Changing to a rapidly absorbed preparation will give predictable blood levels.

Summary: Absorption of digoxin may be significantly increased by concomitant administration of propantheline.

Related Drugs: Undocumented risk may be anticipated with all the anticholinergics. All slow-dissolving digitalis glycoside preparations may be expected to interact similarly.

Mechanism: Medication in a slow-dissolving tablet will be more extensively absorbed if the time spent in the intestine is increased. Propantheline prolongs intestinal emptying time, facilitating more complete absorption.

Detailed Information: See *EDI*, 12/43.00

Digoxin-Psyllium

Significance: 3—minimally clinically significant

Recommendations: Although information is limited, the interaction seems to produce some degree of reduced digoxin absorption. If long-term psyllium and digoxin cotherapy is undertaken, patients should be monitored for decreasing digoxin serum concentrations. A two-hour interval between dosage with these drugs may prevent any problem.

Summary: Coadministration of psyllium hydrophilic mucilloid has been shown to reduce the bioavailability of digoxin.

Related Drugs: There appear to be no reports that any of the digitalis glycosides interact similarly with other bulk producing laxatives.

Mechanism: Possible physical binding of digoxin to psyllium or other absorptive hindrance may explain this interaction.

Detailed Information: See *EDI*, 12/45.00

Digoxin-Quinidine

Significance: 1—highly clinically significant

Potential Effects: Quinidine will cause an increase in digoxin levels.

Recommendations: Monitor digoxin levels closely when quinidine is added to, or withdrawn from, therapy. Some reports recommend reducing the digoxin dose by 30% to 50% when quinidine is added to therapy. Digoxin toxicity may be enhanced by concomitant quinidine, even at therapeutic serum digoxin levels.

Summary: It is well documented that quinidine alters digoxin pharmacokinetics, causing an approximately twofold increase in plasma digoxin concentration.

Related Drugs: Conflicting results make it difficult to determine whether a similar interaction would occur between quinidine and other digitalis glycosides. Quinine was found to increase plasma digoxin concentration.

Mechanism: Reduction in digoxin renal clearance and displacement from tissue digoxin binding sites, leading to a reduced volume of distribution, appear to be the predominant mechanisms involved in this interaction.

Detailed Information: See *EDI*, 12/47.00

Digoxin-Spironolactone

Significance: 2—moderately clinically significant

Recommendations: Concurrent administration of spironolactone and digoxin should be closely monitored, and potassium and digoxin concentrations should be measured frequently to assess the potential for toxicity. Also, the patient should be monitored for changes in therapeutic effects.

Summary: Simultaneous administration of spironolactone and digoxin has been shown to decrease volume of distribution, plasma clearance, and renal clearance and increase plasma digoxin concentrations. Potassium levels have also been shown to fluctuate.

Related Drugs: Because of conflicting data, whether spironolactone increases or reduces the therapeutic action of digitoxin cannot be documented. Conflicting reports make it difficult to predict whether an interaction would occur between spironolactone and other digitalis glycosides.

Mechanism: Increases in steady-state digoxin concentrations associated with spironolactone have been attributed to reduced renal tubular digoxin clearance caused by competitive blocking by spironolactone.

Detailed Information: See *EDI*, 12/50.10

Digoxin-Succinylcholine

Significance: 2—moderately clinically significant

Recommendations: Succinylcholine should be used with caution in patients receiving digoxin or other digitalis glycosides.

Summary: There have been reports of cardiac arrhythmias occurring after the administration of succinylcholine to patients stabilized on digoxin.

Related Drugs: Administration of digoxin and pancuronium has led to sinus tachycardia and atrial flutter. The other digitalis glycosides may also be expected to interact with succinylcholine.

Mechanism: This interaction may be due to a loss of intracellular potassium, sympathetic postganglionic stimulation, or a direct effect on the myocardium by succinylcholine.

Detailed Information: See *EDI*, 12/51.00

Digoxin-Sulfasalazine

Significance: 2—moderately clinically significant

Recommendations: Careful monitoring of digoxin serum levels is recommended to detect subtherapeutic levels when digoxin is taken concurrently with sulfasalazine. Increasing the digoxin dosage or switching to the elixir form did not increase digoxin levels, nor did separating the times of administration, results suggesting that sulfasalazine may need to be discontinued. In an acute situation, parenteral digoxin may be indicated. No literature is available at this time regarding the interaction of sulfasalazine and the soft gelatin capsule form of digoxin.

Summary: Sulfasalazine has been shown to reduce the serum levels of digoxin.

Related Drugs: No documentation is available indicating sulfasalazine interacts similarly with other digitalis glycosides. There appears to be no evidence that other sulfonamides interact with digoxin.

Mechanism: The mechanism of this interaction is unknown.

Detailed Information: See *EDI*, 12/53.00

Digoxin-Tetracycline

Significance: 1—highly clinically significant

Recommendations: Digoxin serum concentrations should be monitored when initiating or discontinuing concurrent tetracycline therapy. Patients who are receiving tetracycline and being digitalized should be closely monitored for overdigitalization.

Summary: There are data to show that tetracycline administration may increase steady-state serum digoxin concentrations.

Related Drugs: A similar interaction is expected to occur with the tetracycline derivatives and digoxin. There is no documentation that tetracycline undergoes a similar reaction with the other digitalis glycosides.

Mechanism: Antibiotics destroy bacteria and decrease digoxin metabolism, which would account for the increased digoxin serum concentrations.

Detailed Information: See *EDI*, 12/55.00

Digoxin-Thyroid

Significance: 2—moderately clinically significant

Recommendations: Patients stabilized on digoxin should be monitored closely when concurrent thyroid therapy is initiated to avoid a decrease in the therapeutic effect of the digoxin. Conversely, increased digoxin sensitivity may result from withdrawal of thyroid preparations in patients maintained on the digitalis glycoside.

Summary: The therapeutic efficacy of digoxin may be decreased in patients with hyperthyroidism or in patients being treated with thyroid hormones.

Related Drugs: Digitoxin has been shown to be similarly affected by hyperthyroidism. The other digitalis glycosides may interact in a similar manner. The interaction with thyroid hormones may occur primarily with liothyronine, but all other thyroid preparations may be expected to interact.

Mechanism: Hyperthyroidism results in lower serum levels of digoxin and other digitalis glycosides.

Detailed Information: See *EDI*, 12/57.00

Digoxin-Tolbutamide

Significance: 3—minimally clinically significant

Potential Effects: Tolbutamide may cause an increase in digoxin levels, leading to digoxin toxicity.

Recommendations: Concurrent administration of digoxin and tolbutamide should be done with caution, and digoxin levels should be closely monitored. Glyburide may be used instead of tolbutamide.

Summary: There are data to show that administration of tolbutamide may cause an increase in digoxin levels, leading to digoxin toxicity and increased adverse effects.

Related Drugs: Glyburide was shown to not significantly interact with digoxin. Because of conflicting results, it is difficult to determine if an interaction would occur between digoxin and other sulfonylurea hypoglycemic agents. It is not known if tolbutamide would interact with other digitalis glycosides.

Mechanism: The mechanism of this interaction is not known.

Detailed Information: See *EDI,* 12/58.01

Digoxin-Trazodone

Significance: 3—minimally clinically significant

Potential Effects: The addition of trazodone to the therapy of a patient stabilized on digoxin may result in increased digoxin serum levels and toxicity.

Recommendations: Patients receiving these drugs concurrently should be carefully monitored for digoxin toxicity. Because conclusive documentation for this interaction is lacking, the incidence and clinical significance of the concurrent administration of these agents has not been determined.

Summary: The addition of trazodone to the therapy of a patient stabilized on digoxin resulted in increased digoxin serum levels from 0.8ng/ml to 2.8ng/ml (therapeutic range: 1.2–1.7ng/ml) and digoxin toxicity.

Related Drugs: Concurrent nefazodone and digoxin has also resulted in increased digoxin levels, but without clinically significant changes in vital signs. It is not known whether an interaction would occur between either trazodone or nefazodone and the other digitalis glycosides. Trazodone and nefazodone are chemically and pharmacologically unrelated to the tricyclic and tetracyclic antidepressant agents.

Mechanism: The mechanism of this interaction is not known.

Detailed Information: See *EDI,* 12/58.10

Digoxin-Trimethoprim

Significance: 3—minimally clinically significant

Potential Effects: Trimethoprim may cause an increase in digoxin levels.

Recommendations: If these agents are used together, digoxin levels should be monitored.

Summary: There are data to show that trimethoprim administration may cause an increase in digoxin levels.

Related Drugs: The other digitalis glycosides eliminated largely through renal mechanisms would be expected to interact similarly with trimethoprim. Other digitalis glycosides metabolized in the liver would not be expected to interact with trimethoprim. There are no drugs related to trimethoprim.

Mechanism: Trimethoprim may decrease the renal tubular secretion of digoxin.

Detailed Information: See *EDI*, 12/58.30

Digoxin-Verapamil

Significance: 1—highly clinically significant

Potential Effects: Verapamil can significantly increase digoxin levels. Both the therapeutic and toxic effects of digoxin have been increased.

Recommendations: Monitor the patient's cardiac status and digoxin levels when these agents are used together. The dosage of digoxin may need to be decreased.

Summary: Serum digoxin concentrations are increased with concurrent verapamil therapy.

Related Drugs: Nifedipine, nicardipine, isradipine and bepridil have been documented to interact with digoxin; however, the data are conflicting. It is not known if verapamil or other calcium channel blocking agents would interact with other digitalis glycosides.

Mechanism: Verapamil impairs the renal and extrarenal clearance of digoxin. The reduction in renal clearance may result from inhibition of tubular secretion.

Detailed Information: See *EDI*, 12/59.00

Chapter Thirteen

Diuretic Drug Interactions

Acetazolamide-Cyclosporine

Significance: 2—moderately clinically significant

Potential Effects: Acetazolamide may increase cyclosporine levels.

Recommendations: Acetazolamide should be used with caution in patients maintained on cyclosporine. Patients undergoing cotherapy should be monitored for an increase in cyclosporine levels and for nephrotoxicity. The dose of one or both agents may need to be adjusted.

Summary: There are data to show that acetazolamide administration may increase cyclosporine levels.

Related Drugs: Documentation is lacking regarding a similar interaction between cyclosporine and other carbonic anhydrase inhibitors. There are no drugs related to cyclosporine.

Mechanism: This interaction may be due to the alteration of cyclosporine entry into red blood cells or an increase in absorption of cyclosporine.

Detailed Information: See *EDI*, 13/0.05

Bendroflumethiazide-Aminoglutethimide

Significance: 3—minimally clinically significant

Potential Effects: The concurrent use of these agents may result in hyponatremia.

Recommendations: Patients taking these agents together should have serum sodium monitored. Fludrocortisone may need to be added or the bendroflumethiazide discontinued if hyponatremia occurs.

Summary: There are data to show that coadministration of these agents may result in reversible hyponatremia.

Related Drugs: A similar interaction may occur between aminoglutethimide and other thiazide diuretics and thiazide-related diuretics.

Mechanism: A synergistic effect may occur with concurrent diuretic therapy and aminoglutethimide, resulting in hyponatremia.

Detailed Information: See *EDI*, 13/0.10

Bendroflumethiazide-Indomethacin

Significance: 2—moderately clinically significant

Potential Effects: Indomethacin may decrease the hypotensive effects of bendroflumethiazide.

Recommendations: Patients' blood pressure should be closely monitored during concurrent therapy of these agents. The dose of bendroflumethiazide may need to be increased.

Summary: Indomethacin has been shown to reduce the hypotensive effects of concurrent bendroflumethiazide.

Related Drugs: Hydrochlorothiazide and indomethacin were shown to exhibit a similar interaction; however, the data are conflicting. Indomethacin may blunt the antihypertensive effect of chlorthalidone. Because of conflicting results, it is difficult to determine whether an interaction would occur between indomethacin and other thiazide diuretics or other thiazide-related diuretics and between bendroflumethiazide and other NSAIAs.

Mechanism: Indomethacin may inhibit prostaglandin synthesis responsible for vasodilation, causing an increase in blood pressure. Indomethacin has been shown to acutely reduce sodium and water excretion.

Detailed Information: See *EDI*, 13/1.00

Chlorothiazide-Calcium Carbonate

Significance: 2—moderately clinically significant

Potential Effects: Concurrent use of these agents may result in hypercalcemia, metabolic alkalosis, and renal failure.

Recommendations: Use these agents together with caution. If milk-alkali syndrome develops, the calcium carbonate and chlorothiazide should be discontinued and electrolyte and fluid abnormalities corrected.

Summary: There are data to show that coadministration of these agents may result in milk-alkali syndrome, characterized by hypercalcemia, metabolic alkalosis, and renal failure.

Related Drugs: An interaction may occur with the other thiazide diuretics and calcium carbonate. It is not known if a similar interaction would occur between chlorothiazide and other calcium salts.

Mechanism: Many factors contribute to the development of milk-alkali syndrome: the blockage of renal excretory capacity, bicarbonate reabsorption, increased calcium intake, volume depletion and decreased glomerular filtration rate.

Detailed Information: See *EDI,* 13/2.10

Chlorothiazide-Colestipol

Significance: 3—minimally clinically significant

Recommendations: If concurrent use of colestipol and chlorothiazide is necessary, it may be advisable to separate their administration by as much time as possible. However, patients should still be closely monitored since an increased dose of the thiazide diuretic may be necessary.

Summary: Chlorothiazide and colestipol resulted in a significant reduction in the excretion of chlorothiazide.

Related Drugs: A similar interaction was documented with cholestyramine. A similar interaction is expected to occur between chlorothiazide and cholestyramine. Similar results may be expected between colestipol and other thiazide diuretics and thiazide-related diuretics.

Mechanism: Colestipol and cholestyramine have been shown to bind chlorothiazide and hydrochlorothiazide.

Detailed Information: See *EDI,* 13/3.00

Chlorothiazide-Metoclopramide

Significance: 3—minimally clinically significant

Recommendations: Although the bioavailability of chlorothiazide, when administered as a solution, is decreased by metoclopramide, it was not determined if the pharmacologic activity of chlorothiazide decreased as well. Based on this limited information, the concurrent use of these agents need not be avoided, and it seems that no special precautions are necessary.

Summary: Metoclopramide has been documented to reduce the recovery of chlorothiazide.

Related Drugs: The other thiazide diuretics and thiazide-related diuretics may undergo a similar interaction with metoclopramide. There are no drugs related to metoclopramide.

Mechanism: Metoclopramide causes thiazides to have less time for dissolution and/or shorter contact time with the intestinal membrane.

Detailed Information: See *EDI,* 13/4.10

Chlorothiazide-Probenecid

Significance: 3—minimally clinically significant

Potential Effects: Probenecid may increase the diuretic effect of chlorothiazine.

Recommendations: If serum uric acid concentrations become elevated, an increase in the dose of probenecid should be considered.

Summary: Probenecid may increase the diuretic effect of chlorothiazide. Chlorothiazide has the potential to elevate serum uric acid concentrations and diminish the uricosuric effect of probenecid.

Related Drugs: Bendroflumethiazide, hydrochlorothiazide, methyclothiazide, chlorthalidone, diazoxide, triamterene, indapamide, trichlormethiazide, cyclopenthiazide, and quinethazone cause serum uric acid elevation and may be expected to antagonize the uricosuric effect of probenecid. Probenecid has been shown to increase the activity of metolazone. Other thiazide diuretics may be expected to interact similarly, although no documentation on such interactions exists. Loop diuretics exhibit a similar reaction.

Mechanism: Probenecid blocks the secretion of chlorothiazide at the proximal renal tubule, resulting in enhancement, through prolongation, of the diuretic effect of chlorothiazide. Hyperuricemia from the thiazide diuretics is attributed to either competitive inhibition of uric acid secretion within the kidney or to indirect enhancement of renal reabsorption of uric acid through redistribution of blood flow.

Detailed Information: See *EDI,* 13/5.00

Chlorothiazide-Propantheline

Significance: 3—minimally clinically significant

Recommendations: Although the bioavailability of chlorothiazide, when administered as a solution, is increased by propantheline, it was not determined if the pharmacologic activity of chlorothiazide increased as well. Based on this limited information, the concurrent use of these agents need not be avoided, and no special precautions are necessary.

Summary: Propantheline was shown to double the bioavailability of chlorothiazide.

Related Drugs: Hydrochlorothiazide bioavailability was increased with propantheline. The other thiazide diuretics and the thiazide-related diuretics may undergo a similar interaction. The other anticholinergics may be expected to enhance the bioavailability of chlorothiazide.

Mechanism: Propantheline delays gastric emptying rate and motility, allowing more time for thiazide dissolution and greater contact time with the intestinal membrane.

Detailed Information: See *EDI,* 13/6.10

Ethacrynic Acid-Cisplatin

Significance: 2—moderately clinically significant

Recommendations: Although this interaction is based on animal studies only, the ototoxicity of each agent is well documented. Therefore, it is important to monitor eighth cranial nerve function during and after concurrent therapy. The use of lower doses of ethacrynic acid may also avoid, or lessen, the potential for an interaction.

Summary: The concurrent use of ethacrynic acid and cisplatin has been shown to produce prolonged and permanent ototoxic effects in animals.

Related Drugs: There are no drugs related to cisplatin. A similar interaction is expected to occur between cisplatin and other loop diuretics.

Mechanism: The mechanism appears to be related to the synergistic toxicity of each agent.

Detailed Information: See *EDI*, 13/7.00

Furosemide-Aspirin

Significance: 3—minimally clinically significant

Recommendations: During concurrent administration of these agents, the dose of furosemide may need to be adjusted if the diuretic effect decreases. However, whether this interaction occurs in all patients or only those with renal insufficiency remains to be determined.

Summary: There are data to show that coadministration of these agents suppresses hemodynamic effects of furosemide and reduces the diuretic effect. Signs of renal insufficiency were abolished when furosemide was added.

Related Drugs: Because of conflicting results, it is difficult to determine whether a similar interaction would occur between the other loop diuretics and other salicylates.

Mechanism: It has been suggested that aspirin and furosemide have opposing effects on renal prostaglandin synthesis.

Detailed Information: See *EDI*, 13/9.00

Furosemide-Charcoal

Significance: 2—moderately clinically significant

Potential Effects: Concurrent furosemide and charcoal administration may decrease the absorption and diuretic effect of furosemide.

Recommendations: If charcoal and furosemide must be given concurrently, it is recommended that furosemide be administered two to three hours prior to charcoal to minimize the effect of charcoal.

Summary: Charcoal reduced the absorption and diuretic effect of furosemide.

Related Drugs: An interaction may occur between charcoal and other loop diuretics because of the high adsorptive capacity of activated charcoal.

Mechanism: The high adsorptive capacity of activated charcoal results in reduced absorption of drugs from the gastrointestinal tract.

Detailed Information: See *EDI*, 13/10.50

Furosemide-Chloral Hydrate

Significance: 3—minimally clinically significant

Recommendations: In patients with acute coronary disease, the concurrent use of these agents may need to be avoided. However, since this interaction does not occur in all patients, concomitant administration should at least be used with caution. If the interaction does occur, the discontinuation of chloral hydrate has been shown to lead to a reversal of the symptoms. Alternatively, the use of flurazepam or another benzodiazepine may be considered as a nocturnal sedative.

Summary: Furosemide and chloral hydrate have resulted in uneasiness, diaphoresis, hot flashes, and blood pressure changes, including hypertension.

Related Drugs: A similar interaction is expected to occur between the loop diuretics and tricoflos.

Mechanism: Furosemide may displace a metabolite of chloral hydrate from plasma protein binding sites, which displaces thyroxine. This can result in a hypermetabolic state.

Detailed Information: See *EDI*, 13/11.00

Furosemide-Cholestyramine

Significance: 2—moderately clinically significant

Potential Effects: The concurrent use of cholestyramine and furosemide may result in decreased furosemide bioavailability and diuretic effect.

Recommendations: The administration of furosemide and cholestyramine should be separated by two to three hours to help avoid a decrease in furosemide bioavailability and diuretic effect.

Summary: The absorption and diuretic effect of furosemide were decreased by concurrent cholestyramine.

Related Drugs: Colestipol has resulted in a decrease in furosemide bioavailability. An interaction may occur between other anionic exchange resins and other loop diuretics.

Mechanism: Furosemide is adsorbed to cholestyramine, an anionic exchange resin, because of the acidic nature of the furosemide molecule.

Detailed Information: See *EDI*, 13/12.10

Furosemide-Indomethacin

Significance: 3—minimally clinically significant

Potential Effects: Indomethacin may decrease the effects of furosemide, possibly by inhibition of prostaglandin synthesis.

Recommendations: If a decrease in furosemide's diuretic or natriuretic effects occurs with indomethacin cotherapy, indomethacin may need to be discontinued.

Summary: Indomethacin has been shown to decrease the diuretic and natriuretic effects and to block the acute audiologic effect and the rise in plasma renin activity associated with furosemide therapy. Furosemide has been reported to reduce indomethacin plasma concentrations; however, not all data support this.

Related Drugs: Indomethacin has reportedly produced a similar attenuation of the effects of ethacrynic acid and bumetanide. Furosemide has been shown to interact with many NSAIAs, and a similar interaction is expected to occur with the NSAIAs and furosemide.

Mechanism: Indomethacin inhibits prostaglandin synthesis and decreases sodium diuresis, and this may vary with the individual NSAIA used.

Detailed Information: See *EDI*, 13/13.00

Furosemide-Phenytoin

Significance: 3—minimally clinically significant

Recommendations: Patients should be monitored for a decreased effect of furosemide when phenytoin (and/or phenobarbital) is administered concurrently. The dose of furosemide may need to be increased.

Summary: There are data to show that phenytoin may significantly delay the diuretic response, and the dose of furosemide may need to be increased.

Related Drugs: It is difficult to relate whether or not other hydantoin anticonvulsants or other barbiturates would interact in a similar manner with other loop diuretics.

Mechanism: This interaction may be due to the decrease in absorption of furosemide or the increase in the reabsorption of sodium in the renal tubules.

Detailed Information: See *EDI,* 13/14.10

Furosemide-Probenecid

Significance: 3—minimally clinically significant

Potential Effects: Concomitant furosemide and probenecid may increase furosemide serum levels and its diuretic effect.

Recommendations: Since probenecid may enhance the actions of furosemide, doses may need to be decreased in patients. Also, since furosemide has the potential to increase uric acid levels, probenecid doses may need to be increased.

Summary: Studies show concomitant use of furosemide and probenecid may increase furosemide serum levels and its diuretic effect. Furosemide may also elevate serum uric acid concentrations which may diminish the uricosuric effects of probenecid.

Related Drugs: Probenecid blocks the secretion of bumetanide and torsemide at the proximal renal tubule. This reduces both drugs' effects. Bumetanide, torsemide, and ethacrynic acid may also increase uric acid levels, antagonizing the effect of probenecid. Thiazide diuretics exhibit a similar reaction with probenecid.

Mechanism: Probenecid blocks the secretion of furosemide at the proximal renal tubule, resulting in enhancement, through prolongation, of the diuretic effect of furosemide. Another possible mechanism includes the displacement of furosemide from plasma protein binding sites by probenecid, resulting in the increased glomerular filtration of unbound furosemide. Hyperuricemia from the loop diuretics may be due to enhanced reabsorption of uric acid through redistribution of blood flow or competitive inhibition of uric acid secretion in the kidney.

Detailed Information: See *EDI,* 13/14.50

Hydrochlorothiazide-Fenfluramine

Significance: 3—minimally clinically significant

Recommendations: Because of the combined anorectic and hypotensive effects of fenfluramine, it may be useful in combination with a thiazide diuretic in the hypertensive obese patient. Caution should be used when prescribing fenfluramine and a thiazide diuretic in a normotensive patient because of the possibility of hypotension.

Summary: Fenfluramine with hydrochlorothiazide has been shown to reduce blood pressure in patients previously unresponsive to hydrochlorothiazide.

Related Drugs: A similar interaction is expected to occur between fenfluramine and other thiazide diuretics and thiazide-related diuretics as well as between hydrochlorothiazide and other anorexiants.

Mechanism: The mechanism of action of fenfluramine in lowering plasma norepinephrine levels and in enhancing the hypotensive effects of hydrochlorothiazide is not clear.

Detailed Information: See *EDI,* 13/15.00

Hydrochlorothiazide, Triamterene-Amantadine

Significance: 3—minimally clinically significant

Recommendations: The concurrent use of these agents should be approached with caution. If symptoms of amantadine toxicity occur, the dose of amantadine may need to be decreased.

Summary: There are data to show that one or both agents of the combination drug (hydrochlorothiazide and triamterene) reduced the clearance and produced higher plasma levels and toxic effects of amantadine.

Related Drugs: Because it is not known which agent was responsible for the interaction, it is not known how other thiazide-related diuretics or other potassium-sparing diuretics would interact with amantadine. There are no drugs related to amantadine.

Mechanism: It has been postulated that one or both of the components of the combination diuretic reduces the tubular secretion of amantadine.

Detailed Information: See *EDI,* 13/17.00

Spironolactone-Aspirin

Significance: 3—minimally clinically significant

Recommendations: The concurrent usage of spironolactone and aspirin need not be avoided, unless additional study establishes a clinically significant effect.

Summary: Concurrent usage of aspirin and spironolactone showed a decrease in the natriuretic effect of spironolactone.

Related Drugs: Further studies are needed to determine any possible effects caused by other salicylates. There is a lack of documentation regarding a similar interaction between aspirin and other potassium-sparing diuretics.

Mechanism: The mechanism of this interaction is controversial and unclear. Aspirin may block the renal tubular secretion of the active metabolite of spironolactone.

Detailed Information: See *EDI,* 13/19.00

Spironolactone-Captopril

Significance: 3—minimally clinically significant

Potential Effects: The concurrent use of these agents may cause an increase in potassium levels.

Recommendations: Monitor potassium levels when using these agents together. The dose of either may need to be decreased or discontinued.

Summary: There are data to show that coadministration of these agents may cause an increase in potassium levels; the clinical signs may or may not be present.

Related Drugs: Captopril may interact similarly with other potassium-sparing diuretics. Enalapril has been shown to increase potassium levels.

Mechanism: Captopril causes potassium retention, and administration of these agents results in an additive interaction, increasing serum potassium concentrations.

Detailed Information: See *EDI,* 13/20.10

Spironolactone-Potassium Chloride

Significance: 1—highly clinically significant

Summary: In the presence of a potassium-sparing diuretic, an added source of potassium can result in serious symptoms of hyperkalemia, which may lead to cardiac failure and arrest.

Related Drugs: Other potassium-sparing diuretics may interact in a similar manner with all absorbable forms of potassium.

Mechanism: Spironolactone produces retention of potassium ions, and a potassium supplement will increase the accumulation of potassium.

Detailed Information: See *EDI*, 13/21.00

Triamterene-Cimetidine

Significance: 3—minimally clinically significant

Potential Effects: Cimetidine decreases the clearance of triamterene.

Recommendations: The use of these agents together need not to be avoided; however, if they are used together, the effects of triamterene should be monitored.

Summary: There are data to show that cimetidine administration will decrease the clearance of triamterene.

Related Drugs: The pharmacokinetics of other potassium-sparing diuretics differ from that of triamterene; therefore, it is not known if a similar interaction would occur with cimetidine. It is not known to what extent an interaction would occur between triamterene and the other H_2-receptor antagonists.

Mechanism: Cimetidine has reduced hepatic hydroxylation, reduced renal tubular secretion and reduced the absorption of triamterene.

Detailed Information: See *EDI*, 13/22.10

Triamterene-Indomethacin

Significance: 2—moderately clinically significant

Potential Effects: The concurrent use of triamterene and indomethacin may lead to reversible acute renal failure.

Recommendations: The concurrent use of these agents requires caution. If renal function deteriorates during concomitant therapy, one or both agents may need to be discontinued.

Summary: A study and four case reports showed the concurrent use of triamterene and indomethacin may lead to reversible acute renal failure.

Related Drugs: Similar interactions have been reported with triamterene and ibuprofen, diclofenac, and fluribrofen. Reports cite the development of acute renal failure with amiloride and indomethacin or ibuprofen. Sulindac, prioxicam and naproxen have been reported not to interact with amiloride. Both indomethacin and diflunisal decreased the diuretic effect of spironolactone, and diflunisal decreased creatinine clearance.

Mechanism: Prostaglandin inhibition by nonsteroidal anti-inflammatory agents may unmask triamterene or amiloride toxicity and contribute to the pathogenesis of the renal failure observed.

Detailed Information: See *EDI*, 13/23.00

Trichlormethiazide-Diazoxide

Significance: 3—minimally clinically significant

Recommendations: Patients should be monitored for blood glucose changes, and dosage adjustments should be made in one or both agents as indicated. The combination may be beneficial in elevating blood glucose in refractory patients or lowering blood pressure, since both agents share those pharmacologic activities.

Summary: Trichlormethiazide and diazoxide alone have been shown to produce hyperglycemia.

Related Drugs: Hyperglycemia has been reported when diazoxide is given with hydrochlorothiazide or bendroflumethiazide. Because of conflicting reports, it is not possible to determine whether hyperglycemia will occur when diazoxide is administered with other thiazide diuretics or thiazide-related diuretics.

Mechanism: Diazoxide and thiazide diuretics act synergistically to inhibit insulin secretion from the pancreas. Diuretics have been reported to precipitate latent diabetes or increase blood glucose levels.

Detailed Information: See *EDI,* 13/25.00

Chapter Fourteen

Hypoglycemic Drug Interactions

Chlorpropamide-Alcohol, Ethyl

Significance: 1—highly clinically significant

Potential Effects: Alcohol consumed while receiving chlorpropamide may result in hypoglycemia.

Recommendations: A disulfiram-like reaction may also occur. Although abstinence from alcohol would be ideal for patients receiving antidiabetic therapy, practical management will more often involve recommending reduced alcohol intake and cautioning the patient regarding potential effects of alcohol while taking antidiabetic agents.

Summary: The combination of alcohol and antidiabetic agents can result in mild flushing to severe hypoglycemic reactions. A disulfiram-type reaction to alcohol has been produced by chlorpropamide.

Related Drugs: Ample documentation exists of an interaction between tolbutamide and alcohol. A similar interaction is expected to occur between alcohol and other first generation sulfonylureas. Glipizide and glyburide have been reported to have a very low incidence of disulfiram-like reactions with concurrent alcohol.

Mechanism: Alcohol, by means of its intrinsic hypoglycemic activity, can induce hypoglycemia and interfere with gluconeogenesis in the liver.

Detailed Information: See *EDI,* 14/1.00

Chlorpropamide-Allopurinol

Significance: 3—minimally clinically significant

Recommendations: Because of the extremely limited evidence of this drug interaction, the clinical significance must be considered minimal. It would be prudent to monitor patients on oral hypoglycemic agents for increases in pharmacologic effect or serum half-life if allopurinol is administered concurrently.

Summary: The half-life of chlorpropamide may be increased by concurrent administration of allopurinol.

Related Drugs: A similar interaction is expected to occur with other sulfonylurea hypoglycemic drugs and allopurinol. Glyburide and glipizide may not interact to the same extent as the other sulfonylureas. There are no drugs related to allopurinol.

Mechanism: The suggested mechanism between chlorpropamide and allopurinol is a competition for renal tubular secretion.

Detailed Information: See *EDI,* 14/3.00

Chlorpropamide-Aspirin

Significance: 2—moderately clinically significant

Recommendations: An individual receiving both chlorpropamide and aspirin may need to have the chlorpropamide dose adjusted downward. The patient should be carefully monitored. Blood or urinary glucose levels will facilitate proper management of such patients. Upon discontinuation of aspirin administration, the requirement for chlorpropamide will increase. It may be beneficial to consider switching to insulin or dietary control in patients requiring aspirin therapy, particularly those who exhibit poor response with the oral hypoglycemic drug. Cases of hypoglycemia can be treated by traditional methods or by the use of glucose plus diazoxide.

Summary: There is an increased risk of chlorpropamide toxicity with concurrent aspirin administration, and use of these agents may result in severe hypoglycemia.

Related Drugs: Insulin response to tolbutamide has been significantly augmented after aspirin. The other first generation sulfonylurea hypoglycemic agents may also interact with aspirin. Glyburide and glipizide may not interact to the same degree as other sulfonylureas. A similar interaction is expected to occur with other salicylates and chlorpropamide.

Mechanism: Sulfonylureas bind extensively to plasma protein where aspirin may cause a displacement and increased concentrations of free drug.

Detailed Information: See *EDI,* 14/5.00

Chlorpropamide-Clofibrate

Significance: 2—moderately clinically significant

Recommendations: When clofibrate is added to the regimen of diabetic patients receiving chlorpropamide or other sulfonylureas, blood glucose levels should be monitored closely for hypoglycemia; it may be necessary to decrease the dose of the sulfonylurea in some patients. Conversely, when clofibrate is discontinued in patients receiving chlorpropamide concurrently, blood glucose levels should be monitored closely for deterioration in diabetic control.

Summary: The hypoglycemic activity of chlorpropamide may be enhanced by concurrent administration of clofibrate.

Related Drugs: Other sulfonylureas have demonstrated a similar interaction with clofibrate. Glyburide and glipizide may interact in a similar manner. Halofenate enhances the hypoglycemic effect of the sulfonylureas.

Mechanism: Clofibrate may increase half-life, decrease excretion, decrease insulin resistance, or displace chlorpropamide and other sulfonylureas from protein binding sites.

Detailed Information: See *EDI,* 14/7.00

Chlorpropamide-Cortisone

Significance: 2—moderately clinically significant

Recommendations: Occurrence of glycosuria should not be an important factor in the decision to discontinue corticosteroid therapy or to initiate it in diabetic patients. However, patients on antidiabetic therapy should be monitored for decreased hypoglycemic action while on concurrent glucocorticoid treatment. To maintain diabetic control during high dose or long-term corticosteroid treatment, increased dosage of chlorpropamide may be required.

Summary: The intrinsic hyperglycemic activity of cortisone may decrease the hypoglycemic effects of concurrently administered chlorpropamide.

Related Drugs: Prolonged treatment with glucocorticoids has been found to elevate plasma glucagon. Other sulfonylurea hypoglycemics and other corticosteroids may be expected to interact similarly.

Mechanism: Chlorpropamide and other sulfonylureas acutely increase sensitivity to glucose, and chlorpropamide may inhibit gluconeogenesis and augment insulin-mediated suppression of hepatic glucose release.

Detailed Information: See *EDI,* 14/9.00

Chlorpropamide-Hydrochlorothiazide

Significance: 2—moderately clinically significant

Recommendations: Diabetic patients controlled by diet with oral hypoglycemic agents or by insulin should be monitored closely for hyperglycemia before and after thiazide or thiazide-like diuretics are initiated. Also, patients who have been maintained on such combination therapy should be observed for symptoms of hypoglycemia when the diuretic is withdrawn from the regimen. Since the development of hypokalemia may be responsible for the pathogenesis of the interaction, therapy should be directed toward preventing abnormal potassium loss. Additionally, the dose of the hypoglycemic drug may be increased, or insulin therapy may be substituted in sufficient dosage to control the diabetic state.

Summary: Diabetic patients regulated by chlorpropamide may exhibit impaired diabetic control when hydrochlorothiazide is added to the drug regimen.

Related Drugs: This drug interaction may occur with other sulfonylurea hypoglycemics. All thiazide diuretics have the potential of producing hypokalemia, and there are ample data exhibiting interactions between chlorpropamide and agents related to hydrochlorothiazide.

Mechanism: Thiazides inhibit the release of insulin by the pancreas. Hypokalemia is believed to be a contributing factor in the pathogenesis of this interaction.

Detailed Information: See *EDI,* 14/11.00

Chlorpropamide-Probenecid

Significance: 3—minimally clinically significant

Recommendations: No changes are necessary during combined therapy; however, patients should be observed for excessive hypoglycemic effects. Neither chlorpropamide nor probenecid should be used in patients with impaired renal function.

Summary: Probenecid was reported to increase the half-life of chlorpropamide.

Related Drugs: Probenecid was reported to prolong the half-life of tolbutamide. It is not known whether other sulfonylurea hypoglycemic agents would interact with probenecid in a similar manner.

Mechanism: Probenecid inhibits the renal excretion of chlorpropamide.

Detailed Information: See *EDI,* 14/13.00

Chlorpropamide-Sucralfate

Significance: 4—not clinically significant

Potential Effects: Sucralfate does not affect the absorption of chlorpropamide.

Recommendations: Although multiple dose studies are needed, the concurrent use of these agents need not be avoided. Sucralfate may be an alternative to cimetidine, which has been shown to interact with glipizide and tolbutamide (see Glipizide-Cimetidine, page 268).

Summary: There are data to show sucralfate does not affect the absorption of chlorpropamide.

Related Drugs: It is not known if a similar lack of interaction would occur between sucralfate and other sulfonylureas. There are no drugs related to sucralfate.

Mechanism: Sucralfate does not appear to affect the pharmacokinetics of chlorpropamide.

Detailed Information: See *EDI,* 14/14.10

Glipizide-Cimetidine

Significance: 2—moderately clinically significant

Recommendations: Caution should be exercised when cimetidine or ranitidine is administered concurrently with glipizide. If a hypoglycemic response occurs, the dose of glipizide may need to be decreased. Although clinical studies are lacking, famotidine may be an alternative to cimetidine. Sucralfate, which was shown not to interact with chlorpropamide (see Chlorpropamide-Sucralfate, page 298), may also be an alternative to cimetidine for ulcer therapy when concurrent sulfonylurea therapy is required.

Summary: There are data to show that cimetidine increases the glipizide area- under-curve, suggesting that some patients are at risk of developing significant hypoglycemia.

Related Drugs: Tolbutamide and glyburide have been shown to interact similarly; however, all data do not support this. A similar interaction may occur between cimetidine and other sulfonylurea hypoglycemic agents. Ranitidine did not seem to significantly alter the pharmacokinetics of glipizide and glyburide. Documentation is lacking regarding an interaction between glipizide and other H_2-receptor antagonists.

Mechanism: It was suggested that cimetidine inhibits the hepatic metabolism of glipizide and tolbutamide, or there may be a reduction in hepatic blood flow.

Detailed Information: See *EDI,* 14/14.30

Glipizide-Charcoal

Significance: 2—moderately clinically significant

Potential Effects: Charcoal adsorbs glipizide, resulting in decreased absorption.

Recommendations: Separating administration times may not avoid this interaction because of glipizide enterohepatic recirculation. Charcoal may be useful in glipizide overdose treatment.

Summary: Concurrent administration of glipizide and charcoal results in a decrease in glipizide absorption.

Related Drugs: A similar interaction would be expected to occur between charcoal and other sulfonylureas.

Mechanism: Glipizide is adsorbed onto the surface of activated charcoal.

Detailed Information: See *EDI,* 14/14.44

Glipizide-Cholestyramine

Significance: 2—moderately clinically significant

Potential Effects: Cholestyramine may bind to glipizide, resulting in decreased absorption of glipizide.

Recommendations: Monitor patients for signs of decreased glipizide absorption with concurrent cholestyramine administration. Separation of administration may not avoid the interaction because of enterohepatic circulation of glipizide.

Summary: Concurrent glipizide and cholestyramine may result in decreased glipizide serum levels.

Related Drugs: It is not known whether an interaction would occur between cholestyramine and other sulfonylureas or between glipizide and colestipol.

Mechanism: Cholestyramine interferes with the absorption of acidic drugs, and glipizide may bind to cholestyramine, preventing absorption.
Detailed Information: See *EDI*, 14/14.45

Glyburide-Gemfibrozil

Significance: 2—moderately clinically significant
Potential Effects: The effect of glyburide may be increased when gemfibrozil is added to therapy.
Recommendations: Patients maintained on glyburide should be closely monitored for a change in blood glucose levels if gemfibrozil is added to, or withdrawn from, therapy. The dose of glyburide may need to be adjusted. Gemfibrozil may be effective as an aid to glycemic control in some patients maintained on sulfonylureas.
Summary: The effect of glyburide may be increased when gemfibrozil is added to therapy.
Related Drugs: A similar interaction may occur between gemfibrozil and other sulfonylureas. There are no drugs related to gemfibrozil.
Mechanism: Gemfibrozil is strongly bound to plasma proteins, and glyburide may be displaced from its binding sites by gemfibrozil.
Detailed Information: See *EDI*, 14/14.46

Glyburide-Rifampin

Significance: 3—minimally clinically significant
Potential Effects: Rifampin may increase the metabolism of glyburide, resulting in decreased levels.
Recommendations: Patients should be monitored for changes in blood glucose concentration if rifampin is added to, or withdrawn from, cotherapy.
Summary: Addition of rifampin to a stable glyburide regimen necessitated an increase in glyburide dosage to maintain blood glucose levels.
Related Drugs: An interaction may occur between rifampin and other sulfonylurea hypoglycemics. There are no drugs related to rifampin.
Mechanism: Rifampin may cause metabolic induction, which may result in an increase in the metabolism of glyburide.
Detailed Information: See *EDI*, 14/14.47

Glipizide-Heparin

Significance: 3—minimally clinically significant
Potential Effects: Heparin may decrease the protein binding of glipizide or inhibit its metabolism/excretion, leading to an increased hypoglycemic effect.
Recommendations: Patients receiving concurrent administration of glipizide and heparin should be monitored for potential hypoglycemia. The dose of glipizide may need to be decreased, or the drug may need to be discontinued.
Summary: There are data to show that heparin may decrease the protein binding of glipizide or inhibit its metabolism and excretion, potentiating an increased hypoglycemic effect.
Related Drugs: Glyburide may interact with heparin similarly to glipizide. Because of differences in protein binding and activity of metabolites, it is not known if other sulfonylureas would interact with heparin. There are no drugs related to heparin.

Mechanism: Heparin may decrease the binding of glipizide, which is highly protein bound and may have inhibited the metabolism or excretion of glipizide.

Detailed Information: See *EDI*, 14/14.50

Insulin-Aspirin

Significance: 3—minimally clinically significant

Recommendations: Patients should be monitored for a change in their blood glucose levels during concurrent use of these agents. If necessary, a lower dose of insulin may be administered.

Summary: The hypoglycemic activity of insulin may be potentiated by concurrent use of aspirin or other salicylates.

Related Drugs: A similar interaction may occur with other salicylates.

Mechanism: Aspirin may reduce plasma glucose, affect pancreatic islet cell function, change hepatic glucose production, inhibit intestinal glucose production, or increase peripheral glucose uptake and oxidation.

Detailed Information: See *EDI*, 14/15.00

Insulin-Chlorpromazine

Significance: 3—minimally clinically significant

Recommendations: Patients receiving hypoglycemic therapy with insulin or sulfonylureas should be observed for loss of diabetic control if high doses of phenothiazines are added to their medication regimen.

Summary: Chlorpromazine may produce a dose- and duration-dependent increase in plasma glucose concentrations that may lead to loss of diabetic control in predisposed individuals.

Related Drugs: Other phenothiazines, thioxanthenes, butyrophenones, dihydroindolones, and dibenzoxazepines may interact with insulin in a similar manner. Because of the mechanism of this interaction, sulfonylurea hypoglycemic agents may also be affected.

Mechanism: This interaction is a result of the inhibition of insulin release from the pancreas.

Detailed Information: See *EDI*, 14/17.00

Insulin-Clofibrate

Significance: 2—moderately clinically significant

Recommendations: It is important to monitor blood glucose levels during concurrent therapy with these agents. The dose of insulin may need to be adjusted.

Summary: Clofibrate has been shown to lower blood glucose levels in insulin-dependent diabetics.

Related Drugs: There are no drugs related to clofibrate. An interaction involving clofibrate and the oral sulfonylureas is discussed in another monograph (see Chlorpropamide-Clofibrate, page 297).

Mechanism: The mechanism of this interaction is unknown. Clofibrate may cause a change in tissue sensitivity to insulin and/or glucose.

Detailed Information: See *EDI*, 14/19.00

Insulin-Diltiazem

Significance: 3—minimally clinically significant

Potential Effects: Diltiazem may increase insulin requirements.

Recommendations: Patients stabilized on insulin should be monitored for increases in insulin requirements if diltiazem therapy is initiated. The insulin dosage may need to be adjusted.

Summary: Insulin resistance was reported when diltiazem was administered to a patient. Diltiazem may increase insulin requirements.

Related Drugs: A similar interaction is expected to occur between insulin and other calcium channel blocking agents.

Mechanism: Calcium antagonists impair insulin-mediated glucose transport, and chelation of intracellular calcium can block insulin action in cells. Diltiazem may cause insulin resistance by its effect on intracellular calcium.

Detailed Information: See *EDI,* 14/20.10

Insulin-Epinephrine

Significance: 3—minimally clinically significant

Recommendations: Patients stabilized on insulin should be monitored for possible increases in blood glucose levels with sympathomimetic administration. Since the parenteral administration of sympathomimetics usually occurs in emergency clinical situations, the elevation of blood glucose may not be of clinical importance. There is no evidence, however, that supports an interaction between epinephrine and exogenously administered insulin.

Summary: Epinephrine raises blood glucose levels and may increase insulin requirements.

Related Drugs: Other sympathomimetic agents may have the same hyperglycemic effect with insulin.

Mechanism: Epinephrine may act synergistically with glucagon to antagonize the effects of insulin.

Detailed Information: See *EDI,* 14/21.00

Insulin-Fenfluramine

Significance: 2—moderately clinically significant

Recommendations: This interaction may be beneficial in certain diabetic patients, and this effect is most marked when fenfluramine is administered immediately before a meal. However, patients must be closely monitored when fenfluramine is added to, or withdrawn from, diabetic therapy.

Summary: The intrinsic hypoglycemic effect of fenfluramine may increase the effects of insulin and result in hypoglycemia when the agents are used concurrently.

Related Drugs: A similar interaction is expected to occur between insulin and other anorexiants. A similar interaction may be expected with other sulfonylureas.

Mechanism: Fenfluramine lowers blood sugar levels as a result of the increased uptake of glucose into skeletal muscle. This hypoglycemic effect is additive in combination with insulin.

Detailed Information: See *EDI,* 14/23.00

Insulin-Guanethidine

Significance: 1—highly clinically significant

Recommendations: Diabetic patients should be closely observed when guanethidine is added to, or deleted from, the drug regimen. A decrease in insulin dose may be required when guanethidine is added, or an increase in insulin dose may be necessitated when guanethidine is withdrawn.

Summary: Long-term guanethidine therapy may improve glucose tolerance, necessitating a reduction in insulin dose.

Related Drugs: A similar interaction is expected to occur between insulin and other drugs related to guanethidine.

Mechanism: The exact mechanism is unknown. Long-term guanethidine depletes tissue catecholamines involved with raising blood sugar levels and may improve glucose tolerance.

Detailed Information: See *EDI,* 14/25.00

Insulin-Isoniazid

Significance: 3—minimally clinically significant

Recommendations: Patients on concurrent therapy with antidiabetic agents and isoniazid should be monitored for possible increases in blood glucose levels. This may be of greater clinical significance in patients with hepatic dysfunction or in those who are slow acetylators of isoniazid.

Summary: Isoniazid antagonizes the hypoglycemic action of insulin by elevating blood sugar levels.

Related Drugs: Because of conflicting results, it is difficult to determine whether an interaction occurs between isoniazid and other sulfonylurea hypoglycemics. There are no drugs related to isoniazid.

Mechanism: By causing disturbances in carbohydrate metabolism, isoniazid may increase blood glucose levels and impair glucose tolerance.

Detailed Information: See *EDI,* 14/27.00

Insulin-Oxytetracycline

Significance: 2—moderately clinically significant

Recommendations: Patients whose diabetes is controlled on insulin therapy who receive oxytetracycline should be monitored closely because of the possibility of hypoglycemia.

Summary: Several cases have been reported in which the administration of oxytetracycline to diabetic patients receiving insulin caused hypoglycemia, necessitating a decrease in insulin dosage.

Related Drugs: A similar interaction is expected to occur with other sulfonylurea hypoglycemics and oxytetracycline. A similar interaction is expected to occur with other tetracyclines.

Mechanism: Oxytetracycline exerts a hypoglycemic effect by increasing the half-life of insulin or by interfering with the action of epinephrine.

Detailed Information: See *EDI,* 14/29.00

Insulin-Phenelzine

Significance: 2—moderately clinically significant

Recommendations: Concurrent MAO inhibitor therapy for depression in a diabetic patient will often require reduction in dosage of the hypoglycemic agent because of enhanced hypoglycemic effects. Since the extent of the reaction is highly unpredictable, any diabetic patients receiving MAO inhibitors should be monitored for possible excessive hypoglycemia.

Summary: Phenelzine can potentiate the action of insulin, resulting in an enhanced hypoglycemic state.

Related Drugs: It is well documented that agents that possess MAOI activity may interact similarly with insulin. A similar interaction is expected to occur with other sulfonylurea hypoglycemics.

Mechanism: A diminution in the epinephrine response following insulin-induced hypoglycemia has been proposed.

Detailed Information: See *EDI*, 14/31.00

Insulin-Phenytoin

Significance: 3—minimally clinically significant

Recommendations: Diabetic patients receiving phenytoin should be closely monitored for elevation of serum glucose levels and symptoms of hyperglycemia. Dosage reduction of phenytoin may prevent or alleviate the symptoms, since some adverse reactions have occurred at high phenytoin dosages. Also, adjusting the sulfonylurea dose whenever phenytoin is added to, or withdrawn from, therapy may be advisable.

Summary: Phenytoin may inhibit endogenous insulin secretion, resulting in clinically significant symptoms of hyperglycemia

Related Drugs: The other hydantoin anticonvulsants may be expected to produce the same hyperglycemic effect as phenytoin. Oral sulfonylurea hypoglycemic agents may be affected by phenytoin.

Mechanism: Phenytoin can induce hyperglycemia through inhibition of endogenous insulin secretion.

Detailed Information: See *EDI*, 14/33.00

Insulin-Propranolol

Significance: 1—highly clinically significant

Potential Effects: Propranolol can delay recovery from hypoglycemia as well as modify the normal cardiovascular response to hypoglycemia.

Recommendations: When use of a beta-blocking agent is indicated in a diabetic patient, particularly one prone to hypoglycemic attacks, one of the cardioselective agents (acebutolol, atenolol, or metoprolol), rather than propranolol, should be used, both to decrease the risk of a hypertensive response to hypoglycemia and to permit more rapid recovery from low blood glucose levels. The danger of unrecognized hypoglycemia in the insulin-dependent diabetic who is taking propranolol can be reduced if the patient is aware of the associated diaphoretic response.

Summary: Propranolol can delay recovery from hypoglycemia and mask hypoglycemic symptoms.

Related Drugs: The cardioselective beta-blocking agents do not seem to prolong the effect on insulin-induced hypoglycemia. A similar interaction is expected to occur between insulin and other noncardioselective beta-blocking agents. Effects of beta-adrenergic blockers on long-term sulfonylurea therapy have not been determined. Because of conflicting reports, it is difficult to determine whether an interaction would occur with other sulfonylurea hypoglycemics.

Mechanism: The mechanism is complicated and unclear, but it is known that propranolol does not affect plasma glucose or insulin concentrations or the rate or magnitude of the fall of plasma glucose.

Detailed Information: See *EDI*, 14/35.00

Insulin-Thyroid

Significance: 2—moderately clinically significant

Recommendations: The management of patients on this combination requires attention to both diabetic control and thyroid function, especially at initiation of therapy.

Summary: The initiation of thyroid replacement therapy may cause an increase in insulin or oral hypoglycemic requirements. Insulin administration may affect thyroid hormone binding and disrupt thyroid function.

Related Drugs: There are no reports of an interaction between hypoglycemic therapy and thyroid replacement therapy. Based on the available evidence, it would seem that any thyroid hormone can interact with any hypoglycemic therapy.

Mechanism: Levothyroxine increases the rate of carbohydrate absorption from the gastrointestinal tract, and both liothyronine and thyroxine suppress insulin secretion from the pancreas.

Detailed Information: See *EDI,* 14/37.00

Insulin-Tobacco

Significance: 3—minimally clinically significant

Recommendations: Because of conflicting results and limited data, it is difficult to determine if diabetic smokers will need a change in their insulin requirements. However, patients' blood glucose should be monitored regularly, and the insulin dose adjusted if necessary.

Summary: Insulin absorption may be decreased in patients who smoke tobacco.

Related Drugs: There are no drugs related to insulin.

Mechanism: The increased insulin requirement in diabetic smokers may be secondary to elevated catecholamine levels, or there may be a decreased absorption because of peripheral vasoconstriction.

Detailed Information: See *EDI,* 14/38.10

Metformin-Iodinated Contrast Media

Significance: 1—highly clinically significant

Potential Effects: Concurrent metformin and iodinated contrast media administration may result in an increased risk of metformin-induced lactic acidosis levels.

Recommendations: Coadministration of parenteral iodinated contrast media and metformin is contraindicated. The manufacturer product information states, "Glucophage (metformin) should be withheld for at least 48 hours prior to, and 48 hours subsequent to, the procedure and reinstituted only after renal function has been re-evaluated and found to be normal."

Summary: Concurrent metformin and iodinated contrast media administration may result in an increased risk of metformin-induced lactic acidosis. Metformin does not react with the iodine, causing renal failure and lactic acidosis. If the parenteral administration of iodinated contrast media causes decreased renal function, metformin may accumulate and result in higher serum lactate levels, thus resulting in an increased risk of lactic acidosis.

Related Drugs: There are no drugs related to metformin.

Mechanism: Metformin does not undergo hepatic metabolism or biliary excretion and is excreted unchanged in the urine. Iodinated contrast media-induced renal failure may interfere with the renal elimination of metformin. Contrast materials may lead to acute renal failure, particularly in diabetic patients, and have been associated with lactic acidosis in patients receiving metformin. This association has been attributed to accumulation of high blood concentrations of metformin resulting from impairment of the renal clearance of metformin during acute renal failure.

Detailed Information: See *EDI,* 14/38.20

Tolazamide-Doxepin

Significance: 2—moderately clinically significant

Potential Effects: Concurrent use of these agents may result in hypoglycemia.

Recommendations: Patients receiving doxepin and tolazamide concurrently should be monitored for low blood glucose levels. If hypoglycemia occurs, the patient should be appropriately treated with dextrose or glucagon, and the sulfonylurea may need to be discontinued or the dose decreased.

Summary: There are data to show that coadministration of these agents may result in hypoglycemia, necessitating a decreased tolazamide dosage.

Related Drugs: Documentation is lacking regarding a similar interaction between tolazamide and other tricyclic antidepressants or between doxepin and other sulfonylureas.

Mechanism: The mechanism of this interaction is not known.

Detailed Information: See *EDI,* 14/38.30

Tolbutamide-Chloramphenicol

Significance: 2—moderately clinically significant

Recommendations: Reduction in the sulfonylurea dose may be necessary if concurrent chloramphenicol administration is indicated. Frequent monitoring of serum glucose levels may enable control during this time. Temporary use of insulin may be required if serum glucose levels cannot be controlled with the oral agent. Since some studies have shown higher serum tolbutamide levels in morning measurements than those later in the day, patients can be monitored for symptoms and cautioned accordingly.

Summary: Chloramphenicol and tolbutamide may cause prolonged hypoglycemic responses because of an increased tolbutamide half-life. Patients with renal insufficiency may be at greater risk for this interaction.

Related Drugs: Chlorpropamide half-life has been increased by chloramphenicol. Tolazamide, acetohexamide, glyburide and glipizide may be affected. There are no drugs related to chloramphenicol.

Mechanism: Interference with renal elimination has been proposed as a mechanism for the increased half-life and elevated serum levels of the sulfonylurea.

Detailed Information: See *EDI,* 14/39.00

Tolbutamide-Diazoxide

Significance: 3—minimally clinically significant

Recommendations: Diabetic patients receiving diazoxide should be monitored for an increase in blood glucose levels. Should hyperglycemia occur, an appropriate adjustment in dosage of one or both drugs is necessary. Treatment with insulin should be considered in patients with severe hyperglycemia resulting from diazoxide administration.

Summary: Hyperglycemia has occurred in patients receiving diazoxide for treatment of severe hypertension, or after long-term administration in the treatment of hypoglycemia.

Related Drugs: The other sulfonylurea hypoglycemics may interact similarly with diazoxide. There are no drugs related to diazoxide.

Mechanism: Diazoxide has been shown to inhibit the release of insulin.

Detailed Information: See *EDI,* 14/41.00

Tolbutamide-Dicumarol

Significance: 2—moderately clinically significant

Recommendations: If dicumarol and a sulfonylurea must be given concurrently, serum glucose concentrations should be closely monitored, and the sulfonylurea dose should be adjusted accordingly when dicumarol is added to, or withdrawn from, the drug regimen. Also, it is prudent to closely monitor prothrombin times since the dose of dicumarol may need to be adjusted.

Summary: Dicumarol may significantly increase the serum half-life of tolbutamide and prolong prothrombin time.

Related Drugs: Dicumarol may interact with other sulfonylurea hypoglycemics. The other coumarin anticoagulants and the indandione derivatives do not interact with tolbutamide.

Mechanism: It has been suggested that dicumarol inhibits the hepatic metabolism of tolbutamide and chlorpropamide. Dicumarol may displace the sulfonylureas from their plasma protein binding sites.

Detailed Information: See *EDI,* 14/43.00

Tolbutamide-Fluconazole

Significance: 3—minimally clinically significant

Potential Effects: Concomitant tolbutamide and fluconazole administration may result in increased tolbutamide levels and possible hypoglycemia symptoms.

Recommendations: Patients should be carefully monitored for changes in blood glucose levels and symptoms of hypoglycemia with concurrent administration of these agents. The dose of tolbutamide may need to be adjusted.

Summary: Concomitant administration of tolbutamide and fluconazole resulted in increased tolbutamide levels.

Related Drugs: An interaction would be expected to occur between fluconazole and other sulfonylureas and between tolbutamide and other imidazole antifungal agents.

Mechanism: Tolbutamide is metabolized by cytochrome P450 isozymes. Fluconazole has been shown to have an inhibitory effect on cytochrome P450 isozymes.

Detailed Information: See *EDI,* 14/44.05

Tolbutamide-Methyldopa

Significance: 3—minimally clinically significant

Recommendations: Although the concurrent use of these agents need not be avoided, blood glucose levels should be monitored, and the dose of tolbutamide may need to be decreased.

Summary: The half-life of tolbutamide was found to be prolonged with coadministration of methyldopa.

Related Drugs: A similar interaction is expected to occur between methyldopa and other sulfonylureas. There are no drugs related to methyldopa.

Mechanism: Methyldopa may decrease the metabolism of tolbutamide by inhibiting the hepatic microsomal enzymes.

Detailed Information: See *EDI,* 14/44.10

Tolbutamide-Phenylbutazone

Significance: 1—highly clinically significant

Potential Effects: Phenylbutazone displaces tolbutamide from its binding sites, resulting in enhanced hypoglycemia.

Recommendations: Because of the possibility that a severe, or even fatal, hypoglycemic reaction can result, use of this combination requires intense monitoring of serum glucose levels and probable dosage reduction of the sulfonylurea. If concurrent long-term therapy is necessary, agents other than phenylbutazone or oxyphenbutazone (e.g., sulindac) should be used whenever possible.

Summary: There are data to show that severe hypoglycemic reactions have occurred after phenylbutazone administration to patients on long-term tolbutamide therapy.

Related Drugs: Tolbutamide has been shown to interact with many NSAIAs; however, the data are conflicting. A similar interaction is expected to occur between tolbutamide and other NSAIAs.

Mechanism: Phenylbutazone may inhibit the excretion or delay the metabolism of tolbutamide or displace tolbutamide from plasma and tissue proteins.

Detailed Information: See *EDI,* 14/45.00

Tolbutamide-Sulfamethizole

Significance: 2—moderately clinically significant

Potential Effects: Sulfamethizole may inhibit the metabolism of tolbutamide or displace it from protein binding sites, leading to enhanced hypoglycemic activity.

Recommendations: Concurrent use of these agents should be done with caution. Patients should be monitored for enhanced hypoglycemic effects. Glyburide or possible glipizide may be alternatives to tolbutamide.

Summary: Tolbutamide-treated patients have developed enhanced hypoglycemic effects after administration of sulfamethizole.

Related Drugs: There are contradictory reports regarding the effect of sulfisoxazole or sulfadiazine on serum glucose or serum tolbutamide. Because of conflicting results, it is difficult to determine whether an interaction would occur between tolbutamide and other sulfonamides. Glyburide and glipizide have been shown not to significantly interact.

Mechanism: Sulfamethizole may inhibit hepatic oxidation, carboxylation and the aromatic ring hydroxylating enzyme system of tolbutamide.

Detailed Information: See *EDI,* 14/47.00

Chapter Fifteen

Sedative-Hypnotic Drug Interactions

Alcohol, Ethyl-Amitriptyline

Significance: 2—moderately clinically significant

Recommendations: The most hazardous of the possible interactions is the enhanced central nervous system depression of alcohol while the patient is on amitriptyline. Patients receiving amitriptyline should be informed that concurrent ingestion of alcohol may produce a greater than expected impairment of the ability to drive an automobile or operate dangerous machinery. The impairment in psychomotor skills caused by the combination of alcohol and amitriptyline may become less harmful with continued amitriptyline administration.

Summary: The effects of the concurrent use of amitriptyline and alcohol are unpredictable. Various studies have reported that amitriptyline can enhance, antagonize, or have no effect on CNS effects.

Related Drugs: Other tricyclic antidepressants and the tetracyclic antidepressants may interact similarly with alcohol.

Mechanism: Enhanced sedation seen with the combination of amitriptyline and alcohol may result from an additive effect.

Detailed Information: See *EDI,* 15/1.00

Alcohol, Ethyl-Bromocriptine

Significance: 3—minimally clinically significant

Recommendations: If side effects of bromocriptine occur or become severe, patients should abstain from the use of alcohol. This interaction may be of benefit in alcoholic patients with severe alcohol withdrawal symptoms.

Summary: Alcohol may potentiate the side effects of bromocriptine.

Related Drugs: There are no drugs related to alcohol or bromocriptine.

Mechanism: Alcohol may enhance the sensitivity of the dopamine receptors, and bromocriptine is a dopamine receptor agonist.

Detailed Information: See *EDI,* 15/2.10

Alcohol, Ethyl-Cimetidine

Significance: 3—minimally clinically significant

Potential Effects: Cimetidine may increase ethyl alcohol serum levels, leading to increased side effects.

Recommendations: Patients should be aware that alcohol blood levels may be increased during concurrent cimetidine, and an increased level of intoxication may result.

Summary: There are data to show that administration of cimetidine may increase alcohol levels, leading to increased side effects; however, it has been shown that cimetidine has no effect on alcohol blood levels.

Related Drugs: Ranitidine and famotidine, when given at recommended doses, do not affect alcohol metabolism. It is not known whether an interaction will occur between nizatidine and alcohol.

Mechanism: Alcohol absorption may be increased with concurrent cimetidine.

Detailed Information: See *EDI,* 15/3.00

Alcohol, Ethyl-Diphenhydramine

Significance: 2—moderately clinically significant

Recommendations: Patients receiving diphenhydramine or other antihistamines should be advised that the concurrent use of alcohol may result in increased mental and motor impairment and may impair their ability to drive an automobile or operate dangerous equipment.

Summary: Concurrent administration of diphenhydramine and alcohol may result in a greater impairment of motor and mental performance.

Related Drugs: Evidence indicates that tripelennamine also interacts with alcohol. Other antihistamines may also interact with alcohol.

Mechanism: The mechanism is unknown.

Detailed Information: See *EDI,* 15/5.00

Alcohol, Ethyl-Disulfiram

Significance: 1—highly clinically significant

Recommendations: Consumption of even small doses (e.g., 15ml) of alcohol leads to this interaction; therefore, concomitant administration should be avoided. Patients have suffered this interaction from taking cough mixtures and using topical preparations such as aftershave lotions and antipsoriatic preparations that contained alcohol. However, the quantity of alcohol required to elicit the interaction varies with individuals. This reaction has also been reported in patients who came in contact with other organic solvents (e.g., paint, "mineral spirits") through inhalation; therefore, patients should be advised of this potential hazard as well.

Summary: Patients ingesting alcohol or using topical preparations that contain alcohol while taking disulfiram will experience throbbing in the head and neck, palpitations, tachycardia, hypotension, sweating, nausea, and vomiting.

Related Drugs: There are no drugs related to alcohol or disulfiram.

Mechanism: Disulfiram alters the intermediary metabolism of alcohol, causing an accumulation of acetaldehyde which is responsible for this unpleasant reaction.

Detailed Information: See *EDI,* 15/7.00

Alcohol, Ethyl-Fluoxetine

Significance: 4—not clinically significant

Potential Effects: Concurrent use of these agents does not result in any alterations in the concentrations or effects of either agent.

Recommendations: Fluoxetine may be considered as an alternative antidepressant agent to the tricyclic or tetracyclic antidepressant agents in patients who consume alcohol. Also, fluoxetine may be beneficial in the treatment of alcoholism.

Summary: The concurrent use of these agents did not alter the plasma or blood concentrations of either drug. Psychomotor activity and subjective effects of alcohol were not affected.

Related Drugs: There are no drugs related to fluoxetine.

Mechanism: Please see summary.

Detailed Information: See *EDI,* 15/8.01

Alcohol, Ethyl-Furazolidone

Significance: 2—moderately clinically significant

Recommendations: If disulfiram-like reactions (e.g., facial flushing, lightheadedness, tachycardia, dyspnea, nausea, vomiting) occur in a patient receiving furazolidone who ingests alcohol, the use of alcohol should be avoided.

Summary: The ingestion of alcohol in patients receiving furazolidone has been shown to result in acute alcohol intolerance similar to a disulfiram reaction.

Related Drugs: There is no evidence of alcohol interacting with nitrofurantoin.

Mechanism: The mechanism of this interaction is unknown.
Detailed Information: See *EDI,* 15/8.10

Alcohol, Ethyl-Glutethimide

Significance: 2—moderately clinically significant
Recommendations: Concurrent ingestion of alcohol and glutethimide (or other central nervous system depressants previously mentioned) may result in an increased depressant activity. Patients should be warned of this possible enhancement of the depressant effects and also that this combination may produce a greater impairment of their ability to drive or operate hazardous machinery.
Summary: Concurrent ingestion of alcohol and glutethimide may result in a greater CNS depression than when either agent is taken alone.
Related Drugs: Methyprylon may interact with alcohol in a manner similar to that of glutethimide. Other drugs that possess CNS depressant activity, such as ethchlorvynol and methaqualone, may interact with alcohol.
Mechanism: The mechanism of this interaction is not documented. The CNS depressant effects result from synergism.
Detailed Information: See *EDI,* 15/9.00

Alcohol, Ethyl-Ketoconazole

Significance: 3—minimally clinically significant
Potential Effects: The ingestion of alcohol with concurrent ketoconazole may result in a "sunburn-like" rash.
Recommendations: Patients should avoid alcohol if a rash develops when also taking ketoconazole.
Summary: A patient taking ketoconazole developed a "sunburn-like" rash that was confined to the face, upper chest, and back shortly after ingesting alcohol.
Related Drugs: There are no drugs related to ketoconazole.
Mechanism: Although the mechanism is unknown, ketoconazole is similar to metronidazole, and metronidazole has been shown to result in a disulfiram-like reaction with alcohol ingestion (see Alcohol, Ethyl-Metronidazole, below).
Detailed Information: See *EDI,* 15/10.10

Alcohol, Ethyl-Metoclopramide

Significance: 3—minimally clinically significant
Recommendations: The clinical significance of the interaction is not completely documented. However, administration of these agents together led to an enhanced alcohol sedation, suggesting that concurrent use should be avoided.
Summary: Concurrent administration of metoclopramide and alcohol has significantly increased the rate of alcohol absorption and sedation.
Related Drugs: There are no drugs related to metoclopramide.
Mechanism: Metoclopramide hastens gastric emptying which results in a quicker absorption onset.
Detailed Information: See *EDI,* 15/11.00

Alcohol, Ethyl-Metronidazole

Significance: 2—moderately clinically significant

Potential Effects: Metronidazole may inhibit the metabolism of alcohol, leading to an increase in acetaldehyde, which is responsible for the disulfiram-like reaction that may occur.

Recommendations: Patients receiving metronidazole should be advised of the potential for this interaction with alcohol ingestion.

Summary: Concurrent use of metronidazole with alcohol has been associated with a disulfiram-type reaction resulting in symptoms of hypotension, nausea, facial flushing, headache, and sweating.

Related Drugs: There are no drugs related to metronidazole.

Mechanism: Metronidazole may produce an inhibition of aldehyde dehydrogenase, and the resultant accumulation of acetaldehyde is responsible for the disulfiram-like reaction.

Detailed Information: See *EDI,* 15/13.00

Amobarbital-Tranylcypromine

Significance: 3—minimally clinically significant

Recommendations: Amobarbital, and possibly other barbiturates, should be used with caution in patients receiving tranylcypromine, other monoamine oxidase inhibitors, or other drugs that possess monoamine oxidase inhibitor activity, such as furazolidone or procarbazine. If concurrent administration is required, the dosage interval of the barbiturate may need to be lengthened because of the prolongation of CNS depression.

Summary: Pretreatment with tranylcypromine may prolong the CNS depressant effect of amobarbital.

Related Drugs: Other MAOIs may prolong the CNS depressant effects of other barbiturates.

Mechanism: MAOIs produce this effect by interference with the metabolism of barbiturates rather than through the effect on monoamine oxidase.

Detailed Information: See *EDI,* 15/15.00

Chloral Hydrate-Alcohol, Ethyl

Significance: 2—moderately clinically significant

Recommendations: All patients taking chloral hydrate should be warned that the CNS depressant effects of both chloral hydrate and alcohol are increased by concurrent ingestion. Patients with cardiovascular disease who receive chloral hydrate long-term should be especially careful about ingesting alcohol in view of the tachycardia and hypotension that can result from the vasodilation reaction.

Summary: Concurrent ingestion of chloral hydrate and alcohol results in greater CNS depression than when either agent is taken alone.

Related Drugs: Based on the mechanism, triclofos and other products metabolized to yield trichloroethanol may be expected to interact with alcohol.

Mechanism: Enhanced CNS depression occurs because of an altered production of active metabolites of chloral hydrate and alcohol.

Detailed Information: See *EDI,* 15/17.00

Chloral Hydrate-Furazolidone

Significance: 4—not clinically significant

Recommendations: Since the drug interaction between chloral hydrate and furazolidone is based on theoretic considerations and has not been documented in humans, the clinical significance of this drug interaction is unsubstantiated, and no special precautions are advised with concurrent use.

Summary: Furazolidone or its metabolite may inhibit the metabolism of chloral hydrate, enhancing the CNS depressant effect.

Related Drugs: Other MAOIs (e.g., procarbazine) may be expected to interact with chloral hydrate in a manner analogous to that of furazolidone.

Mechanism: Chloral hydrate could show exaggerated effects in the presence of monoamine oxidase inhibitors, primarily CNS depression.

Detailed Information: See *EDI,* 15/19.00

Chlormethiazole-Cimetidine

Significance: 3—minimally clinically significant

Potential Effects: Concurrent cimetidine and chlormethiazole may result in a decreased clearance of chlormethiazole.

Recommendations: Patients being administered concurrent cimetidine and chlormethiazole should be monitored for excess sedation and respiratory depression.

Summary: Cimetidine administration resulted in a decreased clearance of chlormethiazole, potentiating sedation and respiratory depression.

Related Drugs: Ranitidine did not appear to interact similarly to cimetidine. An interaction may not occur with famotidine and nizatidine since they do not inhibit mixed function oxidase activity.

Mechanism: The decrease in chlormethiazole is because of cimetidine's inhibition of hepatic mixed function oxidase activity.

Detailed Information: See *EDI,* 15/20.50

Hexobarbital-Rifampin

Significance: 3—minimally clinically significant

Recommendations: A reduction in the effectiveness of hexobarbital may be expected with concurrent rifampin and may necessitate an increased hexobarbital dosage. Whether this occurs with other barbiturates is unknown at this time.

Summary: There are data to show that a reduction in the effectiveness of hexobarbital may occur with concurrent rifampin.

Related Drugs: Because of conflicting results, it is difficult to determine whether an interaction would occur between rifampin and the other barbiturates. There are no drugs related to rifampin.

Mechanism: Rifampin appears to significantly stimulate the metabolism of hexobarbital, reducing its effectiveness.

Detailed Information: See *EDI,* 15/21.00

Meprobamate-Alcohol, Ethyl

Significance: 2—moderately clinically significant

Recommendations: Patients receiving meprobamate should be cautioned regarding the enhancement of the CNS depressant effects of this drug when alcohol is ingested concurrently, because more pronounced and possibly dangerous effects (impairment of driving ability) have been observed when meprobamate was administered to some patients on a long-term basis. If either drug is taken in large doses, these agents can enhance CNS depression, resulting in death. Habitual use of alcohol while taking meprobamate should likewise be avoided.

Summary: Acute alcohol intoxication in patients receiving meprobamate can lead to an additive or synergistic CNS depression as well as an increase in the half-life of meprobamate.

Related Drugs: Propanediol derivatives are related to meprobamate and may interact with alcohol.

Mechanism: The effects of this interaction may be described as enhanced CNS depression produced by two agents having sedative-hypnotic properties.

Detailed Information: See *EDI,* 15/23.00

Meprobamate-Imipramine

Significance: 3—minimally clinically significant

Recommendations: Although one study suggested drowsiness and dizziness in humans were enhanced by the combination of meprobamate and a tricyclic antidepressant, it appears that this interaction is of minor clinical significance. However, patients should be aware that the combination of these drugs may result in enhanced drowsiness and dizziness.

Summary: Imipramine has been shown to enhance the CNS effect of meprobamate in animals.

Related Drugs: Propanediol derivatives are related to meprobamate and may interact with imipramine. Other tricyclic antidepressants and the tetracyclic antidepressants may also interact with meprobamate.

Mechanism: The enhanced sedative effects of meprobamate are mediated by hepatic microsomal enzyme inhibition rather than additive central depression.

Detailed Information: See *EDI,* 15/25.00

Phenobarbital-Alcohol, Ethyl

Significance: 2—moderately clinically significant

Recommendations: The effects of this interaction are dose-related. Relatively moderate amounts of alcohol (90 to 120ml of 100-proof whiskey ingested during one hour) may impair a patient's ability to drive or operate machinery, and this danger is increased when barbiturates are taken concurrently. Large amounts of alcohol (150 to 200ml of 100-proof whiskey) should be avoided while the patient is receiving barbiturates. Although benzodiazepines also interact with alcohol, they may be preferred over barbiturates for treatment of alcohol withdrawal since they result in less respiratory depression and do not disturb sleep patterns.

Summary: Concurrent use of alcohol and barbiturates may result in enhanced CNS depressant effects.

Related Drugs: Pentobarbital has been shown to decrease half-life and action. Other barbiturates may interact with alcohol similarly to phenobarbital.

Mechanism: The CNS depression of this interaction is caused by a synergistic effect of phenobarbital and alcohol.
Detailed Information: See *EDI*, 15/27.00

Phenobarbital-Charcoal

Significance: 3—minimally clinically significant
Recommendations: Activated charcoal may be an effective treatment in an acute phenobarbital overdose. It should be administered as soon as possible, and subsequent doses should be given to increase phenobarbital elimination. However, if charcoal is not used for phenobarbital overdose, the administration of these agents should be separated by as much time as possible.
Summary: Activated charcoal has been shown to reduce the absorption and increase the elimination of phenobarbital.
Related Drugs: Other barbiturates may also be adsorbed by activated charcoal. There are no drugs related to charcoal.
Mechanism: Activated charcoal adsorbs phenobarbital, limiting its absorption, and it may increase the nonrenal clearance of phenobarbital.
Detailed Information: See *EDI*, 15/28.10

Phenobarbital-Chlorcyclizine

Significance: 3—minimally clinically significant
Recommendations: Patients receiving both antihistamines and barbiturates should be cautioned about the combined CNS depressant effects, particularly when driving or operating hazardous machinery. Patients should be reminded that antihistamines occur widely in nonprescription formulas, especially cough and cold remedies.
Summary: Concurrent administration of chlorcyclizine and phenobarbital may enhance CNS depression.
Related Drugs: Other antihistamines and other barbiturates may cause a similar additive depressant action.
Mechanism: The probable mechanism for this interaction is the additive synergistic CNS depressant effect of each agent.
Detailed Information: See *EDI*, 15/29.00

Phenobarbital-Cimetidine

Significance: 3—minimally clinically significant
Recommendations: Although the concurrent use of these agents need not be avoided, the dose of cimetidine may need to be increased if lower cimetidine efficacy occurs.
Summary: There are data to show that coadministration of these agents may necessitate an increased cimetidine dosage secondary to decreased efficacy.
Related Drugs: A similar interaction may occur between cimetidine and other barbiturates. A similar interaction is expected to occur between phenobarbital and other H_2-receptor antagonists.
Mechanism: Phenobarbital may increase the hepatic metabolism of cimetidine through enzyme induction.
Detailed Information: See *EDI*, 15/30.10

Phenobarbital-Cyclosporine

Significance: 2—moderately clinically significant
Potential Effects: Phenobarbital reduces cyclosporine serum levels by hepatic enzyme induction.

Recommendations: Monitor cyclosporine serum levels when these agents are used concurrently. The dose of cyclosporine may need to be adjusted if phenobarbital is added to, or withdrawn from, therapy.

Summary: Concurrent administration of phenobarbital and cyclosporine may decrease cyclosporine serum levels.

Related Drugs: Cyclosporine may interact similarly with other barbiturates. There are no drugs related to cyclosporine.

Mechanism: Phenobarbital, a known inducer of hepatic microsomal enzymes, enhances the metabolism of cyclosporine.

Detailed Information: See *EDI*, 15/30.30

Phenobarbital-Dexamethasone

Significance: 2—moderately clinically significant

Recommendations: Current evidence reveals that if barbiturates, such as phenobarbital, are taken in high doses (120mg/day or more) by patients dependent on steroid therapy, these patients should be observed for clinical evidence of decreased corticosteroid effectiveness. Alternative therapy should be considered in these patients, or a higher dose of the corticosteroid during concomitant therapy may be necessary. For treatment of anxiety and sedation, a benzodiazepine such as diazepam could be utilized. This agent has been shown not to significantly interact with steroids. Patients requiring physiologic replacement doses of steroids should be assessed for adrenal function and pharmacologic response to steroid treatment after initiation of barbiturate therapy. Barbiturates should be given with care to patients with borderline hypoadrenal function, whether of pituitary or adrenal origin.

Summary: Phenobarbital may act to decrease the systemic effects of corticosteroids such as dexamethasone.

Related Drugs: Other corticosteroids may interact with barbiturates. Other barbiturates have not been documented in the literature to interact with corticosteroids.

Mechanism: Barbiturates can induce the activity of hepatic microsomes responsible for drug metabolism and have been shown to influence the metabolism of testosterone and cortisol.

Detailed Information: See *EDI*, 15/31.00

Phenobarbital-Felbamate

Significance: 3-minimally clinically significant

Potential Effects: The addition of felbamate to the therapy of a patient maintained on phenobarbital may result in an increase in phenobarbital serum levels.

Recommendations: Monitor patients carefully for changes in phenobarbital serum levels when felbamate is added to or withdrawn from concurrent therapy. The dose of one or both agents may need to be adjusted.

Summary: In a single case report of a patient with a history of seizures who had been receiving sodium valproate, phenobarbital, and thioridazine for three months before institution of felbamate therapy, the phenobarbital serum level increased.

Related Drugs: It is not known whether an interaction would be expected to occur between felbamate and the other barbiturates or between meprobamate and phenobarbital.

Mechanism: Although the mechanism of this interaction is not known, it is postulated that felbamate may interfere with the metabolism of phenobarbital or that phenobarbital may induce felbamate clearance.

Detailed Information: See EDI, 15/32.50

Phenobarbital-Oral Contraceptive Agents

Significance: 2—moderately clinically significant

Recommendations: Although the incidence of oral contraceptive failure is not known, a sign of developing failure is intermediate breakthrough bleeding or spotting. Two courses of action have been suggested. The first is to increase the ethinyl estradiol content of the oral contraceptive to 50µg, or to 80µg if bleeding persists. The second is to use a mechanical form of contraception. Patients receiving phenobarbital as an anticonvulsant should be monitored for changes in seizure control when oral contraceptive agents are added to, or withdrawn from, therapy.

Summary: Concurrent administration of phenobarbital may result in the failure of oral contraceptive agents.

Related Drugs: Phenobarbital treatment enhanced the metabolism of estrone, progesterone, estradiol, ethinyl estradiol, testosterone, and androsterone. Other barbiturates also induce hepatic enzymes and may interact similarly with oral contraceptive agents.

Mechanism: Phenobarbital is a potent inducer of microsomal enzyme systems, and hormonal steroids have their metabolism increased by this mechanism. Phenobarbital decreases the unbound serum concentration of the steroid. Fluid retention can cause changes in seizure frequency.

Detailed Information: See *EDI,* 15/33.00

Phenobarbital-Pyridoxine

Significance: 3—minimally clinically significant

Recommendations: Although the concurrent use of these agents need not be avoided, serum phenobarbital levels should be monitored. If an increased frequency of seizures occurs in patients receiving phenobarbital and high doses of pyridoxine, the dose of phenobarbital may need to be increased. It is not known if a smaller dose of pyridoxine (e.g., a multivitamin preparation) would interact with phenobarbital.

Summary: The concurrent use of pyridoxine and phenobarbital may decrease phenobarbital plasma levels.

Related Drugs: A similar interaction may occur between pyridoxine and other barbiturates. An interaction would be expected to occur between pyridoxine and primidone. There are no drugs related to pyridoxine.

Mechanism: The reduced serum concentration of phenobarbital could result from increased activity of pyridoxal-phosphate dependent enzymes.

Detailed Information: See *EDI,* 15/35.00

Chapter Sixteen

Vitamin/Nutrient/Food Drug Interactions

Ascorbic Acid-Aspirin

Significance: 4—not clinically significant

Recommendations: Since there is no conclusive evidence that large doses of ascorbic acid will reduce the excretion of aspirin, or that aspirin causes a deficiency of ascorbic acid, the concurrent use of these agents need not be avoided.

Summary: There is no conclusive evidence that ascorbic acid reduces the excretion of aspirin, since ascorbic acid does not consistently acidify the urine.

Related Drugs: The administration of other salicylates, alone or in combination products, may produce a similar interaction. The ability of other NSAIAs to alter ascorbic acid leukocyte levels has not been sufficiently determined.

Mechanism: Aspirin has been reported to alter the uptake of ascorbic acid into the leukocytes. Aspirin may displace ascorbic acid from albumin binding sites. Ascorbic acid in large doses may cause a uricosuric effect.

Detailed Information: See *EDI,* 16/1.00

Ascorbic Acid-Ethinyl Estradiol

Significance: 3—minimally clinically significant

Recommendations: Patients should be advised that starting and stopping ascorbic acid may lead to contraceptive failure. It has been suggested that the increase in plasma ethinyl estradiol during treatment with ascorbic acid might be of some benefit in permitting wider use of the very low dose ethinyl estradiol preparations.

Summary: There are data to show that coadministration of these agents may increase plasma ethinyl estradiol concentrations, and breakthrough bleeding has been documented with the withdrawal of ascorbic acid.

Related Drugs: The use of oral contraceptives may lower concurrent ascorbic acid levels in both leukocytes and platelets. A similar interaction may occur between ascorbic acid and other estrogenic substances. There are no drugs related to ascorbic acid.

Mechanism: This interaction may result from competition for sulfate, increasing the bioavailability and plasma concentrations of ethinyl estradiol. The breakthrough bleeding may be a withdrawal effect of the ascorbic acid, causing sudden falls in the ethinyl estradiol levels.

Detailed Information: See *EDI,* 16/3.00

Cholecalciferol-Aluminum Hydroxide

Significance: 2—moderately clinically significant

Potential Effects: Concurrent administration of cholecalciferol (vitamin D3) and aluminum hydroxide may result in an increase in plasma aluminum levels, possibly leading to toxicity.

Recommendations: Patients taking concurrent aluminum hydroxide and cholecalciferol should be closely monitored for signs of aluminum toxicity. If possible, plasma aluminum concentrations should be monitored.

Summary: The concurrent administration of aluminum hydroxide and cholecalciferol resulted in elevated plasma aluminum concentrations.

Related Drugs: An interaction may occur between cholecalciferol and other aluminum salts. An interaction may occur between aluminum hydroxide and other vitamin D analogues.

Mechanism: The increase in plasma aluminum may be the result of increased intestinal absorption of aluminum and not tissue redistribution.

Detailed Information: See *EDI,* 16/4.50

Cyanocobalamin-Omeprazole

Significance: 3—minimally clinically significant

Potential Effects: Concurrent cyanocobalamin and omeprazole resulted in a decrease in protein-bound cyanocobalamin absorption.

Recommendations: Cyanocobalamin levels should be monitored in patients maintained on long-term omeprazole therapy (it has been shown that cyanocobalamin malabsorption would not be detectable by the standard Schilling test). Because decreased cyanocobalamin levels can cause hematopoietic and irreversible neurologic and cognitive effects, it may be prudent to institute adjunctive cyanocobalamin supplementation.

Summary: The concurrent administration of cyanocobalamin and omeprazole resulted in a decrease in protein-bound cyanocobalamin absorption.

Related Drugs: There are no drugs related to omeprazole. Cimetidine and ranitidine were shown to cause a decrease in cyanocobalamin absorption. A similar interaction may occur between protein-bound cyanocobalamin and other H_2-receptor antagonists.

Mechanism: Decreased absorption of protein-bound cyanocobalamin may be a result of drug-induced achlorhydria. Cyanocobalamin absorption may be inhibited in patients following vagotomy and patients with achlorhydria. Protein-bound cyanocobalamin absorption may be increased by acidic drinks such as cranberry juice.

Detailed Information: See *EDI,* 16/4.70

Ergocalciferol-Phenytoin

Significance: 2—moderately clinically significant

Recommendations: Patients receiving phenytoin with risk factors for the development of osteomalacia (e.g., inadequate dietary vitamin D intake, limited sunlight exposure, relative inactivity) should be monitored periodically for decreased serum calcium levels and evidence of bone demineralization. Adequate nutrition, with the ingestion of foods rich in vitamin D such as milk, fish, and eggs, and sufficient sunlight exposure are necessary for patients receiving phenytoin and other anticonvulsants. Ergocalciferol therapy, at an individualized dosage, may be required in certain high-risk patients to prevent development of osteomalacia and rickets, and in patients with evidence of impaired bone and mineral metabolism. Vitamin D may be given in a daily dose of 400-800IU. If phenytoin-induced demineralization is identified, 2000IU of vitamin D may be given daily.

Summary: Phenytoin may increase the metabolic inactivation of ergocalciferol and decrease the half-life of the vitamin in the body, potentiating hypocalcemia, osteomalacia or rickets.

Related Drugs: A similar interaction may occur with other hydantoin derivatives.

Mechanism: Phenytoin may cause an increase in hydroxylation and hepatic glucuronidation of cholecalciferol, decreasing serum calcium and increasing serum alkaline phosphatase levels.

Detailed Information: See *EDI,* 16/5.00

Ferrous Sulfate-Allopurinol

Significance: 4—not clinically significant

Recommendations: Clinical studies do not support the existence of this interaction; therefore, no additional precautions are required when these drugs are given together.

Summary: Studies do not support an interaction between allopurinol and ferrous ion preparations.

Related Drugs: Other ferrous salts are not expected to interact with allopurinol. There are no drugs related to allopurinol.

Mechanism: Please refer to summary.

Detailed Information: See *EDI*, 16/7.00

Ferrous Sulfate-Aluminum Hydroxide, Magnesium Carbonate, Magnesium Hydroxide

Significance: 3—minimally clinically significant

Potential Effects: The antacids may decrease the absorption of ferrous sulfate.

Recommendations: The administration of antacids and ferrous salts should be separated by several hours.

Summary: There are data to show that antacids may decrease the absorption of ferrous sulfate, reducing the hematologic response expected with ferrous sulfate iron therapy.

Related Drugs: A similar interaction may occur between ferrous sulfate and other antacids. There are data supporting an interaction; however, conflicting data are available.

Mechanism: The mechanism of this potential interaction is not fully known.

Detailed Information: See *EDI*, 16/9.00

Ferrous Sulfate-Ascorbic Acid

Significance: 3—minimally clinically significant

Recommendations: Since the absorption of ferrous salts alone has been shown to be adequate in most humans, there is little justification for concurrent use of ascorbic acid in the treatment of uncomplicated iron deficiency states.

Summary: It has been reported that ferrous ion absorption is facilitated by concurrent administration of ascorbic acid.

Related Drugs: The absorption of other iron salts may also be enhanced in the presence of ascorbic acid.

Mechanism: Ascorbic acid is thought to increase the absorption of ferrous ion by its ability to lower pH, reducing the ferric ion to a more soluble ferrous ion.

Detailed Information: See *EDI*, 16/11.00

Ferrous Sulfate-Cimetidine

Significance: 3—minimally clinically significant

Recommendations: If altered iron metabolism occurs because of impaired absorption during concurrent use of cimetidine and ferrous sulfate, it may be necessary to give iron parenterally.

Summary: There are data to show that coadministration of these agents may alter iron metabolism secondary to impaired absorption with concurrent use of cimetidine and ferrous sulfate.

Related Drugs: A similar interaction may occur with other iron salts. It is not known whether a similar interaction would occur between ferrous sulfate and other H_2-receptor antagonists.

Mechanism: The prolonged reduction of gastric acid secretion induced by high doses of cimetidine may decrease the gastrointestinal absorption of ferrous sulfate.
Detailed Information: See *EDI,* 16/12.01

Ferrous Sulfate-Penicillamine

Significance: 2—moderately clinically significant
Recommendations: The concomitant administration of penicillamine and ferrous salts should be avoided. If both need to be administered, they should be separated by as much time as possible. One report suggests the ferrous salt should be taken two hours after penicillamine. If patients stabilized on a combination of penicillamine and ferrous salts discontinue the ferrous salt, they should be observed for signs and symptoms of penicillamine toxicity and the penicillamine dose decreased if necessary.
Summary: Concomitant administration of ferrous sulfate with penicillamine has been shown to reduce the absorption of penicillamine.
Related Drugs: Ferrous fumarate has been shown to interact similarly to ferrous sulfate. Other ferrous salts may interact similarly. There are no drugs related to penicillamine.
Mechanism: It is proposed that the ferrous ion chelates to the penicillamine, reducing the absorption of penicillamine.
Detailed Information: See *EDI,* 16/12.10

Folic Acid-Sulfasalazine

Significance: 3—minimally clinically significant
Recommendations: In patients with inflammatory bowel disease who require sulfasalazine and folic acid, the administration of folic acid by the parenteral route may avoid this interaction.
Summary: There are data to show that sulfasalazine administration may reduce folate absorption in patients with inflammatory bowel disease.
Related Drugs: A similar interaction may occur between folic acid and other sulfonamides. There are no drugs related to folic acid.
Mechanism: It is not known how the use of sulfasalazine further decreases the absorption of folic acid.
Detailed Information: See *EDI,* 16/13.00

Grapefruit Juice-Quinidine

Significance: 3—minimally clinically significant
Potential Effects: Concurrent quinidine and grapefruit juice administration may result in changes in the rate-corrected QT interval (QT_c) and delayed quinidine absorption.
Recommendations: Patients maintained on quinidine should be monitored for changes in the QT_c interval and delayed absorption of quinidine if grapefruit juice is given concurrently. Further study is needed to determine how these changes may affect clinically unstable patients or stabilized patients on long-term therapy.
Summary: The concurrent administration of quinidine with grapefruit juice delayed the absorption of quinidine and led to a delayed maximal effect on the QT_c.
Related Drugs: It is not known whether a similar interaction would occur between grapefruit juice and quinine, a stereoisomer of quinidine.

Mechanism: Grapefruit juice reduced the area-under-curve and maximum concentration of 3-hydroxyquinidine. This may suggest inhibition of gut wall metabolism by grapefruit juice during absorption of the drug from the gastrointestinal tract. The absorption of quinidine by grapefruit juice appears to be delayed only with concomitant administration because quinidine, a weak base, is likely to remain in the ionized form with concurrent grapefruit juice administration since grapefruit juice has a pH of approximately 4. Previous *in vitro* studies have suggested that, in grapefruit juice, the flavonoids quercetin, kaempferol, and naringenin, which are potent inhibitors of cytochrome P450 metabolism, may increase the bioavailability of quinidine by inhibition of cytochrome $P450_{3A4}$ isozymes.

Detailed Information: See *EDI*, 16/13.50

Grapefruit Juice-Terfenadine

Significance: 2—moderately clinically significant

Potential Effects: The concurrent administration of terfenadine and grapefruit juice may result in increased terfenadine serum levels and associated cardiac changes.

Recommendations: Caution is advised for the consumption of grapefruit juice with terfenadine administration. An effect of QT prolongation can be demonstrated even with a two-hour separation in the administration of these two agents. Because of the variability of terfenadine pharmacokinetics and pharmacodynamics among individuals, further study is needed. Because of the absence of cardiac effects with increased serum levels of loratadine or fexofenadine, these agents could be considered as possible therapy alternatives to terfenadine.

Summary: Concurrent administration of grapefruit juice resulted in increased terfenadine levels by as much as fivefold and increases in the mean QT interval.

Related Drugs: It is not known whether a similar interaction would occur with grapefruit juice and the other nonsedating H1 receptor antagonists. Two studies have shown no effect on electrocardiogram parameters when either loratadine or fexofenadine were given with grapefruit juice.

Mechanism: Naringenin, quercetin, and kaempferol, flavonoids found in grapefruit, are potent inhibitors of cytochrome P450 metabolism. Studies suggest that grapefruit juice inhibits cytochrome $P450_{3A}$ activity *in vitro* and that neither naringin nor naringenin is primarily responsible for this effect. Further studies are needed.

Detailed Information: See *EDI*, 16/14.00

Niacin-Aspirin

Significance: 3—minimally clinically significant

Potential Effects: Niacin induces prostaglandin-mediated vascular dilatation of the skin which can be ameliorated by aspirin.

Recommendations: One aspirin taken 30 minutes before a scheduled niacin dose may be helpful in patients in whom flushing is bothersome. Alternatively, one morning dose of aspirin for fourteen days may suffice.

Summary: The administration of aspirin before niacin administration effectively reduces the flushing response, a common side effect of niacin.

Related Drugs: A similar interaction may occur with other salicylates if the mechanism is related to prostaglandin synthesis inhibition. There are no drugs related to niacin.

Mechanism: The flushing response seen with niacin administration may be related to prostaglandin liberation; if so, then aspirin would be expected to antagonize this effect of niacin.

Detailed Information: See *EDI,* 16/15.00

Pyridoxine-Levodopa

Significance: 1—highly clinically significant

Recommendations: Patients receiving levodopa therapy should avoid products containing more than the pyridoxine dietary allowance (2mg per day). Patients with conditions causing pyridoxine deficiency (diabetes mellitus, chronic alcoholism, malnutrition, and malignancy) may be exceptions to this recommendation. Also included as possible exceptions are patients requiring pyridoxine supplementation because of other drug therapy (those taking isoniazid, cycloserine, or penicillamine, and those with cystinuria or heavy metal poisoning). Concurrent use of carbidopa, a peripheral decarboxylase inhibitor, prevents the inhibitory effect of pyridoxine on levodopa and is recommended for use in patients receiving pyridoxine supplementation.

Summary: Pyridoxine may reduce or abolish the beneficial effects of levodopa in parkinsonism.

Related Drugs: There are no drugs related to pyridoxine and levodopa.

Mechanism: Pyridoxine may alter levodopa metabolism, increase transamination of levodopa or accelerate peripheral nonenzymatic conversion of levodopa to dopamine.

Detailed Information: See *EDI,* 16/17.00

Vitamin A-Neomycin

Significance: 3—minimally clinically significant

Recommendations: It may be advisable to monitor patients on concurrent vitamin A and oral neomycin therapy for a decrease in vitamin A levels. An increased vitamin A dose may be necessary.

Summary: There are data to show that coadministration of these agents may potentiate a decrease in vitamin A levels, necessitating an increased vitamin A dose.

Related Drugs: Isotretinoin, which is chemically related to vitamin A, may also decrease levels with concurrent neomycin. A similar interaction is expected to occur between vitamin A and other oral aminoglycosides.

Mechanism: Neomycin is thought to interfere with activity of bile acids, reducing uptake of vitamin A, and neomycin may cause morphologic changes in the small intestine, interfering with vitamin A absorption.

Detailed Information: See *EDI,* 16/19.00

Chapter Seventeen

Xanthine
Drug Interactions

Aminophylline-Halothane

Significance: 1—highly clinically significant

Recommendations: Although some believe there is a wide margin of safety associated with the concurrent use of these agents, caution should be observed since arrhythmias have been reported. It appears that the use of aminophylline after halothane anesthesia reduces the incidence of this interaction. Alternatively, the use of a noninteracting anesthetic agent such as enflurane may be considered.

Summary: The concurrent use of halothane and aminophylline may lead to cardiac arrhythmias.

Related Drugs: A similar interaction may occur between halothane and other theophylline derivatives. Enflurane anesthesia has been shown to not induce cardiac arrhythmias. Documentation is lacking regarding an interaction between aminophylline and other halogenated inhalation anesthetics.

Mechanism: The exact mechanism of this interaction is unknown. Halothane may potentiate the arrhythmogenic effects of aminophylline by the same metabolic pathway.

Detailed Information: See *EDI,* 17/1.00

Aminophylline-Imipenem

Significance: 3—minimally clinically significant

Potential Effects: Concurrent administration of these agents may result in central nervous system (CNS) toxicity and seizures.

Recommendations: Patients should be carefully monitored for signs of CNS toxicity and seizures with concurrent administration of these agents.

Summary: The concomitant administration of aminophylline and imipenem may have resulted in seizures.

Related Drugs: Concurrent theophylline and imipenem therapy has also caused generalized seizures. It is not known whether an interaction would occur between aminophylline and the other carbapenem antibiotic agent, meropenem, or between imipenem and the other theophylline derivatives.

Mechanism: CNS toxicity is an adverse effect of theophylline. Theophylline-induced seizures are often not predictable because they are often not preceded by other signs of theophylline toxicity, they often occur in the presence of therapeutic theophylline concentrations (10–20µg/ml), and they may occur during oral theophylline therapy. Imipenem has been associated with seizures in approximately 1% of patients during clinical trials. It is postulated that an interaction occurs between imipenem and theophylline based on the temporal relationship of seizures and on the absence of seizures during therapy with either imipenem or theophylline alone. Further studies are needed.

Detailed Information: See *EDI,* 17/1.05

Aminophylline-Interferon

Significance: 2—moderately clinically significant

Potential Effects: Interferon inhibits the metabolism of theophylline (from aminophylline), leading to increased theophylline levels.

Recommendations: Patients receiving aminophylline should be monitored for increased theophylline levels when interferon is administered concurrently. The dose of aminophylline may need to be decreased.

Summary: There are data to show that coadministration of these agents may lead to increased theophylline levels.

Related Drugs: A similar interaction may occur between interferon and other theophylline derivatives that are hepatically metabolized. Dyphylline may not interact with interferon. There are no drugs related to interferon.

Mechanism: Interferon inhibited the metabolism of theophylline by decreasing the activity of the hepatic cytochrome P450 mixed oxidase enzyme system.

Detailed Information: See *EDI*, 17/2.01

Aminophylline-Isoproterenol

Significance: 3—minimally clinically significant

Potential Effects: Data show that isoproterenol may decrease theophylline levels.

Recommendations: In patients maintained on theophylline and in whom isoproterenol is initiated, serum theophylline concentrations should be monitored. While decreased levels of theophylline have been reported, dosing modifications may not be necessary.

Summary: Data show that isoproterenol may decrease serum theophylline concentrations.

Related Drugs: Interactions between isoproterenol and other theophylline derivatives have not been reported. Dyphylline may not interact if the mechanism involves altered hepatic metabolism of aminophylline. There are data available regarding an interaction between albuterol or terbutaline and aminophylline; however, data are conflicting. Documentation is lacking regarding an interaction between aminophylline and other direct-acting sympathomimetics.

Mechanism: The mechanism of the interaction is unknown.

Detailed Information: See *EDI*, 17/2.10

Aminophylline-Ketamine

Significance: 3—minimally clinically significant

Recommendations: The concurrent use of these agents need not be avoided; however, caution should be used. The administration of succinylcholine was successful in resolving the interaction.

Summary: Aminophylline administration and ketamine given before surgery could precipitate convulsive seizures.

Related Drugs: There are no drugs related to ketamine. Documentation is lacking regarding a similar interaction with the other theophylline derivatives.

Mechanism: The mechanism of this interaction is unknown. However, neither drug significantly lowers seizure threshold.

Detailed Information: See *EDI*, 17/3.00

Aminophylline-Levothyroxine

Significance: 3—minimally clinically significant

Potential Effects: Levothyroxine, by altering thyroid function, may increase theophylline clearance. This interaction may result from the correction of a disease state rather than a direct effect of levothyroxine on theophylline.

Recommendations: Patients' theophylline levels should be monitored while establishing a euthyroid state with thyroid replacement therapy. Similarly, patients receiving aminophylline should be monitored for a change in theophylline levels or signs of toxicity if they develop hypothyroidism. The dose of aminophylline may need to be adjusted.

Summary: Levothyroxine, by correcting thyroid function, may increase theophylline clearance.

Related Drugs: A similar interaction may occur between levothyroxine and other theophylline derivatives that are hepatically metabolized. Dyphylline may not interact with levothyroxine. The other thyroid hormones may interact similarly with aminophylline.

Mechanism: Thyroid function may alter the hepatic metabolism of some drugs via the microsomal mixed function oxidase system.

Detailed Information: See *EDI,* 17/4.10

Aminophylline-Oral Contraceptive Agents

Significance: 3—minimally clinically significant

Potential Effects: Oral contraceptive agents may decrease aminophylline clearance, resulting in increased aminophylline levels.

Recommendations: Theophylline levels should be monitored when these agents are used together.

Summary: There are data to show that administration of oral contraceptive agents may decrease aminophylline clearance, resulting in increased aminophylline levels; however, all data do not support this.

Related Drugs: Theophylline has been shown to interact similarly with oral contraceptive agents. Dyphylline may not interact with oral contraceptive agents.

Mechanism: It has been suggested that oral contraceptive agents inhibit the metabolism of aminophylline.

Detailed Information: See *EDI,* 17/5.00

Aminophylline-Tacrine

Significance: 2—moderately clinically significant

Potential Effects: Concurrent administration of tacrine and aminophylline may result in an increase in theophylline elimination half-life and mean plasma concentrations.

Recommendations: Patients receiving concurrent tacrine and aminophylline should be monitored for increases in theophylline concentration and possible associated toxicity. The theophylline dose may need to be adjusted.

Summary: The concurrent administration of tacrine and aminophylline may result in a significant increase in theophylline elimination half-life and mean plasma concentrations.

Related Drugs: A similar interaction may occur between tacrine and other theophylline derivatives that are hepatically metabolized. Caffeine would be expected to interact with tacrine; dyphylline would not. There are no drugs related to tacrine.

Mechanism: It has been postulated that tacrine inhibits theophylline clearance.

Detailed Information: See *EDI,* 17/6.50

Aminophylline-Thiabendazole

Significance: 2—moderately clinically significant

Recommendations: Theophylline levels should be closely monitored during concomitant use of these agents. The dose of aminophylline may need to be decreased, or another anthelmintic may be considered.

Summary: There are data to show that coadministration of these agents may cause an increase in aminophylline levels, causing nausea, lethargy, and general malaise.

Related Drugs: A similar interaction may occur between thiabendazole and other theophylline derivatives. Dyphylline would not be expected to interact similarly. There are no drugs related to thiabendazole.

Mechanism: Thiabendazole may inhibit the hepatic microsomal enzymes responsible for aminophylline's metabolism.

Detailed Information: See *EDI*, 17/7.00

Caffeine-Adenosine

Significance: 3—minimally clinically significant

Potential Effects: Caffeine may inhibit the pharmacologic effects of adenosine.

Recommendations: The concurrent use of these two agents need not be avoided. In patients who regularly take in large amounts of caffeine, the dosage of adenosine may need to be reduced.

Summary: Caffeine has been reported to inhibit the pharmacologic effects of adenosine.

Related Drugs: Theophylline has been shown to interact with adenosine; however, data are conflicting. It is not known whether an interaction would occur between adenosine and other xanthine derivatives that are hepatically metabolized. There are no drugs related to adenosine.

Mechanism: The cardiovascular effects of caffeine and theophylline may result from the antagonism of exogenous adenosine.

Detailed Information: See *EDI*, 17/8.05

Caffeine-Methoxsalen

Significance: 3—minimally clinically significant

Potential Effects: Methoxsalen may inhibit the metabolism of caffeine.

Recommendations: Concurrent use of these agents may need to be avoided. Also, it may be prudent to monitor patients receiving other xanthine derivatives (e.g., theophylline) with methoxsalen.

Summary: There are data to show that administration of methoxsalen will reduce the clearance of caffeine and increase its half-life. The potential for increased adverse effects of caffeine may exist in patients receiving methoxsalen.

Related Drugs: A similar interaction may occur between methoxsalen and other xanthine derivatives that are hepatically metabolized. Dyphylline would not be expected to interact with methoxsalen. A similar interaction may occur between caffeine and the other psoralen, trioxsalen.

Mechanism: Methoxsalen therapy may cause selective induction of hepatic metabolism, inhibiting metabolism of caffeine.

Detailed Information: See *EDI*, 17/8.10

Caffeine-Oral Contraceptive Agents

Significance: 3—minimally clinically significant

Recommendations: The concurrent use of these agents need not be avoided. However, if central nervous system stimulation appears, the dose of caffeine may need to be decreased.

Summary: The total plasma clearance of a single dose of caffeine was reduced and its elimination half-life prolonged in women taking oral contraceptive agents.

Related Drugs: There are no drugs related to caffeine.

Mechanism: Oral contraceptive agents may inhibit the hepatic metabolism of caffeine.

Detailed Information: See *EDI*, 17/9.00

Caffeine-Phenylpropanolamine

Significance: 3—minimally clinically significant

Potential Effects: Phenylpropanolamine may inhibit the metabolism of caffeine resulting in increased caffeine levels and side effects.

Recommendations: Monitor patients for increased side effects when these agents are administered concurrently. Caffeine-containing beverages may also interact with phenylpropanolamine.

Summary: Phenylpropanolamine may increase caffeine serum levels.

Related Drugs: A similar interaction may occur between phenylpropanolamine and other xanthine derivatives that are hepatically metabolized. It is not known whether an interaction would occur between phenylpropanolamine and dyphylline or between caffeine and other indirect-acting sympathomimetics.

Mechanism: The increased plasma levels of caffeine may be the result of inhibition of caffeine metabolism by phenylpropanolamine.

Detailed Information: See *EDI,* 17/10.50

Dyphylline-Probenecid

Significance: 2—moderately clinically significant

Recommendations: If a patient is currently on dyphylline therapy and probenecid is added, the patient should be monitored for increased dyphylline levels (not detectable by theophylline assays); a decrease in the dosage of dyphylline may be necessary. This interaction may be of greater clinical importance in aminophylline-sensitive patients.

Summary: The concurrent administration of probenecid and dyphylline has been shown to increase the half-life, decrease the elimination rate constant and decrease the total body clearance of dyphylline.

Related Drugs: The same results may be expected when probenecid is used with theophylline and oxtriphylline. The concurrent use of sulfinpyrazone and theophylline has resulted in an increase in total plasma theophylline clearance.

Mechanism: Probenecid, which inhibits the renal transport of some compounds, may also inhibit the renal elimination of dyphylline.

Detailed Information: See *EDI,* 17/11.00

Theophylline-Allopurinol

Significance: 2—moderately clinically significant

Recommendations: Large daily doses of allopurinol may decrease theophylline clearance when both drugs are used for longer than two weeks. Since increases in serum theophylline concentrations of 25% have been reported, some patients may require monitoring for signs of possible theophylline toxicity and may need lower doses during concurrent allopurinol therapy.

Summary: Allopurinol may decrease theophylline clearance and increase the risk of toxicity.

Related Drugs: A similar interaction may occur between allopurinol and other theophylline derivatives. Dyphylline is not expected to interact with allopurinol. There are no drugs related to allopurinol.

Mechanism: Allopurinol may inhibit the hepatic drug metabolizing enzymes.

Detailed Information: See *EDI,* 17/13.00

Theophylline-Aluminum Hydroxide, Magnesium Hydroxide

Significance: 3—minimally clinically significant

Potential Effects: Some antacid preparations may increase theophylline absorption.

Recommendations: These agents may be given together; however, theophylline levels should be monitored when initiating therapy.

Summary: There are data to show that coadministration of some antacid preparations may increase theophylline absorption; however, all data do not support this interaction.

Related Drugs: There are data to show that other antacid products may interact with theophylline; however, data are conflicting. Because of conflicting results, it is not known if other theophylline derivatives would interact with an aluminum and magnesium hydroxide combination antacid.

Mechanism: Factors such as gastrointestinal fluid pH may influence the degradation and/or absorption of some slow release theophylline formulations.

Detailed Information: See *EDI,* 17/14.01

Theophylline-Aminoglutethimide

Significance: 3—minimally clinically significant

Recommendations: Although concurrent use of these agents need not be avoided, theophylline levels should be monitored and the theophylline dosage increased if necessary.

Summary: There are data to show that aminoglutethimide administration increases theophylline clearance, possibly decreasing the pharmacologic effects of theophylline.

Related Drugs: A similar interaction may occur between aminoglutethimide and other theophylline derivatives. Dyphylline is not expected to interact with aminoglutethimide. A similar interaction may occur between glutethimide and theophylline.

Mechanism: Aminoglutethimide may increase the metabolism of theophylline.

Detailed Information: See *EDI,* 17/14.10

Theophylline-Caffeine

Significance: 2—moderately clinically significant

Potential Effects: The addition of caffeine to a theophylline regimen may result in increased serum theophylline levels.

Recommendations: Patients receiving theophylline should be carefully monitored for changes in theophylline serum levels when changes in caffeine consumption occur.

Summary: Concurrent caffeine and theophylline may result in an increase in theophylline serum levels.

Related Drugs: It is not known whether an interaction would occur between caffeine and oxtriphylline. Dyphylline would not be expected to interact with caffeine, if the mechanism of this interaction results from an interference of theophylline hepatic metabolism.

Mechanism: Saturation of theophylline metabolism and/or competition between caffeine and theophylline may result in the delay of theophylline elimination.

Detailed Information: See *EDI,* 17/14.50

Theophylline-Carbamazepine

Significance: 2—moderately clinically significant

Potential Effects: The concomitant use of these agents may result in increased or decreased theophylline levels as well as decreased carbamazepine levels. The patient's clinical condition may also worsen.

Recommendations: Patients should be monitored for changes in the levels of both theophylline and carbamazepine, and the dosage of each agent may need to be adjusted until therapeutic levels are maintained and efficacy is achieved.

Summary: Concurrent administration of theophylline and carbamazepine resulted in decreased levels of theophylline in one patient and increased carbamazepine levels in another.

Related Drugs: Concurrent administration of aminophylline has resulted in a decrease in carbamazepine levels and bioavailability. A similar interaction may be expected to occur between carbamazepine and oxtriphylline, which, like theophylline, is hepatically metabolized. Dyphylline is not converted to theophylline in vivo, is not metabolized by the liver, and is rapidly removed from the blood by glomerular filtration, active secretion, or both, and approximately 82% is excreted unchanged in the urine. If the mechanism of this interaction results from increased hepatic metabolism of theophylline, dyphylline would not be expected to interact with carbamazepine. No interaction has been seen between carbamazepine and caffeine. There are no drugs related to carbamazepine.

Mechanism: The mechanism of this interaction is not known. However, it has been suggested that the hepatic metabolism of theophylline is increased by carbamazepine, and theophylline increases the hepatic metabolism of carbamazepine. It is not known why theophylline levels were elevated in one study.

Detailed Information: See *EDI,* 17/15.00

Theophylline-Cefaclor

Significance: 3—minimally clinically significant

Potential Effects: Cefaclor may increase theophylline levels.

Recommendations: Theophylline dosage may need to be decreased if toxicity or increased levels occur. Cefaclor may need to be discontinued.

Summary: The addition of cefaclor to a stabilized theophylline regimen has been shown to result in an increase in theophylline serum levels.

Related Drugs: It is not known whether an interaction would occur between theophylline and other cephalosporins or between cefaclor and other theophylline derivatives.

Mechanism: The mechanism of this interaction is not known. The presence of an acute viral illness has been associated with decreased hepatic cytochrome P450 activity and decreased theophylline clearance, but the patient was afebrile in this case report.

Detailed Information: See *EDI,* 17/16.10

Theophylline-Charcoal

Significance: 1—highly clinically significant

Potential Effects: Charcoal adsorbs theophylline, reducing absorption and increasing clearance.

Recommendations: Charcoal should be administered as soon as possible to decrease theophylline absorption; however, continued administration will increase theophylline clearance. Sorbitol will increase the effectiveness of charcoal. If charcoal is not being used to treat a theophylline overdose, a higher dose of theophylline or separating the administration times is necessary.

Summary: Activated charcoal administration has been shown to decrease the absorption of oral theophylline.

Related Drugs: Other oral theophylline derivatives may also be adsorbed by activated charcoal.

Mechanism: Activated charcoal adsorbs oral theophylline, limiting its absorption from the gastrointestinal tract, and decreases enterohepatic recirculation, increasing theophylline clearance.

Detailed Information: See *EDI,* 17/17.00

Theophylline-Cimetidine

Significance: 1—highly clinically significant

Potential Effects: Cimetidine can inhibit the metabolism of theophylline, resulting in increased theophylline levels.

Recommendations: If these agents are used together, theophylline serum levels should be closely monitored. Antacids, famotidine, or possibly ranitidine may be used as an alternative to cimetidine.

Summary: It is well documented that cimetidine impairs the elimination of theophylline, resulting in increased theophylline levels.

Related Drugs: Aminophylline, caffeine, pentoxifylline and oxtriphylline may also be involved in a similar interaction. Dyphylline is not expected to interact with cimetidine. Ranitidine and famotidine do not appear to significantly influence theophylline disposition.

Mechanism: Cimetidine inhibits the hepatic microsomal mono-oxygenase system, and this inhibition may cause cimetidine to bind to an enzyme system or to theophylline, forming a complex that interrupts metabolism.

Detailed Information: See *EDI,* 17/19.00

Theophylline-Ciprofloxacin

Significance: 2—moderately clinically significant

Potential Effects: Ciprofloxacin or its metabolite may inhibit the hepatic metabolism of theophylline, resulting in increased theophylline levels.

Recommendations: Theophylline levels should be monitored when these agents are used concomitantly. The theophylline dose may need to be decreased or the ciprofloxacin discontinued. Norfloxacin may be substituted for ciprofloxacin; however, indications for the different quinolones may vary. Theophylline levels should still be monitored.

Summary: Several cases have been reported in which ciprofloxacin or its metabolite inhibited the hepatic metabolism of theophylline, resulting in increased theophylline levels and theophylline toxicity.

Related Drugs: Concurrent administration of aminophylline and ciprofloxacin has also been shown to affect theophylline levels, leading to theophylline toxicity. A similar interaction may be expected to occur between ciprofloxacin and the other theophylline derivative that is hepatically metabolized, oxtriphylline. Dyphylline, a theophylline derivative that is not converted to theophylline in vivo and is not metabolized by the liver, would not be expected to interact with ciprofloxacin. Norfloxacin and lomefloxacin have shown conflicting results when administered with theophylline. Enoxacin has increased theophylline levels in several studies, but conflicting data are available. Temafloxacin, nalidixic acid, fleroxacin, and ofloxacin have not been shown to interact with theophylline. Clinafloxacin interacted in a similar fashion as ciprofloxacin. The quinolone antibiotics have also been shown to affect caffeine pharmacokinetics similarly, although conflicting data are available. An interaction would not be expected to occur between theophylline and the other quinolone that is not hepatically metabolized, cinoxacin.

Mechanism: Ciprofloxacin may inhibit the hepatic metabolism of theophylline via the cytochrome P450 enzyme system, the site at which both agents are metabolized. The specific sites within the cytochrome P450 enzyme may be the CYP_{1A2} and CYP_{3A4} sites, and the interindividual variation in the expression of the CYP_{1A2} site may be responsible for the interindividual response seen during concurrent administration of theophylline and ciprofloxacin. There is evidence that this interaction is not caused by the parent drug, ciprofloxacin, but by its 4-oxo metabolite.

Detailed Information: See *EDI,* 17/20.21

Theophylline-Disulfiram

Significance: 2—moderately clinically significant

Potential Effects: Disulfiram may inhibit the metabolism of theophylline, increasing its half-life and serum levels. The metabolism of caffeine may also be inhibited by disulfiram.

Recommendations: Patients receiving disulfiram and theophylline concurrently should be monitored for increased theophylline levels. The dose of theophylline may need to be decreased by as much as 50% depending on the dose of disulfiram. Caffeine should be avoided in patients receiving disulfiram.

Summary: There are data to show that disulfiram administration may inhibit the metabolism of theophylline, increasing its half-life and serum levels.

Related Drugs: A similar interaction may occur between disulfiram and other theophylline derivatives that are hepatically metabolized. Dyphylline is not expected to interact with disulfiram. There are no drugs related to disulfiram.

Mechanism: Disulfiram may inhibit the hepatic metabolism of theophylline by its inhibitory effect on the cytochrome P450 enzyme system.

Detailed Information: See *EDI,* 17/20.30

Theophylline-Erythromycin

Significance: 1—highly clinically significant

Potential Effects: Erythromycin decreases the elimination of theophylline, leading to increased theophylline levels. Theophylline may also decrease erythromycin levels.

Recommendations: Monitor theophylline levels when erythromycin is added to, or withdrawn from, therapy. Also, monitor erythromycin efficacy when these agents are used together.

Summary: Erythromycin and theophylline administration increased serum theophylline concentrations twofold; however, there are conflicting data

Related Drugs: Troleandomycin, erythromycin and clarithromycin have been documented to interact with theophylline. Aminophylline and oxtriphylline have been shown to interact with erythromycin. Caffeine would be expected to interact with erythromycin. Dyphylline is not expected to interact with erythromycin.

Mechanism: The mechanism is not clearly established.

Detailed Information: See *EDI,* 17/21.00

Theophylline-Fluvoxamine

Significance: 3—minimally clinically significant

Potential Effects: The addition of fluvoxamine to a theophylline regimen may result in increased theophylline serum levels and toxicity.

Recommendations: The addition or removal of fluvoxamine from the therapy of a patient maintained on theophylline may result in altered theophylline serum levels. The fluvoxamine may have to be discontinued or the theophylline dose adjusted.

Summary: Fluvoxamine administration may result in increased theophylline levels and toxicity.

Related Drugs: It is not known whether an interaction would occur between fluvoxamine and other theophylline derivatives or between theophylline and other serotonin reuptake inhibitors.

Mechanism: Competitive inhibition of hepatic microsomal enzymes by fluvoxamine may be a factor in the elevated theophylline concentrations.

Detailed Information: See *EDI,* 17/24.50

Theophylline-Furosemide

Significance: 2—moderately clinically significant

Potential Effects: Furosemide may alter theophylline levels.

Recommendations: Monitor theophylline levels when administering these agents together. Separating the dosing of these agents by as much time as possible may avoid this interaction.

Summary: There are data to show that furosemide administration may cause theophylline levels to decrease.

Related Drugs: A similar interaction may occur between furosemide and other theophylline derivatives. Dyphylline is not expected to interact with furosemide. A similar interaction is expected to occur between theophylline and other loop diuretics.

Mechanism: Furosemide may decrease hepatic congestion, increasing theophylline clearance, or displace theophylline from serum proteins.

Detailed Information: See *EDI,* 17/25.00

Theophylline-Hydrocortisone

Significance: 3—minimally clinically significant

Potential Effects: The concurrent administration of these agents may result in increased theophylline levels.

Recommendations: Theophylline levels should be monitored in patients receiving concurrent hydrocortisone. A lower dose of theophylline may be necessary.

Summary: There are data to show that hydrocortisone administration may result in increased theophylline levels; however, there are conflicting data.

Related Drugs: Methylprednisolone and dexamethasone were shown to have no significant effect on theophylline levels. Because of conflicting results, it is difficult to determine if theophylline would interact with other corticosteroids. A similar interaction is expected to occur between hydrocortisone and other theophylline derivatives. Dyphylline would not be expected to interact with hydrocortisone, whereas aminophylline and oxtriphylline would interact similarly.

Mechanism: The mechanism of this interaction is unknown.

Detailed Information: See *EDI*, 17/27.00

Theophylline-Influenza Virus Vaccine

Significance: 3—minimally clinically significant

Potential Effects: Influenza virus vaccine may decrease theophylline metabolism, resulting in increased levels.

Recommendations: Patients maintained on theophylline should be monitored closely for increased theophylline levels if influenza virus vaccine is administered.

Summary: There are data to show that administration of influenza virus vaccine may decrease theophylline metabolism, resulting in increased levels and potentiating increased adverse effects.

Related Drugs: Oxtriphylline has been shown to interact similarly, whereas aminophylline has not. Dyphylline is not expected to interact with influenza virus vaccine.

Mechanism: Influenza vaccine may decrease theophylline biotransformation because of a depression of the cytochrome P450 system.

Detailed Information: See *EDI*, 17/29.00

Theophylline-Isoniazid

Significance: 3—minimally clinically significant

Potential Effects: Concomitant administration of these agents may result in an increase or decrease in theophylline clearance.

Recommendations: Concurrent use of these agents need not be avoided. However, until further clinical studies are done, theophylline levels should be routinely monitored since an adjustment in the dosage of theophylline may be necessary.

Summary: There are data to show that isoniazid administration may result in an increase or decrease in theophylline clearance.

Related Drugs: Isoniazid was shown to decrease the plasma clearance of theophylline and increase its serum concentrations. Because of conflicting results, it is difficult to determine if an interaction would occur between isoniazid and other theophylline derivatives. Dyphylline is not expected to interact with isoniazid. There are no drugs related to isoniazid.

Mechanism: Isoniazid may increase the hepatic metabolism of theophylline by enzyme induction or an unknown mechanism.

Detailed Information: See *EDI*, 17/30.10

Theophylline-Ketoconazole

Significance: 3—minimally clinically significant

Potential Effects: Ketoconazole may decrease theophylline levels.

Recommendations: Theophylline levels should be monitored when ketoconazole is added to or withdrawn from therapy. The dose of theophylline may need to be increased.

Summary: Ketoconazole significantly reduced serum theophylline concentrations.

Related Drugs: Fluconazole has been reported to slightly decrease theophylline clearance. In contrast with oral theophylline, studies failed to show any effect of ketoconazole on theophylline levels following administration of intravenous aminophylline. Because of conflicting results, it is difficult to determine if an interaction would occur between ketoconazole and the other theophylline derivatives or between theophylline and the other imidazole antifungal agents.

Mechanism: The mechanism of this interaction is not known. It is possible that ketoconazole enhanced the metabolism of theophylline since it has been suggested that long-term ketoconazole administration may induce hepatic drug metabolism; however, this would be opposite its expected effect since ketoconazole has been shown to inhibit the hepatic metabolism of other agents.

Detailed Information: See *EDI*, 17/30.30

Theophylline-Methimazole

Significance: 3—minimally clinically significant

Potential Effects: Methimazole, by affecting thyroid function, may decrease theophylline clearance. This interaction may be the result of a correction of a disease state rather than a direct effect of methimazole on theophylline.

Recommendations: Patients' theophylline levels should be monitored while establishing a euthyroid state with antithyroid replacement therapy. Similarly, patients receiving theophylline should be monitored for a change in theophylline levels if they develop hyperthyroidism. The dose of theophylline may need to be adjusted.

Summary: There are data to show that methimazole administration may decrease theophylline clearance. This interaction may be the result of a disease state correction rather than a direct effect on theophylline clearance.

Related Drugs: A similar interaction may occur between methimazole and other theophylline derivatives that are hepatically metabolized. Dyphylline is not expected to interact with methimazole. A similar interaction is expected to occur between theophylline and propylthiouracil.

Mechanism: Hyperthyroidism may increase the activity of the hepatic microsomal enzymes responsible for the metabolism of theophylline.

Detailed Information: See *EDI*, 17/30.50

Theophylline-Mexiletine

Significance: 2—moderately clinically significant

Potential Effects: Concurrent use may result in increased theophylline serum levels.

Recommendations: These agents may be given concurrently, but theophylline levels should be monitored and the theophylline dose reduced if necessary.

Summary: There are data to show that mexiletine administration may cause an increase in theophylline levels, increasing theophylline side effects.

Related Drugs: Mexiletine reduced the clearance of caffeine. A similar interaction may occur between mexiletine and other hepatically metabolized xanthines, if the mechanism involves inhibition of hepatic metabolism. It is not known if dyphylline would interact with mexiletine.

Mechanism: Impaired hepatic metabolism of theophylline by mexiletine may be an explanation.

Detailed Information: See *EDI*, 17/30.70

Theophylline-Moricizine

Significance: 2—moderately clinically significant

Potential Effects: Theophylline serum levels may be decreased with concurrent moricizine.

Recommendations: Theophylline levels should be carefully monitored with concomitant moricizine administration. The dose of theophylline may need to be adjusted.

Summary: Theophylline clearance increased and half-life decreased with concurrent moricizine.

Related Drugs: It is not known whether an interaction would occur between moricizine and other theophylline derivatives or between theophylline and other class I antiarrhythmic agents.

Mechanism: Changes in theophylline clearance are most likely the result of enzyme induction by moricizine.

Detailed Information: See *EDI*, 17/30.85

Theophylline-Omeprazole

Significance: 4—not clinically significant

Potential Effects: Omeprazole does not appear to interact with theophylline to a clinically significant extent.

Recommendations: No special precautions appear necessary with the concurrent use of these agents.

Summary: Omeprazole does not appear to interact with theophylline to a clinically significant extent. Although one study showed increased theophylline absorption when the two drugs were taken concurrently, theophylline serum level changes were not statistically significant.

Related Drugs: Studies on omeprazole's effect on caffeine metabolism are conflicting. The clinical significance of an increase in caffeine metabolism has not been determined. Lansoprazole and pantoprazole have not shown clinically significant effects on the pharmacokinetics of theophylline. Based on the mechanism of omeprazole metabolism, an interaction would not be expected to occur between omeprazole and the other theophylline derivatives.

Mechanism: Although omeprazole is metabolized in the liver by S-mephenytoin hydroxylase in the cytochrome P450 enzyme system, present studies indicate that this agent does not seem to compete with theophylline for metabolism. Omeprazole has been postulated to be an inducer of the cytochrome $P450_{1A2}$ isozyme system both in studies discussed above and in other *in vivo* and *in vitro* studies.

Detailed Information: See *EDI*, 17/30.90

Theophylline-Phenobarbital

Significance: 2—moderately clinically significant

Potential Effects: Phenobarbital may induce the metabolism of theophylline, resulting in decreased theophylline levels.

Recommendations: Theophylline plasma levels should be closely monitored when a barbiturate is added to, or withdrawn from, theophylline therapy. The dose of theophylline may need to be adjusted.

Summary: The concurrent use of phenobarbital and theophylline may reduce theophylline serum levels.

Related Drugs: Secobarbital was shown to interact with theophylline. A similar interaction may occur between theophylline and other barbiturates. A similar interaction is expected to occur between phenobarbital and other theophylline derivatives. Dyphylline is not expected to interact with phenobarbital.

Mechanism: Phenobarbital induces the hepatic microsomal enzymes responsible for theophylline metabolism.

Detailed Information: See *EDI*, 17/31.00

Theophylline-Phenytoin

Significance: 2—moderately clinically significant

Recommendations: It is important to monitor the levels of both phenytoin and theophylline during concurrent therapy. If necessary, the dose of theophylline or phenytoin may need to be increased.

Summary: There are data to show that coadministration may lead to a decrease in theophylline or in phenytoin levels.

Related Drugs: A similar interaction is expected to occur between theophylline and other hydantoin anticonvulsants. Dyphylline is not expected to interact with phenytoin.

Mechanism: Phenytoin may increase the metabolism of theophylline by inducing hepatic microsomal enzymes. Theophylline induces the metabolism of phenytoin or interferes with its absorption.

Detailed Information: See *EDI*, 17/33.00

Theophylline-Propafenone

Significance: 2—moderately clinically significant

Potential Effects: The addition of propafenone to a theophylline regimen may result in increased theophylline serum concentration.

Recommendations: Theophylline levels should be carefully monitored if propafenone is added to, or withdrawn from, concurrent therapy. The dose of theophylline may need to be adjusted.

Summary: The addition of propafenone to the therapy of a patient maintained on theophylline resulted in increased theophylline serum concentrations.

Related Drugs: It is not known if a similar interaction would occur between theophylline and other class IC antiarrhythmic agents. A similar interaction is expected to occur between propafenone and other theophylline derivatives. Dyphylline is not expected to interact with propafenone.

Mechanism: An inhibition of theophylline hepatic metabolism may occur.

Detailed Information: See *EDI*, 17/34.50

Theophylline-Propranolol

Significance: 2—moderately clinically significant

Potential Effects: Propranolol may cause an increase in theophylline serum levels.

Recommendations: Since propranolol may increase bronchial resistance, the patient's clinical status as well as theophylline serum levels should be monitored. The dose of theophylline may need to be adjusted.

Summary: There are data to show that propranolol administration may cause an increase in theophylline serum levels and reduce clearance.

Related Drugs: A similar interaction may occur between propranolol and other theophylline derivatives. Dyphylline is not expected to interact with propranolol. The noncardioselective beta blocking agents that are not extensively hepatically metabolized are expected to interact with theophylline to some degree.

Mechanism: Propranolol and theophylline may have some antagonistic effects that cause this interaction. Propranolol may interfere with the metabolism of theophylline by blocking cyclic AMP in the cytochrome system.

Detailed Information: See *EDI,* 17/35.00

Theophylline-Pyrantel Pamoate

Significance: 2—moderately clinically significant

Potential Effects: Pyrantel pamoate may increase theophylline levels, resulting in toxicity.

Recommendations: The patient should be carefully monitored for changes in theophylline serum levels and for signs of theophylline toxicity when theophylline is administered concomitantly with pyrantel pamoate. The dose of theophylline may need to be adjusted.

Summary: There are data to show that pyrantel pamoate administration may increase theophylline levels, resulting in toxicity and increased adverse effects.

Related Drugs: A similar interaction may occur between pyrantel pamoate and other theophylline derivatives that are hepatically metabolized. Dyphylline is not expected to interact with pyrantel pamoate. There are no drugs related to pyrantel pamoate.

Mechanism: Pyrantel pamoate may inhibit theophylline clearance by inhibition of hepatic enzymes, or it may increase the rate of drug release, increasing the theophylline level.

Detailed Information: See *EDI,* 17/36.05

Theophylline-Rifampin

Significance: 2—moderately clinically significant

Recommendations: Patients maintained on theophylline should have their serum concentrations monitored if rifampin is to be added to, or deleted from, their therapeutic regimen. While most patients may require only monitoring, appropriate dosage adjustments of up to 25% have been suggested.

Summary: Concurrent administration of rifampin and theophylline may result in a more rapid clearance of theophylline.

Related Drugs: Rifampin has been shown to reduce the aminophylline area-under-curve, increase the metabolic clearance and volume of distribution of aminophylline. Dyphylline is not expected to interact with rifampin. There are no drugs related to rifampin.

Mechanism: It is speculated that the increased activity of the hepatic cytochrome P450 enzymes by rifampin is involved in this interaction.
Detailed Information: See *EDI*, 17/36.10

Theophylline-Sucralfate

Significance: 2—moderately clinically significant
Potential Effects: Sucralfate may decrease the absorption of theophylline. This interaction may be clinically significant with the sustained-release dosage form of theophylline.
Recommendations: Although further studies are necessary, theophylline levels should be monitored during concurrent sucralfate administration. The dose of theophylline may need to be adjusted.
Summary: There are data to show that sucralfate administration may decrease the absorption of theophylline; however, there are conflicting data.
Related Drugs: It is not known if sucralfate would affect the absorption of other theophylline derivatives.
Mechanism: Sustained-release theophylline products release drug over a prolonged period, allowing a greater opportunity for an interaction to occur. This may explain the differences in the interaction between sustained-release and immediate-release theophylline products and sucralfate.
Detailed Information: See *EDI*, 17/36.70

Theophylline-Tetracycline

Significance: 3—minimally clinically significant
Potential Effects: Tetracycline may increase theophylline levels. An increased incidence of gastrointestinal complaints may occur from concomitant administration.
Recommendations: These agents may be used together, but theophylline levels should routinely be monitored.
Summary: There are data to show that tetracycline administration may increase theophylline levels and potentiate increased theophylline side effects.
Related Drugs: Doxycycline has not been shown to significantly interact with theophylline. Because of conflicting results, it is difficult to determine if an interaction would occur between theophylline and other tetracyclines and between tetracycline and other theophylline derivatives.
Mechanism: The mechanism of this interaction is unknown. Gastrointestinal complaints may occur with both agents, and this interaction may be a summation response.
Detailed Information: See *EDI*, 17/37.00

Theophylline-Ticlopidine

Significance: 2—moderately clinically significant
Potential Effects: Concurrent administration of theophylline and ticlopidine may result in increased theophylline levels.
Recommendations: Patients should be monitored for increased theophylline levels and signs of theophylline toxicity if ticlopidine is added to therapy.
Summary: Use of ticlopidine resulted in an increase in plasma concentration and half-life of theophylline and a decrease in total plasma clearance and the theophylline elimination rate constant.

Related Drugs: Although documentation is lacking, based on the possible mechanism of action and pharmacologic and structural similarity derivatives of theophylline may be expected to interact with ticlopidine in a similar fashion. If the mechanism involves competition for the N-demethylation metabolic process, dyphylline may not be expected to interact similarly with ticlopidine.

Mechanism: One possible mechanism for this interaction is the interference of theophylline hepatic metabolism by ticlopidine.

Detailed Information: See *EDI,* 17/38.00

Theophylline-Tobacco

Significance: 1—highly clinically significant

Potential Effects: Tobacco use induces the metabolism of theophylline, leading to decreased levels.

Recommendations: Theophylline levels should be monitored if tobacco use is started or stopped.

Summary: There are data to show that tobacco use induces the metabolism of theophylline, leading to decreased levels and necessitating an increase in dosage.

Related Drugs: Aminophylline undergoes the same interaction. Dyphylline is not expected to interact with tobacco.

Mechanism: Smoking is thought to enhance theophylline metabolism by inducing hepatic microsomal enzymes.

Detailed Information: See *EDI,* 17/39.00

Theophylline-Verapamil

Significance: 2—moderately clinically significant

Potential Effects: Verapamil may cause an increase in theophylline serum levels.

Recommendations: Monitor theophylline levels closely when these agents are used together. The dose of theophylline may need to be decreased.

Summary: Verapamil has been shown to cause a doubling of theophylline serum concentrations and clinical manifestations of theophylline toxicity.

Related Drugs: Nifedipine and diltiazem have been documented to interact similarly to verapamil; however, documentation is conflicting. A similar interaction is expected to occur between verapamil and other theophylline derivatives. Dyphylline is not expected to interact similarly with verapamil.

Mechanism: Theophylline clearance has been shown to be affected by substances that may compete with its metabolism, and theophylline and verapamil have a metabolic process in common.

Detailed Information: See *EDI,* 17/41.00

Theophylline-Vidarabine

Significance: 3—minimally clinically significant

Recommendations: Although this interaction has not been clearly established, patients receiving theophylline and vidarabine should be monitored for increasing theophylline serum concentrations. The dose of theophylline may need to be decreased.

Summary: There are data to show that vidarabine administration may potentiate an increase in serum theophylline levels.

Related Drugs: Oxtriphylline would be expected to interact similarly. Dyphylline would not be expected to interact with vidarabine. There are no drugs related to vidarabine.

Mechanism: The major metabolite of vidarabine may compete with theophylline, decreasing theophylline's metabolism and leading to increased serum concentrations.

Detailed Information: See *EDI*, 17/43.00

Chapter Eighteen

Miscellaneous
Drug Interactions

Adenosine-Dipyridamole

Significance: 3—minimally clinically significant

Potential Effects: Dipyridamole may reduce the required dose of adenosine.

Recommendations: Patients maintained on intravenous adenosine should be monitored for increased adenosine effects if dipyridamole is added to cotherapy. The dose of intravenous adenosine may need to be reduced.

Summary: Dipyridamole has been shown to reduce the dose of adenosine necessary to achieve a therapeutic response. There are data to show that concurrent administration of these agents causes an increased reduction in heart rate.

Related Drugs: There are no drugs related to adenosine or dipyridamole.

Mechanism: Dipyridamole in high plasma concentrations may inhibit the uptake of adenosine by erythrocytes or platelets, or by other tissues, inhibiting metabolism of adenosine.

Detailed Information: See *EDI*, 18/0.03

Alteplase-Nitroglycerin

Significance: 2—moderately clinically significant

Potential Effects: Thrombolytic effects of alteplase may be reduced by concurrent nitroglycerin administration.

Recommendations: Caution should be exercised when intravenous nitroglycerin and alteplase are administered concomitantly since nitroglycerin has been shown to decrease the thrombolytic activity of alteplase.

Summary: Decreased thrombolytic effect of alteplase (tissue plasminogen activator) may result with concomitant nitroglycerin administration, studies have shown.

Related Drugs: There is no documentation of an interaction between alteplase and other nitrate derivatives; however, because of the similarity in pharmacologic activity an interaction may be expected to occur.

Mechanism: Nitroglycerin given concomitantly with alteplase may decrease the thrombolytic effect of alteplase by decreasing the plasma alteplase antigen concentrations. It has been postulated that nitroglycerin may enhance hepatic blood flow, thereby facilitating the degradation of alteplase.

Detailed Information: See *EDI*, 18/0.04

Aluminum Hydroxide-Citric Acid

Significance: 3—minimally clinically significant

Potential Effects: Citric acid may increase the absorption of aluminum.

Recommendations: Simultaneous administration of citric acid and aluminum hydroxide should be avoided since significant systemic absorption of aluminum may occur. This may be of additional concern in patients on long-term dialysis or with impaired renal function.

Summary: The systemic absorption of aluminum is enhanced by concomitant citric acid administration.

Related Drugs: An interaction may occur between citric acid or oral citrates and other aluminum salts.

Mechanism: Citric acid and aluminum hydroxide will increase serum levels of a nonionized aluminum-citrate complex which may pass the gastrointestinal barrier.

Detailed Information: See *EDI*, 18/0.05

Amphetamine-Ammonium Chloride

Significance: 3—minimally clinically significant

Recommendations: Since the urinary excretion of amphetamine can be increased by the concurrent administration of ammonium chloride, this interaction may be useful in cases of amphetamine toxicity or overdose. If this effect is not desired, the dose of amphetamine may need to be increased or the ammonium chloride discontinued.

Summary: There are data to show that concurrent ammonium chloride and amphetamine administration may increase the elimination of unchanged amphetamine in the urine, decreasing the pharmacologic effects of amphetamine.

Related Drugs: The other indirect-acting sympathomimetics may interact with ammonium chloride based on a similar metabolic fate. Other agents that acidify the urine may also interact with amphetamine.

Mechanism: The tubular reabsorption of amphetamine is decreased as the pH of the urine becomes more acidic following the administration of ammonium chloride.

Detailed Information: See *EDI*, 18/0.10

Amphetamine-Sodium Bicarbonate

Significance: 3—minimally clinically significant

Recommendations: If increased pharmacologic or toxic effects of amphetamine are observed when sodium bicarbonate is administered concurrently, the dose of amphetamine may need to be decreased or the sodium bicarbonate discontinued.

Summary: Sodium bicarbonate was shown to increase the half-life and metabolism, and decrease the excretion, of amphetamine, potentially causing amphetamine toxicity.

Related Drugs: The other indirect-acting sympathomimetics may interact with sodium bicarbonate. Other agents that alkalinize the urine may interact with amphetamine.

Mechanism: As sodium bicarbonate makes the urine more basic, the tubular reabsorption of amphetamine is increased.

Detailed Information: See *EDI*, 18/0.30

Cimetidine-Aluminum Hydroxide, Magnesium Hydroxide

Significance: 3—minimally clinically significant

Potential Effects: Concomitant antacid administration may decrease the absorption of cimetidine.

Recommendations: If the concomitant use of these agents is necessary, separate the administration of each by as much time as possible, or administer cimetidine with meals followed by the antacid one hour later.

Summary: There are data to show that aluminum hydroxide administration may decrease the absorption of cimetidine; however, data are conflicting.

Related Drugs: Because of conflicting results, it is difficult to determine if an interaction would occur between cimetidine and other antacids. There are data to show that antacids have no effect on ranitidine absorption; however, the data do vary. There are conflicting data regarding the concurrent use of famotidine.

Mechanism: Some component of the antacids may interfere with cimetidine absorption, or the total neutralizing capacity of the antacid may be responsible for the interaction.

Detailed Information: See *EDI*, 18/1.00

Cimetidine-Metoclopramide

Significance: 3—minimally clinically significant

Recommendations: If metoclopramide is administered concurrently with cimetidine, the dose of cimetidine may need to be increased depending on the therapeutic outcome of the combination.

Summary: Metoclopramide and cimetidine administration has resulted in a decreased bioavailability of cimetidine.

Related Drugs: There are no drugs related to metoclopramide. There is a lack of documentation concerning a similar interaction between other H_2-receptor antagonists and metoclopramide.

Mechanism: Metoclopramide increases gastric emptying time, and this may decrease cimetidine absorption.

Detailed Information: See *EDI*, 18/3.00

Cimetidine-Propantheline

Significance: 3—minimally clinically significant

Recommendations: The concurrent use of these agents need not be avoided. However, if both drugs must be used concomitantly, it may be advisable to separate their administration by as much time as possible to avoid a possible interaction.

Summary: There are data to show that propantheline administration may alter cimetidine concentrations; however, these alterations are not very significant.

Related Drugs: A similar interaction may occur between cimetidine and other anticholinergics. Ranitidine was shown to act in contrast with cimetidine when administered with propantheline.

Mechanism: The reduced bioavailability of cimetidine when administered with propantheline may be a consequence of delayed gastric emptying or decreased intestinal motility.

Detailed Information: See *EDI*, 18/4.10

Clofibrate-Oral Contraceptive Agents

Significance: 3—minimally clinically significant

Recommendations: Until further studies are done, the concurrent administration of these agents need not be avoided. However, if the antihyperlipidemic effect of clofibrate decreases in the patient receiving concomitant oral contraceptive agents, the dose of clofibrate may need to be increased.

Summary: Clofibric acid (a form of clofibrate) clearance was found to be greater in those who were receiving oral contraceptive agents.

Related Drugs: There are no drugs related to clofibrate.

Mechanism: The oral contraceptive agents may induce the metabolism of clofibric acid.

Detailed Information: See *EDI*, 18/4.30

Clomiphene-Cimetidine

Significance: 3—minimally clinically significant

Potential Effects: Cimetidine may decrease the ability of clomiphene to stimulate ovulation.

Recommendations: The dose of clomiphene may need to be increased in patients receiving cimetidine.

Summary: Cimetidine has been shown to reduce the ovulation-stimulatory effects of clomiphene during concurrent administration of these agents.

Related Drugs: There is no documentation that other H_2-receptor antagonists would interact similarly with clomiphene. There are no drugs related to clomiphene.

Mechanism: The mechanism of this interaction is not known.

Detailed Information: See *EDI*, 18/4.32

Cyclosporine-Allopurinol

Significance: 2—moderately clinically significant

Potential Effects: The addition of allopurinol to a stable cyclosporine regimen may result in increased cyclosporine serum levels.

Recommendations: Patients should be closely monitored for changes in cyclosporine levels and renal status when allopurinol is added to therapy. The dose of cyclosporine may need to be decreased.

Summary: The addition of allopurinol to the therapy of a patient maintained on cyclosporine resulted in increased cyclosporine levels.

Related Drugs: It is unknown if tacrolimus and allopurinol would exhibit the same interaction.

Mechanism: The mechanism of this interaction is not known.

Detailed Information: See *EDI*, 18/4.38

Cyclosporine-Azathioprine

Significance: 3—minimally clinically significant

Potential Effects: Azathioprine administration may decrease cyclosporine absorption and levels.

Recommendations: Cyclosporine levels should be monitored if azathioprine is added to, or withdrawn from, therapy. The dose of cyclosporine may need to be adjusted.

Summary: Azathioprine and concurrent cyclosporine may result in decreased cyclosporine plasma levels.

Related Drugs: There are no drugs related to cyclosporine or azathioprine.

Mechanism: Azathioprine is not metabolized by hepatic cytochrome P450, and azathioprine may interfere with cyclosporine absorption.

Detailed Information: See *EDI*, 18/4.41

Cyclosporine-Carbamazepine

Significance: 2—moderately clinically significant

Potential Effects: Cyclosporine blood levels may be reduced by concurrent carbamazepine.

Recommendations: Cyclosporine blood levels should be monitored if carbamazepine is added to, or deleted from, concurrent therapy. Carbamazepine may need to be discontinued; sodium valproate may be an acceptable alternative therapy.

Summary: There are data to show that carbamazepine increased cyclosporine whole blood levels when the carbamazepine was discontinued.

Related Drugs: There are no drugs related to carbamazepine or cyclosporine.

Mechanism: The reduction in cyclosporine blood levels may be the result of the induction of hepatic cytochrome P450 by carbamazepine.

Detailed Information: See *EDI*, 18/4.42

Cyclosporine-Cholestyramine

Significance: 4—not clinically significant

Potential Effects: Cholestyramine may reduce cyclosporine absorption, but this has not been documented.

Recommendations: Although no interaction was found, cyclosporine levels should be closely monitored during cholestyramine coadministration.

Summary: Cholestyramine administration may reduce cyclosporine absorption, but this has not been documented.

Related Drugs: Documentation is lacking regarding an interaction between cyclosporine and colestipol. There are no drugs related to cyclosporine.

Mechanism: The effect of cholestyramine on cyclosporine absorption is not known. Cholestyramine could interfere with the oral absorption of cyclosporine.

Detailed Information: See *EDI,* 18/0.70

Cyclosporine-Methyltestosterone

Significance: 2—moderately clinically significant

Potential Effects: Cyclosporine levels may be increased by concurrent methyltestosterone use, and hepatic and renal dysfunction may occur even at low doses of cyclosporine.

Recommendations: Monitor hepatic and renal function and cyclosporine levels closely if these agents are given together. The dose of methyltestosterone may need to be decreased or the drug may need to be discontinued.

Summary: Administration of cyclosporine and methyltestosterone resulted in significant increases in blood levels of cyclosporine. Both severe renal and hepatic dysfunction were reported as a result of this interaction.

Related Drugs: Danazole, norethindrone, and oxymetholone have been reported to cause a similar interaction with cyclosporine. If the mechanism involves inhibition of hepatic metabolism of cyclosporine by methyltestosterone, then the other androgens may be expected to interact similarly based on a similar metabolic fate. There is no information on whether this interaction occurs with tacrolimus.

Mechanism: It has been suggested that methyltestosterone and other sex steroids may inhibit the hepatic microsomal enzymes responsible for the metabolism of cyclosporine. It has also been suggested that since cyclosporine is eliminated mainly through biliary excretion, reduced bile flow may result in increased cyclosporine levels with subsequent toxicity.

Detailed Information: See *EDI,* 18/4.43

Cyclosporine-Metoclopramide

Significance: 2—moderately clinically significant

Potential Effects: Metoclopramide may increase the absorption of cyclosporine.

Recommendations: Monitor cyclosporine levels closely if the agents must be used together. Concurrent cyclosporine and metoclopramide should be avoided if possible.

Summary: There are data to show that metoclopramide may increase bioavailability, peak levels, area-under-curve and absorption, and decrease time to peak of cyclosporine.

Related Drugs: There are no drugs related to cyclosporine or metoclopramide.

Mechanism: By increasing gastric emptying rate, metoclopramide
will increase the delivery of cyclosporine to its absorption site in
the small intestine, resulting in increased absorption of
cyclosporine.

Detailed Information: See *EDI*, 18/4.47

Cyclosporine-Nafcillin

Significance: 2—moderately clinically significant

Potential Effects: Nafcillin may induce the metabolism of
cyclosporine, leading to decreased levels.

Recommendations: Caution should be used when nafcillin therapy
is instituted in a patient maintained on cyclosporine.
Cyclosporine whole-blood levels may be reduced to subtherapeutic levels.

Summary: There are data to show that nafcillin may decrease
cyclosporine blood levels.

Related Drugs: A similar interaction may occur between
cyclosporine and other penicillins that are hepatically metabolized. It is not known whether an interaction would occur between
cyclosporine and other penicillins. There are no drugs related to
cyclosporine.

Mechanism: The enhanced hepatic clearance of cyclosporine may
have resulted from cytochrome P450 enzyme induction.

Detailed Information: See *EDI*, 18/4.49

Cyclosporine-Oral Contraceptive Agents

Significance: 3—minimally clinically significant

Potential Effects: The administration of oral contraceptive agents
concurrently with cyclosporine may lead to an increase in
cyclosporine levels and hepatotoxicity because of decreased
elimination of cyclosporine.

Recommendations: Hepatic function should be monitored in
patients receiving cyclosporine and oral contraceptive agents
concurrently. The cyclosporine serum level and serum creatinine
should also be monitored. The cyclosporine dose may need to be
decreased.

Summary: The concurrent administration of cyclosporine and oral
contraceptive agents may increase cyclosporine levels, potentiating the hepatotoxic effects.

Related Drugs: There are no drugs related to cyclosporine.

Mechanism: Oral contraceptive agents may decrease the elimination of cyclosporine, potentiating the hepatotoxic effect of
cyclosporine.

Detailed Information: See *EDI*, 18/4.45

Cyclosporine-Quinine

Significance: 2—moderately clinically significant

Potential Effects: Quinine may decrease cyclosporine levels by
increasing its clearance.

Recommendations: The addition of quinine to a cyclosporine regimen should be approached with caution. Cyclosporine blood levels should be monitored, and quinine may have to be discontinued.

Summary: The addition of quinine to a cyclosporine regimen may
reduce cyclosporine blood levels.

Related Drugs: Quinidine is expected to interact with cyclosporine in a similar manner. There are no drugs related to cyclosporine.

Mechanism: Quinine could interfere with the bioavailability of cyclosporine or increase its clearance.

Detailed Information: See *EDI*, 18/4.48

Dexamethasone-Aminoglutethimide

Significance: 2—moderately clinically significant

Recommendations: Patients receiving dexamethasone and aminoglute-thimide should be observed and monitored for a decreased effect of dexamethasone. Increasing the dose of dexamethasone or substituting hydrocortisone appears to avoid the interaction.

Summary: Aminoglutethimide may cause an increased metabolism of dexamethasone and a reduction in its half-life and bioavailability. This may lead to a decrease in the therapeutic efficacy of dexamethasone.

Related Drugs: Because of conflicting results, it is difficult to determine if an interaction would occur between aminoglutethimide and other corticosteroids. A similar interaction may occur between glutethimide and dexamethasone.

Mechanism: Aminoglutethimide appears to induce the hepatic enzymes responsible for the metabolism of dexamethasone, reducing the bioavailability of dexamethasone.

Detailed Information: See *EDI*, 18/4.50

Dexamethasone-Ephedrine

Significance: 3—minimally clinically significant

Potential Effects: Ephedrine may cause an increase in the clearance of dexamethasone.

Recommendations: If these agents are used together, the dose of dexamethasone may need to be increased.

Summary: There are data to show that ephedrine administration may decrease plasma half-life and increase the metabolic clearance of dexamethasone, decreasing its therapeutic effect.

Related Drugs: It is not known if an interaction would occur between dexamethasone and other indirect, direct or mixed acting sympathomimetics, if the mechanism involves increased liver perfusion or hepatic enzyme induction. A similar interaction may occur between ephedrine and other corticosteroids.

Mechanism: Ephedrine may increase the hepatic clearance of dexamethasone or induce hepatic microsomal enzymes.

Detailed Information: See *EDI*, 18/4.70

Didanosine-Ganciclovir

Significance: 2—moderately clinically significant

Potential Effects: Concurrent didanosine and ganciclovir may increase didanosine serum levels.

Recommendations: The clinical significance of this interaction has not been determined.

Summary: In a study of 11 HIV patients, concurrent administration of didanosine and ganciclovir resulted in increased didanosine serum levels.

Related Drugs: It is not known if a similar interaction would occur between didanosine and the other antiviral agents pharmaco logically related to ganciclovir (acyclovir, famciclovir, valacyclovir). It is also not known if the other antiretroviral agents will interact with ganciclovir.

Mechanism: It is postulated that ganciclovir may compete with didanosine for tubular secretion in the kidney with resultant increases in didanosine serum concentrations.

Detailed Information: See *EDI*, 18/4.90

Dihydroergotamine-Nitroglycerin

Significance: 2—moderately clinically significant

Recommendations: Patients should be monitored for symptoms of ergotism (e.g., cold, pale, and numb feet and legs, muscle pain, headache, nausea, vomiting) when these agents are used concomitantly. The dosage of dihydroergotamine may need to be reduced in some patients.

Summary: There are data to show that nitroglycerin administration may cause the ergotism, secondary to an increased dihydroergotamine response, necessitating a decrease in dose.

Related Drugs: Ergoloid mesylates may interact with nitroglycerin in a similar manner. Other nitrates may interact similarly with the ergot alkaloids.

Mechanism: Nitroglycerin may decrease the first-pass metabolism of dihydroergotamine and increase its bioavailability.

Detailed Information: See *EDI*, 18/5.00

Dobutamine-Cimetidine

Significance: 3—minimally clinically significant

Potential Effects: The effect of dobutamine may be exaggerated.

Recommendations: Patients maintained on cimetidine should be carefully monitored if dobutamine is administered, since the effect of dobutamine may be increased. The dose of dobutamine may need to be decreased to attain the expected effect.

Summary: Cimetidine has been shown to increase dobutamine response.

Related Drugs: It is not known whether an interaction would occur between cimetidine and other direct-acting sympathomimetics or between dobutamine and other H_2-receptor antagonists.

Mechanism: The exaggerated dobutamine response may be due to impaired dobutamine metabolism, resulting from cimetidine-induced inhibition of the hepatic mixed function oxidase system.

Detailed Information: See *EDI*, 18/6.50

Ergonovine-Dopamine

Significance: 2—moderately clinically significant

Recommendations: Although limited documentation is available, it indicates that concurrent use of these agents should be avoided if possible. Hypertension that resulted from the use of these agents was successfully treated with chlorpromazine.

Summary: An isolated case report suggested that the vasoconstrictive properties of ergonovine and dopamine may be additive, leading to an increased incidence of gangrene.

Related Drugs: Other reports are lacking of similar interactions between other mixed acting sympathomimetic amines and other ergot alkaloids; however, an interaction may be expected to occur.

Mechanism: The interaction probably results from the synergistic peripheral vasoconstriction activity of both agents.

Detailed Information: See *EDI*, 18/7.00

Fat Emulsion, Intravenous-Cyclosporine

Significance: 2—moderately clinically significant

Potential Effects: The addition of intravenous fat emulsion to cyclosporine therapy may result in increased cyclosporine levels and toxicity.

Recommendations: Because of the changes in levels of serum lipoproteins that accompany the intravenous administration of fat emulsions, the use of these agents should be avoided in patients on cyclosporine therapy.

Summary: The addition of intravenous fat emulsion to patients maintained on cyclosporine may result in increased cyclosporine levels and toxicity.

Related Drugs: There are no drugs related to cyclosporine or fat emulsion.

Mechanism: Cyclosporine is lipophilic and it will bind to the components in the intravenous fat emulsion.

Detailed Information: See *EDI,* 18/8.20

Foscarnet-Cyclosporine

Significance: 2—moderately clinically significant

Potential Effects: Concurrent use of cyclosporine and foscarnet may result in reversible acute renal failure.

Recommendations: Patients receiving concurrent therapy with cyclosporine and foscarnet should be monitored for a decrease in renal function. Foscarnet may need to be discontinued.

Summary: In two case reports, concurrent use of cyclosporine and foscarnet may have resulted in reversible acute renal failure without a significant increase in cyclosporine concentration.

Related Drugs: It is not known whether there is an interaction between foscarnet and tacrolimus.

Mechanism: It was proposed that the reversible acute renal failure may be due to additive or synergistic nephrotoxic effects of cyclosporine and foscarnet.

Detailed Information: See *EDI,* 18/8.40

Glycopyrrolate-Ritodrine

Significance: 2—moderately clinically significant

Potential Effects: Ritodrine may potentiate the effect of glycopyrrolate on heart rate, possibly leading to severe tachycardia.

Recommendations: Caution should be exercised in patients who are receiving, or have recently received, ritodrine if glycopyrrolate is to be given.

Summary: There are data to show that ritodrine administration may potentiate the effect of glycopyrrolate on heart rate, possibly leading to severe tachycardia.

Related Drugs: The other anticholinergic agents may interact in a similar manner with ritodrine. Other sympathomimetic agents may potentiate the cardiovascular effect of glycopyrrolate.

Mechanism: Ritodrine has been implicated in tachyarrhythmias, and glycopyrrolate may increase heart rate because of its parasympatholytic effects.

Detailed Information: See *EDI,* 18/8.50

Hydrocortisone-Cholestyramine

Significance: 3—minimally clinically significant

Recommendations: Patients should be observed for a change in their clinical response to the corticosteroid, and an increase in the dose may be necessary.

Summary: Cholestyramine has been shown to cause a reduction in the hydrocortisone plasma concentration area-under-curve.

Related Drugs: Because of conflicting data, it would be difficult to determine if a similar interaction would occur between cholestyramine and other corticosteroids. Documentation is lacking regarding an interaction with colestipol.

Mechanism: Cholestyramine has been demonstrated to bind hydrocortisone and may also decrease and delay the absorption of hydrocortisone.

Detailed Information: See *EDI,* 18/9.00

Levodopa-Aluminum Hydroxide, Magnesium Hydroxide

Significance: 3—minimally clinically significant

Recommendations: The addition of an antacid containing aluminum hydroxide and magnesium hydroxide 30 minutes before levodopa therapy may allow the dosage of levodopa to be decreased in some patients, thus minimizing gastrointestinal side effects. Other patients refractory to levodopa therapy may benefit as well. If this interaction is not desired, separating the dosage of these agents by as much time as possible or decreasing the dose of levodopa may be necessary.

Summary: Antacids containing aluminum hydroxide and magnesium hydroxide may enhance the rate of absorption of levodopa.

Related Drugs: A similar interaction may occur between levodopa and other antacids. There are no drugs related to levodopa.

Mechanism: Antacids may increase gastric emptying time, decreasing levodopa's gastric metabolism and leading to increased levels in the central nervous system.

Detailed Information: See *EDI,* 18/10.10

Levodopa-Domperidone

Significance: 3—minimally clinically significant

Potential Effects: This agent also reduces the incidence of gastrointestinal side effects of levodopa and may enable a higher optimum levodopa dose. Domperidone results in increased levodopa plasma concentrations.

Recommendations: No precautions are necessary regarding the concurrent use of levodopa and domperidone.

Summary: There are data to show that domperidone administration can increase levodopa plasma concentrations.

Related Drugs: There are no drugs related to levodopa or domperidone.

Mechanism: The mechanism of this interaction is unknown.

Detailed Information: See *EDI,* 18/10.21

Levodopa-Ferrous Sulfate

Significance: 2—moderately clinically significant

Potential Effects: Ferrous sulfate may chelate with levodopa, leading to decreased levodopa levels.

Recommendations: Patients should be monitored closely if ferrous sulfate is added to, or withdrawn from, concomitant therapy with levodopa. The dose of levodopa may need to be adjusted.

Summary: There are data to show that ferrous sulfate administration may chelate with levodopa, reducing levodopa bioavailability and levels.

Related Drugs: An interaction would be expected to occur between levodopa and other oral ferrous salts. There are no drugs related to levodopa.

Mechanism: This mechanism is similar to the one that causes a decrease in the absorption of methyldopa with concurrent ferrous sulfate (see Methyldopa-Ferrous Sulfate, page 166). Ferrous sulfate may decrease levodopa absorption by chelation.

Detailed Information: See *EDI*, 18/10.25

Levodopa, Benserazide-Orphenadrine

Significance: 3—minimally clinically significant

Potential Effects: Concurrent levodopa/benserazide and orphenadrine may result in erratic absorption of levodopa, resulting in impaired motor responses.

Recommendations: Therapeutic response to levodopa/benserazide should be carefully evaluated and monitored with concurrent orphenadrine therapy for parkinsonism.

Summary: A study showed that administering orphenadrine with levodopa/benserazide results in variable levodopa absorption and therapeutic response.

Related Drugs: There is no information on whether orphenadrine interacts with carbidopa/levodopa.

Mechanism: The proposed mechanism may be related to anticholinergic effects on gastric motility leading to erratic absorption; however, the exact mechanism is unknown.

Detailed Information: See *EDI*, 18/10.27

Levodopa-Papaverine

Significance: 3—minimally clinically significant

Potential Effects: Papaverine may block the effects of levodopa, causing a worsening of parkinsonism.

Recommendations: Patients should be monitored for worsening of the symptoms of Parkinson's disease when papaverine is added to levodopa therapy. The dose of levodopa may need to be increased.

Summary: There are data to show that concurrent papaverine and levodopa therapy will result in the antagonism of levodopa's pharmacologic effect.

Related Drugs: A similar interaction is expected to occur between levodopa and ethaverine. There are no drugs related to levodopa.

Mechanism: The antagonism in this interaction may be due to papaverine blocking the dopamine receptors in the striatum.

Detailed Information: See *EDI*, 18/10.30

Levodopa-Trihexyphenidyl

Significance: 4—not clinically significant

Potential Effects: Trihexyphenidyl may decrease levodopa levels; however, this has not been demonstrated in humans.

Recommendations: No precautions need be made for patients receiving concurrent levodopa and trihexyphenidyl. Patients maintained on levodopa may need to be monitored if trihexyphenidyl is added to, or withdrawn from, therapy. The dose of levodopa may need to be adjusted.

Summary: The effectiveness of levodopa may be decreased by the addition of trihexyphenidyl; however, this has not been demonstrated in humans.

Related Drugs: It is not known if an interaction would occur between levodopa and other anticholinergic agents. There are no drugs related to levodopa.

Mechanism: When gastric emptying is prolonged, the metabolism of levodopa by gastric mucosa may be increased, and this may decrease the plasma levodopa levels.

Detailed Information: See *EDI*, 18/10.50

Levothyroxine-Calcium Carbonate

Significance: 3—minimally clinically significant

Potential Effects: Simultaneous ingestion of calcium carbonate formulations and sodium levothyroxine may result in increased serum thyroid stimulating hormone levels and reduced levothyroxine efficacy.

Recommendations: If concurrent use of the agents is necessary, separating the administration by at least four hours should maintain levothyroxine efficacy.

Summary: Simultaneous ingestion of calcium carbonate formulations and sodium levothyroxine reduced levothyroxine efficacy. However, conflicting data are available.

Related Drugs: Based on structural and pharmacologic similarity and the proposed mechanism, an interaction may be expected to occur between levothyroxine and the other orally administered calcium compounds and between the other orally administered calcium compounds and other thyroid preparations.

Mechanism: It is thought that calcium carbonate might form insoluble chelates with levothyroxine. This would lead to decreased levothyroxine bioavailability. The formation of insoluble complexes has been shown to occur between levothyroxine and ferrous sulfate.

Detailed Information: See *EDI*, 18/10.70

Levothyroxine-Ferrous Sulfate

Significance: 3—minimally clinically significant

Potential Effects: Concurrent ferrous sulfate and levothyroxine may result in a reduction in levothyroxine efficacy.

Recommendations: If concurrent therapy with these two agents is necessary, it may be possible to reduce the extent of the iron-levothyroxine interaction by separating the administration times of the medications by two or more hours. Routine thyroid function monitoring should also be undertaken.

Summary: There are data to show that ferrous sulfate may cause a reduction in levothyroxine efficacy.

Related Drugs: An interaction may occur between levothyroxine and other orally administered iron compounds and between ferrous sulfate and other thyroid drugs.

Mechanism: The formation of an insoluble ferric-levothyroxine complex may reduce the absorption of levothyroxine.

Detailed Information: See *EDI*, 18/11.05

Levothyroxine-Lovastatin

Significance: 3—minimally clinically significant

Potential Effects: The addition of lovastatin to, or withdrawal from, levothyroxine therapy may result in a change in serum thyroxine levels.

Recommendations: A patient maintained on levothyroxine should be carefully monitored for changes in serum thyroxine levels if lovastatin is added to, or deleted from, cotherapy.

Summary: There are data to show that increases in the serum thyroxine levels have been documented when lovastatin is given concomitantly with levothyroxine.

Related Drugs: All thyroid compounds structurally similar to levothyroxine may interact with lovastatin. A similar interaction would be expected to occur between levothyroxine and the other HMG-CoA reductase inhibitors, although documentation is lacking.

Mechanism: A synergism may occur between lovastatin and levothyroxine, causing myolysis mediated by the thyrotoxic state.

Detailed Information: See *EDI,* 18/11.00

Levothyroxine-Sucralfate

Significance: 3—minimally clinically significant

Potential Effects: Administration of sucralfate and levothyroxine at the same time may decrease the absorption of levothyroxine.

Recommendations: Patients receiving concurrent levothyroxine and sucralfate should be monitored for decreased response to thyroid hormone replacement therapy. Adjustment of levothyroxine dosage, separating the administration of these agents by several hours, or alternative therapy for sucralfate may need to be considered.

Summary: Three case reports and a follow-up study describe concurrent levothyroxine and sucralfate administration that resulted in decreased levothyroxine absorption. However, other reports in the literature dispute these findings.

Related Drugs: An aluminum hydroxide-containing antacid caused elevated levels of thyroid stimulating hormone (TSH) in a patient stabilized for five years on levothyroxine. Discontinuation returned TSH levels to normal, but two individual rechallenges with the antacid produced similar results. An interaction would be expected to occur between levothyroxine and other aluminum-containing compounds.

Mechanism: The exact mechanism for this interaction is unknown. One possible mechanism is the interference of either intraluminal or transintestinal transport of the levothyroxine by sucralfate. Another possible mechanism is the binding of levothyroxine to sucralfate or aluminum. Sucralfate has been shown to bind levothyroxine *in vitro,* and other studies have reported that aluminum hydroxide has a considerable nonspecific absorptive capacity for levothyroxine.

Detailed Information: See *EDI,* 18/11.20

Lovastatin-Cyclosporine

Significance: 3—minimally clinically significant

Potential Effects: Concurrent use of these agents may result in myolysis.

Recommendations: Use these agents together with caution. Monitor lova-statin levels if possible. Patients should report any unexplained muscle pain, tenderness, or weakness.

Summary: Concurrent administration of lovastatin and cyclosporine may result in myolysis.

Related Drugs: There are no drugs related to cyclosporine. A similar interaction would be expected to occur between cyclosporine and the other HMG-CoA reductase inhibitors, although documentation is lacking.

Mechanism: Cyclosporine may increase lovastatin levels, resulting in an increased incidence of myolysis.

Detailed Information: See *EDI,* 18/12.01

Lovastatin-Erythromycin

Significance: 1—highly clinically significant

Potential Effects: Concurrent administration of lovastatin and erythromycin may result in increased lovastatin levels and rhabdomyolysis.

Recommendations: Extreme caution should be exercised when administering these two agents concurrently. If alternative antimicrobials or temporary discontinuation of lovastatin is not possible, patients should be instructed to report any unexplained muscle pain, tenderness, or weakness.

Summary: Concurrent administration of lovastatin and erythromycin may result in increased lovastatin levels to as high as 97.6ng equivalent/ml (normal: approximately 12.2ng equivalent/ml) and rhabdomyolysis.

Related Drugs: Similar interactions have been reported between lovastatin and clarithromycin and between atorvastatin and erythromycin. *In vitro,* the metabolism of cerivastatin was inhibited in the presence of troleandomycin. Since pravastatin is not metabolized by the cytochrome $P450_{3A}$ system, it would not be expected to interact with the macrolide antibiotics. An interaction would be expected between atorvastatin, lovastatin, simvastatin, or cerivastatin and the other macrolide antibiotics as well as between the macrolides and the other HMG-CoA reductase inhibitors.

Mechanism: Atorvastatin, cerivastatin, lovastatin, and simvastatin are metabolized by the cytochrome $P450_{3A}$ isoenzyme system. Erythromycin may affect the metabolism of these agents either by competitive or noncompetitive inhibition.

Detailed Information: See *EDI,* 18/12.05

Lovastatin-Gemfibrozil

Significance: 2—moderately clinically significant

Potential Effects: Concurrent use of these agents may result in myolysis.

Recommendations: Concurrent use of lovastatin and gemfibrozil should be approached with caution. Patients should be instructed to report any unexplained muscle pain, tenderness, weakness, or discolored urine. Alternative therapy may need to be considered.

Summary: Concurrent administration of lovastatin and gemfibrozil may result in rhabdomyolysis and acute renal failure.

Related Drugs: Subjects receiving combined therapy with pravastatin and gemfibrozil had creatine kinase elevations and musculoskeletal symptoms; severe myopathies did not occur. Rhabdomyolosis has been related to the concurrent use of gemfibrozil and atorvastatin, simvastatin, and pravastatin. No interaction has been seen between gemfibrozil and fluvastatin. An interaction would be expected to occur between gemfibrozil and cerivastatin or between lovastatin and the other fibric acid derivatives.

Mechanism: Although lovastatin administration alone has been reported to cause myolysis and increased creatine kinase, gemfibrozil may increase the incidence by an unknown mechanism.

Detailed Information: See *EDI*, 18/12.03

Lovastatin-Grapefruit Juice

Significance: 1—highly clinically significant

Potential Effects: The concurrent administration of lovastatin and grapefruit juice may result in increased serum concentrations of lovastatin and its active metabolite.

Recommendations: The administration of grapefruit juice during therapy with lovastatin should be avoided.

Summary: Concurrent administration of lovastatin and grapefruit juice resulted in greatly increased serum concentrations of lovastatin and lovastatin acid, its active metabolite.

Related Drugs: Based on the postulated mechanism and pharmacologic similarity, an interaction may be expected to occur between grapefruit juice and the HMG-CoA reductase inhibitors simvastatin, atorvastatin, and cerivastatin provided the metabolism of these agents involves cytochrome $P450_{3A4}$ inhibition. It is not known whether an interaction would occur between grapefruit juice and pravastatin or fluvastatin.

Mechanism: The mechanism probably involves bioflavonoids present in grapefruit juice. Grapefruit juice selectively down-regulates cytochrome $P450_{3A4}$ in the small intestine, where this isoenzyme is extensively expressed. This prevents presystemic metabolism mediated by cytochrome $P450_{3A4}$. Even though the hydrolysis of lovastatin to lovastatin acid is not mediated by cytochrome $P450_{3A4}$, the concentration of lovastatin acid increases with the level of lovastatin. Cytochrome $P450_{3A4}$ also plays an important role in the metabolism of the HMG-CoA reductase inhibitors simvastatin and atorvastatin. However, other enzymes are mainly responsible for the metabolism of pravastatin and fluvastatin. It has been demonstrated that the metabolic pathways involved in cerivastatin first-pass metabolism are insensitive to those cytochrome P450 isozymes induced by cimetidine (2C8-10, 2D6, 3A3); however, other investigators have found that cytochrome P450 isoenzymes play a major role in cerivastatin metabolism.

Detailed Information: See *EDI*, 18/12.04

Lovastatin-Nicotinic Acid

Significance: 2—moderately clinically significant

Potential Effects: Concurrent use of these agents may result in myolysis.

Recommendations: If concurrent therapy of these agents is required, patients should be monitored for signs of myolysis.

Summary: The concurrent use of these agents may result in an increased incidence of myolysis.

Related Drugs: There are no drugs related to lovastatin or nicotinic acid.

Mechanism: Lovastatin has been reported to cause myolysis and increased creatine kinase; however, the mechanism of this interaction is not known.

Detailed Information: See *EDI*, 18/12.07

Magnesium Hydroxide-Sodium Polystyrene Sulfonate

Significance: 2—moderately clinically significant

Recommendations: The concurrent use of magnesium hydroxide-containing antacids and sodium polystyrene sulfonate should be avoided, if possible, in patients with renal disease. However, if the combined use of these agents is necessary, separate their administration by several hours.

Summary: It has been documented in two patients with renal disease that metabolic alkalosis occurred in one patient and metabolic acidosis was reversed in the other after concurrent administration of sodium polystyrene sulfonate and an antacid containing magnesium hydroxide.

Related Drugs: The concurrent use of other combination antacids and sodium polystyrene sulfonate has been documented to result in a rapid alkalinization of the blood. There are no drugs related to sodium polystyrene sulfonate.

Mechanism: In the presence of sodium polystyrene sulfonate, the magnesium chloride interacts and bicarbonate is secreted in the small bowel and reabsorbed, leading to metabolic alkalosis.

Detailed Information: See *EDI*, 18/12.10

Medroxyprogesterone-Aminoglutethimide

Significance: 3—minimally clinically significant

Recommendations: Patients receiving these agents concurrently should be monitored for a decrease in the therapeutic efficacy of medroxyprogesterone. A high dose of medroxyprogesterone may be necessary.

Summary: There are data to show that aminoglutethimide may decrease the therapeutic efficacy of medroxyprogesterone; however, there are conflicting data.

Related Drugs: An interaction may occur between amino-glutethimide and other progestins. A similar interaction is expected to occur between medroxyprogesterone and glutethimide.

Mechanism: Aminoglutethimide may induce the hepatic enzymes responsible for medroxyprogesterone metabolism.

Detailed Information: See *EDI*, 18/12.30

Metoclopramide-Atropine

Significance: 3—minimally clinically significant

Recommendations: Since these agents antagonize the pharmacologic effect of one another, their concurrent use should be avoided. If the two drugs are to be used, metoclopramide should precede atropine by two hours.

Summary: These agents are antagonists. When metoclopramide was given first, atropine reversed metoclopramide. When atropine was given first, metoclopramide reversed the atropine-induced depression of sphincter pressure.

Related Drugs: A similar interaction is expected to occur between metoclopramide and other anticholinergics. There are no drugs related to metoclopramide.

Mechanism: It is postulated that metoclopramide may lead to an increase in lower esophageal sphincter pressure, which may be antagonized or potentiated by effects on cholinergic receptors.

Detailed Information: See *EDI*, 18/13.00

Metoclopramide-Levodopa

Significance: 3—minimally clinically significant

Recommendations: The evidence suggests that a competitive antagonism is possible with the coadministration of these two agents. Therefore, patients should be monitored for such an interaction, with an appropriate adjustment made in the dosage of levodopa if necessary.

Summary: There is evidence that the concurrent use of levodopa will reverse some of the pharmacologic activities of metoclopramide.

Related Drugs: There are no drugs related to metoclopramide or levodopa.

Mechanism: Metoclopramide is a dopaminergic antagonist and levodopa, the precursor of dopamine, apparently antagonizes by inhibiting the action of metoclopramide.

Detailed Information: See *EDI*, 18/15.00

Metyrapone-Phenytoin

Significance: 3—minimally clinically significant

Potential Effects: The addition of oral metyrapone may elicit a subnormal response resulting from decreased metyrapone blood levels in subjects maintained on phenytoin.

Recommendations: Invalid results for the metapyrone test may occur in patients maintained on phenytoin. Doubling the metyrapone dose has produced valid results.

Summary: The addition of oral metyrapone elicited a subnormal response resulting from decreased metyrapone blood levels in subjects maintained on phenytoin.

Related Drugs: Although no documentation exists for a similar interaction between metyrapone and the other hydantoin anticonvulsants, one would be expected based on structural and pharmacologic similarity. There are no drugs related to metyrapone.

Mechanism: It is postulated that phenytoin induced hepatic enzymes, resulting in an increased metyrapone metabolism.

Detailed Information: See *EDI*, 18/15.50

Misoprostol-Aluminum Hydroxide, Magnesium Hydroxide

Significance: 3—minimally clinically significant

Potential Effects: The antacid may decrease the bioavailability of misoprostol.

Recommendations: The concurrent use of misoprostol and an aluminum/magnesium hydroxide antacid should be approached with caution. The efficacy of misoprostol may be decreased.

Summary: There are data to show that administration of misoprostol with an aluminum-magnesium hydroxide antacid will result in the reduced bioavailability of misoprostol.

Related Drugs: It is not known whether an interaction would occur between misoprostol and other antacids that contain aluminum or magnesium. There are no drugs related to misoprostol.

Mechanism: This interaction is believed to result from the decreased bioavailability of misoprostol.

Detailed Information: See *EDI*, 18/16.03

Nizatidine-Charcoal

Significance: 3—minimally clinically significant

Potential Effects: Charcoal adsorbs nizatidine, reducing its absorption.

Recommendations: Separate administration time as much as possible, unless the charcoal is being used to treat nizatidine overdose.

Summary: There are data to show that charcoal adsorbs nizatidine and reduces its absorption.

Related Drugs: There is no documentation of an interaction between charcoal and other H_2-receptor antagonists. There are no drugs related to charcoal.

Mechanism: Charcoal adsorbs nizatidine in the gastrointestinal tract, preventing the absorption of nizatidine.

Detailed Information: See *EDI*, 18/16.05

Omeprazole-Clarithromycin

Significance: 3—minimally clinically significant

Potential Effects: The concurrent use of omeprazole and clarithromycin may result in increased serum levels for both agents.

Recommendations: The concurrent use of these agents may be advantageous, leading to increased tissue levels of the antibiotic. This combination may be especially effective against Helicobacter pylori infection.

Summary: Concurrent administration of omeprazole and clarithromycin resulted in increased serum levels for both agents.

Related Drugs: Lansoprazole has also been reported to interact with clarithromycin, causing glossitis, stomatitis, and/or black tongue. Although there is no documentation regarding an interaction between omeprazole and the other macrolide antibiotics that form inactive cytochrome P450 metabolite complexes to some extent (erythromycin, troleandomycin, josamycin), if the mechanism involves inhibition of the cytochrome $P450_{3A}$ isozyme, then an interaction would be expected to occur that may result in increased levels of one or both interacting agents. The macrolides that form inactive cytochrome P450 metabolite complexes (spiramycin, dirithromycin, azithromycin) would not be expected to affect the serum level of omeprazole based on the postulated mechanism, but it is not known whether omeprazole would affect the macrolide serum level. An interaction would be expected to occur between clarithromycin and the other proton pump inhibitor, pantoprazole.

Mechanism: It has been postulated that clarithromycin inhibits the cytochrome $P450_{3A}$ isozyme, that this isozyme makes a significant contribution to the metabolism of omeprazole *in vivo*, and that clarithromycin may have an inhibitory effect on omeprazole metabolism.

Detailed Information: See *EDI*, 18/16.07

Omeprazole-Cyclosporine

Significance: 2—moderately clinically significant

Potential Effects: Omeprazole may inhibit cyclosporine metabolism, resulting in increased levels.

Recommendations: When omeprazole is added to, or withdrawn from, a cyclosporine regimen, the patient should be carefully monitored for changes in cyclosporine levels. The dose of cyclosporine may need to be adjusted.

Summary: There are data to show that omeprazole will inhibit cyclosporine metabolism and increase its levels.

Related Drugs: There are no drugs related to cyclosporine or omeprazole.

Mechanism: These agents may compete for the cytochrome P450 system, which may result in an inhibition of cyclosporine metabolism.

Detailed Information: See *EDI*, 18/16.08

Penicillamine-Aluminum Hydroxide, Magnesium Hydroxide

Significance: 3—minimally clinically significant

Recommendations: The concomitant administration of penicillamine with an aluminum hydroxide-magnesium hydroxide antacid should be avoided. Although documentation is lacking, if both preparations need to be administered, separate administration by as much time as possible.

Summary: There are data to show that administration of a combination antacid product containing aluminum hydroxide and magnesium hydroxide with penicillamine will reduce penicillamine bioavailability and absorption.

Related Drugs: A similar interaction is expected to occur between penicillamine and other antacids if the mechanism involves chelation of penicillamine.

Mechanism: Aluminum and magnesium ions are thought to chelate penicillamine, limiting its absorption.

Detailed Information: See *EDI*, 18/16.10

Penicillamine-Chloroquine

Significance: 3—minimally clinically significant

Potential Effects: Chloroquine may increase penicillamine levels.

Recommendations: Patients maintained on penicillamine therapy should be monitored for penicillamine toxicity if chloroquine is added to therapy. The dose of penicillamine may need to be reduced.

Summary: There are data to show that chloroquine administration will increase plasma penicillamine concentrations.

Related Drugs: It is not known whether an interaction would occur between penicillamine and other aminoquinolones. There are no drugs related to penicillamine.

Mechanism: The mechanism of this interaction is not known.

Detailed Information: See *EDI*, 18/16.27

Penicillamine-Indomethacin

Significance: 3—minimally clinically significant

Potential Effects: Indomethacin may increase penicillamine levels.

Recommendations: Patients maintained on penicillamine therapy should be monitored for penicillamine toxicity if indomethacin is added to therapy. The dose of penicillamine may need to be reduced.

Summary: There are data to show that indomethacin administration will increase plasma penicillamine concentrations.

Related Drugs: It is not known whether an interaction would occur between penicillamine and other NSAIAs. There are no drugs related to penicillamine.

Mechanism: The mechanism of this interaction is not known.

Detailed Information: See *EDI*, 18/16.25

Prednisolone-Cyclosporine

Significance: 2—moderately clinically significant

Potential Effects: The concurrent use of these agents may result in increased levels of either agent.

Recommendations: If increased levels of prednisolone (e.g., cushingoid symptoms) or cyclosporine (e.g., nephrotoxicity) occur, the dose of one or both agents may need to be decreased.

Summary: There are data to show that coadministration of these agents may result in increased levels of either agent.

Related Drugs: Prednisolone has been shown to decrease cyclosporine levels. Methylprednisolone has been shown to increase cyclosporine levels. The concurrent use of cyclosporine and other corticosteroids may result in increased levels of either agent. However, which drug would be affected is difficult to determine.

Mechanism: Prednisolone may decrease cyclosporine clearance by a hepatotoxic effect, cyclosporine may reduce the hepatic cytochrome P450 needed for prednisolone metabolism, or there may be a competitive inhibition of these agents.

Detailed Information: See *EDI,* 18/16.30

Prednisolone-Oral Contraceptive Agents

Significance: 2—moderately clinically significant

Potential Effects: Oral contraceptive agents may decrease the clearance of prednisolone.

Recommendations: Patients taking these agents together should be monitored for increased corticosteroid effects. The dose of prednisolone may need to be reduced.

Summary: There are data to show that oral contraceptive agents may inhibit the elimination of oral or intravenous prednisolone.

Related Drugs: A similar interaction is expected to occur between oral contraceptive agents and other corticosteroids.

Mechanism: Oral contraceptives may inhibit the hepatic metabolism of prednisolone and other corticosteroids. Oral contraceptives may also decrease endogenous cortisol clearance, competitively inhibiting prednisolone metabolism.

Detailed Information: See *EDI,* 18/17.00

Prednisone-Aluminum Hydroxide

Significance: 3—minimally clinically significant

Recommendations: Patients should be observed for a change in their clinical response to the corticosteroid. The dose of the corticosteroid may need to be increased.

Summary: Study results conflict as to whether administration of prednisone and an aluminum hydroxide antacid preparation may decrease the oral bioavailability of prednisone.

Related Drugs: An antacid preparation containing aluminum and magnesium hydroxide interacted similarly. A similar interaction is expected to occur between other corticosteroids and other antacid preparations.

Mechanism: Antacid preparations may physically adsorb prednisone.

Detailed Information: See *EDI,* 18/19.00

Probucol-Cyclosporine

Significance: 2—moderately clinically significant

Potential Effects: Concurrent cyclosporine and probucol may result in a decrease in cyclosporine levels.

Recommendations: Patients on cyclosporine therapy in whom probucol therapy is added or discontinued should be monitored for changes in cyclosporine levels. The dosage of cyclosporine may need to be adjusted.

Summary: In two studies, concurrent administration of cyclosporine and probucol resulted in a decrease in cyclosporine levels.

Related Drugs: It is not known if there is an interaction between probucol and tacrolimus.

Mechanism: It is speculated that probucol may have inhibited the absorption of cyclosporine by increasing the excretion of bile acid in the feces, or it may have altered the disposition of cyclosporine by altering lipid concentrations.
Detailed Information: See *EDI*, 18/20.00

Pyridostigmine-Methylprednisolone

Significance: 3—minimally clinically significant
Recommendations: If severe muscle weakness occurs during concurrent use of these agents, ventilatory assistance should be provided. It may also be necessary to discontinue the corticosteroid.
Summary: The concurrent administration of methylprednisolone and pyridostigmine may decrease muscle strength, possibly necessitating mechanical ventilation.
Related Drugs: Neostigmine administration resulted in the same interaction. Documentation is lacking regarding an interaction between other anticholinesterases and other corticosteroids.
Mechanism: The mechanism of this interaction is unknown.
Detailed Information: See *EDI*, 18/21.00

Ranitidine-Sucralfate

Significance: 3—minimally clinically significant
Potential Effects: Ranitidine may bind to sucralfate, resulting in decreased absorption of ranitidine.
Recommendations: Until further multiple dose studies are done, the concurrent administration of these agents need not be avoided. It may be best to separate the administration of these agents by as much time as possible.
Summary: There are data to show that ranitidine may bind to sucralfate, resulting in decreased absorption of ranitidine; however, there are some conflicting data.
Related Drugs: Because of conflicting results, it is difficult to determine if an interaction would occur between sucralfate and other H_2-receptor antagonists. There are no drugs related to sucralfate.
Mechanism: The mechanism of the potential interaction between ranitidine and sucralfate is not known. Ranitidine may bind to the sucralfate paste in the gastrointestinal fluids.
Detailed Information: See *EDI*, 18/22.10

Simvastatin-Nefazodone

Significance: 3—minimally clinically significant
Potential Effects: Concurrent administration of simvastatin and nefazodone may result in rhabdomyolysis and myositis.
Recommendations: Concurrent use of simvastatin and nefazodone should be approached with caution. Patients should be monitored for signs of myositis and rhabdomyolysis. One or both agents may need to be discontinued.
Summary: Concurrent administration of simvastatin and nefazodone may have resulted in rhabdomyolysis and myositis.
Related Drugs: Although documentation is lacking, based on the proposed mechanism a similar interaction would be expected to occur between nefazodone and the other HMG-CoA reductase inhibitors. There are no drugs related to nefazodone.
Mechanism: Nefazodone is an inhibitor of the cytochrome $P450_{3A4}$ isoenzyme system. Simvastatin is thought to be metabolized by $P450_{3A4}$ isoenzyme. It is postulated that nefazodone inhibits

the metabolism of simvastatin.
Detailed Information: See *EDI*, 18/22.20

Tacrolimus-Erythromycin

Significance: 2—moderately clinically significant
Potential Effects: Concurrent use of tacrolimus and erythromycin may result in increased tacrolimus plasma levels.
Recommendations: Concurrent tacrolimus and erythromycin may result in increased tacrolimus plasma levels with possible associated central nervous system toxicity or nephrotoxicity. Tacrolimus plasma levels should be carefully monitored. The dose of tacrolimus may need to be adjusted, and consideration should be given to an alternative for erythromycin.
Summary: There are data to show that concurrent tacrolimus and erythromycin may result in increased tacrolimus plasma levels.
Related Drugs: An interaction would be expected to occur between tacrolimus and other macrolide antibiotics that form inactive cytochrome P450 metabolite complexes. Azithromycin and spiramycin would not be expected to interact with tacrolimus.
Mechanism: This interaction may result from inhibition of hepatic cytochrome P450 metabolism.
Detailed Information: See *EDI*, 18/22.70

Tacrolimus-Fluconazole

Significance: 2—moderately clinically significant
Potential Effects: Concurrent tacrolimus and fluconazole administration may result in increased tacrolimus plasma levels, possibly resulting in nephrotoxicity.
Recommendations: Patients maintained on tacrolimus should be carefully monitored for increased tacrolimus levels and possible associated nephrotoxicity if fluconazole is added to therapy. The dose of tacrolimus may need to be adjusted.
Summary: An increase in the plasma concentration of tacrolimus (by as much as threefold) with coadministration of fluconazole may lead to the development of acute renal failure. It is important to note that tacrolimus alone is nephrotoxic; therefore, the combination of these agents may lead to an increased risk of nephrotoxicity.
Related Drugs: Increased tacrolimus concentrations after coadministration of clotrimazole troches with oral tacrolimus have been reported. Concomitant administration of ketoconazole with tacrolimus has also resulted in increased tacrolimus plasma concentrations.
Mechanism: The mechanism of this interaction is not known, but two possible mechanisms have been postulated. First, intestinal metabolism of tacrolimus may be reduced in the presence of fluconazole. There is evidence of abundant cytochrome P450 in the enterocytes of the human jejunal mucosa. Since metabolism of tacrolimus in the intestinal microsomes may occur, an alteration of the kinetics of tacrolimus may result. Second, it has also been shown *in vivo* and *in vitro* that fluconazole may inhibit the hepatic P450$_{3A}$ enzymes responsible for tacrolimus metabolism.
Detailed Information: See *EDI*, 18/22.30

Tacrolimus-Nifedipine

Significance: 3—minimally clinically significant

Potential Effects: Concurrent administration of nifedipine and tacrolimus may result in increased tacrolimus levels requiring decreased tacrolimus dosages.

Recommendations: Tacrolimus blood levels should be carefully monitored in patients receiving concurrent nifedipine therapy, especially when nifedipine is initiated or discontinued. The dosage of tacrolimus may need to be adjusted.

Summary: Concurrent administration of nifedipine and tacrolimus resulted in increased tacrolimus levels by as much as 55%, requiring decreased tacrolimus dosages.

Related Drugs: An *in vitro* study in human liver microsomes found verapamil to be a competitive inhibitor of tacrolimus metabolism. Conflicting data are available on the effect of diltiazem. A similar interaction may be expected to occur between tacrolimus and the other calcium channel blockers. There are no agents related to tacrolimus.

Mechanism: Tacrolimus is metabolized by cytochrome $P450_{3A4}$ in the small intestine and liver. *In vivo* studies using isolated human liver and intestinal microsomes with high cytochrome $P450_{3A4}$ content have found nifedipine to be a competitive inhibitor of tacrolimus metabolism. Elevated concentrations of tacrolimus have been associated with an increased incidence of nephrotoxicity, neurotoxicity, and diabetogenicity.

Detailed Information: See *EDI*, 18/22.80

Thyroid-Cholestyramine

Significance: 2—moderately clinically significant

Recommendations: Thyroxine and cholestyramine should be administered as far apart as possible (optimally four to six hours). When these drugs are used concurrently, the patient should be observed for symptoms of hypothyroidism (e.g., weakness, fatigue, cold intolerance, and dry, puffy skin). If possible, before cholestyramine is added to the drug regimen of a patient maintained on a thyroid preparation, baseline thyroid status should be determined. Periodic evaluation of thyroid status should be performed to detect changes in thyroid response.

Summary: Cholestyramine has been shown to cause a clinically significant decrease in the absorption of thyroid hormones.

Related Drugs: All thyroid compounds are expected to interact with cholestyramine. Colestipol may bind thyroid.

Mechanism: Cholestyramine forms strong ionic bonds with thyroid in the gastrointestinal tract, decreasing its absorption.

Detailed Information: See *EDI*, 18/23.00

Zidovudine-Atovaquone

Significance: 3—minimally clinically significant

Potential Effects: Concurrent administration of zidovudine and atovaquone may result in an increase in zidovudine serum levels.

Recommendations: The increase reported in zidovudine area-under-curve (AUC) by itself may not be clinically significant. However, this interaction may be clinically significant in those patients who are also receiving agents that may produce bone marrow toxicity. The dose of zidovudine may need to be decreased by one-third in those patients.

Summary: Concurrent administration of zidovudine and atovaquone resulted in increased zidovudine serum levels. Atovaquone pharmacokinetics were unaffected.

Related Drugs: It is not known whether an interaction would occur between atovaquone and the other reverse transcriptase inhibitors. There are no drugs related to atovaquone.

Mechanism: Atovaquone decreases the zidovudine-glucuronide AUC and the ratio of zidovudine-glucuronide AUC to zidovudine AUC. It is postulated that zidovudine glucuronidation is inhibited by atovaquone. It is also postulated that this elevated zidovudine concentration may allow a larger amount of the parent to be metabolized by the cytochrome P450 system. This would be important because formation of the 3'-amino-3'-deoxythymidine zidovudine metabolite is mediated by the cytochrome P450 system and has been shown to be five-fold to seven-fold more toxic to bone marrow cells than zidovudine.

Detailed Information: See *EDI*, 18/24.50

Zidovudine-Rifampin

Significance: 2—moderately clinically significant

Potential Effects: Concomitant zidovudine and rifampin may result in an increased clearance of zidovudine, which may lead to decreased effectiveness of antiretroviral therapy.

Recommendations: Zidovudine serum levels should be carefully monitored if rifampin is added to, or withdrawn from, concurrent therapy. The dose of zidovudine may need to be adjusted. This interaction may have clinical implications for optimal antiretroviral therapy.

Summary: There are data to show that concomitant zidovudine and rifampin may increase zidovudine clearance.

Related Drugs: Rifabutin was shown to interact similarly with zidovudine. There are no drugs related to zidovudine.

Mechanism: The interaction between rifampin or rifabutin and zidovudine may be caused by the induction of hepatic glucuronidation enzymes.

Detailed Information: See *EDI*, 18/25.00

Appendices

RELATED DRUGS

For the purpose of uniformity and consistency, the following groups of drugs have been arranged based on pharmacologic and chemical relationships. This appendix contains a complete list of the agents in a specific related drug class. If any of these agents are specifically implicated in a monograph by documentation or the mechanism of action of the primary drug interaction, a statement discussing their involvement appears in the Related Drugs section of the monograph.

Agents to Treat Shock
Dobutamine
Dopamine
Ephedrine
Epinephrine
Isoproterenol
Mephentermine
Metaraminol
Methoxamine
Norepinephrine
Phenylephrine

Aminoglycosides
Amikacin
Gentamicin
Kanamycin
Neomycin
Netilmicin
Streptomycin
Tobramycin

Androgen Derivatives

All Inclusive
Danazol
Dromostanolone
Ethylestrenol
Fluoxymesterone
Methandrostenolone
Methyltestosterone
Nandrolone
Oxandrolone
Oxymetholone
Stanozolol
Testolactone
Testosterone

C-17 Alkylated
Danazol
Ethylestrenol
Fluoxymesterone
Methandrostenolone
Methyltestosterone
Oxandrolone
Oxymetholone
Stanozolol

~ngiotensin Converting ~me Inhibitors
~zepril
~ril

Enalapril
Enalaprilat
Fosinopril
Lisinopril
Moexipril
Perindopril
Quinapril
Ramipril
Trandolapril
Trandolaprilat

Angiotensin II Receptor Antagonists
Candesartan
Eprosartan
Irbesartan
Losartan
Valsartan

Anorexiants
Benzphetamine
Diethylpropion
Fenfluramine
Mazindol
Phendimetrazine
Phenmetrazine
Phentermine
Phenylpropanolamine

Antacids
Aluminum Carbonate Gel, Basic
Aluminum Hydroxide Gel
Aluminum Phosphate Gel
Calcium Carbonate
Dihydroxyaluminum Aminoacetate
Dihydroxyaluminum Sodium Carbonate
Magaldrate
Magnesium Carbonate
Magnesium Hydroxide
Magnesium Oxide
Magnesium Trisilicate
Sodium Bicarbonate

Antiarrhythmics, Class I

(Subclass)
Disopyramide (*A*)
Encainide (*C*)

Flecainide (*C*)
Indecainide (*C*)
Lidocaine (*B*)
Mexiletine (*B*)
Moricizine
Procainamide (*A*)
Propafenone (*C*)
Quinidine *(A)*
Tocainide (*B*)

Anticholinergics
Anisotropine
Atropine
Belladonna
Benztropine
Biperiden
Clidinium
Dicyclomine
Emepronium
Ethopropazine
Glycopyrrolate
Hexocyclium
Hyoscyamine
Isopropamide
Mepenzolate
Methantheline
Methscopolamine
Oxybutynin
Oxyphencyclimine
Oxyphenonium
Procyclidine
Propantheline
Scopolamine
Tridihexethyl
Trihexyphenidyl

Anticoagulants, Oral
Coumarins
Acenocoumarol
Dicumarol
Nicoumalone
Phenprocoumon
Warfarin
Indandiones
Anisindione
Phenindione

Antihistamines
Nonsedating
Astemizole
Fexofenadine
Levocabastine
Loratadine
Terfenadine
Sedating
Astemizole
Azatadine
Azelastine
Bromodiphenhydramine

Brompheniramine
Buclizine
Carbinoxamine
Cetirizine
Chlorcyclizine
Chlorpheniramine
Clemastine
Cyclizine
Cyproheptadine
Dexchlorpheniramine
Dimethindene
Diphenhydramine
Hydroxyzine
Mebhydrolin
Meclizine
Mequitazine
Phenindamine
Pheniramine
Phenyltoloxamine
Pyrilamine
Tripelennamine
Triprolidine

Antineoplastic Alkylating Agents
Nitrogen Mustards
Chlorambucil
Cyclophosphamide
Ifosfamide
Mechlorethamine
Melphalan
Treosulfan
Nitrosoureas
Busulfan
Carmustine
Lomustine
Pipobroman
Streptozocin
Thiotepa
Uracil Mustard

Antineoplastic Antimetabolites
Cytarabine
Floxuridine
Fluorouracil
Mercaptopurine
Methotrexate
Thioguanine

Antiparkinsonism Anticholinergics
Belladonna
Benztropine
Biperiden
Cycrimine
Ethopropazine
Orphenadrine
Procyclidine
Trihexyphenidyl

Antipsychotics, Miscellaneous
Benperidol
Chlorprothixene
Clozapine
Flupenthixol
Haloperidol
Loxapine
Molindone
Pimozide
Reboxetine
Risperidone
Sertindole
Thiothixene
Trifluperidol

Barbiturates
General
Amobarbital
Aprobarbital
Barbital
Butabarbital
Butalbital
Butobarbitone
Hexobarbital
Mephobarbital
Metharbital
Pentobarbital
Phenobarbital
Primidone
Secobarbital
Talbutal
Anesthesia
Methohexital
Thiamylal
Thiopental

Benzodiazepines
Alprazolam
Bromazepam
Brotizolam
Chlordiazepoxide
Clobazam
Clonazepam
Clorazepate
Diazepam
Estazolam
Flunitrazepam
Flurazepam
Halazepam
Ketazolam
Lorazepam
Lormetazepam
Medazepam
Midazolam
Oxazepam
ʿazepam
ʿepam
ʾᵐam

Beta-Blocking Agents
Cardioselective (β_1)
Acebutolol
Atenolol
Betaxolol
Bisoprolol
Esmolol
Metoprolol
Noncardioselective (β_1 and β_2)

Carteolol
Carvedilol
Celiprolol
Labetalol
Levobunolol
Nadolol
Oxprenolol
Penbutolol
Pindolol
Propranolol
Sotalol
Tertatolol
Timolol
Ophthalmic
Betaxolol
Carteolol
Levobunolol
Metipranolol
Timolol

Bulk Producing Laxatives
Hemicellulose
Malt Extract
Methylcellulose
Psyllium

Calcium Channel Blockers
Amlodipine
Bepridil
Diltiazem
Felodipine
Isradipine
Lacidipine
Mibefradil
Nicardipine
Nifedipine
Nimodipine
Nilvadipine
Nisoldipine
Terodiline
Verapamil

Carbonic Anhydrase Inhibitors
Acetazolamide
Brinzolamide, Ophthalmic
Dichlorphenamide
Dorzolamide, Ophthalmic
Methazolamide

Central Nervous System Depressants
Acetylcarbromal
Alcohol, Ethyl
Chloral Hydrate
Ethchlorvynol
Ethinamate
Glutethimide
Meprobamate
Methyprylon
Paraldehyde

Cephalosporins
Cefaclor
Cefadroxil
Cefamandole
Cefazaflur
Cefazolin
Cefibuten
Cefdinir
Cefepime
Cefixime
Cefmetazole
Cefodizime
Cefonicid
Cefoperazone
Ceforanide
Cefotaxime
Cefotetan
Cefoxitin
Cefpirome
Cefpodoxime
Cefprozil
Cefsulodin
Ceftazidime
Ceftizoxime
Ceftriaxone
Cefuroxime
Cephalexin
Cephaloglycin
Cephalothin
Cephapirin
Cephradine
Loracarbef
Moxalactam

Corticosteroids
Beclomethasone
Betamethasone
Corticotropin
Cortisone
Cosyntropin
Desoxycorticosterone
Dexamethasone
Fludrocortisone
Fluocinolone
Fluocortolone
Flunisolide
Hydrocortisone
Methylprednisolone

Paramethasone
Prednisolone
Prednisone
Triamcinolone

Digitalis Glycosides
Deslanoside
Digitalis
Digitoxin
Digoxin

Ergot Alkaloids
Bromocriptine
Cabergoline
Dihydroergotamine
Ergoloid Mesylates
Ergonovine
Ergotamine
Methylergonovine
Methysergide

Estrogenic Substances
Chlorotrianisene
Conjugated Estrogens
Diethylstilbestrol
Esterified Estrogens
Estradiol
Estrone
Estropipate
Ethinyl Estradiol
Mestranol
Polyestradiol
Quinestrol

Fibric Acid Derivatives
Bezafibrate
Cifrofibrate
Clofibrate
Fenofibrate
Gemfibrozil

H_2-Receptor Antagonists
Cimetidine
Famotidine
Nizatidine
Ranitidine

Heparin, Low Molecular Weight
Ardeparin
Certoparin
Dalteparin
Enoxaparin
Tinzaparin

HMG-CoA Reductase Inhibitors
Atorvastatin
Fluvastatin
Lovastatin

Pravastatin
Simvastatin

Hydantoin Anticonvulsants
Ethotoin
Fosphenitoin
Mephenytoin
Phenytoin

Hydroxytryptamine (5HT$_1$)
Receptor Agonists
Naratriptan
Rizatriptan
Sumatriptan
Zolmitriptan

Imidazole Antifungal Agents
Butoconazole
Clotrimazole
Econazole
Fenliconazole
Fluconazole
Isoconazole
Itraconazole
Ketoconazole
Miconazole
Oxiconazole
Terconazole
Tioconazole

Inhalation Anesthetic Agents
General
Cyclopropane
Ether
Nitrous Oxide
Halogenated
Desflurane
Enflurane
Halothane
Isoflurane
Methoxyflurane

Local Anesthetics
Benzocaine
Bupivacaine
Chloroprocaine
Dibucaine
Etidocaine
Lidocaine
Mepivacaine
Piperocaine
Prilocaine
Procaine
Propoxycaine
Ropivacaine
Tetracaine

Loop Diuretics
Bumetanide
Ethacrynic Acid
Furosemide
Piretanide
Torsemide

Macrolide Antibiotics
Azithromycin
Clarithromycin
Dirithromycin
Erythromycin
Josamycin
Spiramycin
Troleandomycin

Monoamine Oxidase Inhibitors
Furazolidone
Hypericum
Isocarboxazid
Moclobemide
Pargyline
Phenelzine
Procarbazine
Selegiline
Tranylcypromine

Narcotics
Alfentanil
Buprenorphine
Codeine
Dextromoramide
Dezocine
Diamorphine
Diphenoxylate
Diphenoxin
Ethoheptazine
Fentanyl
Hydrocodone
Hydromorphone
Levorphanol
Meperidine
Meptazinol
Methadone
Morphine
Nalbuphine
Oxycodone
Oxymorphone
Pentazocine
Phenoperidine
Propoxyphene
Sufentanil
Tramadol

Neuromuscular Blocking Agents
Depolarizing
Succinylcholine
Nondepolarizing
Alcuronium
Atracurium
Cisatracurium

Doxacurium
Gallamine
Metocurine
Mivacurium
Pancuronium
Pipecuronium
Rocuronium
Tubocurarine
Vecuronium

Nitrate Derivatives
Amyl Nitrite
Erythrityl Tetranitrate
Isosorbide Dinitrate
Isosorbide Mononitrate
Nitroglycerin
Pentaerythritol Tetranitrate

Nonsteroidal Anti-inflammatory Agents
Acemetacin
Diclofenac
Etodolac
Felbinac
Fenoprofen
Flurbiprofen
Ibuprofen
Indomethacin
Ketoprofen
Ketorolac
Meclofenamate
Mefenamic Acid
Nabumetone
Naproxen
Nimesulide
Oxaprozin
Oxyphenbutazone
Phenylbutazone
Piroxicam
Sulindac
Suprofen
Tiaprofenic Acid
Tolmetin

Ophthalmic
Diclofenac
Flurbiprofen
Ketorolac
Oxyphenbutazone
Suprofen

Topical
Diclofenac
Felbinac
Ketoprofen
Naproxen
Piroxicam

Penicillins
Amoxicillin
Ampicillin
Azlocillin
Bacampicillin
Benethamine Penicillin
Carbenicillin
Carfecillin
Cloxacillin
Cyclacillin
Dicloxacillin
Mecillinam
Methicillin
Mezlocillin
Nafcillin
Oxacillin
Penicillin G
Penicillin V
Piperacillin
Pivampicillin
Pivmecillinam
Temocillin
Ticarcillin

Phenothiazines
Acetophenazine
Carphenazine
Chlorpromazine
Flupenthixol
Fluphenazine
Mesoridazine
Methdilazine
Pericyazine
Perphenazine
Piperacetazine
Pipotiazine
Prochlorperazine
Promazine
Promethazine
Propiomazine
Thiethylperazine
Thioproperazine
Thioridazine
Trifluoperazine
Triflupromazine
Trimeprazine
Zuclopenthixol

Polypeptide Antibiotics
Bacitracin
Capreomycin
Colistimethate
Colistin
Polymyxin B

Potassium-Sparing Diuretics
Amiloride
Potassium Canrenoate
Spironolactone
Triamterene

Progestins
Allylestrenol
Hydroxyprogesterone
Medroxyprogesterone

Megestrol
Norethindrone
Norgestimate
Norgestrel
Progesterone

Propanediol Derivatives
Carisoprodol
Chlorphenesin
Mephenesin
Meprobamate
Methocarbamol

Quinolone Antibacterials
Alatrovafluxocin
Cinoxacin
Ciprofloxacin
Clinafloxacin
Enoxacin
Fleroxacin
Grepafloxacin
Levofloxacin
Lomefloxacin
Nalidixic Acid
Norfloxacin
Ofloxacin
Rosoxacin
Sparfloxacin
Temafloxacin
Trovafloxacin

Ophthalmic
Ciprofloxacin
Norfloxacin
Ofloxacin

Rauwolfia Alkaloids
Alseroxylon
Deserpidine
Rauwolfia Serpentina
Rescinnamine
Reserpine

Retinoic Acid Derivatives
Acitretin
Isotretinoin
Retinol (Vitamin A)
Tretinoin

Salicylates
Aloxiprin
Aspirin
Calcium Carbaspirin
Choline Salicylate
Diflunisal
Magnesium Salicylate
Salicylamide
Salsalate
Sodium Salicylate
Sodium Thiosalicylate

Serotonin Reuptake Inhibitors

Selective
Citalopram
Fluoxetine
Fluvoxamine
Paroxetine
Sertraline

Nonselective
Nefazodone
Venlafaxine

Sulfonamides
Sulfacytine
Sulfadiazine
Sulfadoxine
Sulfamerazine
Sulfamethazine
Sulfamethizole
Sulfamethoxazole
Sulfapyridine
Sulfasalazine
Sulfisoxazole

Sulfonylureas
Acetohexamide
Chlorpropamide
Gliclazide
Glimepiride
Glipizide
Gliquidone
Glyburide
Tolazamide
Tolbutamide

Sympathomimetics
(a = alpha agonist activity,
b = beta agonist activity)

Direct Acting
Albuterol - b
Bitolterol - b
Dobutamine - a, b
Eformoterol - b
Epinephrine - a, b
Ethylnorepinephrine - b
Isoetharine - b
Isoproterenol - b
Metaproterenol - b
Methoxamine - a
Midodrine - a
Norepinephrine - a, b
Pirbuterol - b
Procaterol - b
Rimiterol - b
Ritodrine
Salmeterol - b
Terbutaline - b

Indirect Acting
Amphetamine - a, b
Benzphetamine - a, b

Dexfenfluramine - a, b
Dextroamphetamine - a, b
Diethylpropion - a, b
Ephedrine - a, b
Etafedrine - a, b
Fenfluramine - a, b
Isometheptene - a, b
Mazindol - a, b
Mephentermine - a, b
Methamphetamine - a, b
Methylphenidate - a, b
Phendimetrazine - a, b
Phenmetrazine - a, b
Phentermine - a, b
Phenylpropanolamine - a, b
Prolintane - a, b
Pseudoephedrine - a, b
Tyramine - a, b
Mixed Acting
Dopamine - a, b
Metaraminol - a, b
Phenylephrine - a, b

Tetracyclines
Chlortetracycline
Demeclocycline
Doxycycline
Methacycline
Minocycline
Oxytetracycline
Tetracycline

Theophylline Derivatives
Aminophylline
Dyphylline
Oxtriphylline
Theophylline

Thiazide Diuretics
Bendroflumethiazide
Benzthiazide
Chlorothiazide
Cyclopenthiazide
Cyclothiazide
Flumethiazide
Hydrochlorothiazide
Hydroflumethiazide
Methyclothiazide
Polythiazide
Trichlormethiazide
Xipamide

Thiazide-Related Diuretics
Chlorthalidone
Indapamide
Metolazone
Quinethazone

Thyroid Drugs
Dextrothyroxine

Levothyroxine
Liothyronine
Liotrix
Thyroglobulin
Thyrotropin
Thyroid

Tricyclic Antidepressants
Amitriptyline
Amoxapine
Butryptyline
Clomipramine
Desipramine
Dothiepin
Doxepin
Imipramine
Iprindole
Lofepramine
Nortriptyline
Protriptyline
Trimipramine

Urinary Acidifiers
Ammonium Biphosphate
Ammonium Chloride
Ascorbic Acid
Potassium Acid Phosphate
Sodium Acid Phosphate
Sodium Acid Pyrophosphate

Urinary Alkalinizers
Potassium Citrate
Sodium Acetate
Sodium Bicarbonate
Sodium Citrate
Sodium Lactate
Tromethamine

Vitamin D Analogues
Alfacalcidol
Calcifediol
Calcitriol
Cholecalciferol
Dihydrotachysterol
Ergocalciferol

CODE 1 INTERACTIONS

The following is an alphabetical listing of those drug-drug interactions that are classified in *Pocket Guide to EDI* as Code 1, or highly clinically significant, interactions. Receiving a Code 1 significance rating are interactions that are of great potential harm to the patient, that are predictable or frequent, and that are well documented. The page numbers of their respective monographs follow.

Alcohol, Ethyl-Disulfiram 311
Aminophylline-Halothane 327
Carbamazepine-Charcoal 103
Carbamazepine-Erythromycin 104
Chlorpropamide-Alcohol, Ethyl 296
Clonidine-Propranolol 160
Clozapine-Carbamazepine 230
Dicumarol-Allopurinol 69
Digitoxin-Rifampin 269
Digoxin-Amiodarone 271
Digoxin-Erythromycin Base 273
Digoxin-Propantheline 280
Digoxin-Quinidine 280
Digoxin-Tetracycline 282
Digoxin-Verapamil 284
Diltiazem-Cyclosporine 46
Erythromycin-Cyclosporine 183
Erythromycin-Terfenadine 184
Ether-Neomycin 25
Fluoxetine-Tranylcypromine 141
Furazolidone-Amphetamine 185
Gentamicin-Carbenicillin 185
Gentamicin-Cephalothin 185
Guanethidine-Chlorpromazine 162
Guanethidine-Desipramine 162
Halothane-Epinephrine 26
Heparin-Aspirin 71
Insulin-Guanethidine 302
Insulin-Propranolol 304
Kanamycin-Ethacrynic Acid 191
Ketoconazole-Cyclosporine 193
Ketoconazole-Terfenadine 195
Lidocaine-Cimetidine 53
Lincomycin-Kaolin 196
Lithium Carbonate-Acetazolamide 238
Lithium Carbonate-Chlorothiazide 239
Lovastatin-Erythromycin 359
Lovastatin-Grapefruit Juice 360
Meperidine-Phenelzine 14
Mercaptopurine-Allopurinol 215
Metformin-Iodinated Contrast Media 305
Methotrexate-Aspirin 216
Methotrexate-Leucovorin 218
Methotrexate-Probenecid 219
Methotrexate-Sulfamethoxazole, Trimethoprim 220
Phenelzine-Levodopa 152
Phenytoin-Cimetidine 115
Phenytoin-Disulfiram 118

Phenytoin-Dopamine 118
Phenytoin-Fluconazole 119
Propranolol-Cimetidine 258
Propranolol-Epinephrine 260
Pyridoxine-Levodopa 325
Quinidine-Amiodarone 61
Quinidine-Verapamil 65
Rifampin-Cyclosporine 202
Rifampin-Oral Contraceptive Agents 202
Spironolactone-Potassium Chloride 292
Tetracycline-Aluminum Hydroxide 205
Tetracycline-Ferrous Sulfate 205
Theophylline-Charcoal 333
Theophylline-Cimetidine 334
Theophylline-Erythromycin 335
Theophylline-Tobacco 343
Tolbutamide-Phenylbutazone 307
Tranylcypromine-Phenylpropanolamine 153
Triazolam-Ketoconazole 250
Tubocurarine-Gentamicin 40
Warfarin-Amiodarone 75
Warfarin-Aspirin 76
Warfarin-Cimetidine 79
Warfarin-Clofibrate 80
Warfarin-Disulfiram 81
Warfarin-Erythromycin 82
Warfarin-Glucagon 86
Warfarin-Glutethimide 86
Warfarin-Methyltestosterone 90
Warfarin-Nalidixic Acid 92
Warfarin-Phenobarbital 94
Warfarin-Phenylbutazone 94
Warfarin-Phytonadione 95
Warfarin-Rifampin 97
Warfarin-Sulfamethoxazole 98
Warfarin-Sulfinpyrazone 98
Warfarin-Thyroid 100

Index

The *Pocket Guide* index, an abbreviated version of the one found in *Evaluations of Drug Interactions*, includes all drugs mentioned in a monograph title and all other drugs involved in highly significant interactions. Drugs related to those mentioned in a monograph title that are involved in minimally significant interactions are not indexed.

Some of the index entries contain, in addition to page numbers, a boldface number. This refers to the significance code of a drug interaction. Significance codes are included only for drugs mentioned in a monograph title, not for other drugs that may be mentioned in a monograph.

For an explanation of the significance coding, see How to Use *Pocket Guide to Evaluations of Drug Interactions*, page vii.

Acarbose,
    digoxin **3,** 269
    warfarin **3,** 74
Acebutolol hydrochloride,
    epinephrine, 260
    insulin, 302
Acenocoumarol,
    allopurinol, 69
    aloxiprin, 76
    aminoglutethimide, 86
    amiodarone hydrochloride, 75
    amobarbital, 94
    aprobarbital, 94
    aspirin, 76
    barbital, 94
    butabarbital sodium, 94
    butalbital, 94
    butobarbitone, 94
    calcium carbaspirin, 76
    cetirizine **3,** 69
    clarithromycin, 82
    clofibrate, 80
    danazol, 90
    dextrothyroxine sodium, 100
    diflunisal, 76
    disulfiram, 81
    erythromycin, 82
    erythromycin estolate, 82
    erythromycin ethylsuccinate, 82
    erythromycin gluceptate, 82
    erythromycin lactobionate, 82
    erythromycin stearate, 82
    ethylestrenol, 90
    feprazone, 94
    fluoxymesterone, 90
    gemfibrozil, 80
    glucagon, 86
    glucagon, recombinant, 86
    glutethimide, 86
    levothyroxine sodium, 100
    liothyronine sodium, 100
    menadiol sodium diphosphate,
        vitamin K4, 95
    menadione, 95
    mephobarbital, 94
    methandrostenolone, 90
    metharbital, 94
    methohexital sodium, 94
    methyltestosterone, 90
    methyprylon, 86
    nalidixic acid, 92
    norfloxacin, 92
    oxandrolone, 90
    oxymetholone, 90
    oxyphenbutazone, 94
    pentobarbital sodium, 94
    phenobarbital, 94
    phenylbutazone, 94
    phytonadione, vitamin K1, 95
    primidone, 94
    rifabutin, 97
    rifampin, 97
    secobarbital, 94
    sodium salicylate, 76
    stanozolol, 90
    talbutal, 94
    thiamylal sodium, 94
    thiopental sodium, 94
    thyroglobulin, 100
    thyroid desiccated, 100
    thyroid strong, 100
Acetaminophen,
    alcohol, ethyl-oral/injectable **3,** 2
    charcoal **3,** 2
    chloramphenicol **3,** 176
    isoniazid **3,** 2
    lamotrigine **3,** 110
    oral contraceptive agents **3,** 2
    oral contraceptives,
        low-dose **3,** 2
    phenobarbital **3,** 3
    phenytoin **3,** 3
    propranolol hydrochloride **3,** 3
    sulfinpyrazone **3,** 4
    terfenadine **2,** 4
    warfarin **3,** 75
    zidovudine **3,** 208
Acetazolamide,
    aspirin **2,** 6
    cyclosporine **2,** 286
    lithium **1,** 238
    phenytoin **4,** 111

primidone **3,** 129
timolol maleate, ophthalmic **3,** 264
Acetohexamide,
alcohol, ethyl - oral/injectable, 296
feprazone, 307
oxyphenbutazone, 307
phenylbutazone, 307
Acetophenazine maleate,
guanethidine, 162
Acetylcysteine,
bacampicillin hydrochloride **3,** 173
Acyclovir, oral,
probenecid **3,** 173
zidovudine **3,** 208
Acyclovir, parenteral,
lithium **3,** 238
Adenosine, parenteral,
caffeine **3,** 330
Albuterol sulfate,
chloroform, 26
enflurane, 26
halothane, 26
methoxyflurane, 26
metoprolol tartrate, 260
timolol maleate, oral, 260
Alcohol, ethyl - oral/injectable,
acetaminophen **3,** 2
acetohexamide, 296
amitriptyline hydrochloride **2,** 310
aspirin **2,** 6
bromocriptine mesylate **3,** 310
calcium carbimide, 311
cefoperazone sodium 2, 174
chloral hydrate **2,** 313
chlorpromazine hydrochloride **2,** 225
chlorpropamide **1,** 296
cimetidine, oral **3,** 310
diazepam **2,** 232
diphenhydramine **2,** 310
disopyramide phosphate **3,** 47
disulfiram **1,** 311
fluoxetine hydrochloride **4**, 311
furazolidone **2,** 311
gliclazide, 296
glimepiride, 296
glipizide, 296
gliquidone, 296
glutethimide **2,** 312
glyburide, 296
guanethidine **2,** 161
ketoconazole **3,** 312
lithium **3,** 239
meprobamate **2,** 315
methotrexate **3,** 216
metoclopramide hydrochloride **3,** 312
metronidazole, systemic **2,** 313

monosulfiram, 311
nifedipine **3,** 57
nitric oxide, inhalation **2,** 29
phenobarbital **2,** 315
phenytoin **2,** 112
procainamide hydrochloride **3,** 59
propoxyphene **2,** 20
propranolol hydrochloride **3,** 256
thiram, topical, 311
tolazamide, 296
tolbutamide, 296
warfarin **3,** 75
Alcuronium chloride,
amikacin sulfate, 40
bacitracin, 40
colistin sulfate, 40
demeclocycline hydrochloride, 40
doxycycline hyclate, parenteral, 40
doxycycline hydrochloride, 40
gentamicin sulfate, 40
kanamycin sulfate, oral, 40
kanamycin sulfate, parenteral, 40
lymecycline, 40
methacycline hydrochloride, 40
minocycline hydrochloride pellets, 40
minocycline hydrochloride, 40
minocycline, parenteral, 40
neomycin sulfate, oral, 40
neomycin sulfate, parenteral, 40
netilmicin, 40
oxytetracycline, 40
oxytetracycline, parenteral, 40
paromomycin sulfate, 40
polymyxin B sulfate, 40
polymyxin B sulfate, vaccine use, 40
rolitetracycline, injectable, 40
streptomycin sulfate, 40
tetracycline, 40
tetracycline hydrochloride, parenteral, 40
tobramycin, 40
Aldesleukin, interleukin-2 human,
dexamethasone **2,** 214
Alfentanil hydrochloride,
erythromycin **2,** 5
isocarboxazid, 14
pargyline hydrochloride, 14
phenelzine sulfate, 14
selegiline hydrochloride, 14
tranylcypromine sulfate, 14
Allergenic extract,
propranolol hydrochloride **3,** 256
Allopurinol,
acenocoumarol, 69
aluminum hydroxide **3,** 5
ampicillin sodium **3,** 173
anisindione, 69

azathioprine sodium, 215
captopril **3,** 156
chlorpropamide **3,** 296
cyclophosphamide **2,** 211
cyclosporine **2,** 349
dicumarol **1,** 69
ferrous sulfate **4,** 322
mercaptopurine **1,** 215
nicoumalone, 69
phenytoin **2,** 112
probenecid **3,** 5
theophylline **2,** 331
vidarabine **2,** 208
warfarin, 69
Aloxiprin,
    acenocoumarol, 76
    anisindione, 76
    dicumarol, 76
    heparin, 71
    methotrexate, 215
    methotrexate sodium, parenteral,
        216
    nicoumalone, 76
    phenindione, 76
    warfarin, 76
Alprazolam,
    fluoxetine hydrochloride **2,** 224
    itraconazole, 250
    ketoconazole, 250
Alteplase, recombinant,
    nitroglycerin **2,** 346
Aluminum carbonate, basic,
    demeclocycline hydrochloride,
        205
    doxycycline hydrochloride, 205
    methacycline hydrochloride, 205
    oxytetracycline, 205
    tetracycline, 205
Aluminum hydroxide,
    allopurinol **3,** 5
    aspirin **2,** 7
    captopril **3,** 156
    chlorpromazine hydrochloride **3,**
        225
    cholecalciferol, vitamin D3 **2,** 320
    cimetidine, oral **3,** 347
    ciprofloxacin hydrochloride **2,** 178
    citric acid **3,** 346
    clorazepate dipotassium **3,** 229
    demeclocycline hydrochloride,
        205
    digoxin **2,** 270
    doxycycline hydrochloride, 205
    ethambutol hydrochloride **3,** 184
    ferrous sulfate **3,** 322
    indomethacin **3,** 12
    isoniazid **3,** 188
    ketoconazole 2, 191
    levodopa **3,** 355
    methacycline hydrochloride, 204
    mexiletine hydrochloride **3,** 54

misoprostol **3,** 362
oxytetracycline, 205
penicillamine **3,** 364
phenytoin **3,** 112
prednisone **3,** 365
propranolol hydrochloride **3,** 257
quinidine **3,** 64
tetracycline **1,** 205
theophylline **3,** 332
ticlopidine hydrochloride **3,** 73
valproic acid **3,** 130
vitamin D3, prenatal multivitamin
    use **2,** 320
Aluminum oxide,
    demeclocycline hydrochloride,
        205
    doxycycline hydrochloride, 205
    methacycline hydrochloride, 205
    oxytetracycline, 205
    tetracycline, 205
Aluminum phosphate,
    demeclocycline hydrochloride,
        205
    doxycycline hydrochloride, 205
    methacycline hydrochloride, 205
    oxytetracycline, 205
    tetracycline, 205
Amantadine hydrochloride,
    triamterene **3,** 292
Amikacin sulfate,
    alcuronium chloride, 40
    amoxicillin, 185
    atracurium besylate, 39
    azlocillin sodium, 185
    bacampicillin hydrochloride, 185
    benethamine penicillin, 185
    bumetanide, 191
    bumetanide, injectable, 191
    carbenicillin disodium, 185
    cefprozil, 185
    ceftibuten dihyrate, 185
    cefuroxime, 185
    cephalexin, 185
    cephalothin sodium, 185
    cloxacillin sodium, 185
    cyclacillin, 185
    dicloxacillin, 185
    doxacurium chloride, 40
    enflurane, 25
    ethacrynic acid, 191
    ethacrynic acid, injectable, 191
    ether, 25
    flucloxacillin, 185
    furosemide, 191
    furosemide, injectable, 191
    gallamine triethiodide, 39
    halothane, 25
    isoflurane, 25
    methicillin sodium, 185
    methoxyflurane, 25
    metocurine iodide, 39

mezlocillin sodium, 185
mivacurium chloride, 39
moxalactam disodium, 185
nafcillin sodium, 185
nitrous oxide, 25
oxacillin sodium, 185
pancuronium bromide, 39
penicillin G, 185
penicillin G benzathine, 185
penicillin G procaine, 185
penicillin V, 185
pipecuronium bromide, 39
piperacillin sodium, 185
piretanide, 191
rocuronium bromide, 39
succinylcholine chloride, 39
temocillin sodium, 185
ticarcillin disodium, 185
torsemide, injection, 191
torsemide, oral, 191
tubocurarine chloride, 39
vecuronium bromide, 39
Amiloride hydrochloride,
  potassium acetate, 290
  potassium bicarbonate, 290
  potassium biphosphate, 290
  potassium chloride, 290
  potassium citrate, 290
  potassium gluconate, 290
  potassium iodide, 290
  potassium iodide, prenatal
    multivitamin use, 290
  potassium perchlorate, 290
  potassium phosphate, 290
  potassium salicylate, 290
  potassium, salt unspecified, 290
Aminoglutethimide,
  acenocoumarol, 86
  anisindione, 86
  bendroflumethiazide **3,** 286
  dexamethasone **2,** 352
  dicumarol, 86
  digitoxin **3,** 268
  medroxyprogesterone acetate **3,** 361
  nicoumalone, 86
  propranolol hydrochloride **3,** 257
  theophylline **3,** 332
  warfarin, 86
Aminophylline,
  cimetidine hydrochloride,
    parenteral, 332
  cimetidine, oral, 332
  diazepam **3,** 231
  erythromycin, 333
  erythromycin estolate, 335
  erythromycin ethylsuccinate, 335
  erythromycin gluceptate, 335
  erythromycin lactobionate, 335
  erythromycin stearate, 335
  halothane **1,** 327

imipenem in combination with
  cilastatin **3,** 327
interferon alfa-2a **2,** 327
isoproterenol **3,** 328
ketamine hydrochloride **3,** 328
levothyroxine sodium **3,** 328
oral contraceptive agents **3,** 329
oral contraceptives, low-dose **3,** 329
pancuronium bromide **2,** 30
propofol **3,** 33
tacrine hydrochloride **2,** 329
thiabendazole **2,** 329
tobacco, 343
Aminosalicylic acid,
  digoxin **3,** 270
  rifampin **4,** 201
Amiodarone hydrochloride,
  acenocoumarol, 75
  anisindione, 75
  cholestyramine **3,** 45
  cyclosporine **2,** 45
  deslanoside, 269
  dicumarol, 75
  digitalis, 269
  digitoxin, 269
  digoxin **1,** 271
  digoxin capsule, stabilized, 269
  diltiazem hydrochloride **2,** 45
  flecainide acetate **2,** 51
  lidocaine hydrochloride, systemic **2,** 46
  metoprolol tartrate **2,** 254
  nicoumalone, 75
  phenytoin **2,** 113
  procainamide hydrochloride **2,** 59
  quinidine **1,** 61
  warfarin **1,** 75
Amitriptyline hydrochloride,
  alcohol, ethyl - oral/injectable **2,** 308
  chlordiazepoxide **3,** 135
  disulfiram **3,** 135
  fluconazole **2,** 135
  guanadrel sulfate, 163
  guanethidine, 163
  methyldopa **3,** 165
  morphine **3,** 16
  valproic acid **3,** 130
Ammonium chloride,
  amphetamine **3,** 347
  flecainide acetate **2,** 51
  methadone hydrochloride **3,** 15
  mexiletine hydrochloride **3,** 55
Amobarbital,
  acenocoumarol, 94
  anisindione, 94
  dicumarol, 94
  nicoumalone, 94
  tranylcypromine sulfate **3,** 313
  warfarin, 94

Amoxapine,
  guanethidine, 163
Amoxicillin,
  amikacin sulfate, 185
  gentamicin sulfate, 185
  netilmicin, 185
  tobramycin, 185
Amphetamine,
  ammonium chloride **3,** 347
  chloroform, 26
  chlorpromazine hydrochloride **2,** 226
  enflurane, 26
  furazolidone **1,** 185
  halothane, 26
  isocarboxazid, 184
  methoxyflurane, 26
  pargyline hydrochloride, 184
  phenelzine sulfate, 184
  procarbazine hydrochloride, 184
  propoxyphene **3,** 20
  sodium bicarbonate **3,** 347
  tranylcypromine sulfate, 184
Amphotericin B,
  cyclosporine **2,** 181
Ampicillin sodium,
  allopurinol **3,** 173
  amikacin sulfate, 185
  atenolol **3,** 253
  gentamicin sulfate, 185
  kanamycin sulfate, oral, 185
  kanamycin sulfate, parenteral, 185
  neomycin sulfate, oral, 185
  neomycin sulfate, parenteral, 185
  netilmicin, 185
  oral contraceptive agents **2,** 173
  paromomycin sulfate, 185
  streptomycin sulfate, 185
  sulfasalazine **3,** 204
  tobramycin, 185
Anileridine,
  isocarboxazid, 14
  pargyline hydrochloride, 14
  phenelzine sulfate, 14
  selegiline hydrochloride, 14
  tranylcypromine sulfate, 14
Anisindione,
  allopurinol, 69
  aloxiprin, 76
  aminoglutethimide, 86
  amiodarone hydrochloride, 78
  amobarbital, 94
  aprobarbital, 94
  aspirin, 76
  butabarbital sodium, 94
  butalbital, 94
  butobarbitone, 94
  calcium carbaspirin, 76
  clofibrate, 80
  danazol, 90
  diflunisal, 76

  disulfiram, 81
  erythromycin, 82
  erythromycin estolate, 82
  erythromycin ethylsuccinate, 82
  erythromycin gluceptate, 82
  erythromycin lactobionate, 82
  erythromycin stearate, 82
  feprazone, 94
  glucagon, 86
  glucagon, recombinant, 86
  glutethimide, 86
  levothyroxine sodium, 100
  methyltestosterone, 90
  nalidixic acid, 92
  norfloxacin, 92
  oxymetholone, 90
  oxyphenbutazone, 94
  pentobarbital sodium, 94
  phenobarbital, 94
  phenylbutazone, 94
  rifabutin, 97
  rifampin, 97
  secobarbital, 94
  sodium salicylate, 76
  thyroid desiccated, 100
  thyroid strong, 100
Anisotropine methylbromide,
  digoxin, 278
Aprobarbital,
  acenocoumarol, 94
  anisindione, 94
  dicumarol, 94
  nicoumalone, 94
  warfarin, 94
Arbutamine hydrochloride,
  chloroform, 26
  enflurane, 26
  halothane, 26
  methoxyflurane, 26
Ardeparin sodium,
  certoparin, 71
  dalteparin sodium, 71
  enoxaparin, 71
  sodium salicylate, 76
  tinzaparin sodium, 71
Ascorbic acid, vitamin C,
  aspirin **4,** 320
  ethinyl estradiol **3,** 320
  ferrous sulfate **3,** 322
  warfarin **4,** 76
Aspirin,
  acenocoumarol, 76
  acetazolamide **2,** 6
  alcohol, ethyl - oral/injectable **2,** 6
  aluminum hydroxide **2,** 7
  anisindione, 76
  ascorbic acid, vitamin C **4,** 318
  captopril **2,** 157
  charcoal **3,** 7
  chlorpropamide **2,** 296
  dicumarol, 76

dipyridamole **3,** 7
fluoxetine hydrochloride **3,** 139
furosemide **3,** 289
ginkgo **3,** 8
griseofulvin **3,** 8
heparin **1,** 71
indomethacin **3,** 12
insulin **3,** 301
magnesium hydroxide **2,** 7
methotrexate **1,** 216
methotrexate sodium, parenteral,
  215
methylprednisolone **2,** 8
niacin, vitamin B3 **3,** 324
nicoumalone, 76
nitroglycerin **3,** 9
oral contraceptive agents **3,** 9
penicillin G **3,** 199
phenytoin 4, 113
propranolol hydrochloride **3,** 257
spironolactone **3,** 292
sulfinpyrazone **2,** 21
valproic acid **2,** 131
warfarin **1,** 76
Astemizole,
  clarithromycin, 183
  erythromycin, 183
  erythromycin estolate, 183
  erythromycin ethylsuccinate, 183
  erythromycin gluceptate, 183
  erythromycin lactobionate, 183
  erythromycin stearate, 183
  itraconazole, 194
  ketoconazole, 194
  spiramycin, 183
  troleandomycin, 183
Atenolol,
  ampicillin sodium **3,** 253
  calcium carbonate, oral **3,** 253
  clonidine hydrochloride,
    transdermal, 160
  clonidine hydrochloride, 160
  disopyramide phosphate **3,** 47
  propantheline bromide **3,** 253
Atorvastatin calcium,
  grapefruit juice, 356
Atovaquone,
  zidovudine **2,** 368
Atracurium besylate,
  amikacin sulfate, 40
  colistin sulfate, 40
  kanamycin sulfate, oral, 40
  kanamycin sulfate, parenteral, 40
  neomycin sulfate, oral, 40
  neomycin sulfate, parenteral, 40
  netilmicin, 40
  paromomycin sulfate, 40
  streptomycin sulfate, 40
  tranylcypromine sulfate **3,** 153
Atropine,
  digoxin, 278

metoclopramide hydrochloride **3,**
  361
mexiletine hydrochloride **3,** 55
Attapulgite,
  demeclocycline hydrochloride,
    204
  doxycycline hydrochloride, 204
  kaolin, 204
  lymecycline, 204
  methacycline hydrochloride, 204
  minocycline hydrochloride
    pellets, 204
  minocycline hydrochloride, 204
  oxytetracycline, 204
  tetracycline, 204
Azathioprine sodium,
  allopurinol, 214
  cyclosporine **3,** 349
  enalapril maleate **3,** 160
  pancuronium bromide **3,** 30
  warfarin **2,** 77
Azithromycin,
  cyclosporine, 182
  warfarin, 82
Azlocillin sodium,
  amikacin sulfate, 185
  gentamicin sulfate, 185
  netilmicin, 185
  tobramycin, 185
Bacampicillin hydrochloride,
  acetylcysteine **3,** 173
  amikacin sulfate, 185
  gentamicin sulfate, 185
  netilmicin, 185
  tobramycin, 185
Bacitracin,
  alcuronium chloride, 40
  doxacurium chloride, 40
  ether, 25
  gallamine triethiodide, 40
  methoxyflurane, 25
  metocurine iodide, 40
  mivacurium chloride, 40
  pancuronium bromide, 40
  pipecuronium bromide, 40
  rocuronium bromide, 40
  succinylcholine chloride, 40
  tubocurarine chloride, 40
  vecuronium bromide, 40
Baclofen,
  ibuprofen **3,** 11
Barbital,
  acenocoumarol, 94
  dicumarol, 94
  nicoumalone, 94
  phenindione, 94
  warfarin, 94
Belladonna,
  digoxin, 278
Bellafoline,
  digoxin, 278

Bendroflumethiazide,
  aminoglutethimide **3,** 286
  indomethacin **3,** 286
  lithium, 238
Benethamine penicillin,
  amikacin sulfate, 185
  gentamicin sulfate, 185
  kanamycin sulfate, oral, 185
  kanamycin sulfate, parenteral, 185
  neomycin sulfate, oral, 185
  neomycin sulfate, parenteral, 185
  netilmicin, 185
  paromomycin sulfate, 185
  streptomycin sulfate, 185
  tobramycin, 185
Benserazide,
  orphenadrine citrate **3,** 356
Benzphetamine hydrochloride,
  chloroform, 26
  enflurane, 26
  furazolidone, 184
  halothane, 26
  isocarboxazid, 184
  methoxyflurane, 26
  moclobemide, 153
  pargyline hydrochloride, 153
  phenelzine sulfate, 153
  procarbazine hydrochloride, 153
  tranylcypromine sulfate, 153
Benzthiazide,
  lithium, 238
Benztropine mesylate,
  chlorpromazine hydrochloride **2,** 226
  digoxin, 278
Betaxolol hydrochloride, oral,
  epinephrine, 259
  insulin, 302
Bethanidine sulphate,
  chlorpromazine hydrochloride, 162
  desipramine hydrochloride, 163
  mazindol **2,** 156
Bezafibrate,
  dicumarol, 80
  phenindione, 80
  warfarin, 80
Biperiden,
  digoxin, 278
Bismuth subsalicylate,
  demeclocycline hydrochloride, 204
  doxycycline hydrochloride, 204
  methacycline hydrochloride, 204
  oxytetracycline, 204
  tetracycline, 204
Bisoprolol fumarate,
  epinephrine, 259
  insulin, 302
Bitolterol mesylate,
  chloroform, 26

  enflurane, 26
  halothane, 26
  methoxyflurane, 26
  metoprolol tartrate, 259
  timolol maleate, oral, 259
Bleomycin sulfate,
  cisplatin **3,** 211
Brinzolamide, ophthalmic,
  lithium, 237
Bromocriptine mesylate,
  alcohol, ethyl - oral/injectable **3,** 310
  thioridazine hydrochloride **2,** 250
Bumetanide,
  amikacin sulfate, 191
  gentamicin sulfate, 191
  kanamycin sulfate, oral, 191
  kanamycin sulfate, parenteral, 191
  lithium, 238
  neomycin sulfate, oral, 191
  neomycin sulfate, parenteral, 191
  netilmicin, 191
  probenecid **3,** 291
  streptomycin sulfate, 191
  tobramycin, 191
Bumetanide, injectable,
  amikacin sulfate, 191
  gentamicin sulfate, 191
  kanamycin sulfate, oral, 191
  kanamycin sulfate, parenteral, 191
  lithium, 238
  neomycin sulfate, oral, 191
  neomycin sulfate, parenteral, 191
  netilmicin, 191
  streptomycin sulfate, 191
  tobramycin, 191
Bupivacaine hydrochloride,
  diazepam **3,** 24
  ritodrine hydrochloride **2,** 24
Buprenorphine hydrochloride,
  isocarboxazid, 14
  pargyline hydrochloride, 14
  phenelzine sulfate, 14
  selegiline hydrochloride, 14
  tranylcypromine sulfate, 14
Bupropion hydrochloride,
  carbamazepine **3,** 136
  imipramine **3,** 142
Buspirone hydrochloride,
  cimetidine, oral **4,** 224
  erythromycin **3,** 136
  fluoxetine hydrochloride **3,** 137
  itraconazole **3,** 190
  phenelzine sulfate **3,** 151
Butabarbital sodium,
  acenocoumarol, 94
  anisindione, 94
  dicumarol, 94
  nicoumalone, 94
  warfarin, 94
Butalbital,

acenocoumarol, 94
anisindione, 94
dicumarol, 94
nicoumalone, 94
warfarin, 94
Butobarbitone,
acenocoumarol, 94
anisindione, 94
dicumarol, 94
nicoumalone, 94
phenindione, 94
warfarin, 94
Butoconazole nitrate,
cyclosporine, 192
phenytoin, 119
Butorphanol tartrate,
pargyline hydrochloride, 14
phenelzine sulfate, 14
selegiline hydrochloride, 14
tranylcypromine sulfate, 14
Butriptyline hydrochloride,
guanadrel sulfate, 163
guanethidine, 163
Caffeine,
adenosine, parenteral **3,** 330
cimetidine hydrochloride,
parenteral, 332
cimetidine, oral, 332
clozapine, 230
erythromycin, 335
erythromycin estolate, 335
erythromycin ethylsuccinate, 335
erythromycin gluceptate, 335
erythromycin lactobionate, 335
erythromycin stearate, 335
methoxsalen **3,** 330
oral contraceptive agents **3,** 330
oral contraceptives, low-dose **3,**
330
phenylpropanolamine **3,** 331
theophylline **2,** 332
Calcium acetate,
demeclocycline hydrochloride,
205
doxycycline hydrochloride, 205
methacycline hydrochloride, 205
oxytetracycline, 205
tetracycline, 205
Calcium ascorbate,
demeclocycline hydrochloride,
205
doxycycline hydrochloride, 205
methacycline hydrochloride, 205
oxytetracycline, 205
tetracycline, 205
Calcium carbaspirin,
acenocoumarol, 76
anisindione, 76
heparin, 71
methotrexate, 215
methotrexate sodium,

parenteral, 215
nicoumalone, 76
phenindione, 76
warfarin, 76
Calcium carbimide,
alcohol, ethyl - oral/injectable, 309
warfarin, 81
Calcium carbonate, oral,
atenolol **3,** 253
chlorothiazide **2,** 287
demeclocycline hydrochloride,
205
doxycycline hydrochloride, 205
levothyroxine sodium **3,** 357
methacycline hydrochloride, 205
oxytetracycline, 205
tetracycline, 205
Calcium chloride, injectable,
digitalis **2,** 267
Calcium chloride, oral,
demeclocycline hydrochloride,
205
doxycycline hydrochloride, 205
methacycline hydrochloride, 205
oxytetracycline, 205
tetracycline, 205
Calcium citrate, oral,
demeclocycline hydrochloride,
205
doxycycline hydrochloride, 205
methacycline hydrochloride, 205
oxytetracycline, 205
tetracycline, 205
Calcium glubionate, oral,
demeclocycline hydrochloride,
205
doxycycline hydrochloride, 205
methacycline hydrochloride, 205
oxytetracycline, 205
tetracycline, 205
Calcium glucoheptonate,
demeclocycline hydrochloride,
205
doxycycline hydrochloride, 205
methacycline hydrochloride, 205
oxytetracycline, 205
tetracycline, 205
Calcium gluconate, oral,
demeclocycline hydrochloride,
205
doxycycline hydrochloride, 205
methacycline hydrochloride, 205
oxytetracycline, 205
tetracycline, 205
verapamil hydrochloride **2,** 65
Calcium glycerophosphate, oral,
demeclocycline hydrochloride,
205
doxycycline hydrochloride, 205
methacycline hydrochloride, 205
oxytetracycline, 205

tetracycline, 205
Calcium iodate,
 demeclocycline hydrochloride, 205
 doxycycline hydrochloride, 205
 metformin hydrochloride **1,** 305
 methacycline hydrochloride, 205
 oxytetracycline, 205
 tetracycline, 205
Calcium lactate gluconate,
 demeclocycline hydrochloride, 205
 doxycycline hydrochloride, 205
 methacycline hydrochloride, 205
 oxytetracycline, 205
 tetracycline, 205
Calcium lactate, oral,
 demeclocycline hydrochloride, 205
 doxycycline hydrochloride, 205
 methacycline hydrochloride, 205
 oxytetracycline, 205
 tetracycline, 205
Calcium lactobionate, oral,
 demeclocycline hydrochloride, 205
 doxycycline hydrochloride, 205
 lymecycline, 205
 methacycline hydrochloride, 205
 minocycline hydrochloride pellets, 205
 minocycline hydrochloride, 205
 oxytetracycline, 205
 tetracycline, 205
Calcium phosphate, oral,
 demeclocycline hydrochloride, 205
 doxycycline hydrochloride, 205
 methacycline hydrochloride, 205
 oxytetracycline, 205
 tetracycline, 205
Calcium, oral salt unspecified,
 demeclocycline hydrochloride, 205
 doxycycline hydrochloride, 205
 methacycline hydrochloride, 205
 oxytetracycline, 205
 tetracycline, 205
Captopril,
 allopurinol **3,** 156
 aluminum hydroxide **3,** 156
 aspirin **2,** 157
 chlorpromazine hydrochloride **2,** 157
 digoxin **2,** 271
 furosemide **2,** 157
 indomethacin **2,** 157
 magnesium carbonate **3,** 156
 magnesium hydroxide **3,** 156
 naloxone hydrochloride **3,** 158
 nitroprusside sodium **3,** 168
 potassium chloride **3,** 158
 probenecid **3,** 159
 spironolactone **3,** 292
Carbamazepine,
 bupropion hydrochloride **3,** 136
 charcoal **1,** 103
 cimetidine, oral **2,** 103
 clarithromycin, 104
 clonazepam **3,** 108
 clozapine **1,** 230
 cyclosporine **2,** 349
 danazol **2,** 103
 desipramine hydrochloride **3,** 104
 doxycycline hydrochloride **2,** 182
 erythromycin **1,** 104
 erythromycin estolate, 104
 erythromycin ethylsuccinate, 104
 erythromycin gluceptate, 104
 erythromycin lactobionate, 104
 erythromycin stearate, 104
 ethosuximide **3,** 109
 felbamate **2,** 104
 haloperidol **2,** 237
 hydrochlorothiazide **3,** 105
 isoniazid **2,** 105
 isotretinoin **3,** 105
 lithium **2,** 239
 metoclopramide hydrochloride **3,** 106
 metronidazole, systemic **2,** 106
 niacinamide (nicotinamide) **3,** 106
 oral contraceptive agents **3,** 107
 oral contraceptives, low-dose **3,** 107
 pancuronium bromide **3,** 30
 phenobarbital **3,** 107
 phenytoin **3,** 113
 propoxyphene **2,** 107
 terfenadine **3,** 108
 theophylline **2,** 333
 troleandomycin, 104
 valproic acid **2,** 131
 verapamil hydrochloride **2,** 108
Carbenicillin disodium,
 amikacin sulfate, 185
 gentamicin sulfate **1,** 185
 heparin **2,** 72
 kanamycin sulfate, oral, 185
 kanamycin sulfate, parenteral, 185
 neomycin sulfate, oral, 185
 neomycin sulfate, parenteral, 185
 netilmicin, 185
 paromomycin sulfate, 185
 streptomycin sulfate, 185
 tobramycin, 185
Carbonyl iron,
 doxycycline hydrochloride, 205
 lymecycline, 205
 methacycline hydrochloride, 205
 minocycline hydrochloride pellets, 205

minocycline hydrochloride, 205
oxytetracycline, 205
tetracycline, 205
Carfecillin,
    gentamicin sulfate, 185
Carmustine,
    cimetidine, oral **2,** 211
    phenytoin **2,** 114
Carteolol hydrochloride,
    ophthalmic,
    clonidine hydrochloride,
        transdermal, 160
    clonidine hydrochloride, 160
Carteolol hydrochloride,
    clonidine hydrochloride,
        transdermal, 160
    clonidine hydrochloride, 160
    epinephrine, 259
    insulin, 302
Carvedilol,
    cimetidine hydrochloride,
        parenteral, 257
    cimetidine, oral, 257
    clonidine hydrochloride,
        transdermal, 160
    clonidine hydrochloride, 160
    epinephrine, 259
    insulin, 302
Cefaclor,
    gentamicin sulfate, 185
    theophylline **3,** 333
    tobramycin, 185
Cefadroxil monohydrate,
    gentamicin sulfate, 185
    tobramycin, 185
Cefamandole nafate,
    gentamicin sulfate, 185
    tobramycin, 185
    warfarin **2,** 77
Cefazolin sodium,
    gentamicin sulfate, 185
    tobramycin, 185
Cefdinir,
    gentamicin sulfate, 185
    tobramycin, 185
Cefepime hydrochloride,
    gentamicin sulfate, 185
    tobramycin, 185
Cefmetazole sodium,
    gentamicin sulfate, 185
    tobramycin, 185
Cefonicid sodium,
    gentamicin sulfate, 185
    tobramycin, 185
Cefoperazone sodium,
    alcohol, ethyl - oral/injectable **2,**
    174
    gentamicin sulfate, 185
    tobramycin, 185
Ceforanide,
    gentamicin sulfate, 185

tobramycin, 185
Cefotaxime sodium,
    cimetidine, oral **3,** 174
    gentamicin sulfate, 185
    tobramycin, 185
Cefotetan disodium,
    gentamicin sulfate, 185
    tobramycin, 185
Cefoxitin sodium,
    gentamicin sulfate, 185
    tobramycin, 185
Cefpirome sulfate,
    gentamicin sulfate, 185
    tobramycin, 185
Cefpodoxime proxetil,
    gentamicin sulfate, 185
    tobramycin, 185
Cefprozil,
    amikacin sulfate, 185
    gentamicin sulfate, 185
    kanamycin sulfate, oral, 185
    kanamycin sulfate, parenteral, 185
    neomycin sulfate, oral, 185
    neomycin sulfate, parenteral, 185
    netilmicin, 185
    paromomycin sulfate, 185
    streptomycin sulfate, 185
    tobramycin, 185
Ceftazidime,
    gentamicin sulfate, 185
    tobramycin, 185
Ceftibuten dihyrate,
    amikacin sulfate, 185
    gentamicin sulfate, 185
    kanamycin sulfate, oral, 185
    kanamycin sulfate, parenteral, 185
    neomycin sulfate, oral, 185
    neomycin sulfate, parenteral, 185
    netilmicin, 185
    paromomycin sulfate, 185
    streptomycin sulfate, 185
    streptomycin sulfate, vaccine
        use, 185
    tobramycin, 185
Ceftizoxime sodium,
    gentamicin sulfate, 185
    tobramycin, 185
Ceftriaxone sodium,
    gentamicin sulfate, 185
    tobramycin, 185
Cefuroxime,
    amikacin sulfate, 185
    gentamicin sulfate, 185
    kanamycin sulfate, oral, 185
    kanamycin sulfate, parenteral, 185
    neomycin sulfate, oral, 185
    neomycin sulfate, parenteral, 185
    netilmicin, 185
    paromomycin sulfate, 185
    streptomycin sulfate, 185
    tobramycin, 185

Index

Celiprolol hydrochloride,
  clonidine hydrochloride,
    transdermal, 160
  clonidine hydrochloride, 160
  epinephrine, 259
  insulin, 302
Cephalexin,
  amikacin sulfate, 185
  gentamicin sulfate, 185
  kanamycin sulfate, oral, 185
  kanamycin sulfate, parenteral, 185
  neomycin sulfate, oral, 185
  neomycin sulfate, parenteral, 185
  netilmicin, 185
  paromomycin sulfate, 185
  streptomycin sulfate, 185
  tobramycin, 185
Cephalothin sodium,
  amikacin sulfate, 185
  colistimethate sodium **2,** 175
  gentamicin sulfate **1,** 185
  kanamycin sulfate, oral, 185
  kanamycin sulfate, parenteral, 185
  neomycin sulfate, oral, 185
  neomycin sulfate, parenteral, 185
  netilmicin, 185
  paromomycin sulfate, 185
  probenecid **2,** 175
  streptomycin sulfate, 185
  tobramycin, 185
Cephapirin sodium,
  gentamicin sulfate, 185
  tobramycin, 185
Cephradine,
  gentamicin sulfate, 185
  tobramycin, 185
Cerivastatin,
  grapefruit juice, 356
Certoparin,
  ardeparin sodium, 71
  dalteparin sodium, 71
  enoxaparin, 71
  sodium salicylate, 76
  tinzaparin sodium, 71
Cetirizine,
  acenocoumarol **3,** 69
Charcoal,
  acetaminophen **3,** 2
  aspirin **3,** 7
  carbamazepine **1,** 103
  digoxin **3,** 271
  disopyramide phosphate **2,** 48
  flecainide acetate **3,** 51
  furosemide **2,** 289
  glipizide **2,** 299
  nizatidine **3,** 362
  nortriptyline hydrochloride **3,** 146
  phenobarbital **3,** 316
  phenylbutazone **3,** 18
  phenytoin **2,** 114
  promazine hydrochloride **3,** 249

propoxyphene **3,** 21
  theophylline **1,** 333
Chloral hydrate,
  alcohol, ethyl - oral/injectable **2,**
    313
  furazolidone **4,** 311
  furosemide **3,** 289
  warfarin **2,** 78
Chloramphenicol,
  acetaminophen **3,** 176
  cyclophosphamide **2,** 212
  dicumarol **2,** 69
  penicillin G **4,** 199
  phenobarbital **3,** 176
  phenytoin **2,** 114
  rifampin **2,** 176
  tolbutamide **2,** 306
Chlorcyclizine hydrochloride,
  phenobarbital **3,** 316
Chlordiazepoxide,
  amitriptyline hydrochloride **3,** 135
  ketoconazole **3,** 224
  warfarin **4,** 78
Chlormethiazole,
  cimetidine, oral **3,** 314
Chloroform,
  albuterol sulfate, 26
  amphetamine, 26
  arbutamine hydrochloride, 26
  benzphetamine hydrochloride, 26
  bitolterol mesylate, 26
  dexfenfluramine hydrochloride, 26
  dextroamphetamine, 26
  diethylpropion hydrochloride, 26
  dobutamine hydrochloride, 26
  dopamine hydrochloride, 26
  eformoterol fumarate, 26
  ephedrine, 26
  epinephrine, 26
  etafedrine hydrochloride, 26
  ethylnorepinephrine
    hydrochloride, 26
  fenfluramine hydrochloride, 26
  fenoterol hydrobromide, 26
  isoetharine, 26
  isometheptene, 26
  isoproterenol, 26
  mazindol, 26
  mephentermine sulfate, 26
  metaproterenol sulfate, 26
  metaraminol bitartrate, 26
  methamphetamine hydrochloride,
    26
  methoxamine hydrochloride, 26
  methylphenidate hydrochloride, 26
  norepinephrine bitartrate, 26
  phendimetrazine tartrate, 26
  phenmetrazine hydrochloride, 26
  phentermine hydrochloride, 26
  phenylephrine, 26
  phenylpropanolamine, 26

pirbuterol acetate, 26
procaterol hydrochloride, 26
pseudoephedrine, 26
rimiterol hydrobromide, 26
salmeterol hydroxynaphthoate, 26
salmeterol xinafoate, 26
terbutaline sulfate, 26
Chloroquine,
  cimetidine, oral **3,** 177
  cyclosporine **3,** 177
  kaolin **3,** 177
  levothyroxine sodium **3,** 178
  metronidazole, systemic **2,** 196
  penicillamine **3,** 364
Chlorothiazide,
  calcium carbonate, oral **2,** 287
  colestipol hydrochloride **3,** 287
  lithium **1,** 239
  metoclopramide hydrochloride **3,** 287
  probenecid **3,** 288
  propantheline bromide **3,** 288
Chlorotrianisene,
  rifampin, 202
Chlorpheniramine,
  phenytoin **2,** 115
  propranolol hydrochloride **4,** 257
Chlorphenoxamine hydrochloride,
  digoxin, 278
  digoxin capsule, stabilized, 278
Chlorpromazine hydrochloride,
  alcohol, ethyl - oral/injectable **2,** 225
  aluminum hydroxide **3,** 225
  amphetamine **2,** 226
  benztropine mesylate **2,** 226
  bethanidine sulphate, 162
  captopril **2,** 157
  diazoxide, oral **2,** 227
  guanadrel sulfate, 162
  guanethidine **1,** 162
  insulin **3,** 301
  levodopa **3,** 227
  lithium **2,** 227
  magnesium hydroxide **3,** 225
  meperidine hydrochloride **2,** 14
  phenobarbital **3,** 228
  phenytoin **3,** 115
  piperazine **3,** 228
  propranolol hydrochloride **2,** 258
  tobacco **3,** 229
  valproic acid **3,** 131
Chlorpropamide,
  alcohol, ethyl - oral/injectable **1,** 296
  allopurinol **3,** 296
  aspirin **2,** 296
  clofibrate **2,** 297
  cortisone acetate **2,** 297
  feprazone, 306
  hydrochlorothiazide **2,** 298

oxyphenbutazone, 306
phenylbutazone, 306
probenecid **3,** 298
sucralfate **4,** 298
Chlorprothixene,
  guanethidine, 162
Chlortetracycline hydrochloride,
  penicillin G **2,** 200
Chlorthalidone,
  lithium, 238
  warfarin **3,** 78
Cholecalciferol, vitamin D3,
  aluminum hydroxide **2,** 320
Cholestyramine,
  amiodarone hydrochloride **3,** 45
  cyclosporine **4,** 350
  digitoxin **2,** 268
  doxepin hydrochloride **3,** 138
  furosemide **2,** 290
  glipizide **2,** 299
  hydrocortisone acetone injection **3,** 354
  hydrocortisone sodium succinate **3,** 354
  hydrocortisone sodium phosphate **3,** 354
  hydrocortisone, oral/systemic **3,** 354
  naproxen **3,** 17
  propranolol hydrochloride **3,** 258
  spironolactone **2,** 170
  thyroid strong **2,** 368
  warfarin **2,** 79
Choline salicylate,
  methotrexate, 215
  methotrexate sodium, parenteral, 215
Cimetidine hydrochloride,
  parenteral,
  aminophylline, 332
  caffeine, 332
  carvedilol, 257
  ethotoin, 115
  fosphenytoin sodium, parenteral, 115
  labetalol hydrochloride, 257
  lidocaine hydrochloride, local-injectable, 53
  lidocaine hydrochloride, systemic, 53
  mephenytoin, 115
  metoprolol tartrate, 257
  oxtriphylline, 332
  pentoxifylline, 332
  phenindione, 79
  phenytoin, 115
  propranolol hydrochloride, 257
  theophylline, 332
  warfarin, 79
Cimetidine, oral,
  alcohol, ethyl - oral/injectable **3,**

Index

310
aluminum hydroxide **3,** 347
aminophylline, 332
buspirone hydrochloride **4,** 224
caffeine, 332
carbamazepine **2,** 103
carmustine **2,** 211
carvedilol, 257
cefotaxime sodium **3,** 174
chlormethiazole **3,** 314
chloroquine **3,** 177
clomiphene citrate **3,** 348
clozapine **2,** 231
diazepam **2,** 233
digoxin **3,** 272
dobutamine hydrochloride **3,** 353
erythromycin stearate **3,** 182
ethotoin, 115
ferrous sulfate **3,** 322
flecainide acetate **2,** 52
fluorouracil **3,** 214
fosphenytoin sodium, parenteral, 115
glipizide **2,** 299
imipramine **2,** 142
indomethacin **3,** 12
ketoconazole **2,** 192
labetalol hydrochloride, 258
lidocaine hydrochloride, local-injection, 53
lidocaine hydrochloride, systemic **1,** 53
magnesium hydroxide **3,** 347
mephenytoin, 115
metoclopramide hydrochloride **3,** 348
metoprolol tartrate, 258
metronidazole, parenteral **3,** 197
moricizine hydrochloride **3,** 57
morphine **2,** 17
nifedipine **2,** 57
oxtriphylline, 334
paroxetine hydrochloride **3,** 149
pentoxifylline, 334
phenindione, 79
phenobarbital **3,** 316
phenytoin **1,** 115
procainamide hydrochloride **2,** 59
propantheline bromide **3,** 348
propranolol hydrochloride **1,** 258
quinidine **2,** 62
succinylcholine chloride **2,** 34
tetracycline **3,** 205
theophylline **1,** 334
triamterene **3,** 293
valproic acid **3,** 129
venlafaxine hydrochloride **3,** 154
warfarin **1,** 79
Cinoxacin,
warfarin, 92
Ciprofibrate,

phenindione, 80
Ciprofloxacin hydrochloride,
aluminum hydroxide **2,** 178
cyclosporine **2,** 179
enteral nutrition **3,** 180
ferrous sulfate **2,** 179
magnesium hydroxide **2,** 178
phenytoin **3,** 116
theophylline **2,** 334
warfarin, 92
Cisapride,
diltiazem hydrochloride **2,** 46
warfarin, 80
Cisplatin,
bleomycin sulfate **3,** 211
ethacrynic acid **2,** 288
lithium **3,** 240
methotrexate **2,** 216
paclitaxel **2,** 221
Citalopram hydrobromide,
fentanyl citrate, 14
isocarboxazid, 141
moclobemide, 141
pargyline hydrochloride, 141
phenelzine sulfate, 141
remifentanil hydrochloride, 14
selegiline hydrochloride, 141
tranylcypromine sulfate, 141
Citric acid,
aluminum hydroxide **3,** 346
Clarithromycin,
acenocoumarol, 82
astemizole, 184
carbamazepine, 104
cyclosporine, 183
digoxin, 273
fluoxetine hydrochloride **3,** 139
omeprazole **3,** 363
simvastatin, 359
terfenadine, 184
theophylline, 335
warfarin, 82
Clidinium bromide,
digoxin, 280
Clindamycin,
enflurane, 25
ether, 25
halothane, 25
methoxyflurane, 25
nitrous oxide, 25
pancuronium bromide **2,** 31
Clindamycin phosphate, injectable,
enflurane, 25
ether, 25
halothane, 25
methoxyflurane, 25
nitrous oxide, 25
pancuronium bromide **2,** 31
Clofibrate,
acenocoumarol, 80
anisindione, 80

chlorpropamide **2,** 297
dicumarol, 80
insulin **2,** 301
nicoumalone, 80
oral contraceptives, low-dose **3,** 348
probenecid **3,** 19
rifampin **3,** 202
warfarin **1,** 80
Clomiphene citrate,
  cimetidine, oral **3,** 348
Clomipramine hydrochloride,
  guanethidine, 162
Clonazepam,
  carbamazepine **3,** 108
  phenelzine sulfate **3,** 151
  primidone **4,** 109
  valproic acid **3,** 132
Clonidine hydrochloride,
  transdermal,
  atenolol, 160
  carteolol hydrochloride,
    ophthalmic, 160
  carteolol hydrochloride, 160
  carvedilol, 160
  celiprolol hydrochloride, 160
  metoprolol tartrate, 160
  nadolol, 160
  penbutolol sulfate, 160
  pindolol, 160
  propranolol hydrochloride, 160
  tertatolol hydrochloride, 160
  timolol maleate, oral, 160
Clonidine hydrochloride,
  atenolol, 160
  carteolol hydrochloride,
    ophthalmic, 160
  carteolol hydrochloride, 160
  carvedilol, 160
  celiprolol hydrochloride, 160
  cyclosporine **2,** 159
  fluphenazine **3,** 236
  metoprolol tartrate, 160
  nadolol, 160
  naloxone hydrochloride **3,** 159
  penbutolol sulfate, 160
  pindolol, 160
  propranolol hydrochloride **1,** 160
  rifampin **4,** 160
  tertatolol hydrochloride, 160
  timolol maleate, oral, 160
Clorazepate dipotassium,
  aluminum hydroxide **3,** 229
  influenza virus vaccine, split
    virion **3,** 229
  magnesium hydroxide **3,** 229
Clotrimazole,
  cyclosporine, 193
  fosphenytoin sodium, parenteral,
    119
  phenytoin, 119

Cloxacillin sodium,
  amikacin sulfate, 185
  gentamicin sulfate, 185
  netilmicin, 185
  tobramycin, 185
Clozapine,
  caffeine **3,** 229
  carbamazepine **1,** 230
  cimetidine, oral **2,** 231
  erythromycin stearate **2,** 231
  fluvoxamine maleate **2,** 231
Cocaine hydrochloride,
  propranolol hydrochloride **2,** 259
Codeine,
  isocarboxazid, 14
  pargyline hydrochloride, 14
  phenelzine sulfate, 14
  selegiline hydrochloride, 14
  tranylcypromine sulfate, 14
Colestipol hydrochloride,
  chlorothiazide **3,** 287
Colistimethate sodium,
  cephalothin sodium **2,** 175
Colistin sulfate,
  alcuronium chloride, 40
  atracurium besylate, 40
  doxacurium chloride, 40
  enflurane, 25
  ether, 25
  gallamine triethiodide, 40
  halothane, 25
  methoxyflurane, 25
  metocurine iodide, 40
  mivacurium chloride, 40
  nitrous oxide, 25
  pancuronium bromide, 40
  pipecuronium bromide, 40
  rocuronium bromide, 40
  succinylcholine chloride, 40
  tubocurarine chloride, 40
  vecuronium bromide, 40
Conjugated estrogens,
  rifampin, 202
Corticotropin,
  dicumarol **2,** 70
Cortisone acetate,
  chlorpropamide **2,** 297
Cyanocobalamin, vitamin B12,
  omeprazole **3,** 321
Cyclacillin,
  amikacin sulfate, 185
  gentamicin sulfate, 185
  netilmicin, 185
  tobramycin, 185
Cyclobenzaprine hydrochloride,
  guanadrel sulfate, 162
  guanethidine, 162
Cyclopenthiazide,
  lithium, 239
Cyclophosphamide,
  allopurinol **2,** 211

chloramphenicol **2,** 212
digoxin **2,** 272
hydrochlorothiazide **3,** 212
indomethacin **3,** 212
methotrexate **3,** 212
prednisone **3,** 213
succinylcholine chloride **2,** 34
Cyclosporine,
    acetazolamide **2,** 286
    allopurinol **2,** 349
    amiodarone hydrochloride **2,** 45
    amphotericin B **2,** 181
    azathioprine sodium **3,** 349
    azithromycin, 183
    butoconazole nitrate, 193
    carbamazepine **2,** 349
    chloroquine **2,** 177
    cholestyramine **4,** 350
    ciprofloxacin hydrochloride **2,** 179
    clarithromycin, 183
    clonidine hydrochloride **2,** 159
    clotrimazole, 193
    diclofenac **2,** 9
    digoxin **2,** 272
    diltiazem hydrochloride **1,** 46
    dirithromycin, 183
    disopyramide phosphate **3,** 48
    erythromycin **1,** 183
    erythromycin estolate, 183
    erythromycin ethylsuccinate, 183
    erythromycin gluceptate, 183
    erythromycin lactobionate, 183
    erythromycin stearate, 183
    etoposide **2,** 213
    fat emulsion, intravenous **2,** 354
    fenticonazole nitrate, 193
    fluconazole, 193
    fluoxetine hydrochloride **3,** 140
    foscarnet sodium **2,** 354
    griseofulvin **3,** 187
    imipenem in combination with
        cilastatin **2,** 188
    itraconazole, 193
    ketoconazole **1,** 193
    lercanidipine hydrochloride, 46
    lovastatin **3,** 358
    melphalan **2,** 215
    methyltestosterone **2,** 350
    metoclopramide hydrochloride **2,**
        350
    miconazole nitrate, 193
    nafcillin sodium **2,** 351
    nicardipine hydrochloride,
        parenteral use, 46
    nicardipine hydrochloride, 46
    nifedipine, 46
    nisoldipine, 46
    omeprazole **2,** 363
    oral contraceptive agents **3,** 351
    oral contraceptives, low-dose **3,**
        351

oxiconazole nitrate, 193
pancuronium bromide **2,** 31
phenobarbital **2,** 316
phenytoin **2,** 116
prednisolone **2,** 364
probucol **2,** 365
propafenone hydrochloride **2,** 61
quinine **2,** 351
rifabutin, 202
rifampin **1,** 202
sulfadiazine **2,** 203
terbinafine hydrochloride **2,** 204
terconazole, 193
ticlopidine hydrochloride **2,** 74
tioconazole, 193
trimethoprim **3,** 203
troleandomycin, 183
verapamil hydrochloride pellets,
    46
verapamil hydrochloride,
    sustained-release, 46
verapamil hydrochloride, 46
warfarin **2,** 80
Cyclothiazide,
    lithium, 239
Cyproheptadine hydrochloride,
    fluoxetine hydrochloride **2,** 140
Cytarabine,
    methotrexate **3,** 217
    methotrexate sodium, parenteral
        3, 217
Dalteparin sodium,
    ardeparin sodium, 71
    certoparin, 71
    enoxaparin, 71
    sodium salicylate, 76
    tinzaparin sodium, 71
Danazol,
    acenocoumarol, 90
    anisindione, 90
    carbamazepine **2,** 103
    dicumarol, 90
    nicoumalone, 90
    warfarin, 90
Dantrolene sodium,
    vecuronium bromide **3,** 42
    verapamil hydrochloride **2,** 65
Dapsone,
    rifampin **3,** 181
    trimethoprim **3,** 181
Demeclocycline hydrochloride,
    alcuronium chloride, 40
    aluminum carbonate, basic, 205
    aluminum hydroxide, 205
    aluminum oxide, 205
    aluminum phosphate, 205
    attapulgite, 205
    bismuth subsalicylate, 205
    calcium acetate, 205
    calcium ascorbate, 205
    calcium carbonate, oral, 205

calcium chloride, oral, 205
calcium citrate, oral, 205
calcium glubionate, oral, 205
calcium glucoheptonate, 205
calcium gluconate, oral, 205
calcium glycerophosphate, oral, 205
calcium iodate, 205
calcium lactate gluconate, 205
calcium lactate, oral, 205
calcium lactobionate, oral, 205
calcium phosphate, oral, 205
calcium, oral salt unspecified, 205
digoxin, 282
digoxin capsule, stabilized, 282
dihydroxyaluminum, 205
doxacurium chloride, 40
ferric ammonium citrate, 205
ferrous fumarate, 205
ferrous gluconate, 205
ferrous glycine sulfate, 205
ferrous hydroxide polymaltose, 205
ferrous ions, salt unspecified, 205
ferrous succinate, 205
ferrous sulfate, 205
gallamine triethiodide, 40
iron dextran complex, 205
iron peptonized, 205
kaolin, 205
magaldrate, 205
magnesium carbonate, 205
magnesium chloride, oral, 205
magnesium hydroxide, 205
magnesium oxide, 205
magnesium salicylate, 205
magnesium sulfate, 205
magnesium trisilicate, 205
metocurine iodide, 40
mivacurium chloride, 40
pancuronium bromide, 40
pipecuronium bromide, 40
rocuronium bromide, 40
succinylcholine chloride, 40
sucralfate, 205
tubocurarine chloride, 40
vecuronium bromide, 40
Desflurane,
epinephrine, 26
Desipramine hydrochloride,
bethanidine sulphate, 162
carbamazepine **3,** 104
guanadrel sulfate, 162
guanethidine **1,** 162
phenylbutazone **3,** 19
propranolol hydrochloride **3,** 259
quinidine **3,** 137
thioridazine hydrochloride **2,** 138
Deslanoside,
amiodarone hydrochloride, 271
propantheline bromide, 280

rifampin, 269
Dexamethasone,
aldesleukin, interleukin-2 human **2,** 214
aminoglutethimide **2,** 352
ephedrine **3,** 352
phenobarbital **2,** 317
phenytoin **2,** 117
Dexfenfluramine hydrochloride,
chloroform, 26
enflurane, 26
furazolidone, 185
halothane, 26
isocarboxazid, 153
methoxyflurane, 26
metoprolol tartrate, 260
moclobemide, 153
pargyline hydrochloride, 153
phenelzine sulfate, 153
procarbazine hydrochloride, 153
propranolol hydrochloride, 260
selegiline hydrochloride, 153
timolol maleate, ophthalmic, 260
timolol maleate, oral, 260
tranylcypromine sulfate, 153
venlafaxine hydrochloride, 153
Dexpanthenol,
succinylcholine chloride **4,** 35
Dextran 40,
heparin **2,** 72
Dextran 70,
heparin **2,** 72
Dextroamphetamine,
chloroform, 26
enflurane, 26
furazolidone, 185
guanethidine **2,** 163
halothane, 26
isocarboxazid, 153
methoxyflurane, 26
moclobemide, 153
pargyline hydrochloride, 153
phenelzine sulfate, 153
procarbazine hydrochloride, 153
tranylcypromine sulfate, 153
Dextromethorphan hydrobromide
isocarboxazid, 14
moclobemide, 14
pargyline hydrochloride, 14
paroxetine hydrochloride **2,** 150
phenelzine sulfate, 14
selegiline hydrochloride, 14
tranylcypromine sulfate, 14
Dextrothyroxine sodium,
acenocoumarol, 100
dicumarol, 100
nicoumalone, 100
warfarin, 100
Dezocine,
selegiline hydrochloride, 14
Diatrizoate meglumine,

metformin hydrochloride, 305
Diatrizoate sodium,
  metformin hydrochloride, 305
  propranolol hydrochloride **3,** 259
Diazepam,
  alcohol, ethyl - oral/injectable **2,**
    232
  aminophylline **3,** 232
  bupivacaine hydrochloride **3,** 24
  cimetidine, oral **2,** 233
  digoxin **2,** 272
  disulfiram **3,** 233
  gallamine triethiodide **3,** 25
  isoniazid, 234
  ketamine hydrochloride, **2,** 27
  levodopa **3,** 234
  lithium **3,** 240
  methadone hydrochloride **3,** 15
  omeprazole **3,** 234
  oral contraceptive agents **3,** 235
  oral contraceptives, low-dose **3,**
    235
  phenytoin **3,** 117
  propofol **3,** 34
  propranolol hydrochloride **3,** 235
  rifampin **3,** 236
  tobacco **3,** 236
Diazoxide, oral,
  chlorpromazine hydrochloride **2,**
    227
  phenytoin **2,** 117
  tolbutamide **3,** 306
  trichlormethiazide **3,** 293
  warfarin **3,** 81
Dicalcium phosphate,
  tetracycline, 205
Dichlorphenamide,
  lithium, 238
Diclofenac,
  cyclosporine **2,** 9
Dicloxacillin,
  amikacin sulfate, 185
  gentamicin sulfate, 185
  netilmicin, 185
  tobramycin, 185
Dicumarol,
  allopurinol **1,** 69
  aloxiprin, 76
  aminoglutethimide, 86
  amiodarone hydrochloride, 75
  amobarbital, 94
  aprobarbital, 94
  aspirin, 76
  barbital, 94
  bezafibrate, 80
  butabarbital sodium, 94
  butalbital, 94
  butobarbitone, 94
  chloramphenicol **2,** 69
  clofibrate, 80
  corticotropin **2,** 70

danazol, 90
dextrothyroxine sodium, 100
diflunisal, 76
disulfiram, 81
erythromycin, 82
erythromycin estolate, 82
erythromycin ethylsuccinate, 82
erythromycin gluceptate, 82
erythromycin lactobionate, 82
erythromycin stearate, 82
ethylestrenol, 90
fenofibrate, micronized, 80
feprazone, 94
fluoxymesterone, 90
gemfibrozil, 80
glucagon, 86
glucagon, recombinant, 86
glutethimide, 86
levothyroxine sodium, 100
liothyronine sodium, 100
menadiol sodium diphosphate,
    vitamin K4, 95
menadione, 95
mephobarbital, 94
methandrostenolone, 90
metharbital, 94
methohexital sodium
    diphosphate, 94
methylphenidate hydrochloride **3,**
    70
methyltestosterone, 90
methyprylon, 86
nalidixic acid, 92
norfloxacin, 92
oral contraceptive agents **2,** 70
oxandrolone, 90
oxymetholone, 90
oxyphenbutazone, 94
pentobarbital sodium, 94
phenobarbital, 94
phenylbutazone, 94
phenytoin **2,** 71
phytonadione, vitamin K1, 95
primidone, 94
rifampin, 97
secobarbital, 94
sodium salicylate, 76
stanozolol, 90
talbutal, 94
thiamylal sodium, 94
thiopental sodium, 94
thyroglobulin, 100
thyroid desiccated, 100
thyroid strong, 100
tolbutamide **2,** 307
Dicyclomine hydrochloride,
  digoxin, 280
Didanosine,
  ganciclovir **2,** 352
  itraconazole **2,** 191
Diethylpropion hydrochloride,

chloroform, 26
enflurane, 26
furazolidone, 185
halothane, 26
isocarboxazid, 153
methoxyflurane, 26
moclobemide, 153
pargyline hydrochloride, 153
phenelzine sulfate, 153
procarbazine hydrochloride, 153
tranylcypromine sulfate, 153
Diethylstilbestrol,
rifampin, 202
succinylcholine chloride **2,** 35
Difenoxin hydrochloride,
isocarboxazid, 14
pargyline hydrochloride, 14
phenelzine sulfate, 14
selegiline hydrochloride, 14
tranylcypromine sulfate, 14
Diflunisal,
acenocoumarol, 76
anisindione, 76
dicumarol, 76
methotrexate, 216
methotrexate sodium, parenteral,
216
nicoumalone, 76
oxazepam **3,** 248
warfarin, 76
Digitalis,
amiodarone hydrochloride, 271
calcium chloride, injectable **2,**
267
phenytoin **2,** 267
propantheline bromide, 280
reserpine **3,** 267
Digitoxin,
aminoglutethimide **3,** 268
amiodarone hydrochloride, 271
cholestyramine **2,** 268
diltiazem hydrochloride, 283
phenobarbital **2,** 269
phenylbutazone **3,** 269
propantheline bromide, 280
quinidine, 280
rifabutin, 269
rifampin **1,** 269
verapamil hydrochloride pellets,
283
verapamil hydrochloride,
sustained-release, 283
verapamil hydrochloride, 283
Digoxin,
acarbose **3,** 269
aluminum hydroxide **2,** 270
aminosalicylic acid **3,** 270
amiodarone hydrochloride **1,** 271
anisotropine methylbromide, 280
atropine, 280
belladonna, 280

bellafoline, 280
benztropine mesylate, 280
biperiden, 280
captopril **2,** 271
charcoal, 271
chlorphenoxamine hydrochloride,
280
cimetidine, oral **3,** 272
clarithromycin, 273
clidinium bromide, 280
cyclophosphamide **2,** 272
cyclosporine **2,** 272
demeclocycline hydrochloride,
282
diazepam **2,** 272
dicyclomine hydrochloride, 280
diltiazem hydrochloride, 283
disopyramide phosphate **3,** 273
doxycycline hyclate, parenteral,
282
doxycycline hydrochloride, 282
erythromycin **1,** 273
erythromycin estolate, 273
erythromycin ethylsuccinate, 273
erythromycin gluceptate, 273
erythromycin lactobionate, 273
erythromycin stearate, 273
esmolol hydrochloride **3,** 273
ethoheptazine citrate, 280
furosemide **2,** 275
ginseng **3,** 275
glycopyrrolate, 280
heparin **3,** 276
hydroxychloroquine sulfate **2,** 276
hyoscyamine, 280
ibuprofen **2,** 276
hexocyclium methylsulfate, 280
isopropamide iodide, 280
itraconazole **2,** 277
kaolin **2,** 277
lymecycline, 282
magnesium hydroxide **2,** 270
magnesium trisilicate **2,** 270
mepenzolate bromide, 280
methacycline hydrochloride, 282
methantheline bromide, 280
methscopolamine bromide, 280
methscopolamine nitrate, 280
methyldopa **3,** 277
metoclopramide hydrochloride **2,**
278
mexiletine hydrochloride **4,** 278
minocycline hydrochloride
pellets, 282
minocycline hydrochloride, 282
minocycline, parenteral, 282
moricizine hydrochloride **4,** 278
neomycin sulfate, oral **2,** 279
nifedipine, 283
oxybutynin chloride, 280
oxyphencyclimine hydrochloride,

280
oxytetracycline, 282
oxytetracycline, parenteral, 282
penicillamine **2,** 279
pirenzepine dihydrochloride, 280
prazosin hydrochloride **2,** 279
prednisone **2,** 272
procarbazine hydrochloride **2,**
  272
procyclidine hydrochloride, 280
propafenone hydrochloride **2,**
  279
propantheline bromide **1,** 280
psyllium **3,** 280
quinidine **1,** 280
rifabutin, 269
rifampin, 269
rolitetracycline, injectable, 282
scopolamine, ophthalmic, 280
scopolamine, systemic, 280
spironolactone **2,** 281
succinylcholine chloride **2,** 281
sulfasalazine **2,** 282
tetracycline **1,** 282
tetracycline hydrochloride,
  parenteral, 282
thyroid strong **2,** 282
tolbutamide **3,** 283
trazodone hydrochloride **3,** 283
tridihexethyl chloride, 280
trihexyphenidyl hydrochloride,
  280
trimethoprim **3,** 283
verapamil hydrochloride pellets,
  284
verapamil hydrochloride,
  sustained-release, 284
verapamil hydrochloride **1,** 284
vincristine sulfate **2,** 272
Digoxin capsule, stabilized,
  amiodarone hydrochloride, 271
  chlorphenoxamine hydrochloride,
    280
  demeclocycline hydrochloride,
    282
  diltiazem hydrochloride, 284
  doxycycline hyclate, parenteral,
    282
  doxycycline hydrochloride, 282
  erythromycin, 273
  erythromycin estolate, 273
  erythromycin ethylsuccinate, 273
  erythromycin gluceptate, 273
  erythromycin lactobionate, 273
  erythromycin stearate, 273
  fluoxetine hydrochloride **2,** 274
  lymecycline, 282
  methacycline hydrochloride, 282
  minocycline hydrochloride, 282
  minocycline, parenteral, 282
  nifedipine, 284

oxytetracycline, 282
oxytetracycline, parenteral, 282
propafenone hydrochloride **2,** 279
quinidine, 280
rifampin, 269
rolitetracycline, injectable, 282
tetracycline, 282
tetracycline hydrochloride,
  parenteral, 282
verapamil hydrochloride pellets,
  284
verapamil hydrochloride,
  sustained-release, 284
verapamil hydrochloride, 284
Dihydrocodeine bitartrate,
  isocarboxazid, 14
  pargyline hydrochloride, 14
  phenelzine sulfate, 14
  selegiline hydrochloride, 14
  tranylcypromine sulfate, 14
Dihydroergotamine mesylate,
  nitroglycerin **2,** 353
Dihydroxyaluminum,
  demeclocycline hydrochloride,
    205
  doxycycline hydrochloride, 205
  methacycline hydrochloride, 205
  oxytetracycline, 205
  tetracycline, 205
Diltiazem hydrochloride,
  amiodarone hydrochloride **2,** 45
  cisapride **2,** 46
  cyclosporine **1,** 46
  digitoxin, 284
  digoxin, 284
  digoxin capsule, stabilized, 284
  insulin **3,** 301
  quinidine, 65
Diphenhydramine,
  alcohol, ethyl - oral/injectable **2,**
    310
  temazepam **2,** 250
  warfarin **4,** 81
Diphenoxylate hydrochloride,
  isocarboxazid, 14
  pargyline hydrochloride, 14
  phenelzine sulfate, 14
  quinidine **3,** 62
  selegiline hydrochloride, 14
  tranylcypromine sulfate, 14
Dipyridamole,
  adenosine, parenteral **3,** 346
  aspirin **3,** 7
Dirithromycin,
  cyclosporine, 183
  warfarin, 82
Disodium hydrogen citrate,
  lithium, 238
Disopyramide phosphate,
  alcohol, ethyl - oral/injectable **3,**
    47

atenolol **3,** 47
charcoal **2,** 48
cyclosporine **3,** 48
digoxin **3,** 273
erythromycin **2,** 48
isosorbide dinitrate, sublingual **2,** 49
phenytoin **2,** 49
quinidine **3,** 50
rifampin **3,** 50
warfarin **3,** 81
Disulfiram,
acenocoumarol, 81
alcohol, ethyl - oral/injectable **1,** 311
amitriptyline hydrochloride **3,** 135
anisindione, 81
diazepam **3,** 233
dicumarol, 81
ethotoin, 118
fosphenytoin sodium, parenteral, 118
isoniazid **3,** 189
mephenytoin, 118
metronidazole, systemic **2,** 197
nicoumalone, 81
perphenazine **3,** 249
phenytoin **1,** 118
theophylline **2,** 335
warfarin **1,** 81
Dobutamine hydrochloride,
chloroform, 26
cimetidine, oral **3,** 353
enflurane, 26
halothane, 26
methoxyflurane, 26
propranolol hydrochloride, 260
timolol maleate, ophthalmic, 260
timolol maleate, oral, 260
Domperidone,
levodopa **3,** 355
levodopa, combined with carbidopa **3,** 355
Dopamine hydrochloride,
chloroform, 26
enflurane, 26
ergonovine maleate **2,** 353
fosphenytoin sodium, parenteral, 118
furazolidone, 153
halothane, 26
isocarboxazid, 153
methoxyflurane, 26
metoprolol tartrate, 260
moclobemide, 153
pargyline hydrochloride, 153
phenelzine sulfate, 153
phenytoin **1,** 118
procarbazine hydrochloride, 153
propranolol hydrochloride, 260
timolol maleate, ophthalmic, 260

timolol maleate, oral, 260
tranylcypromine sulfate, 153
Dorzolamide hydrochloride, lithium, 238
Dorzolamide hydrochloride, lithium, 238
Dothiepin hydrochloride, guanethidine, 162
Doxacurium chloride,
amikacin sulfate, 40
bacitracin, 40
colistin sulfate, 40
demeclocycline hydrochloride, 40
doxycycline hyclate, parenteral, 40
doxycycline hydrochloride, 40
gentamicin sulfate, 40
kanamycin sulfate, oral, 40
kanamycin sulfate, parenteral, 40
lymecycline, 40
methacycline hydrochloride, 40
minocycline hydrochloride pellets, 40
minocycline hydrochloride, 40
minocycline, parenteral, 40
neomycin sulfate, oral, 40
neomycin sulfate, parenteral, 40
netilmicin, 40
oxytetracycline, 40
oxytetracycline, parenteral, 40
paromomycin sulfate, 40
polymyxin B sulfate, 40
polymyxin B sulfate, vaccine use, 40
streptomycin sulfate, 40
tetracycline, 40
tobramycin, 40
Doxepin hydrochloride,
cholestyramine **3,** 138
guanadrel sulfate, 162
guanethidine, 162
propoxyphene **3,** 139
tolazamide **2,** 306
Doxepin hydrochloride, topical,
guanadrel sulfate, 162
guanethidine, 162
Doxorubicin hydrochloride,
phenobarbital **3,** 213
Doxycycline hyclate, parenteral,
alcuronium chloride, 40
digoxin, 282
digoxin capsule, stabilized, 282
doxacurium chloride, 40
gallamine triethiodide, 40
metocurine iodide, 40
mivacurium chloride, 40
pancuronium bromide, 40
pipecuronium bromide, 40
rocuronium bromide, 40
succinylcholine chloride, 40
tubocurarine chloride, 40

vecuronium bromide, 40
Doxycycline hydrochloride,
alcuronium chloride, 40
aluminum carbonate, basic, 205
aluminum hydroxide, 205
aluminum oxide, 205
aluminum phosphate, 205
attapulgite, 205
bismuth subsalicylate, 205
calcium acetate, 205
calcium ascorbate, 205
calcium carbonate, oral, 205
calcium chloride, oral, 205
calcium citrate, oral, 205
calcium glubionate, oral, 205
calcium glucoheptonate, 205
calcium gluconate, oral, 205
calcium glycerophosphate, oral,
205
calcium iodate, 205
calcium lactate gluconate, 205
calcium lactate, oral, 205
calcium lactobionate, oral, 205
calcium phosphate, oral, 205
calcium, oral salt unspecified,
205
carbamazepine **2,** 182
carbonyl iron, 205
digoxin, 282
digoxin capsule, stabilized, 282
dihydroxyaluminum, 205
doxacurium chloride, 40
ferric ammonium citrate, 205
ferrous fumarate, 205
ferrous gluconate, 205
ferrous glycine sulfate, 205
ferrous hydroxide polymaltose,
205
ferrous ions, salt unspecified, 205
ferrous succinate, 205
ferrous sulfate, 205
gallamine triethiodide, 40
iron dextran complex, 205
iron peptonized, 205
kaolin, 205
magaldrate, 205
magnesium carbonate, 205
magnesium chloride, oral, 205
magnesium hydroxide, 205
magnesium oxide, 205
magnesium sulfate, 205
magnesium trisilicate, 205
metocurine iodide, 40
mivacurium chloride, 40
pancuronium bromide, 40
phenobarbital **2,** 182
phenytoin **2,** 182
pipecuronium bromide, 40
rocuronium bromide, 40
succinylcholine chloride, 40
sucralfate, 205

tubocurarine chloride, 40
vecuronium bromide, 40
Droperidol,
guanethidine, 162
Dyphylline,
halothane, 327
probenecid **2,** 331
Echothiophate iodide,
succinylcholine chloride **2,** 35
Econazole nitrate,
phenytoin, 119
Eformoterol fumarate,
chloroform, 26
enflurane, 26
halothane, 26
methoxyflurane, 26
metoprolol tartrate, 260
timolol maleate, oral, 260
Enalapril maleate,
azathioprine sodium **3,** 160
lithium **2,** 240
rifampin **3,** 161
Enflurane,
albuterol sulfate, 26
amikacin sulfate, 25
amphetamine, 26
arbutamine hydrochloride, 26
benzphetamine hydrochloride, 26
bitolterol mesylate, 26
clindamycin, 25
clindamycin phosphate,
injectable, 25
colistin sulfate, 25
dexfenfluramine hydrochloride, 26
dextroamphetamine, 26
diethylpropion hydrochloride, 26
dobutamine hydrochloride, 26
dopamine hydrochloride, 26
eformoterol fumarate, 26
ephedrine, 26
epinephrine, 26
etafedrine hydrochloride, 26
ethylnorepinephrine
hydrochloride, 26
fenfluramine hydrochloride, 26
fenoterol hydrobromide, 26
gentamicin sulfate, 25
isoetharine, 26
isometheptene, 26
isoniazid **3,** 24
isoproterenol, 26
kanamycin sulfate, oral, 25
kanamycin sulfate, parenteral, 25
mazindol, 26
mephentermine sulfate, 26
metaproterenol sulfate, 26
metaraminol bitartrate, 26
methamphetamine hydrochloride,
26
methoxamine hydrochloride, 26
methylphenidate hydrochloride,

26
norepinephrine bitartrate, 26
phendimetrazine tartrate, 26
phenmetrazine hydrochloride, 26
phentermine hydrochloride, 26
phenylephrine, 26
phenylpropanolamine, 26
pirbuterol acetate, 26
polymyxin B sulfate, 25
polymyxin B sulfate, vaccine use, 25
procaterol hydrochloride, 26
pseudoephedrine, 26
rimiterol hydrobromide, 26
salmeterol hydroxynaphthoate, 26
salmeterol xinafoate, 26
streptomycin sulfate, 25
terbutaline sulfate, 26
tobramycin, 25
Enoxacin,
warfarin, 92
Enoxaparin,
ardeparin sodium, 71
certoparin, 71
dalteparin sodium, 71
sodium salicylate, 76
tinzaparin sodium, 71
Enteral nutrition,
ciprofloxacin hydrochloride **3,** 180
Ephedrine,
chloroform, 26
dexamethasone **3,** 352
enflurane, 26
furazolidone, 185
isocarboxazid, 153
methoxyflurane, 26
moclobemide, 153
pargyline hydrochloride, 153
phenelzine sulfate, 153
procarbazine hydrochloride, 153
reserpine **2,** 169
tranylcypromine sulfate, 153
Epinephrine,
acebutolol hydrochloride, 260
betaxolol hydrochloride, oral, 260
bisoprolol fumarate, 260
carteolol hydrochloride, 260
carvedilol, 260
celiprolol hydrochloride, 260
chloroform, 26
desflurane, 26
enflurane, 26
ether, 26
furazolidone, 185
halothane **1,** 26
imipramine **2,** 143
insulin **3,** 302
isoflurane, 26
isoproterenol, 26
methoxyflurane, 26
nadolol, 260
norepinephrine bitartrate, 26
oxprenolol, 260
penbutolol sulfate, 260
pindolol, 260
propranolol hydrochloride **1,** 260
sevoflurane, 26
sotalol hydrochloride, 260
terbutaline sulfate, 26
tertatolol hydrochloride, 260
timolol maleate, ophthalmic, 260
timolol maleate, oral, 260
Ergocalciferol, vitamin D2,
phenytoin **2,** 321
Ergonovine maleate,
dopamine hydrochloride **2,** 353
Ergotamine tartrate,
erythromycin **2,** 183
propranolol hydrochloride **3,** 260
Erythromycin,
acenocoumarol, 82
alfentanil hydrochloride **2,** 5
aminophylline, 335
anisindione, 82
astemizole, 184
buspirone hydrochloride **3,** 136
caffeine, 335
carbamazepine **1,** 104
cyclosporine **1,** 183
dicumarol, 82
digoxin **1,** 273
digoxin capsule, stabilized, 273
disopyramide phosphate **2,** 48
ergotamine tartrate **2,** 183
felodipine **3,** 50
lincomycin hydrochloride **3,** 196
lovastatin **1,** 359
midazolam hydrochloride **2,** 247
nicoumalone, 82
oxtriphylline, 335
penicillin G **3,** 200
simvastatin, 360
tacrolimus **2,** 367
terfenadine **1,** 184
theophylline **1,** 335
valproic acid **2,** 132
vinblastine sulfate **3,** 222
warfarin **1,** 82
Erythromycin estolate,
acenocoumarol, 82
aminophylline, 335
anisindione, 82
astemizole, 184
caffeine, 335
carbamazepine, 104
cyclosporine, 183
dicumarol, 82
digoxin, 273
digoxin capsule, stabilized, 273
lovastatin, 359
nicoumalone, 82
oxtriphylline, 335

simvastatin, 359
terfenadine, 184
theophylline, 335
warfarin, 82
Erythromycin ethylsuccinate,
  acenocoumarol, 82
  aminophylline, 335
  anisindione, 82
  astemizole, 184
  caffeine, 335
  carbamazepine, 104
  cyclosporine, 183
  dicumarol, 82
  digoxin, 273
  digoxin capsule, stabilized, 273
  lovastatin, 359
  nicoumalone, 82
  oxtriphylline, 335
  simvastatin, 359
  terfenadine, 184
  theophylline, 335
  valproic acid **2,** 132
  warfarin, 82
Erythromycin gluceptate,
  acenocoumarol, 82
  aminophylline, 335
  anisindione, 82
  astemizole, 184
  caffeine, 335
  carbamazepine, 104
  cyclosporine, 183
  dicumarol, 82
  digoxin, 273
  digoxin capsule, stabilized, 273
  lovastatin, 359
  nicoumalone, 82
  oxtriphylline, 335
  simvastatin, 359
  terfenadine, 184
  theophylline, 335
  warfarin, 82
Erythromycin lactobionate,
  acenocoumarol, 82
  aminophylline, 335
  anisindione, 82
  astemizole, 184
  caffeine, 335
  carbamazepine, 104
  cyclosporine, 183
  dicumarol, 82
  digoxin, 273
  digoxin capsule, stabilized, 273
  lovastatin, 359
  nicoumalone, 82
  oxtriphylline, 335
  simvastatin, 359
  terfenadine, 184
  theophylline, 335
  warfarin, 82
Erythromycin stearate,
  acenocoumarol, 82

aminophylline, 335
anisindione, 82
astemizole, 184
caffeine, 335
carbamazepine, 104
cimetidine, oral **3,** 182
clozapine **2,** 231
cyclosporine, 183
dicumarol, 82
digoxin, 273
digoxin capsule, stabilized, 273
lovastatin, 359
nicoumalone, 82
oxtriphylline, 335
simvastatin, 359
terfenadine, 184
theophylline, 335
warfarin, 82
Esmolol hydrochloride,
  digoxin **3,** 273
  nitroprusside sodium **3,** 170
Esterified estrogens,
  rifampin, 202
Estradiol,
  rifabutin, 202
  rifampin, 202
Estradiol, transdermal,
  rifabutin, 202
  rifampin, 202
Estriol,
  rifampin, 202
Estrogen,
  rifampin, 202
Estrone,
  rifampin, 202
Estropipate,
  rifampin, 202
Etafedrine hydrochloride,
  chloroform, 26
  enflurane, 26
  furazolidone, 185
  isocarboxazid, 153
  methoxyflurane, 26
  metoprolol tartrate, 260
  pargyline hydrochloride, 153
  phenelzine sulfate, 153
  procarbazine hydrochloride, 153
  propranolol hydrochloride, 260
  timolol maleate, ophthalmic, 260
  timolol maleate, oral, 260
  tranylcypromine sulfate, 153
Ethacrynic acid,
  amikacin sulfate, 191
  cisplatin **2,** 153
  gentamicin sulfate, 191
  kanamycin sulfate, oral **1,** 191
  kanamycin sulfate, parenteral, 191
  lithium, 239
  neomycin sulfate, oral, 191
  neomycin sulfate, parenteral, 191
  netilmicin, 191

streptomycin sulfate, 191
tobramycin, 191
warfarin **2,** 82
Ethacrynic acid, injectable,
  amikacin sulfate, 191
  gentamicin sulfate, 191
  kanamycin sulfate, oral, 191
  kanamycin sulfate, parenteral, 191
  lithium, 239
  neomycin sulfate, oral, 191
  neomycin sulfate, parenteral, 191
  netilmicin, 191
  streptomycin sulfate, 191
  tobramycin, 191
Ethambutol hydrochloride,
  aluminum hydroxide **3,** 184
Ethchlorvynol,
  warfarin **2,** 83
Ether,
  amikacin sulfate, 25
  bacitracin, 25
  clindamycin, 25
  clindamycin phosphate,
    injectable, 25
  colistin sulfate, 25
  epinephrine, 26
  gentamicin sulfate, 25
  isoproterenol, 26
  kanamycin sulfate, oral, 25
  kanamycin sulfate, parenteral, 25
  neomycin sulfate, oral **1,** 25
  neomycin sulfate, parenteral, 25
  norepinephrine bitartrate, 26
  oxytetracycline, 25
  oxytetracycline, parenteral, 25
  polymyxin B sulfate, 25
  polymyxin B sulfate, vaccine use,
    25
  rolitetracycline, injectable, 25
  streptomycin sulfate, 25
  terbutaline sulfate, 26
  tetracycline, 25
  tetracycline hydrochloride,
    parenteral, 25
  tobramycin, 25
Ethinyl estradiol,
  ascorbic acid, vitamin C **3,** 320
  imipramine **3,** 143
  rifabutin, 202
  rifampin, 202
Ethoheptazine citrate,
  digoxin, 280
Ethosuximide,
  carbamazepine **3,** 109
  isoniazid **3,** 109
  phenytoin **3,** 119
  valproic acid **3,** 110
Ethotoin,
  cimetidine hydrochloride,
    parenteral, 115
  cimetidine, oral, 115
disulfiram, 118
fluconazole, 119
ofloxacin, 92
ranitidine hydrochloride,
  parenteral, 115
ranitidine hydrochloride, oral, 115
Ethylestrenol,
  acenocoumarol, 90
  dicumarol, 90
  nicoumalone, 90
  warfarin, 90
Ethylnorepinephrine hydrochloride,
  chloroform, 26
  enflurane, 26
  halothane, 26
  methoxyflurane, 26
  metoprolol tartrate, 260
  timolol maleate, oral, 260
Etomidate,
  verapamil hydrochloride **3,** 25
Etoposide,
  cyclosporine **2,** 213
  mitomycin **3,** 220
  warfarin **3,** 83
Etretinate,
  methotrexate **2,** 217
  warfarin **2,** 83
Fat emulsion, intraveneous,
  cyclosporine **2,** 354
Felbamate,
  carbamazepine **2,** 104
  phenobarbital **3,** 317
  phenytoin **2,** 119
  valproic acid **2,** 133
  warfarin **2,** 84
Felodipine,
  erythromycin **3,** 50
Fenfluramine hydrochloride,
  chloroform, 26
  enflurane, 26
  furazolidone, 185
  halothane, 26
  hydrochlorothiazide **3,** 291
  insulin **2,** 302
  isocarboxazid, 153
  methoxyflurane, 26
  moclobemide, 153
  pargyline hydrochloride, 153
  phenelzine sulfate, 153
  procarbazine hydrochloride, 153
  tranylcypromine sulfate, 153
Fenofibrate, micronized,
  dicumarol, 80
  phenindione, 80
  warfarin, 80
  phenobarbital **3,** 10
Fenoterol hydrobromide,
  chloroform, 26
  enflurane, 26
  halothane, 26
  methoxyflurane, 26

metoprolol tartrate, 260
timolol maleate, oral, 260
Fentanyl citrate,
  citalopram hydrobromide, 14
  pargyline hydrochloride, 14
  phenelzine sulfate, 14
  propranolol hydrochloride **3,** 10
  selegiline hydrochloride, 14
  tranylcypromine sulfate, 14
Fenticonazole nitrate,
  cyclosporine, 193
  fosphenytoin sodium, parenteral, 119
  phenytoin, 119
Feprazone,
  acenocoumarol, 94
  acetohexamide, 182
  anisindione, 94
  chlorpropamide, 182
  dicumarol, 94
  gliclazide, 182
  glimepiride, 182
  gliquidone, 182
  nicoumalone, 94
  tolazamide, 182
  tolbutamide, 182
  warfarin, 94
Ferric ammonium citrate,
  demeclocycline hydrochloride, 205
  doxycycline hydrochloride, 205
  lymecycline, 205
  methacycline hydrochloride, 205
  minocycline hydrochloride pellets, 205
  minocycline hydrochloride, 205
  oxytetracycline, 205
  tetracycline, 205
Ferrous fumarate,
  demeclocycline hydrochloride, 205
  doxycycline hydrochloride, 205
  lymecycline, 205
  methacycline hydrochloride, 205
  minocycline hydrochloride pellets, 205
  minocycline hydrochloride, 205
  oxytetracycline, 205
  tetracycline, 205
Ferrous gluconate,
  demeclocycline hydrochloride, 205
  doxycycline hydrochloride, 205
  lymecycline, 205
  methacycline hydrochloride, 205
  minocycline hydrochloride pellets, 205
  minocycline hydrochloride, 205
  oxytetracycline, 205
  tetracycline, 205
Ferrous glycine sulfate,

demeclocycline hydrochloride, 205
doxycycline hydrochloride, 205
lymecycline, 205
methacycline hydrochloride, 205
minocycline hydrochloride pellets, 205
minocycline hydrochloride, 205
oxytetracycline, 205
tetracycline, 205
Ferrous hydroxide polymaltose,
  demeclocycline hydrochloride, 205
  doxycycline hydrochloride, 205
  lymecycline, 205
  methacycline hydrochloride, 205
  minocycline hydrochloride pellets, 205
  minocycline hydrochloride, 205
  oxytetracycline, 205
  tetracycline, 205
Ferrous ions, salt unspecified,
  demeclocycline hydrochloride, 205
  doxycycline hydrochloride, 205
  lymecycline, 205
  methacycline hydrochloride, 205
  minocycline hydrochloride pellets, 205
  minocycline hydrochloride, 205
  oxytetracycline, 205
  tetracycline, 205
Ferrous succinate,
  demeclocycline hydrochloride, 205
  doxycycline hydrochloride, 205
  lymecycline, 205
  methacycline hydrochloride, 205
  minocycline hydrochloride pellets, 205
  minocycline hydrochloride, 205
  oxytetracycline, 205
  tetracycline, 205
Ferrous sulfate,
  allopurinol **4,** 322
  aluminum hydroxide **3,** 322
  ascorbic acid, vitamin C **3,** 322
  cimetidine, oral **3,** 322
  ciprofloxacin hydrochloride **2,** 179
  demeclocycline hydrochloride, 205
  doxycycline hydrochloride, 205
  levodopa **2,** 355
  levothyroxine sodium **3,** 357
  lymecycline, 205
  magnesium carbonate **3,** 322
  magnesium hydroxide **3,** 322
  methacycline hydrochloride, 205
  methyldopa **2,** 166
  minocycline hydrochloride pellets, 205

minocycline hydrochloride, 205
oxytetracycline, 205
penicillamine **2,** 323
tetracycline **1,** 205
Flecainide acetate,
amiodarone hydrochloride **2,** 51
ammonium chloride **2,** 51
charcoal **3,** 51
cimetidine, oral **2,** 52
isoproterenol **2,** 52
propranolol hydrochloride **3,** 261
quinine **3,** 52
sodium bicarbonate **2,** 53
Flosequinan,
warfarin, 92
Flucloxacillin,
amikacin sulfate, 185
gentamicin sulfate, 185
netilmicin, 185
tobramycin, 185
Fluconazole,
amitriptyline hydrochloride **2,** 135
cyclosporine, 193
ethotoin, 119
fosphenytoin sodium, parenteral,
119
mephenytoin, 119
phenytoin **1,** 119
tacrolimus **2,** 367
tolbutamide **3,** 307
warfarin **2,** 84
Flumethiazide,
lithium, 239
Fluorouracil,
cimetidine, oral **3,** 214
hydrochlorothiazide **3,** 212
Fluoxetine hydrochloride,
alcohol, ethyl - oral/injectable **4,**
311
alprazolam **2,** 224
aspirin **3,** 139
buspirone hydrochloride **3,** 137
clarithromycin **3,** 139
cyclosporine **3,** 140
cyproheptadine hydrochloride **2,**
140
digoxin capsule, stabilized **2,** 274
furazolidone, 141
haloperidol **3,** 237
isocarboxazid, 141
lithium **2,** 241
marijuana **2,** 141
moclobemide, 141
nortriptyline hydrochloride **2,** 147
pargyline hydrochloride, 141
phenelzine sulfate, 141
phenytoin **2,** 120
pimozide **3,** 249
procarbazine hydrochloride, 141
propranolol hydrochloride **2,** 261
selegiline hydrochloride, 141

tranylcypromine sulfate **1,** 141
trazodone hydrochloride **3,** 154
tryptophan **3,** 142
valproic acid **3,** 133
warfarin **3,** 85
Fluoxymesterone,
acenocoumarol, 90
dicumarol, 90
nicoumalone, 90
warfarin, 90
Flupenthixol decanoate, injectable
guanethidine, 162
Flupenthixol dihydrochloride, oral,
guanethidine, 162
Fluphenazine,
clonidine hydrochloride **3,** 236
guanethidine, 162
Fluvoxamine maleate,
clozapine **2,** 231
furazolidone, 141
moclobemide, 141
olanzapine **3,** 248
pargyline hydrochloride, 141
phenelzine sulfate, 141
procarbazine hydrochloride, 141
selegiline hydrochloride, 141
theophylline **3,** 336
tranylcypromine sulfate, 141
Folic acid,
phenytoin **2,** 120
sulfasalazine **3,** 323
Foscarnet sodium,
cyclosporine **2,** 354
Fosphenytoin sodium, parenteral,
cimetidine hydrochloride,
parenteral, 115
cimetidine, oral, 115
clotrimazole, 119
disulfiram, 118
dopamine hydrochloride, 118
fenticonazole nitrate, 119
fluconazole, 119
isoconazole nitrate, 119
itraconazole, 119
ketoconazole, 119
miconazole nitrate, 119
oxiconazole nitrate, 119
ranitidine hydrochloride,
parenteral, 115
ranitidine hydrochloride, oral, 115
terconazole, 119
tioconazole, 119
Furazolidone,
alcohol, ethyl - oral/injectable **2,**
311
amphetamine **1,** 185
benzphetamine hydrochloride,
185
chloral hydrate **4,** 314
dexfenfluramine hydrochloride,
185

Index

dextroamphetamine, 185
diethylpropion hydrochloride, 185
dopamine hydrochloride, 153
ephedrine, 185
epinephrine, 185
etafedrine hydrochloride, 185
fenfluramine hydrochloride, 185
fluoxetine hydrochloride, 141
fluvoxamine maleate, 141
isometheptene, 153
levodopa, 152
mazindol, 185
meperidine hydrochloride, 14
mephentermine sulfate, 185
metaraminol bitartrate, 153
methamphetamine hydrochloride, 185
methylphenidate hydrochloride, 185
nalbuphine hydrochloride, 14
naphazoline hydrochloride, 153
oxymetazoline hydrochloride, 153
phendimetrazine tartrate, 185
phenmetrazine hydrochloride, 185
phentermine hydrochloride, 185
phenylephrine, 153
phenylpropanolamine, 185
pseudoephedrine, 185
tetrahydrozoline hydrochloride, 153
venlafaxine hydrochloride, 141
xylometazoline hydrochloride, 153
Furosemide,
  amikacin sulfate, 191
  aspirin **3,** 289
  captopril **2,** 157
  charcoal **2,** 289
  chloral hydrate **3,** 289
  cholestyramine **2,** 290
  digoxin **2,** 275
  gentamicin sulfate, 191
  indomethacin **3,** 290
  kanamycin sulfate, oral, 191
  kanamycin sulfate, parenteral, 191
  lithium, 239
  neomycin sulfate, oral, 191
  neomycin sulfate, parenteral, 191
  netilmicin, 191
  pancuronium bromide **3,** 31
  phenytoin **3,** 290
  probenecid **3,** 291
  propranolol hydrochloride **2,** 262
  streptomycin sulfate, 191
  theophylline **2,** 336
  tobramycin, 191
Furosemide, injectable,
  amikacin sulfate, 191
  gentamicin sulfate, 191
  kanamycin sulfate, oral, 191

kanamycin sulfate, parenteral, 191
lithium, 239
neomycin sulfate, oral, 191
neomycin sulfate, parenteral, 191
netilmicin, 191
streptomycin sulfate, 191
tobramycin, 191
Gallamine triethiodide,
  amikacin sulfate, 40
  bacitracin, 40
  colistin sulfate, 40
  demeclocycline hydrochloride, 40
  diazepam **3,** 25
  doxycycline hyclate, parenteral, 40
  doxycycline hydrochloride, 40
  gentamicin sulfate, 40
  kanamycin sulfate, oral, 40
  kanamycin sulfate, parenteral, 40
  lymecycline, 40
  methacycline hydrochloride, 40
  minocycline hydrochloride pellets, 40
  minocycline hydrochloride, 40
  minocycline, parenteral, 40
  neomycin sulfate, oral, 40
  neomycin sulfate, parenteral, 40
  netilmicin, 40
  oxytetracycline, 40
  oxytetracycline, parenteral, 40
  paromomycin sulfate, 40
  polymyxin B sulfate, 40
  polymyxin B sulfate, vaccine use, 40
  rolitetracycline, injectable, 40
  streptomycin sulfate, 40
  tetracycline, 40
  tetracycline hydrochloride, parenteral, 40
  tobramycin, 40
Ganciclovir,
  didanosine **2,** 352
Gemfibrozil,
  acenocoumarol, 80
  dicumarol, 80
  glyburide **2,** 300
  lovastatin **2,** 359
  nicoumalone, 80
  phenindione, 80
  warfarin, 80
Gentamicin sulfate,
  alcuronium chloride, 40
  amoxicillin, 185
  ampicillin sodium, 185
  azlocillin sodium, 185
  bacampicillin hydrochloride, 185
  benethamine penicillin, 185
  bumetanide, 191
  bumetanide, injectable, 191
  carbenicillin disodium **1,** 185
  carfecillin, 185

cefaclor, 185
cefadroxil monohydrate, 185
cefamandole nafate, 185
cefazolin sodium, 185
cefdinir, 185
cefepime hydrochloride, 185
cefmetazole sodium, 185
cefonicid sodium, 185
cefoperazone sodium, 185
ceforanide, 185
cefotaxime sodium, 185
cefotetan disodium, 185
cefoxitin sodium, 185
cefpirome sulfate, 185
cefpodoxime proxetil, 185
cefprozil, 185
ceftazidime, 185
ceftibuten dihyrate, 185
ceftizoxime sodium, 185
ceftriaxone sodium, 185
cefuroxime, 185
cephalexin, 185
cephalothin sodium **1,** 185
cephapirin sodium, 185
cephradine, 185
cloxacillin sodium, 185
cyclacillin, 185
dicloxacillin, 185
doxacurium chloride, 40
enflurane, 25
ethacrynic acid, 191
ethacrynic acid, injectable, 191
ether, 25
flucloxacillin, 185
furosemide, 191
furosemide, injectable, 191
gallamine triethiodide, 40
halothane, 25
indomethacin **2,** 186
isoflurane, 25
mecillinam, 185
methicillin sodium, 185
methoxyflurane, 25
metocurine iodide, 40
mezlocillin sodium, 185
mivacurium chloride, 40
moxalactam disodium, 185
nafcillin sodium, 185
nitrous oxide, 25
oxacillin sodium, 185
pancuronium bromide, 40
penicillin G, 185
penicillin G benzathine, 185
penicillin G procaine, 185
penicillin V, 185
pipecuronium bromide, 40
piperacillin sodium, 185
piretanide, 191
polymyxin B sulfate **2,** 186
rocuronium bromide, 40
succinylcholine chloride, 40

temocillin sodium, 185
ticarcillin disodium, 185
torsemide, injection, 191
torsemide, oral, 191
tubocurarine chloride **1,** 40
vancomycin hydrochloride **3,** 187
vecuronium bromide, 40
Ginkgo,
    aspirin **3,** 8
    warfarin **3,** 85
Ginseng,
    digoxin **3,** 275
    warfarin **3,** 85
Gliclazide,
    alcohol, ethyl - oral/injectable, 296
    feprazone, 182
    oxyphenbutazone, 182
    phenylbutazone, 182
Glimepiride,
    alcohol, ethyl - oral/injectable, 296
    feprazone, 182
    oxyphenbutazone, 182
    phenylbutazone, 182
Glipizide,
    alcohol, ethyl - oral/injectable, 296
    charcoal **2,** 299
    cholestyramine **2,** 299
    cimetidine, oral **2,** 299
    heparin **3,** 300
Gliquidone,
    alcohol, ethyl - oral/injectable, 296
    feprazone, 182
    oxyphenbutazone, 182
    phenylbutazone, 182
Glucagon,
    acenocoumarol, 86
    anisindione, 86
    dicumarol, 86
    nicoumalone, 86
    warfarin **1,** 86
Glucagon, recombinant,
    acenocoumarol, 86
    anisindione, 86
    dicumarol, 86
    nicoumalone, 86
    warfarin, 86
Glutethimide,
    acenocoumarol, 86
    alcohol, ethyl - oral/injectable **2,**
        312
    anisindione, 86
    dicumarol, 86
    labetalol hydrochloride **3,** 253
    nicoumalone, 86
    warfarin **1,** 86
Glyburide,
    alcohol, ethyl - oral/injectable, 296
    gemfibrozil **2,** 300
    rifampin **3,** 300
Glycopyrrolate,
    digoxin, 280

ritodrine hydrochloride **2,** 354
Gold sodium thiomalate,
  naproxen **2,** 10
  tobacco **3,** 11
Grapefruit juice,
  atorvastatin calcium, 360
  cerivastatin, 360
  lovastatin **1,** 360
  quinidine **3,** 323
  simvastatin, 360
  terfenadine **2,** 324
Griseofulvin,
  aspirin **3,** 8
  cyclosporine **3,** 187
  oral contraceptive agents **2,** 187
  phenobarbital **3,** 188
  warfarin **2,** 87
Guanadrel sulfate,
  amitriptyline hydrochloride, 162
  butriptyline hydrochloride, 162
  chlorpromazine hydrochloride,
    162
  cyclobenzaprine hydrochloride,
    162
  desipramine hydrochloride, 162
  doxepin hydrochloride, 162
  imipramine, 162
  maprotiline hydrochloride, 162
  nortriptyline hydrochloride, 162
  opipramol, 162
  protriptyline hydrochloride, 162
Guanethidine,
  acetophenazine maleate, 162
  alcohol, ethyl - oral/injectable **2,**
    161
  amitriptyline hydrochloride, 162
  amoxapine, 162
  butriptyline hydrochloride, 162
  chlorpromazine hydrochloride **1,**
    162
  chlorprothixene, 162
  clomipramine hydrochloride, 162
  cyclobenzaprine hydrochloride,
    162
  desipramine hydrochloride **1,** 162
  dextroamphetamine **2,** 163
  dothiepin hydrochloride, 162
  doxepin hydrochloride, 162
  doxepin hydrochloride, topical,
    162
  droperidol, 162
  flupenthixol decanoate,
    injectable, 162
  flupenthixol dihydrochloride, oral,
    162
  fluphenazine, 162
  haloperidol, 162
  hydrochlorothiazide **2,** 163
  imipramine, 162
  insulin **1,** 302
  loxapine, 162

maprotiline hydrochloride, 162
mequitazine, 162
mesoridazine besylate, 162
methdilazine, 162
methotrimeprazine, 162
minoxidil **2,** 164
nortriptyline hydrochloride, 162
opipramol, 162
oxypertine, 162
pericyazine, 162
perphenazine, 162
phenelzine sulfate **2,** 164
phenylephrine **2,** 164
piperacetazine, 162
prochlorperazine, 162
promazine hydrochloride, 162
promethazine, 162
protriptyline hydrochloride, 162
thiethylperazine maleate, 162
thioproperazine mesylate, 162
thioridazine hydrochloride, 162
thiothixene, 162
trifluoperazine hydrochloride, 162
triflupromazine hydrochloride, 162
trimeprazine tartrate, 162
trimipramine maleate, 162
zuclopenthixol, 162
Guanfacine hydrochloride,
  phenobarbital **3,** 164
Haloperidol,
  carbamazepine **2,** 237
  fluoxetine hydrochloride **3,** 237
  guanethidine, 162
  lithium **2,** 241
  methyldopa **3,** 166
  phenindione **3,** 73
  rifampin **2,** 237
  tacrine hydrochloride **2,** 238
Halothane,
  albuterol sulfate, 26
  amikacin sulfate, 25
  aminophylline **1,** 327
  amphetamine, 26
  arbutamine hydrochloride, 26
  benzphetamine hydrochloride, 26
  bitolterol mesylate, 26
  clindamycin, 25
  clindamycin phosphate,
    injectable, 25
  colistin sulfate, 25
  dexfenfluramine hydrochloride, 26
  dextroamphetamine, 26
  diethylpropion hydrochloride, 26
  dobutamine hydrochloride, 26
  dopamine hydrochloride, 26
  dyphylline, 327
  eformoterol fumarate, 26
  epinephrine **1,** 26
  ethylnorepinephrine
    hydrochloride, 26
  fenfluramine hydrochloride, 26

fenoterol hydrobromide, 26
gentamicin sulfate, 25
isoetharine, 26
isometheptene, 26
isoproterenol, 26
kanamycin sulfate, oral, 25
kanamycin sulfate, parenteral, 25
ketamine hydrochloride **2,** 27
labetalol hydrochloride **2,** 254
mazindol, 26
mephentermine sulfate, 26
metaproterenol sulfate, 26
metaraminol bitartrate, 26
methamphetamine hydrochloride, 26
methoxamine hydrochloride, 26
methylphenidate hydrochloride, 26
neomycin sulfate, oral, 25
neomycin sulfate, parenteral, 25
nifedipine **3,** 58
norepinephrine bitartrate, 26
oxtriphylline, 327
phendimetrazine tartrate, 26
phenmetrazine hydrochloride, 26
phentermine hydrochloride, 26
phenylephrine, 26
phenylpropanolamine, 26
phenytoin **3,** 26
pirbuterol acetate, 26
polymyxin B sulfate, 25
polymyxin B sulfate, vaccine use, 25
procaterol hydrochloride, 26
pseudoephedrine, 26
reserpine **2,** 169
rifampin **2,** 27
rimiterol hydrobromide, 26
salmeterol hydroxynaphthoate, 26
salmeterol xinafoate, 26
streptomycin sulfate, 25
terbutaline sulfate, 26
theophylline, 327
tobramycin, 25
Heparin,
aloxiprin, 71
aspirin **1,** 71
calcium carbaspirin, 71
carbenicillin disodium **2,** 72
dextran 40 **2,** 72
dextran 70 **2,** 72
digoxin **3,** 276
glipizide **2,** 300
nitroglycerin **2,** 72
sodium salicylate, 76
tobacco **3,** 73
Hexocyclium methylsulfate,
digoxin, 280
Hydralazine hydrochloride,
indomethacin **3,** 165
propranolol hydrochloride **3,** 262
Hydrochlorothiazide,

carbamazepine **3,** 105
chlorpropamide **2,** 298
cyclophosphamide **3,** 212
fenfluramine hydrochloride **3,** 291
fluorouracil **3,** 212
guanethidine **2,** 163
lithium, 239
methotrexate **3,** 212
Hydrocodone bitartrate,
isocarboxazid, 14
pargyline hydrochloride, 14
phenelzine sulfate, 14
selegiline hydrochloride, 14
tranylcypromine sulfate, 14
Hydrocortisone acetate, injectable,
cholestyramine **3,** 354
pancuronium bromide **3,** 32
theophylline **3,** 336
Hydrocortisone sodium succinate,
cholestyramine **3,** 354
pancuronium bromide **3,** 32
theophylline **3,** 336
Hydrocortisone sodium phosphate,
cholestyramine **3,** 354
pancuronium bromide **3,** 32
theophylline **3,** 336
Hydrocortisone, oral/systemic,
cholestyramine **3,** 354
pancuronium bromide **3,** 32
theophylline **3,** 336
Hydroflumethiazide,
lithium, 239
Hydromorphone hydrochloride,
isocarboxazid, 14
pargyline hydrochloride, 14
phenelzine sulfate, 14
selegiline hydrochloride, 14
tranylcypromine sulfate, 14
Hydroxychloroquine sulfate,
digoxin **2,** 276
Hyoscyamine,
digoxin, 280
Ibuprofen,
baclofen **3,** 11
digoxin **2,** 276
phenytoin **2,** 120
warfarin **2,** 87
Ifosfamide,
warfarin **2,** 87
Imipenem combined with cilastatin,
aminophylline **3,** 327
cyclosporine **2,** 188
Imipramine,
bupropion hydrochloride **3,** 142
cimetidine, oral **2,** 142
epinephrine **2,** 143
ethinyl estradiol **3,** 143
guanadrel sulfate, 162
guanethidine, 162
levodopa **3,** 144

liothyronine sodium **2,** 144
lithium **3,** 144
meprobamate **3,** 315
methyltestosterone **3,** 145
nitroglycerin, sublingual **2,** 145
phenytoin **3,** 121
reserpine **3,** 145
tobacco **3,** 146
tranylcypromine sulfate **2,** 146
Indapamide,
lithium, 239
Indomethacin,
aluminum hydroxide **3,** 12
aspirin **3,** 12
bendroflumethiazide **2,** 286
captopril **2,** 157
cimetidine, oral **3,** 12
cyclophosphamide **3,** 212
furosemide **3,** 290
gentamicin sulfate **2,** 186
hydralazine hydrochloride **3,** 165
lithium **2,** 241
nitroglycerin **3,** 13
penicillamine **3,** 364
phenylpropanolamine **2,** 13
prazosin hydrochloride **2,** 168
probenecid **2,** 13
propranolol hydrochloride **2,** 262
triamterene **2,** 293
warfarin **2,** 88
Influenza virus vaccine, split virion,
clorazepate dipotassium **3,** 229
phenytoin **3,** 121
theophylline **3,** 337
warfarin **3,** 88
Influenza virus vaccine, whole virion,
theophylline **3,** 337
Insulin,
acebutolol hydrochloride, 304
aspirin **3,** 301
betaxolol hydrochloride, oral, 304
bisoprolol fumarate, 304
carteolol hydrochloride, 304
carvedilol, 304
celiprolol hydrochloride, 304
chlorpromazine hydrochloride **3,**
301
clofibrate **2,** 301
diltiazem hydrochloride **3,** 301
epinephrine **3,** 175
fenfluramine hydrochloride **2,** 302
guanethidine **1,** 302
isoniazid **3,** 303
labetalol hydrochloride, 304
nadolol, 304
oxprenolol, 304
oxytetracycline **2,** 303
penbutolol sulfate, 304
phenelzine sulfate **2,** 303
phenytoin **3,** 304
pindolol, 304

propranolol hydrochloride **1,** 304
sotalol hydrochloride, 304
tertatolol hydrochloride, 304
thyroid desiccated **2,** 304
timolol maleate, ophthalmic, 304
timolol maleate, oral, 304
tobacco **3,** 305
Interferon alfa-2a,
aminophylline **2,** 327
Iocetamic acid, 62% iodine,
metformin hydrochloride, 305
Iodamide,
metformin hydrochloride, 305
Iodipamide meglumine,
metformin hydrochloride, 305
Iodoquinol,
metformin hydrochloride, 305
Iodoxamine meglumine,
metformin hydrochloride, 305
Iopamidol,
metformin hydrochloride, 305
Iopanoic acid, 66.68% iodine,
metformin hydrochloride, 305
Iopodic acid,
metformin hydrochloride, 305
Iopydol,
metformin hydrochloride, 305
Iopydone,
metformin hydrochloride, 305
Iothalamate meglumine,
metformin hydrochloride, 305
Iothalamate sodium,
metformin hydrochloride, 305
Iotrolan,
metformin hydrochloride, 305
Ioversol,
metformin hydrochloride, 305
Ioxaglate meglumine,
metformin hydrochloride, 305
Ioxaglate sodium,
metformin hydrochloride, 305
Ipodate calcium, 61.7% iodine,
metformin hydrochloride, 305
Ipodate sodium, 61.4% iodine,
metformin, hydrochloride, 305
Iron dextran complex,
demeclocycline hydrochloride, 205
doxycycline hydrochloride, 205
lymecycline, 205
methacycline hydrochloride, 205
minocycline hydrochloride
pellets, 205
minocycline hydrochloride, 205
oxytetracycline, 205
tetracycline, 205
Iron peptonized,
demeclocycline hydrochloride, 205
doxycycline hydrochloride, 205
lymecycline, 205
methacycline hydrochloride, 205
minocycline hydrochloride

pellets, 205
minocycline hydrochloride, 205
oxytetracycline, 205
tetracycline, 205
Isocarboxazid,
alfentanil hydrochloride, 14
amphetamine, 185
anileridine, 14
benzphetamine hydrochloride, 185
buprenorphine hydrochloride, 14
citalopram hydrobromide, 141
codeine, 14
dexfenfluramine hydrochloride, 153
dextroamphetamine, 153
dextromethorphan hydrobromide, 14
diethylpropion hydrochloride, 153
difenoxin hydrochloride, 14
dihydrocodeine bitartrate, 14
diphenoxylate hydrochloride, 14
dopamine hydrochloride, 153
ephedrine, 153
etafedrine hydrochloride, 153
fenfluramine hydrochloride, 153
fluoxetine hydrochloride, 141
fluvoxamine maleate, 141
hydrocodone bitartrate, 14
hydromorphone hydrochloride, 14
isometheptene, 153
levodopa, 152
levorphanol tartrate, 14
mazindol, 153
meperidine hydrochloride, 14
mephentermine sulfate, 153
meptazinol, 14
metaraminol bitartrate, 153
methamphetamine hydrochloride, 153
methylphenidate hydrochloride, 153
nalbuphine hydrochloride, 14
naphazoline hydrochloride, 153
opium, 14
oxycodone, 14
oxymetazoline hydrochloride, 153
oxymorphone hydrochloride, 14
paroxetine hydrochloride, 141
phendimetrazine tartrate, 153
phenmetrazine hydrochloride, 153
phenoperidine hydrochloride, 14
phentermine hydrochloride, 153
phenylephrine, 153
phenylpropanolamine, 153
pseudoephedrine, 153
sertraline hydrochloride, 141
sufentanil citrate, 14
tetrahydrozoline hydrochloride, 153
venlafaxine hydrochloride, 141

xylometazoline hydrochloride, 153
Isoconazole nitrate,
fosphenytoin sodium, parenteral, 119
phenytoin, 119
Isoetharine,
chloroform, 26
enflurane, 26
halothane, 26
methoxyflurane, 26
metoprolol tartrate, 260
timolol maleate, oral, 260
Isoflurane,
amikacin sulfate, 25
epinephrine, 26
gentamicin sulfate, 25
kanamycin sulfate, oral, 25
kanamycin sulfate, parenteral, 25
streptomycin sulfate, 25
succinylcholine chloride **2,** 36
tobramycin, 25
Isometheptene,
chloroform, 26
enflurane, 26
furazolidone, 153
halothane, 26
isocarboxazid, 153
moclobemide, 153
pargyline hydrochloride, 153
phenelzine sulfate, 153
procarbazine hydrochloride, 153
tranylcypromine sulfate, 153
Isoniazid,
acetaminophen **3,** 2
aluminum hydroxide **3,** 188
carbamazepine **2,** 105
diazepam **3,** 234
disulfiram **3,** 189
enflurane **3,** 24
ethosuximide **3,** 109
insulin **3,** 303
meperidine hydrochloride **3,** 189
phenytoin **2,** 122
prednisolone **3,** 189
propranolol hydrochloride **3,** 189
pyridoxine hydrochloride **3,** 190
rifampin **2,** 190
theophylline **3,** 337
valproic acid **3,** 133
warfarin **3,** 89
Isopropamide iodide,
digoxin, 280
Isoproterenol,
aminophylline **3,** 328
chloroform, 26
enflurane, 26
epinephrine, 26
ether, 26
flecainide acetate **2,** 52
halothane, 26
methoxyflurane, 26

Isosorbide dinitrate, sublingual,
  disopyramide phosphate **2,** 49
Isotretinoin,
  carbamazepine **3,** 105
Itraconazole,
  alprazolam, 250
  astemizole, 195
  buspirone hydrochloride **3,** 190
  cyclosporine, 193
  didanosine **2,** 191
  digoxin **2,** 277
  fosphenytoin sodium, parenteral,
    119
  phenytoin, 119
  terfenadine, 195
  triazolam, 250
Kanamycin sulfate, oral,
  alcuronium chloride, 40
  ampicillin sodium, 185
  atracurium besylate, 40
  benethamine penicillin, 185
  bumetanide, 191
  bumetanide, injectable, 191
  carbenicillin disodium, 185
  cefprozil, 185
  ceftibuten dihyrate, 185
  cefuroxime, 185
  cephalexin, 185
  cephalothin sodium, 185
  doxacurium chloride, 40
  enflurane, 25
  ethacrynic acid **1,** 191
  ethacrynic acid, injectable, 191
  ether, 25
  furosemide, 191
  furosemide, injectable, 191
  gallamine triethiodide, 40
  halothane, 25
  isoflurane, 25
  methoxyflurane, 25
  metocurine iodide, 40
  mivacurium chloride, 40
  moxalactam disodium, 185
  nitrous oxide, 25
  pancuronium bromide, 40
  penicillin G, 185
  penicillin G benzathine, 185
  penicillin G procaine, 185
  penicillin V, 185
  pipecuronium bromide, 40
  piretanide, 191
  rocuronium bromide, 40
  succinylcholine chloride, 40
  temocillin sodium, 185
  ticarcillin disodium, 185
  torsemide, injection, 191
  torsemide, oral, 191
  tubocurarine chloride, 40
  vecuronium bromide, 40
Kanamycin sulfate, parenteral,
  alcuronium chloride, 40

  ampicillin sodium, 185
  atracurium besylate, 40
  benethamine penicillin, 185
  bumetanide, 191
  bumetanide, injectable, 191
  carbenicillin disodium, 185
  cefprozil, 185
  ceftibuten dihyrate, 185
  cefuroxime, 185
  cephalexin, 185
  cephalothin sodium, 185
  doxacurium chloride, 40
  enflurane, 25
  ethacrynic acid, 191
  ethacrynic acid, injectable, 191
  ether, 25
  furosemide, 191
  furosemide, injectable, 191
  gallamine triethiodide, 40
  halothane, 25
  isoflurane, 25
  methoxyflurane, 25
  metocurine iodide, 40
  mivacurium chloride, 40
  moxalactam disodium, 185
  nitrous oxide, 25
  pancuronium bromide, 40
  penicillin G, 185
  penicillin G benzathine, 185
  penicillin G procaine, 185
  penicillin V, 185
  pipecuronium bromide, 40
  piretanide, 191
  rocuronium bromide, 40
  succinylcholine chloride, 40
  temocillin sodium, 185
  ticarcillin disodium, 185
  torsemide, injection, 191
  torsemide, oral, 191
  tubocurarine chloride, 40
  vecuronium bromide, 40
Kaolin,
  attapulgite, 205
  chloroquine **3,** 177
  demeclocycline hydrochloride,
    205
  digoxin **2,** 277
  doxycycline hydrochloride, 205
  lincomycin hydrochloride **1,** 196
  lymecycline, 205
  methacycline hydrochloride, 205
  minocycline hydrochloride
    pellets, 205
  minocycline hydrochloride, 205
  oxytetracycline, 205
  tetracycline, 205
Ketamine hydrochloride,
  aminophylline **3,** 328
  diazepam **2,** 27
  halothane **2,** 27
  thyroid strong **3,** 28

tubocurarine chloride **2,** 40
Ketoconazole,
  alcohol, ethyl - oral/injectable **3,** 312
  alprazolam, 250
  aluminum hydroxide **2,** 192
  astemizole, 195
  chlordiazepoxide **3,** 244
  cimetidine, oral **2,** 192
  cyclosporine **1,** 193
  fosphenytoin sodium, parenteral, 119
  magnesium hydroxide **2,** 192
  methylprednisolone **2,** 193
  omeprazole **2,** 194
  phenytoin, 119
  quinidine **2,** 62
  rifampin **2,** 194
  sucralfate **3,** 195
  terfenadine **1,** 195
  theophylline **3,** 338
  triazolam **1,** 250
Ketoprofen,
  methotrexate **2,** 217
Labetalol hydrochloride,
  cimetidine hydrochloride, parenteral, 258
  cimetidine, oral, 258
  glutethimide **3,** 253
  halothane **2,** 254
  insulin, 304
Lamotrigine,
  acetaminophen **3,** 110
  valproic acid **3,** 110
Lercanidipine hydrochloride,
  cyclosporine, 46
  quinidine, 292
Leucovorin calcium,
  methotrexate **1,** 218
  methotrexate sodium, parenteral, 218
Levodopa,
  aluminum hydroxide **3,** 355
  chlorpromazine hydrochloride **3,** 227
  diazepam **3,** 234
  domperidone **3,** 355
  ferrous sulfate **2,** 355
  furazolidone, 152
  imipramine **3,** 144
  isocarboxazid, 152
  magnesium hydroxide **3,** 355
  methyldopa **3,** 166
  metoclopramide hydrochloride **3,** 361
  moclobemide, 152
  papaverine hydrochloride **3,** 356
  pargyline hydrochloride, 152
  phenelzine sulfate **1,** 152
  phenytoin **3,** 122
  procarbazine hydrochloride, 152

pyridoxine hydrochloride **1,** 325
  tranylcypromine sulfate, 152
  trihexyphenidyl hydrochloride **4,** 356
Levodopa, combined with benserazide,
  orphenadrine citrate **3,** 356
Levodopa, combined with carbidopa,
  domperidone **3,** 355
Levorphanol tartrate,
  isocarboxazid, 14
  pargyline hydrochloride, 14
  phenelzine sulfate, 14
  selegiline hydrochloride, 14
  tranylcypromine sulfate, 14
Levothyroxine sodium,
  acenocoumarol, 100
  aminophylline **3,** 328
  anisindione, 100
  calcium carbonate, oral **3,** 357
  chloroquine **3,** 178
  dicumarol, 100
  ferrous sulfate **3,** 357
  lovastatin **3,** 357
  nicoumalone, 100
  phenytoin **3,** 122
  sucralfate **3,** 358
  warfarin, 100
Lidocaine hydrochloride, local-injectable,
  cimetidine hydrochloride, parenteral, 53
  cimetidine, oral, 53
Lidocaine hydrochloride, systemic,
  amiodarone hydrochloride **2,** 46
  cimetidine hydrochloride, parenteral, 53
  cimetidine, oral **1,** 53
  phenobarbital **3,** 53
  procainamide hydrochloride **3,** 54
  propranolol hydrochloride **2,** 54
  succinylcholine chloride **2,** 36
Lincomycin hydrochloride,
  erythromycin **3,** 196
  kaolin **1,** 196
Liothyronine sodium,
  acenocoumarol, 100
  dicumarol, 100
  imipramine **2,** 144
  nicoumalone, 100
  warfarin, 100
Lithium,
  acetazolamide **1,** 238
  acyclovir, parenteral **3,** 238
  alcohol, ethyl - oral/injectable **3,** 239
  bendroflumethiazide, 239
  benzthiazide, 239
  brinzolamide, ophthalmic, 238
  bumetanide, 239

Index

bumetanide, injectable, 239
carbamazepine **2,** 239
chlorothiazide **1,** 239
chlorpromazine hydrochloride **2,** 227
chlorthalidone, 239
cisplatin **3,** 240
cyclopenthiazide, 239
cyclothiazide, 239
diazepam **3,** 240
dichlorphenamide, 238
disodium hydrogen citrate, 238
dorzolamide hydrochloride, 238
dorzolamide hydrochloride, 238
enalapril maleate **2,** 240
ethacrynic acid, 239
ethacrynic acid, injectable, 239
flumethiazide, 239
fluoxetine hydrochloride **2,** 241
furosemide, 239
furosemide, injectable, 239
haloperidol **2,** 241
hydrochlorothiazide, 239
hydroflumethiazide, 239
imipramine **3,** 144
indapamide, 239
indomethacin **2,** 241
mazindol **2,** 242
methazolamide, 238
methyclothiazide, 239
methyldopa **2,** 242
metolazone, 239
metoprolol tartrate **2,** 243
metronidazole, systemic **2,** 243
norepinephrine bitartrate **3,** 243
pancuronium bromide **3,** 32
phenytoin **3,** 244
piretanide, 239
polythiazide, 239
potassium citrate, 238
potassium iodide **2,** 244
quinethazone, 239
sodium acetate, 238
sodium bicarbonate, 238
sodium bicarbonate, parenteral, 238
sodium citrate, 238
sodium lactate, 238
tetracycline **2,** 244
theophylline **2,** 245
thioridazine hydrochloride **2,** 245
torsemide, injection, 239
torsemide, oral, 239
trichlormethiazide, 239
tromethamine, 238
verapamil hydrochloride **2,** 246
xipamide, 239
Lofexidine hydrochloride,
propranolol hydrochloride, 160
Lomefloxacin hydrochloride,
warfarin, 92

Lomustine,
theophylline **3,** 215
Lorazepam,
probenecid **3,** 246
Lovastatin,
cyclosporine **3,** 358
erythromycin **1,** 359
erythromycin estolate, 359
erythromycin ethylsuccinate, 359
erythromycin glucephate, 359
erythromycin lactobionate, 359
erythromycin stearate, 359
gemfibrozil **2,** 359
grapefruit juice **1,** 360
levothyroxine sodium **3,** 357
niacin, vitamin B3 **2,** 360
warfarin **2,** 89
Loxapine,
guanethidine, 162
sumatriptan succinate, injection **3,** 247
Lymecycline,
alcuronium chloride, 40
attapulgite, 205
calcium lactobionate, oral, 205
carbonyl iron, 205
digoxin, 282
digoxin capsule, stabilized, 282
doxacurium chloride, 40
ferric ammonium citrate, 205
ferrous fumarate, 205
ferrous gluconate, 205
ferrous glycine sulfate, 205
ferrous hydroxide polymaltose, 205
ferrous ions, salt unspecified, 205
ferrous succinate, 205
ferrous sulfate, 205
gallamine triethiodide, 40
iron dextran complex, 205
iron peptonized, 205
kaolin, 205
magaldrate, 205
metocurine iodide, 40
minocycline hydrochloride
pellets, 282
mivacurium chloride, 40
pancuronium bromide, 40
pipecuronium bromide, 40
rocuronium bromide, 40
succinylcholine chloride, 40
tubocurarine chloride, 40
vecuronium bromide, 40
Magaldrate,
demeclocycline hydrochloride, 205
doxycycline hydrochloride, 205
lymecycline, 205
methacycline hydrochloride, 205
minocycline hydrochloride
pellets, 205

minocycline hydrochloride, 205
oxytetracycline, 205
tetracycline, 205
ticlopidine hydrochloride **3,** 73
Magnesium aspartate,
tetracycline, 205
Magnesium carbonate,
captopril **3,** 156
demeclocycline hydrochloride,
205
doxycycline hydrochloride, 205
ferrous sulfate **3,** 322
methacycline hydrochloride, 205
oxytetracycline, 205
tetracycline, 205
Magnesium chloride, oral,
demeclocycline hydrochloride,
205
doxycycline hydrochloride, 205
methacycline hydrochloride, 205
oxytetracycline, 205
tetracycline, 205
Magnesium citrate,
tetracycline, 205
Magnesium glucoheptonate,
tetracycline, 205
Magnesium gluconate,
tetracycline, 205
Magnesium hydroxide,
aspirin **2,** 7
captopril **3,** 156
chlorpromazine hydrochloride **3,**
225
cimetidine, oral **3,** 347
ciprofloxacin hydrochloride **2,** 178
clorazepate dipotassium **3,** 229
demeclocycline hydrochloride,
205
digoxin **2,** 270
doxycycline hydrochloride, 205
ferrous sulfate **3,** 322
ketoconazole **2,** 192
levodopa **3,** 355
methacycline hydrochloride, 205
mexiletine hydrochloride **3,** 54
misoprostol **3,** 362
oxytetracycline, 205
penicillamine **3,** 364
sodium polystyrene sulfonate **2,**
361
tetracycline, 205
theophylline **3,** 332
ticlopidine hydrochloride **3,** 73
warfarin **4,** 89
Magnesium lactate,
tetracycline, 205
Magnesium oxide,
demeclocycline hydrochloride,
205
doxycycline hydrochloride, 205
methacycline hydrochloride, 205

oxytetracycline, 205
tetracycline, 205
Magnesium salicylate,
demeclocycline hydrochloride,
205
methotrexate, 216
methotrexate sodium, parenteral,
216
Magnesium sulfate,
demeclocycline hydrochloride,
205
doxycycline hydrochloride, 205
methacycline hydrochloride, 205
nifedipine **3,** 58
oxytetracycline, 205
tetracycline, 205
Magnesium sulfate, parenteral,
vecuronium bromide **3,** 42
Magnesium trisilicate,
demeclocycline hydrochloride,
205
digoxin **2,** 270
doxycycline hydrochloride, 205
methacycline hydrochloride, 205
nitrofurantoin **3,** 198
oxytetracycline, 205
phenytoin **3,** 112
tetracycline, 205
Magnesium, salt unspecified,
tetracycline, 205
Maprotiline hydrochloride,
guanadrel sulfate, 162
guanethidine, 162
Marijuana,
fluoxetine hydrochloride **2,** 141
nortriptyline hydrochloride **2,** 147
Mazindol,
bethanidine sulphate **2,** 156
chloroform, 26
enflurane, 26
furazolidone, 185
halothane, 26
isocarboxazid, 153
lithium **2,** 242
methoxyflurane, 26
metoprolol tartrate, 260
pargyline hydrochloride, 185
phenelzine sulfate, 185
procarbazine hydrochloride, 185
propranolol hydrochloride, 260
timolol maleate, ophthalmic, 260
timolol maleate, oral, 260
tranylcypromine sulfate, 153
Mecillinam,
gentamicin sulfate, 185
Medroxyprogesterone acetate,
aminoglutethimide **3,** 361
Meglumine iotroxiate,
metformin hydrochloride, 305
Melphalan,
cyclosporine **2,** 215

Menadiol sodium disphos, vitamin
K4,
    acenocoumarol, 95
    dicumarol, 95
    nicoumalone, 95
    warfarin, 95
Menadione,
    acenocoumarol, 95
    dicumarol, 95
    nicoumalone, 95
    phenindione, 95
    warfarin, 95
Mepenzolate bromide,
    digoxin, 280
Meperidine hydrochloride,
    chlorpromazine hydrochloride **2,**
        14
    furazolidone, 14
    isocarboxazid, 14
    isoniazid **3,** 189
    moclobemide, 14
    pargyline hydrochloride, 14
    phenelzine sulfate **1,** 14
    phenobarbital **3,** 14
    phenytoin **3,** 15
    procarbazine hydrochloride, 14
    selegiline hydrochloride, 14
    tranylcypromine sulfate, 14
Mephentermine sulfate,
    chloroform, 26
    enflurane, 26
    furazolidone, 185
    halothane, 26
    isocarboxazid, 153
    methoxyflurane, 26
    moclobemide, 153
    pargyline hydrochloride, 153
    phenelzine sulfate, 153
    procarbazine hydrochloride, 153
    tranylcypromine sulfate, 153
Mephenytoin,
    cimetidine hydrochloride,
        parenteral, 115
    cimetidine, oral, 115
    disulfiram, 118
    fluconazole, 119
    ranitidine hydrochloride,
        parenteral, 115
    ranitidine hydrochloride, oral, 115
Mephobarbital,
    acenocoumarol, 94
    dicumarol, 94
    nicoumalone, 94
    warfarin, 94
Meprobamate,
    alcohol, ethyl - oral/injectable **2,**
        315
    imipramine **3,** 315
    warfarin **3,** 90
Meptazinol,
    isocarboxazid, 14

pargyline hydrochloride, 14
phenelzine sulfate, 14
selegiline hydrochloride, 14
tranylcypromine sulfate, 14
Mequitazine,
    guanethidine, 162
Mercaptopurine,
    allopurinol **1,** 215
Mesoridazine besylate,
    guanethidine, 162
Mestranol,
    rifampin, 202
Metaproterenol sulfate,
    chloroform, 26
    enflurane, 26
    halothane, 26
    methoxyflurane, 26
    metoprolol tartrate, 260
    timolol maleate, oral, 260
Metaraminol bitartrate,
    chloroform, 26
    enflurane, 26
    furazolidone, 153
    halothane, 26
    isocarboxazid, 153
    methoxyflurane, 26
    metoprolol tartrate, 260
    pargyline hydrochloride, 153
    phenelzine sulfate, 153
    procarbazine hydrochloride, 153
    propranolol hydrochloride, 260
    timolol maleate, ophthalmic, 260
    timolol maleate, oral, 260
    tranylcypromine sulfate, 153
Metformin hydrochloride,
    calcium iodate, 305
    diatrizoate meglumine, 305
    diatrizoate sodium, 305
    iocetamic acid, 62% iodine, 305
    iodamide, 305
    iodipamide meglumine, 305
    iodoquinol, 305
    iodoxamine meglumine, 305
    iopamidol, 305
    iopanoic acid, 66.68% iodine,
        305
    iopodic acid, 305
    iopydol, 305
    iopydone, 305
    iothalamate meglumine, 305
    iothalamate sodium, 305
    iotrolan, 305
    ioversol, 305
    ioxaglate meglumine, 305
    ioxaglate sodium, 305
    ipodate calcium, 61.7% iodine,
        305
    ipodate sodium, 61.4% iodine,
        305
    meglumine iotroxiate, 305
    metrizamide, 305

propyliodine, 305
radioactive iodine-131, 305
tyropanoate sodium, 57.4%
  iodine, 305
Methacycline hydrochloride,
  alcuronium chloride, 40
  aluminum carbonate, basic, 205
  aluminum hydroxide, 205
  aluminum oxide, 205
  aluminum phosphate, 205
  attapulgite, 205
  bismuth subsalicylate, 205
  calcium acetate, 205
  calcium ascorbate, 205
  calcium carbonate, oral, 205
  calcium chloride, oral, 205
  calcium citrate, oral, 205
  calcium glubionate, oral, 205
  calcium glucoheptonate, 205
  calcium gluconate, oral, 205
  calcium glycerophosphate, oral,
    205
  calcium iodate, 205
  calcium lactate gluconate, 205
  calcium lactate, oral, 205
  calcium lactobionate, oral, 205
  calcium phosphate, oral, 205
  calcium, oral salt unspecified,
    205
  carbonyl iron, 205
  digoxin, 282
  digoxin capsule, stabilized, 282
  dihydroxyaluminum, 205
  doxacurium chloride, 40
  ferric ammonium citrate, 205
  ferrous fumarate, 205
  ferrous gluconate, 205
  ferrous glycine sulfate, 205
  ferrous hydroxide polymaltose,
    205
  ferrous ions, salt unspecified, 205
  ferrous succinate, 205
  ferrous sulfate, 205
  gallamine triethiodide, 40
  iron dextran complex, 205
  iron peptonized, 205
  kaolin, 205
  magaldrate, 205
  magnesium carbonate, 205
  magnesium chloride, oral, 205
  magnesium hydroxide, 205
  magnesium oxide, 205
  magnesium sulfate, 205
  magnesium trisilicate, 205
  metocurine iodide, 40
  mivacurium chloride, 40
  pancuronium bromide, 40
  pipecuronium bromide, 40
  rocuronium bromide, 40
  succinylcholine chloride, 40
  sucralfate, 205

tubocurarine chloride, 40
vecuronium bromide, 40
Methadone hydrochloride,
  ammonium chloride **3,** 15
  diazepam **3,** 15
  rifampin **2,** 16
Methamphetamine hydrochloride,
  chloroform, 26
  enflurane, 26
  furazolidone, 185
  halothane, 26
  isocarboxazid, 153
  methoxyflurane, 26
  moclobemide, 153
  pargyline hydrochloride, 153
  phenelzine sulfate, 153
  procarbazine hydrochloride, 153
  tranylcypromine sulfate, 153
Methandrostenolone,
  acenocoumarol, 90
  dicumarol, 90
  nicoumalone, 90
  oxyphenbutazone **3,** 18
  warfarin, 90
Methantheline bromide,
  digoxin, 280
Metharbital,
  acenocoumarol, 94
  dicumarol, 94
  nicoumalone, 94
  warfarin, 94
Methazolamide,
  lithium, 238
Methdilazine,
  guanethidine, 162
Methicillin sodium,
  amikacin sulfate, 185
  gentamicin sulfate, 185
  neomycin sulfate, oral, 185
  netilmicin, 185
  tobramycin, 185
Methimazole,
  theophylline **3,** 338
Methohexital sodium,
  acenocoumarol, 94
  dicumarol, 94
  nicoumalone, 94
  warfarin, 94
Methotrexate,
  alcohol, ethyl - oral/injectable **3,**
    216
  aloxiprin, 216
  aspirin **1,** 216
  calcium carbaspirin, 216
  choline salicylate, 216
  cisplatin **2,** 216
  cyclophosphamide **3,** 212
  cytarabine **3,** 217
  diflunisal, 216
  etretinate **2,** 217
  hydrochlorothiazide **3,** 212

ketoprofen **2,** 217
leucovorin calcium **1,** 218
magnesium salicylate, 216
neomycin sulfate, oral **2,** 218
phenytoin **2,** 114
probenecid **1,** 219
procarbazine hydrochloride **2,**
    219
proguanil hydrochloride, 220
salicylamide, 216
salsalate, 216
sodium bicarbonate **3,** 219
sodium salicylate, 216
sodium thiosalicylate, 216
sulfacytine, 220
sulfadiazine, 220
sulfadoxine, 220
sulfamerazine, 220
sulfamethazine, 220
sulfamethizole, 220
sulfamethoxazole **1,** 220
sulfapyridine, 220
sulfasalazine, 220
sulfisoxazole, 220
trimethoprim **1,** 220
Methotrexate sodium, parenteral,
    aloxiprin, 216
    aspirin, 216
    calcium carbaspirin, 216
    choline salicylate, 216
    cytarabine **3,** 217
    diflunisal, 216
    leucovorin calcium, 218
    magnesium salicylate, 216
    omeprazole **2,** 218
    probenecid, 219
    proguanil hydrochloride, 220
    salicylamide, 216
    salsalate, 216
    sodium salicylate, 216
    sodium thiosalicylate, 216
    sulfacytine, 220
    sulfadiazine, 220
    sulfadoxine, 220
    sulfamerazine, 220
    sulfamethazine, 220
    sulfamethizole, 220
    sulfamethoxazole, 220
    sulfapyridine, 220
    sulfasalazine, 220
    sulfisoxazole, 220
    trimethoprim, 220
Methotrimeprazine,
    guanethidine, 162
Methoxamine hydrochloride,
    chloroform, 26
    enflurane, 26
    halothane, 26
    methoxyflurane, 26
    metoprolol tartrate, 260
    propranolol hydrochloride, 260

timolol maleate, ophthalmic, 260
timolol maleate, oral, 260
Methoxsalen,
    caffeine **3,** 330
    phenytoin **2,** 123
Methoxyflurane,
    albuterol sulfate, 26
    amikacin sulfate, 25
    amphetamine, 26
    arbutamine hydrochloride, 26
    bacitracin, 25
    benzphetamine hydrochloride, 26
    bitolterol mesylate, 26
    clindamycin, 25
    clindamycin phosphate, injectable
        25
    colistin sulfate, 25
    dexfenfluramine hydrochloride,
        26
    dextroamphetamine, 26
    diethylpropion hydrochloride, 26
    dobutamine hydrochloride, 26
    dopamine hydrochloride, 26
    eformoterol fumarate, 26
    ephedrine, 26
    epinephrine, 26
    etafedrine hydrochloride, 26
    ethylnorepinephrine
        hydrochloride, 26
    fenfluramine hydrochloride, 26
    fenoterol hydrobromide, 26
    gentamicin sulfate, 25
    isoetharine, 26
    isoproterenol, 26
    kanamycin sulfate, oral, 25
    kanamycin sulfate, parenteral, 25
    mazindol, 26
    mephentermine sulfate, 26
    metaproterenol sulfate, 26
    metaraminol bitartrate, 26
    methamphetamine hydrochloride,
        26
    methoxamine hydrochloride, 26
    methylphenidate hydrochloride,
        26
    neomycin sulfate, oral, 25
    neomycin sulfate, parenteral, 25
    norepinephrine bitartrate, 26
    phendimetrazine tartrate, 26
    phenmetrazine hydrochloride, 26
    phentermine hydrochloride, 26
    phenylephrine, 26
    phenylpropanolamine, 26
    pirbuterol acetate, 26
    polymyxin B sulfate, 25
    polymyxin B sulfate, vaccine use,
        25
    procaterol hydrochloride, 26
    pseudoephedrine, 26
    rimiterol hydrobromide, 26
    salmeterol hydroxynaphthoate, 26

salmeterol xinafoate, 26
secobarbital **2,** 28
streptomycin sulfate, 25
terbutaline sulfate, 26
tetracycline **2,** 29
tobramycin, 25
Methscopolamine bromide,
  digoxin, 280
Methscopolamine nitrate,
  digoxin, 280
Methyclothiazide,
  lithium, 239
Methyldopa,
  amitriptyline hydrochloride **3,** 165
  digoxin **3,** 277
  ferrous sulfate **2,** 166
  haloperidol **3,** 166
  levodopa **3,** 166
  lithium **2,** 242
  norepinephrine bitartrate **2,** 167
  pargyline hydrochloride **3,** 149
  phenobarbital **4,** 167
  phenoxybenzamine hydrochloride
    3, 167
  propranolol hydrochloride **2,** 168
  tolbutamide **3,** 307
Methylphenidate hydrochloride,
  chloroform, 26
  dicumarol **3,** 70
  enflurane, 26
  furazolidone, 185
  halothane, 26
  isocarboxazid, 153
  methoxyflurane, 26
  moclobemide, 153
  pargyline hydrochloride, 153
  phenelzine sulfate, 153
  phenytoin **3,** 123
  procarbazine hydrochloride, 153
  tranylcypromine sulfate, 153
Methylprednisolone,
  aspirin **2,** 8
  ketoconazole **2,** 193
  pyridostigmine **3,** 366
  troleandomycin **2,** 207
Methyltestosterone,
  acenocoumarol, 90
  anisindione, 90
  cyclosporine **2,** 350
  dicumarol, 90
  imipramine **3,** 145
  nicoumalone, 90
  warfarin **1,** 90
Methyprylon,
  acenocoumarol, 86
  dicumarol, 86
  nicoumalone, 86
  warfarin, 86
Metoclopramide hydrochloride,
  alcohol, ethyl - oral/injectable **3,**
    312

atropine **3,** 361
carbamazepine **3,** 106
chlorothiazide **3,** 287
cimetidine, oral **3,** 348
cyclosporine **2,** 350
digoxin **2,** 278
levodopa **3,** 361
mexiletine hydrochloride **3,** 56
morphine **3,** 17
quinidine **3,** 63
succinylcholine chloride **3,** 36
Metocurine iodide,
  amikacin sulfate, 40
  bacitracin, 40
  colistin sulfate, 40
  demeclocycline hydrochloride, 40
  doxycycline hyclate, parenteral,
    40
  doxycycline hydrochloride, 40
  gentamicin sulfate, 40
  kanamycin sulfate, oral, 40
  kanamycin sulfate, parenteral, 40
  lymecycline, 40
  methacycline hydrochloride, 40
  minocycline hydrochloride pellets,
    40
  minocycline hydrochloride, 40
  minocycline, parenteral, 40
  neomycin sulfate, oral, 40
  neomycin sulfate, parenteral, 40
  netilmicin, 40
  oxytetracycline, 40
  oxytetracycline, parenteral, 40
  paromomycin sulfate, 40
  phenytoin **2,** 29
  polymyxin B sulfate, 40
  polymyxin B sulfate, vaccine use,
    40
  rolitetracycline, injectable, 40
  streptomycin sulfate, 40
  tetracycline, 40
  tetracycline hydrochloride,
    parenteral, 40
  tobramycin, 40
Metolazone,
  lithium, 239
Metoprolol tartrate,
  albuterol sulfate, 260
  amiodarone hydrochloride **2,** 254
  bitolterol mesylate, 260
  cimetidine hydrochloride,
    parenteral, 258
  cimetidine, oral, 258
  clonidine hydrochloride,
    transdermal, 160
  clonidine hydrochloride, 160
  dexfenfluramine hydrochloride,
    260
  dopamine hydrochloride, 260
  eformoterol fumarate, 260
  etafedrine hydrochloride, 260

ethylnorepinephrine
hydrochloride, 260
fenoterol hydrobromide, 260
isoetharine, 260
lithium **2,** 243
mazindol, 260
metaproterenol sulfate, 260
metaraminol bitartrate, 260
methoxamine hydrochloride, 260
oral contraceptive agents **3,** 255
pentobarbital sodium **2,** 255
pirbuterol acetate, 260
procaterol hydrochloride, 260
rifampin **2,** 255
rimiterol hydrobromide, 260
salmeterol xinafoate, 260
terbutaline sulfate, 260
Metrizamide,
metformin hydrochloride, 305
Metronidazole, parenteral,
cimetidine, oral **3,** 197
Metronidazole, systemic,
alcohol, ethyl - oral/injectable **2,**
313
carbamazepine **2,** 106
chloroquine **2,** 196
disulfiram **2,** 197
lithium **2,** 243
phenobarbital **2,** 197
phenytoin **3,** 123
warfarin **2,** 90
Metyrapone,
phenytoin **3,** 362
Mexiletine hydrochloride,
aluminum hydroxide **3,** 54
ammonium chloride **3,** 55
atropine **3,** 55
digoxin **4,** 278
magnesium hydroxide **3,** 54
metoclopramide hydrochloride **3,**
56
phenytoin **3,** 56
rifampin **3,** 56
theophylline **2,** 338
tobacco **3,** 56
Mezlocillin sodium,
amikacin sulfate, 185
gentamicin sulfate, 185
netilmicin, 185
tobramycin, 185
Miconazole nitrate,
cyclosporine, 193
fosphenytoin sodium, parenteral,
119
phenytoin, 119
tobramycin **3,** 207
Midazolam hydrochloride,
erythromycin **2,** 247
thiopental sodium **3,** 247
Minocycline hydrochloride pellets,
alcuronium chloride, 40

attapulgite, 205
calcium lactobionate, oral, 205
carbonyl iron, 205
digoxin, 282
doxacurium chloride, 40
ferric ammonium citrate, 205
ferrous fumarate, 205
ferrous gluconate, 205
ferrous glycine sulfate, 205
ferrous hydroxide polymaltose,
205
ferrous ions, salt unspecified, 205
ferrous succinate, 205
ferrous sulfate, 205
gallamine triethiodide, 40
iron dextran complex, 205
iron peptonized, 205
kaolin, 205
lymecycline, 282
magaldrate, 205
metocurine iodide, 40
mivacurium chloride, 40
pancuronium bromide, 40
pipecuronium bromide, 40
rocuronium bromide, 40
succinylcholine chloride, 40
tubocurarine chloride, 40
vecuronium bromide, 40
Minocycline hydrochloride,
alcuronium chloride, 40
attapulgite, 205
calcium lactobionate, oral, 205
carbonyl iron, 205
digoxin, 282
digoxin capsule, stabilized, 282
doxacurium chloride, 40
ferric ammonium citrate, 205
ferrous fumarate, 205
ferrous gluconate, 205
ferrous glycine sulfate, 205
ferrous hydroxide polymaltose,
205
ferrous ions, salt unspecified, 205
ferrous succinate, 205
ferrous sulfate, 205
gallamine triethiodide, 40
iron dextran complex, 205
iron peptonized, 205
kaolin, 205
magaldrate, 205
metocurine iodide, 40
mivacurium chloride, 40
pancuronium bromide, 40
pipecuronium bromide, 40
rocuronium bromide, 40
succinylcholine chloride, 40
tubocurarine chloride, 40
vecuronium bromide, 40
Minocycline, parenteral,
alcuronium chloride, 40
digoxin, 282

digoxin capsule, stabilized, 282
doxacurium chloride, 40
gallamine triethiodide, 40
metocurine iodide, 40
mivacurium chloride, 40
pancuronium bromide, 40
pipecuronium bromide, 40
rocuronium bromide, 40
succinylcholine chloride, 40
tubocurarine chloride, 40
vecuronium bromide, 40
Minoxidil,
  guanethidine **2,** 164
Misoprostol,
  aluminum hydroxide **3,** 362
  magnesium hydroxide **3,** 362
  phenylbutazone **3,** 19
  propranolol hydrochloride **3,** 263
Mitomycin,
  etoposide **3,** 220
  vinblastine sulfate **2,** 220
Mitotane,
  spironolactone **3,** 221
  warfarin **2,** 91
Mivacurium chloride,
  amikacin sulfate, 40
  bacitracin, 40
  colistin sulfate, 40
  demeclocycline hydrochloride, 40
  doxycycline hyclate, parenteral, 40
  doxycycline hydrochloride, 40
  gentamicin sulfate, 40
  kanamycin sulfate, oral, 40
  kanamycin sulfate, parenteral, 40
  lymecycline, 40
  methacycline hydrochloride, 40
  minocycline hydrochloride pellets, 40
  minocycline hydrochloride, 40
  minocycline, parenteral, 40
  neomycin sulfate, oral, 40
  neomycin sulfate, parenteral, 40
  netilmicin, 40
  oxytetracycline, 40
  oxytetracycline, parenteral, 40
  paromomycin sulfate, 40
  polymyxin B sulfate, 40
  polymyxin B sulfate, vaccine use, 40
  rolitetracycline, injectable, 40
  streptomycin sulfate, 40
  tetracycline, 40
  tetracycline hydrochloride, parenteral, 40
  tobramycin, 40
Moclobemide,
  benzphetamine hydrochloride, 153
  citalopram hydrobromide, 141
  dexfenfluramine hydrochloride, 153
  dextroamphetamine, 153
  dextromethorphan hydrobromide, 14
  diethylpropion hydrochloride, 153
  dopamine hydrochloride, 153
  ephedrine, 153
  fenfluramine hydrochloride, 153
  fluoxetine hydrochloride, 141
  fluvoxamine maleate, 141
  isometheptene, 153
  levodopa, 152
  meperidine hydrochloride, 14
  mephentermine sulfate, 153
  methamphetamine hydrochloride, 153
  methylphenidate hydrochloride, 153
  phendimetrazine tartrate, 153
  phenmetrazine hydrochloride, 153
  phenylpropanolamine, 153
  pseudoephedrine, 153
  venlafaxine hydrochloride, 141
Monosulfiram,
  alcohol, ethyl - oral/injectable, 311
Moricizine hydrochloride,
  cimetidine, oral **3,** 57
  digoxin **4,** 278
  theophylline **3,** 339
  warfarin **2,** 92
Morphine,
  amitriptyline hydrochloride **3,** 16
  cimetidine, oral **2,** 17
  metoclopramide hydrochloride **3,** 17
  thiopental sodium **2,** 38
  tubocurarine chloride **2,** 40
Moxalactam disodium,
  amikacin sulfate, 185
  gentamicin sulfate, 185
  kanamycin sulfate, oral, 185
  kanamycin sulfate, parenteral, 185
  neomycin sulfate, oral, 185
  neomycin sulfate, parenteral, 185
  netilmicin, 185
  paromomycin sulfate, 185
  streptomycin sulfate, 185
  tobramycin, 185
Nadolol,
  clonidine hydrochloride, transdermal, 160
  clonidine hydrochloride, 160
  epinephrine, 260
  insulin, 304
  phenelzine sulfate **3,** 256
Nafcillin sodium,
  amikacin sulfate, 185
  cyclosporine **2,** 351
  gentamicin sulfate, 185
  netilmicin, 185
  tobramycin, 185

warfarin **2,** 92
Nalbuphine hydrochloride,
  furazolidone, 14
  isocarboxazid, 14
  pargyline hydrochloride, 14
  phenelzine sulfate, 14
  selegiline hydrochloride, 14
  tranylcypromine sulfate, 14
Nalidixic acid,
  acenocoumarol, 92
  anisindione, 92
  dicumarol, 92
  nicoumalone, 92
  warfarin **1,** 92
Naloxone hydrochloride,
  captopril **3,** 158
  clonidine hydrochloride **3,** 159
Naphazoline hydrochloride,
  furazolidone, 153
  isocarboxazid, 153
  pargyline hydrochloride, 153
  phenelzine sulfate, 153
  tranylcypromine sulfate, 153
Naproxen,
  cholestyramine **3,** 17
  gold sodium thiomalate **2,** 10
  valproic acid **3,** 130
  simvastatin **3,** 366
Neomycin sulfate, oral,
  alcuronium chloride, 40
  ampicillin sodium, 185
  atracurium besylate, 40
  benethamine penicillin, 185
  bumetanide, 191
  bumetanide, injectable, 191
  carbenicillin disodium, 185
  cefprozil, 185
  ceftibuten dihyrate, 185
  cefuroxime, 185
  cephalexin, 185
  cephalothin sodium, 185
  digoxin **2,** 279
  doxacurium chloride, 40
  ethacrynic acid, 191
  ethacrynic acid, injectable, 191
  ether **1,** 25
  furosemide, 191
  furosemide, injectable, 191
  gallamine triethiodide, 40
  halothane, 25
  methicillin sodium, 185
  methotrexate **2,** 218
  methoxyflurane, 25
  metocurine iodide, 40
  mivacurium chloride, 40
  moxalactam disodium, 185
  nitrous oxide, 25
  pancuronium bromide, 40
  penicillin G, 185
  penicillin G benzathine, 185
  penicillin G procaine, 185

  penicillin V, 185
  pipecuronium bromide, 40
  piretanide, 191
  rocuronium bromide, 40
  succinylcholine chloride, 40
  temocillin sodium, 185
  ticarcillin disodium, 185
  torsemide, injection, 191
  torsemide, oral, 191
  tubocurarine chloride, 40
  vecuronium bromide, 40
  vitamin A **3,** 325
  vitamin A, prenatal multivitamin
    use **3,** 325
  warfarin **3,** 93
Neomycin sulfate, parenteral,
  alcuronium chloride, 40
  ampicillin sodium, 185
  atracurium besylate, 40
  benethamine penicillin, 185
  bumetanide, 191
  bumetanide, injectable, 191
  carbenicillin disodium, 185
  cefprozil, 185
  ceftibuten dihyrate, 185
  cefuroxime, 185
  cephalexin, 185
  cephalothin sodium, 185
  doxacurium chloride, 40
  ethacrynic acid, 191
  ethacrynic acid, injectable, 191
  ether, 25
  furosemide, 191
  furosemide, injectable, 191
  gallamine triethiodide, 40
  halothane, 25
  methoxyflurane, 25
  metocurine iodide, 40
  mivacurium chloride, 40
  moxalactam disodium, 185
  nitrous oxide, 25
  pancuronium bromide, 40
  penicillin G, 185
  penicillin G benzathine, 185
  penicillin G procaine, 185
  penicillin V, 185
  pipecuronium bromide, 40
  piretanide, 191
  rocuronium bromide, 40
  succinylcholine chloride, 40
  temocillin sodium, 185
  ticarcillin disodium, 185
  torsemide, injection, 191
  tubocurarine chloride, 40
  vecuronium bromide, 40
Neostigmine,
  succinylcholine chloride **2,** 37
Netilmicin,
  alcuronium chloride, 40
  amoxicillin, 185
  ampicillin sodium, 185

atracurium besylate, 40
azlocillin sodium, 185
bacampicillin hydrochloride, 185
benethamine penicillin, 185
bumetanide, 191
bumetanide, injectable, 191
carbenicillin disodium, 185
cefprozil, 185
ceftibuten dihyrate, 185
cefuroxime, 185
cephalexin, 185
cephalothin sodium, 185
cloxacillin sodium, 185
cyclacillin, 185
dicloxacillin, 185
doxacurium chloride, 40
ethacrynic acid, 191
ethacrynic acid, injectable, 191
flucloxacillin, 185
furosemide, 191
furosemide, injectable, 191
gallamine triethiodide, 40
methicillin sodium, 185
metocurine iodide, 40
mezlocillin sodium, 185
mivacurium chloride, 40
moxalactam disodium, 185
nafcillin sodium, 185
oxacillin sodium, 185
pancuronium bromide, 40
penicillin G, 185
penicillin G benzathine, 185
penicillin G procaine, 185
penicillin V, 185
pipecuronium bromide, 40
piperacillin sodium, 185
piretanide, 191
rocuronium bromide, 40
succinylcholine chloride, 40
temocillin sodium, 185
ticarcillin disodium, 185
torsemide, injection, 191
torsemide, oral, 191
tubocurarine chloride, 40
vecuronium bromide, 40
Niacin, vitamin B3,
    aspirin **3,** 324
    lovastatin **2,** 360
    sulfinpyrazone **3,** 22
Niacinamide (nicotinamide),
    carbamazepine **3,** 106
Nicardipine hydrochloride,
    parenteral use,
    cyclosporine, 46
    quinidine, 292
Nicardipine hydrochloride,
    cyclosporine, 46
    quinidine, 292
Nicoumalone,
    allopurinol, 69
    aloxiprin, 76

aminoglutethimide, 86
amiodarone hydrochloride, 75
amobarbital, 94
aprobarbital, 94
aspirin, 76
barbital, 94
butabarbital sodium, 94
butalbital, 94
butobarbitone, 94
calcium carbaspirin, 76
clofibrate, 80
danazol, 90
dextrothyroxine sodium, 100
diflunisal, 76
disulfiram, 81
erythromycin, 82
erythromycin estolate, 82
erythromycin ethylsuccinate, 82
erythromycin gluceptate, 82
erythromycin lactobionate, 82
erythromycin stearate, 82
ethylestrenol, 90
feprazone, 94
fluoxymesterone, 90
gemfibrozil, 80
glucagon, 86
glucagon, recombinant, 86
glutethimide, 86
levothyroxine sodium, 100
liothyronine sodium, 100
menadiol sodium diphosphate
    vitamin K4, 95
menadione, 95
mephobarbital, 94
methandrostenolone, 90
metharbital, 94
methohexital sodium, 94
methyltestosterone, 90
methyprylon, 86
nalidixic acid, 92
norfloxacin, 92
oxandrolone, 90
oxymetholone, 90
oxyphenbutazone, 94
pentobarbital sodium, 94
phenobarbital, 94
phenylbutazone, 94
phytonadione, vitamin K1, 95
pirbuterol acetate, 95
primidone, 94
rifabutin, 97
rifampin, 97
secobarbital, 94
sodium salicylate, 76
stanozolol, 90
talbutal, 94
thiamylal sodium, 94
thiopental sodium, 94
thyroglobulin, 100
thyroid desiccated, 100
thyroid strong, 100

Nifedipine,
  alcohol, ethyl - oral/injectable **3,** 57
  cimetidine, oral **2,** 57
  cyclosporine, 46
  digoxin, 284
  digoxin capsule, stabilized, 284
  halothane **3,** 58
  magnesium sulfate **3,** 58
  phenytoin **2,** 124
  quinidine, 292
  tacrolimus **3,** 368
Nimodipine,
  quinidine, 292
Nisoldipine,
  cyclosporine, 46
Nitric oxide, inhalation,
  alcohol, ethyl - oral/injectable **2,** 29
Nitrofurantoin,
  magnesium trisilicate **3,** 198
  phenytoin **3,** 124
  probenecid **3,** 198
  propantheline bromide **3,** 199
Nitroglycerin,
  alteplase, recombinant **2,** 346
  aspirin **3,** 9
  dihydroergotamine mesylate **2,** 353
  heparin **2,** 72
  indomethacin **3,** 13
  pancuronium bromide **3,** 33
Nitroglycerin, sublingual,
  imipramine **2,** 145
  pancuronium bromide **3,** 33
Nitroprusside sodium,
  captopril **3,** 168
  esmolol hydrochloride **3,** 170
Nitrous oxide,
  amikacin sulfate, 25
  clindamycin, 25
  clindamycin phosphate, injectable, 25
  colistin sulfate, 25
  gentamicin sulfate, 25
  kanamycin sulfate, oral, 25
  kanamycin sulfate, parenteral, 25
  neomycin sulfate, oral, 25
  neomycin sulfate, parenteral, 25
  polymyxin B sulfate, 25
  polymyxin B sulfate, vaccine use, 25
  streptomycin sulfate, 25
  tobramycin, 25
Nizatidine,
  charcoal **3,** 362
Norepinephrine bitartrate,
  chloroform, 26
  enflurane, 26
  epinephrine, 26
  ether, 26
  halothane, 26
  lithium **3,** 243
  methoxyflurane, 26
  methyldopa **2,** 167
  timolol maleate, ophthalmic, 260
Norfloxacin,
  acenocoumarol, 92
  anisindione, 92
  dicumarol, 92
  nicoumalone, 92
  sucralfate **2,** 199
  warfarin, 92
Nortriptyline hydrochloride,
  charcoal **3,** 146
  fluoxetine hydrochloride **2,** 147
  guanadrel sulfate, 162
  guanethidine, 162
  marijuana **2,** 147
  phenobarbital **3,** 148
  rifampin **3,** 148
  terbinafine hydrochloride **2,** 148
  warfarin **4,** 93
Ofloxacin,
  ethotoin, 92
  warfarin, 92
Olanzapine,
  fluvoxamine maleate **3,** 248
Omeprazole,
  clarithromycin **3,** 363
  cyanocobalamin, vitamin B12 **3,** 321
  cyclosporine **2,** 363
  diazepam **3,** 234
  ketoconazole **2,** 194
  methotrexate sodium, parenteral **2,** 218
  phenytoin **2,** 124
  theophylline **4,** 339
  warfarin **3,** 93
Opipramol,
  guanadrel sulfate, 162
  guanethidine, 162
Opium,
  isocarboxazid, 14
  pargyline hydrochloride, 14
  phenelzine sulfate, 14
  selegiline hydrochloride, 14
  tranylcypromine sulfate, 14
Oral contraceptive agents,
  acetaminophen **3,** 2
  aminophylline **3,** 329
  ampicillin sodium **2,** 173
  aspirin **3,** 9
  caffeine **3,** 330
  carbamazepine **3,** 107
  cyclosporine **3,** 351
  diazepam **3,** 235
  dicumarol **2,** 70
  griseofulvin **2,** 187
  metoprolol tartrate **3,** 255
  phenobarbital **2,** 318

phenytoin **3,** 125
prednisolone **2,** 365
rifabutin, 202
rifampin **1,** 202
tetracycline **2,** 206
trimethoprim **3,** 204
troleandomycin **2,** 207
Oral contraceptives, low-dose,
acetaminophen **3,** 2
aminophylline **3,** 329
caffeine **3,** 330
carbamazepine **3,** 107
clofibrate **3,** 348
cyclosporine **3,** 351
diazepam **3,** 235
phenobarbital **2,** 318
rifabutin, 202
rifampin, 202
Orphenadrine citrate,
benserazide **3,** 356
levodopa, combined with
benserazide **3,** 356
propoxyphene **4,** 21
Oxacillin sodium,
amikacin sulfate, 185
gentamicin sulfate, 185
netilmicin, 185
tobramycin, 185
Oxandrolone,
acenocoumarol, 90
dicumarol, 90
nicoumalone, 90
warfarin, 90
Oxazepam,
diflunisal **3,** 248
Oxiconazole nitrate,
cyclosporine, 193
fosphenytoin sodium, parenteral,
119
phenytoin, 119
Oxprenolol,
epinephrine, 260
insulin, 304
Oxtriphylline,
cimetidine hydrochloride,
parenteral, 334
cimetidine, oral, 334
erythromycin, 335
erythromycin estolate, 335
erythromycin ethylsuccinate, 335
erythromycin gluceptate, 335
erythromycin lactobionate, 335
erythromycin stearate, 335
halothane, 327
tobacco, 343
Oxybutynin chloride,
digoxin, 280
Oxycodone,
isocarboxazid, 14
pargyline hydrochloride, 14
phenelzine sulfate, 14

selegiline hydrochloride, 14
tranylcypromine sulfate, 14
Oxymetazoline hydrochloride,
furazolidone, 153
isocarboxazid, 153
pargyline hydrochloride, 153
phenelzine sulfate, 153
tranylcypromine sulfate, 153
Oxymetholone,
acenocoumarol, 90
anisindione, 90
dicumarol, 90
nicoumalone, 90
warfarin, 90
Oxymorphone hydrochloride,
isocarboxazid, 14
pargyline hydrochloride, 14
phenelzine sulfate, 14
selegiline hydrochloride, 14
tranylcypromine sulfate, 14
Oxypertine,
guanethidine, 162
Oxyphenbutazone,
acenocoumarol, 94
acetohexamide, 182
anisindione, 94
chlorpropamide, 182
dicumarol, 94
gliclazide, 182
glimepiride, 182
gliquidone, 182
methandrostenolone **3,** 18
nicoumalone, 94
tolazamide, 182
tolbutamide, 182
warfarin, 94
Oxyphencyclimine hydrochloride,
digoxin, 280
Oxytetracycline,
alcuronium chloride, 40
aluminum carbonate, basic, 205
aluminum hydroxide, 205
aluminum oxide, 205
aluminum phosphate, 205
attapulgite, 205
bismuth subsalicylate, 205
calcium acetate, 205
calcium ascorbate, 205
calcium carbonate, oral, 205
calcium chloride, oral, 205
calcium citrate, oral, 205
calcium glubionate, oral, 205
calcium glucoheptonate, 205
calcium gluconate, oral, 205
calcium glycerophosphate, oral,
205
calcium iodate, 205
calcium lactate gluconate, 205
calcium lactate, oral, 205
calcium lactobionate, oral, 205
calcium phosphate, oral, 205

calcium, oral salt unspecified, 205
carbonyl iron, 205
digoxin, 282
digoxin capsule, stabilized, 282
dihydroxyaluminum, 205
doxacurium chloride, 40
ether, 25
ferric ammonium citrate, 205
ferrous fumarate, 205
ferrous gluconate, 205
ferrous glycine sulfate, 205
ferrous hydroxide polymaltose, 205
ferrous ions, salt unspecified, 205
ferrous succinate, 205
ferrous sulfate, 205
gallamine triethiodide, 40
insulin **2,** 303
iron dextran complex, 205
iron peptonized, 205
kaolin, 205
magaldrate, 205
magnesium carbonate, 205
magnesium chloride, oral, 205
magnesium hydroxide, 205
magnesium oxide, 205
magnesium sulfate, 205
magnesium trisilicate, 205
metocurine iodide, 40
mivacurium chloride, 40
pancuronium bromide, 40
pipecuronium bromide, 40
rocuronium bromide, 40
succinylcholine chloride, 40
sucralfate, 205
tubocurarine chloride, 40
vecuronium bromide, 40
Oxytetracycline, parenteral,
    alcuronium chloride, 40
    digoxin, 282
    digoxin capsule, stabilized, 282
    doxacurium chloride, 40
    ether, 25
    gallamine triethiodide, 40
    metocurine iodide, 40
    mivacurium chloride, 40
    pancuronium bromide, 40
    pipecuronium bromide, 40
    rocuronium bromide, 40
    succinylcholine chloride, 40
    tubocurarine chloride, 40
    vecuronium bromide, 40
Paclitaxel,
    cisplatin **2,** 221
Pancuronium bromide,
    amikacin sulfate, 40
    aminophylline **2,** 30
    azathioprine sodium **3,** 30
    bacitracin, 40
    carbamazepine **3,** 30
    clindamycin **2,** 31

clindamycin phosphate,
    injectable **2,** 31
colistin sulfate, 40
cyclosporine **2,** 31
demeclocycline hydrochloride, 40
doxycycline hyclate, parenteral, 40
doxycycline hydrochloride, 40
furosemide **3,** 31
gentamicin sulfate, 40
hydrocortisone acetate, injectable **3,** 32
hydrocortisone sodium succinate **3,** 32
hydrocortisone sodium phosphate **3,** 32
hydrocortisone, oral/systemic **3,** 32
kanamycin sulfate, oral, 40
kanamycin sulfate, parenteral, 40
lithium **3,** 32
lymecycline, 40
methacycline hydrochloride, 40
minocycline hydrochloride pellets, 40
minocycline hydrochloride, 40
minocycline, parenteral, 40
neomycin sulfate, oral, 40
neomycin sulfate, parenteral, 40
netilmicin, 40
nitroglycerin **3,** 33
nitroglycerin, sublingual **3,** 33
oxytetracycline, 40
oxytetracycline, parenteral, 40
paromomycin sulfate, 40
polymyxin B sulfate, 40
polymyxin B sulfate, vaccine use, 40
streptomycin sulfate, 40
tetracycline, 40
tobramycin, 40
triethylene thiophosphoramide **3,** 33
Papaverine hydrochloride,
    levodopa **3,** 356
Para-aminobenzoic acid, paba,
    procainamide hydrochloride **3,** 59
Pargyline hydrochloride,
    alfentanil hydrochloride, 14
    amphetamine, 185
    anileridine, 14
    benzphetamine hydrochloride, 153
    buprenorphine hydrochloride, 14
    butorphanol tartrate, 14
    citalopram hydrobromide, 141
    codeine, 14
    dexfenfluramine hydrochloride, 153
    dextroamphetamine, 153
    dextromethorphan hydrobromide, 14

diethylpropion hydrochloride, 153
difenoxin hydrochloride, 14
dihydrocodeine bitartrate, 14
diphenoxylate hydrochloride, 14
dopamine hydrochloride, 153
ephedrine, 153
etafedrine hydrochloride, 153
fenfluramine hydrochloride, 153
fentanyl citrate, 14
fluoxetine hydrochloride, 141
fluvoxamine maleate, 141
hydrocodone bitartrate, 14
hydromorphone hydrochloride, 14
isometheptene, 153
levodopa, 152
levorphanol tartrate, 14
mazindol, 185
meperidine hydrochloride, 14
mephentermine sulfate, 153
meptazinol, 14
metaraminol bitartrate, 153
methamphetamine hydrochloride, 153
methyldopa **3,** 149
methylphenidate hydrochloride, 153
nalbuphine hydrochloride, 14
naphazoline hydrochloride, 153
opium, 14
oxycodone, 14
oxymetazoline hydrochloride, 153
oxymorphone hydrochloride, 14
paroxetine hydrochloride, 141
phendimetrazine tartrate, 153
phenmetrazine hydrochloride, 153
phenoperidine hydrochloride, 14
phentermine hydrochloride, 185
phenylephrine, 153
phenylpropanolamine, 153
pseudoephedrine, 153
remifentanil hydrochloride, 14
sufentanil citrate, 14
tetrahydrozoline hydrochloride, 153
venlafaxine hydrochloride, 141
xylometazoline hydrochloride, 153
Paromomycin sulfate,
  alcuronium chloride, 40
  ampicillin sodium, 185
  atracurium besylate, 40
  benethamine penicillin, 185
  carbenicillin disodium, 185
  cefprozil, 185
  ceftibuten dihyrate, 185
  cefuroxime, 185
  cephalexin, 185
  cephalothin sodium, 185
  doxacurium chloride, 40
  gallamine triethiodide, 40
  metocurine iodide, 40
  mivacurium chloride, 40
moxalactam disodium, 185
pancuronium bromide, 40
penicillin G, 185
penicillin G benzathine, 185
penicillin G procaine, 185
penicillin V, 185
pipecuronium bromide, 40
rocuronium bromide, 40
succinylcholine chloride, 40
temocillin sodium, 185
ticarcillin disodium, 185
tubocurarine chloride, 40
vecuronium bromide, 40
Paroxetine hydrochloride,
  cimetidine, oral **3,** 149
  dextromethorphan hydrobromide **2,** 150
  isocarboxazid, 141
  pargyline hydrochloride, 141
  phenelzine sulfate, 141
  selegiline hydrochloride, 141
  tranylcypromine sulfate, 141
  zolpidem tartrate **3,** 150
Penbutolol sulfate,
  clonidine hydrochloride, transdermal, 160
  clonidine hydrochloride, 160
  epinephrine, 260
  insulin, 304
Penicillamine,
  aluminum hydroxide **3,** 364
  chloroquine **3,** 364
  digoxin **2,** 279
  ferrous sulfate **2,** 323
  indomethacin **3,** 364
  magnesium hydroxide **3,** 364
  probenecid **3,** 20
Penicillin G,
  amikacin sulfate, 185
  aspirin **3,** 199
  chloramphenicol **4,** 199
  chlortetracycline hydrochloride **2,** 200
  erythromycin **3,** 200
  gentamicin sulfate, 185
  kanamycin sulfate, oral, 185
  kanamycin sulfate, parenteral, 185
  neomycin sulfate, oral, 185
  neomycin sulfate, parenteral, 185
  netilmicin, 185
  paromomycin sulfate, 185
  probenecid **3,** 201
  streptomycin sulfate, 185
  tobramycin, 185
Penicillin G benzathine,
  amikacin sulfate, 185
  gentamicin sulfate, 185
  kanamycin sulfate, oral, 185
  kanamycin sulfate, parenteral, 185
  neomycin sulfate, oral, 185
  neomycin sulfate, parenteral, 185

netilmicin, 185
paromomycin sulfate, 185
streptomycin sulfate, 185
tobramycin, 185
Penicillin G procaine,
amikacin sulfate, 185
gentamicin sulfate, 185
kanamycin sulfate, oral, 185
kanamycin sulfate, parenteral, 185
neomycin sulfate, oral, 185
neomycin sulfate, parenteral, 185
netilmicin, 185
paromomycin sulfate, 185
streptomycin sulfate, 185
tobramycin, 185
Penicillin V,
amikacin sulfate, 185
gentamicin sulfate, 185
kanamycin sulfate, oral, 185
kanamycin sulfate, parenteral, 185
neomycin sulfate, oral, 185
neomycin sulfate, parenteral, 185
netilmicin, 185
paromomycin sulfate, 185
streptomycin sulfate, 185
tobramycin, 185
Pentazocine,
phenelzine sulfate, 14
selegiline hydrochloride, 14
tranylcypromine sulfate, 14
Pentobarbital sodium,
acenocoumarol, 94
anisindione, 94
dicumarol, 94
metoprolol tartrate **2,** 255
nicoumalone, 94
warfarin, 94
Pentoxifylline,
cimetidine hydrochloride,
parenteral, 334
cimetidine, oral, 334
Pericyazine,
guanethidine, 162
Perphenazine,
disulfiram **3,** 249
guanethidine, 162
Phendimetrazine tartrate,
chloroform, 26
enflurane, 26
furazolidone, 185
halothane, 26
isocarboxazid, 153
methoxyflurane, 26
moclobemide, 153
pargyline hydrochloride, 153
phenelzine sulfate, 153
procarbazine hydrochloride, 153
tranylcypromine sulfate, 153
Phenelzine sulfate,
alfentanil hydrochloride, 14
amphetamine, 185

anileridine, 14
benzphetamine hydrochloride,
153
buprenorphine hydrochloride, 14
buspirone hydrochloride **3,** 151
butorphanol tartrate, 14
citalopram hydrobromide, 141
clonazepam **3,** 151
codeine, 14
dexfenfluramine hydrochloride,
153
dextroamphetamine, 153
dextromethorphan hydrobromide,
14
diethylpropion hydrochloride, 153
difenoxin hydrochloride, 14
dihydrocodeine bitartrate, 14
diphenoxylate hydrochloride, 14
dopamine hydrochloride, 153
ephedrine, 153
etafedrine hydrochloride, 153
fenfluramine hydrochloride, 153
fentanyl citrate, 14
fluoxetine hydrochloride, 141
fluvoxamine maleate, 141
guanethidine **3,** 164
hydrocodone bitartrate, 14
hydromorphone hydrochloride, 14
insulin **2,** 303
isometheptene, 153
levodopa **1,** 152
levorphanol tartrate, 14
mazindol, 185
meperidine hydrochloride **1,** 14
mephentermine sulfate, 153
meptazinol, 14
metaraminol bitartrate, 153
methamphetamine hydrochloride,
153
methylphenidate hydrochloride,
153
nadolol **3,** 256
nalbuphine hydrochloride, 14
naphazoline hydrochloride, 153
opium, 14
oxycodone, 14
oxymetazoline hydrochloride, 153
oxymorphone hydrochloride, 14
paroxetine hydrochloride, 141
pentazocine, 14
phendimetrazine tartrate, 153
phenmetrazine hydrochloride, 153
phenoperidine hydrochloride, 14
phentermine hydrochloride, 153
phenylephrine, 153
phenylpropanolamine, 153
propoxyphene, 14
pseudoephedrine, 153
remifentanil hydrochloride, 14
sertraline hydrochloride, 141
sufentanil citrate, 14

sulfisoxazole **3,** 152
tetrahydrozoline hydrochloride, 153
venlafaxine hydrochloride, 141
xylometazoline hydrochloride, 153
Phenindione,
  aloxiprin, 76
  barbital, 94
  bezafibrate, 80
  butobarbitone, 94
  calcium carbaspirin, 76
  cimetidine hydrochloride, parenteral, 79
  cimetidine, oral, 79
  ciprofibrate, 80
  fenofibrate, micronized, 80
  gemfibrozil, 80
  haloperidol **3,** 73
  menadione, 95
  rifabutin, 97
Phenmetrazine hydrochloride,
  chloroform, 26
  enflurane, 26
  furazolidone, 185
  halothane, 26
  isocarboxazid, 153
  methoxyflurane, 26
  moclobemide, 153
  pargyline hydrochloride, 153
  phenelzine sulfate, 153
  procarbazine hydrochloride, 153
  tranylcypromine sulfate, 153
Phenobarbital,
  acenocoumarol, 94
  acetaminophen **3,** 3
  alcohol, ethyl - oral/injectable **2,** 315
  anisindione, 94
  carbamazepine **3,** 107
  charcoal **3,** 316
  chloramphenicol **3,** 176
  chlorcyclizine hydrochloride **3,** 316
  chlorpromazine hydrochloride **3,** 228
  cimetidine, oral **3,** 316
  cyclosporine **2,** 316
  dexamethasone **2,** 317
  dicumarol, 94
  digitoxin **2,** 269
  doxorubicin hydrochloride **3,** 213
  doxycycline hydrochloride **2,** 182
  felbamate **3,** 317
  fenoprofen calcium **3,** 10
  griseofulvin **3,** 188
  guanfacine hydrochloride **3,** 164
  lidocaine hydrochloride, systemic **3,** 53
  meperidine hydrochloride **3,** 14
  methyldopa **4,** 167
  metronidazole, systemic **2,** 197

nicoumalone, 94
nortriptyline hydrochloride **3,** 148
oral contraceptive agents **2,** 318
oral contraceptives, low-dose **2,** 318
phenytoin **3,** 125
pyridoxine hydrochloride **3,** 318
quinidine **2,** 63
theophylline **2,** 340
valproic acid **2,** 111
verapamil hydrochloride **3,** 66
warfarin **1,** 94
Phenoperidine hydrochloride,
  isocarboxazid, 14
  pargyline hydrochloride, 14
  phenelzine sulfate, 14
  selegiline hydrochloride, 14
  tranylcypromine sulfate, 14
Phenoxybenzamine hydrochloride,
  methyldopa **3,** 167
Phentermine hydrochloride,
  chloroform, 26
  enflurane, 26
  furazolidone, 185
  halothane, 26
  isocarboxazid, 153
  methoxyflurane, 26
  pargyline hydrochloride, 185
  phenelzine sulfate, 153
  procarbazine hydrochloride, 153
  tranylcypromine sulfate, 153
Phenylbutazone,
  acenocoumarol, 94
  acetohexamide, 182
  anisindione, 94
  charcoal **3,** 18
  chlorpropamide, 182
  desipramine hydrochloride **3,** 19
  dicumarol, 94
  digitoxin **3,** 269
  gliclazide, 182
  glimepiride, 182
  gliquidone, 182
  misoprostol **3,** 19
  nicoumalone, 94
  phenytoin **2,** 126
  tolazamide, 182
  tolbutamide **1,** 307
  warfarin **1,** 94
Phenylephrine,
  chloroform, 26
  enflurane, 26
  furazolidone, 153
  guanethidine **2,** 164
  halothane, 26
  isocarboxazid, 153
  methoxyflurane, 26
  pargyline hydrochloride, 153
  phenelzine sulfate, 153
  procarbazine hydrochloride, 153
  timolol maleate, ophthalmic, 260

tranylcypromine sulfate, 153
Phenylpropanolamine,
    caffeine **3,** 331
    chloroform, 26
    enflurane, 26
    furazolidone, 185
    halothane, 26
    indomethacin **2,** 13
    isocarboxazid, 153
    methoxyflurane, 26
    moclobemide, 153
    pargyline hydrochloride, 153
    phenelzine sulfate, 153
    procarbazine hydrochloride, 153
    thioridazine hydrochloride **2,** 226
    tranylcypromine sulfate **1,** 153
Phenytoin,
    acetaminophen **3,** 3
    acetazolamide **4,** 111
    alcohol, ethyl - oral/injectable **2,** 112
    allopurinol **2,** 112
    aluminum hydroxide **3,** 112
    amiodarone hydrochloride **2,** 113
    aspirin **4,** 113
    butoconazole nitrate, 119
    carbamazepine **3,** 113
    carmustine **2,** 114
    charcoal **2,** 114
    chloramphenicol **2,** 114
    chlorpheniramine **2,** 115
    chlorpromazine hydrochloride **3,** 115
    cimetidine hydrochloride, parenteral, 115
    cimetidine, oral **1,** 115
    ciprofloxacin hydrochloride **3,** 116
    clotrimazole, 119
    cyclosporine **2,** 116
    dexamethasone **2,** 117
    diazepam **3,** 117
    diazoxide, oral **2,** 117
    dicumarol **2,** 71
    digitalis **3,** 267
    disopyramide phosphate **2,** 49
    disulfiram **1,** 118
    dopamine hydrochloride **1,** 118
    doxycycline hydrochloride **2,** 182
    econazole nitrate, 119
    ergocalciferol, vitamin D2 **2,** 321
    ethosuximide **3,** 119
    felbamate **2,** 119
    fenticonazole nitrate, 119
    fluconazole **1,** 119
    fluoxetine hydrochloride **2,** 120
    folic acid **2,** 120
    furosemide **3,** 290
    halothane **3,** 26
    ibuprofen **2,** 120
    imipramine **3,** 121
    influenza virus vaccine, split

    virion **3,** 121
    insulin **3,** 304
    isoconazole nitrate, 119
    isoniazid **2,** 122
    itraconazole, 119
    ketoconazole, 119
    levodopa **3,** 122
    levothyroxine sodium **3,** 122
    lithium **3,** 244
    magnesium trisilicate **3,** 112
    meperidine hydrochloride **3,** 15
    methotrexate **2,** 114
    methoxsalen **2,** 123
    methylphenidate hydrochloride **3,** 123
    metocurine iodide **2,** 29
    metronidazole, systemic **3,** 123
    metyrapone **3,** 362
    mexiletine hydrochloride **3,** 56
    miconazole nitrate, 119
    nifedipine **2,** 124
    nitrofurantoin **3,** 124
    omeprazole **2,** 124
    oral contraceptive agents **3,** 125
    oxiconazole nitrate, 119
    phenobarbital **3,** 125
    phenylbutazone **2,** 126
    primidone **2,** 129
    pyridoxine hydrochloride **3,** 126
    quinidine **2,** 63
    ranitidine hydrochloride, parenteral, 115
    ranitidine hydrochloride, oral, 115
    rifampin **2,** 126
    sucralfate **2,** 127
    sulfamethizole **2,** 127
    terconazole, 119
    theophylline **2,** 340
    ticlopidine hydrochloride **2,** 127
    tioconazole, 119
    trazodone hydrochloride **3,** 128
    trimethoprim **2,** 128
    valproic acid **2,** 128
    vinblastine sulfate **2,** 114
    vitamin D2, prenatal multivitamin use **2,** 321
Phytonadione, vitamin K1,
    acenocoumarol, 95
    dicumarol, 95
    nicoumalone, 95
    warfarin **1,** 95
Pimozide,
    fluoxetine hydrochloride **3,** 249
    sulfamethoxazole **3,** 152
    trimethoprim **3,** 152
Pindolol,
    clonidine hydrochloride, transdermal, 160
    clonidine hydrochloride, 160
    epinephrine, 260
    insulin, 304

Pipecuronium bromide,
  amikacin sulfate, 40
  bacitracin, 40
  colistin sulfate, 40
  demeclocycline hydrochloride, 40
  doxycycline hyclate, parenteral, 40
  doxycycline hydrochloride, 40
  gentamicin sulfate, 40
  kanamycin sulfate, oral, 40
  kanamycin sulfate, parenteral, 40
  lymecycline, 40
  methacycline hydrochloride, 40
  minocycline hydrochloride pellets, 40
  minocycline hydrochloride, 40
  minocycline, parenteral, 40
  neomycin sulfate, oral, 40
  neomycin sulfate, parenteral, 40
  netilmicin, 40
  oxytetracycline, 40
  oxytetracycline, parenteral, 40
  paromomycin sulfate, 40
  polymyxin B sulfate, 40
  polymyxin B sulfate, vaccine use, 40
  rolitetracycline, injectable, 40
  streptomycin sulfate, 40
  tetracycline, 40
  tetracycline hydrochloride, parenteral, 40
  tobramycin, 40
Piperacetazine,
  guanethidine, 162
Piperacillin sodium,
  amikacin sulfate, 185
  gentamicin sulfate, 185
  netilmicin, 185
  tobramycin, 185
  vecuronium bromide **2,** 42
Piperazine,
  chlorpromazine hydrochloride **3,** 228
Pirbuterol acetate,
  chloroform, 26
  enflurane, 26
  halothane, 26
  methoxyflurane, 26
  metoprolol tartrate, 260
  nicoumalone, 95
  timolol maleate, oral, 260
Pirenzepine dihydrochloride,
  digoxin, 280
Piretanide,
  amikacin sulfate, 191
  gentamicin sulfate, 191
  kanamycin sulfate, oral, 191
  kanamycin sulfate, parenteral, 191
  lithium, 239
  neomycin sulfate, oral, 191
  neomycin sulfate, parenteral, 191

  netilmicin, 191
  streptomycin sulfate, 191
  tobramycin, 191
Polyestradiol phosphate,
  rifampin, 202
Polymyxin B sulfate,
  alcuronium chloride, 40
  doxacurium chloride, 40
  enflurane, 25
  ether, 25
  gallamine triethiodide, 40
  gentamicin sulfate **2,** 186
  halothane, 25
  methoxyflurane, 25
  metocurine iodide, 40
  mivacurium chloride, 40
  nitrous oxide, 25
  pancuronium bromide, 40
  pipecuronium bromide, 40
  prochlorperazine **2,** 201
  rocuronium bromide, 40
  succinylcholine chloride, 40
  tubocurarine chloride, 40
  vecuronium bromide, 40
Polymyxin B sulfate, vaccine use,
  alcuronium chloride, 40
  doxacurium chloride, 40
  enflurane, 25
  ether, 25
  gallamine triethiodide, 40
  halothane, 25
  methoxyflurane, 25
  metocurine iodide, 40
  mivacurium chloride, 40
  nitrous oxide, 25
  pancuronium bromide, 40
  pipecuronium bromide, 40
  rocuronium bromide, 40
  succinylcholine chloride, 40
  tubocurarine chloride, 40
  vecuronium bromide, 40
Polythiazide,
  lithium, 239
Potassium acetate,
  amiloride hydrochloride, 292
  potassium canrenoate, 292
  spironolactone, 292
  triamterene, 292
Potassium bicarbonate,
  amiloride hydrochloride, 292
  potassium canrenoate, 292
  spironolactone, 292
  triamterene, 292
Potassium biphosphate,
  amiloride hydrochloride, 292
  potassium canrenoate, 292
  spironolactone, 292
  triamterene, 292
Potassium canrenoate,
  potassium acetate, 292
  potassium bicarbonate, 292

potassium biphosphate, 292
potassium chloride, 292
potassium citrate, 292
potassium gluconate, 292
potassium iodide, 292
potassium iodide, prenatal
  multivitamin use, 292
potassium perchlorate, 292
potassium phosphate, 292
potassium salicylate, 292
potassium, salt unspecified, 292
Potassium chloride,
  amiloride hydrochloride, 292
  captopril **3,** 158
  potassium canrenoate, 292
  spironolactone **1,** 292
  triamterene, 292
Potassium citrate,
  amiloride hydrochloride, 292
  lithium, 238
  potassium canrenoate, 292
  spironolactone, 292
  triamterene, 292
Potassium gluconate,
  amiloride hydrochloride, 292
  potassium canrenoate, 292
  spironolactone, 292
  triamterene, 292
Potassium iodide,
  amiloride hydrochloride, 292
  lithium **2,** 244
  potassium canrenoate, 292
  spironolactone, 292
  triamterene, 292
Potassium iodide, prenatal
  multivitamin use,
  amiloride hydrochloride, 292
  potassium canrenoate, 292
  spironolactone, 292
  triamterene, 292
Potassium perchlorate,
  amiloride hydrochloride, 292
  potassium canrenoate, 292
  spironolactone, 292
  triamterene, 292
Potassium phosphate,
  amiloride hydrochloride, 292
  potassium canrenoate, 292
  spironolactone, 292
  triamterene, 292
Potassium salicylate,
  amiloride hydrochloride, 292
  potassium canrenoate, 292
  spironolactone, 292
  triamterene, 292
Potassium, salt unspecified,
  amiloride hydrochloride, 292
  potassium canrenoate, 292
  spironolactone, 292
  triamterene, 292
Pravastatin sodium,
  propranolol hydrochloride **3,** 263
Prazosin hydrochloride,
  digoxin **2,** 279
  indomethacin **2,** 168
  propranolol hydrochloride **2,** 169
  verapamil hydrochloride **3,** 169
Prednisolone,
  cyclosporine **2,** 364
  isoniazid **3,** 189
  oral contraceptive agents **2,** 365
  rifampin **2,** 202
Prednisone,
  aluminum hydroxide **3,** 365
  cyclophosphamide **3,** 213
  digoxin **2,** 272
  timolol maleate, ophthalmic **2,**
    265
Primidone,
  acenocoumarol, 94
  acetazolamide **3,** 129
  clonazepam **4,** 109
  dicumarol, 94
  nicoumalone, 94
  phenytoin **2,** 129
  warfarin, 94
Probenecid,
  acyclovir, oral **3,** 173
  allopurinol **3,** 5
  bumetanide **3,** 291
  captopril **3,** 159
  cephalothin sodium **2,** 175
  chlorothiazide **3,** 288
  chlorpropamide **3,** 298
  clofibrate **3,** 19
  dyphylline **2,** 331
  furosemide **3,** 291
  indomethacin **2,** 13
  lorazepam **3,** 246
  methotrexate **1,** 219
  methotrexate sodium, parenteral,
    219
  nitrofurantoin **3,** 198
  penicillamine **3,** 20
  penicillin G **3,** 201
  rifampin **4,** 203
  sulfinpyrazone **4,** 22
  thiopental sodium **3,** 39
  zidovudine **2,** 209
Probucol,
  cyclosporine **2,** 365
Procainamide hydrochloride,
  alcohol, ethyl - oral/injectable **3,**
    59
  amiodarone hydrochloride **2,** 59
  cimetidine, oral **2,** 59
  lidocaine hydrochloride, systemic
    3, 54
  para-aminobenzoic acid, paba **3,**
    59
  propranolol hydrochloride **3,** 60
  quinidine **3,** 60

succinylcholine chloride **3,** 37
trimethoprim **3,** 60
Procarbazine hydrochloride,
  amphetamine, 185
  benzphetamine hydrochloride,
    153
  dexfenfluramine hydrochloride,
    153
  dextroamphetamine, 153
  diethylpropion hydrochloride, 153
  digoxin **2,** 272
  dopamine hydrochloride, 153
  ephedrine, 153
  etafedrine hydrochloride, 153
  fenfluramine hydrochloride, 153
  fluoxetine hydrochloride, 141
  fluvoxamine maleate, 141
  isometheptene, 153
  levodopa, 152
  mazindol, 185
  meperidine hydrochloride, 14
  mephentermine sulfate, 153
  metaraminol bitartrate, 153
  methamphetamine hydrochloride,
    153
  methotrexate **2,** 219
  methylphenidate hydrochloride,
    153
  phendimetrazine tartrate, 153
  phenmetrazine hydrochloride, 153
  phentermine hydrochloride, 153
  phenylephrine, 153
  phenylpropanolamine, 153
  pseudoephedrine, 153
  venlafaxine hydrochloride, 141
Procaterol hydrochloride,
  chloroform, 26
  enflurane, 26
  halothane, 26
  methoxyflurane, 26
  metoprolol tartrate, 260
  timolol maleate, oral, 260
Prochlorperazine,
  guanethidine, 162
  polymyxin B sulfate **2,** 201
Procyclidine hydrochloride,
  digoxin, 280
Proguanil hydrochloride,
  methotrexate, 220
  methotrexate sodium, parenteral,
    220
  warfarin, 98
Promazine hydrochloride,
  charcoal **3,** 249
  guanethidine, 162
  succinylcholine chloride **2,** 37
Promethazine,
  guanethidine, 162
Propafenone hydrochloride,
  cyclosporine **2,** 61
  digoxin **2,** 279

digoxin capsule, stabilized **2,** 279
  quinidine **2,** 61
  theophylline **2,** 340
  warfarin **2,** 95
Propantheline bromide,
  atenolol **3,** 253
  chlorothiazide **3,** 288
  cimetidine, oral **3,** 348
  deslanoside, 280
  digitalis, 280
  digitoxin, 280
  digoxin **1,** 280
  nitrofurantoin **3,** 199
Propofol,
  aminophylline **3,** 33
  diazepam **3,** 34
Propoxyphene,
  alcohol, ethyl - oral/injectable **2,**
    20
  amphetamine **3,** 20
  carbamazepine **2,** 107
  charcoal **3,** 21
  doxepin hydrochloride **3,** 139
  orphenadrine citrate **4,** 21
  phenelzine sulfate, 14
  selegiline hydrochloride, 14
  warfarin **2,** 96
Propranolol hydrochloride,
  acetaminophen **3,** 3
  alcohol, ethyl - oral/injectable **3,**
    256
  allergenic extracts **3,** 256
  aluminum hydroxide **3,** 257
  aminoglutethimide **3,** 257
  aspirin **3,** 257
  chlorpheniramine **4,** 257
  chlorpromazine hydrochloride **2,**
    258
  cholestyramine **3,** 258
  cimetidine hydrochloride,
    parenteral, 258
  cimetidine, oral **1,** 258
  clonidine hydrochloride,
    transdermal, 160
  clonidine hydrochloride **1,** 160
  cocaine hydrochloride **2,** 259
  desipramine hydrochloride **3,** 259
  dexfenfluramine hydrochloride,
    260
  diatrizoate sodium **3,** 259
  diazepam **3,** 235
  dobutamine hydrochloride, 260
  dopamine hydrochloride, 260
  epinephrine **1,** 260
  ergotamine tartrate **3,** 260
  etafedrine hydrochloride, 260
  fentanyl citrate **3,** 10
  flecainide acetate **3,** 261
  fluoxetine hydrochloride **2,** 261
  furosemide **2,** 262
  hydralazine hydrochloride **3,** 262

indomethacin **2,** 262
insulin **1,** 304
isoniazid **3,** 189
lidocaine hydrochloride, systemic **2,** 54
lofexidine hydrochloride, 160
mazindol, 260
metaraminol bitartrate, 260
methoxamine hydrochloride, 260
methyldopa **2,** 168
misoprostol **3,** 263
pravastatin sodium **3,** 263
prazosin hydrochloride **2,** 169
procainamide hydrochloride **3,** 60
quinidine **3,** 263
salmeterol hydroxynaphthoate, 260
theophylline **2,** 341
thyroid strong **2,** 264
tobacco **2,** 264
tranylcypromine sulfate **4,** 153
tubocurarine chloride **2,** 41
verapamil hydrochloride **2,** 66
warfarin **2,** 96
Propyliodine,
    metformin hydrochloride, 305
Propylthiouracil,
    warfarin, 100
Protriptyline hydrochloride,
    guanadrel sulfate, 162
    guanethidine, 162
Pseudoephedrine,
    chloroform, 26
    enflurane, 26
    furazolidone, 185
    halothane, 26
    isocarboxazid, 153
    methoxyflurane, 26
    moclobemide, 153
    pargyline hydrochloride, 153
    phenelzine sulfate, 153
    procarbazine hydrochloride, 153
    tranylcypromine sulfate, 153
Psyllium,
    digoxin **3,** 280
Pyrantel pamoate,
    theophylline **2,** 341
Pyridostigmine,
    methylprednisolone **3,** 366
Pyridoxine hydrochloride,
    isoniazid **3,** 190
    levodopa **1,** 325
    phenobarbital **3,** 318
    phenytoin **3,** 126
Quinestrol,
    rifampin, 202
Quinethazone,
    lithium, 239
Quinidine,
    aluminum hydroxide **3,** 64
    amiodarone hydrochloride **1,** 61

cimetidine, oral **2,** 62
desipramine hydrochloride **3,** 137
digitoxin, 280
digoxin **1,** 280
digoxin capsule, stabilized, 280
diltiazem hydrochloride, 292
diphenoxylate hydrochloride **3,** 62
disopyramide phosphate **3,** 50
grapefruit juice **3,** 323
ketoconazole **2,** 62
lercanidipine hydrochloride, 292
metoclopramide hydrochloride **3,** 63
nicardipine hydrochloride, parenteral use, 292
nicardipine hydrochloride, 292
nifedipine, 292
nimodipine, 292
phenobarbital **2,** 63
phenytoin **2,** 63
procainamide hydrochloride **3,** 60
propafenone hydrochloride **2,** 61
propranolol hydrochloride **3,** 263
reserpine **3,** 64
rifampin **3,** 64
tubocurarine chloride **2,** 41
verapamil hydrochloride pellets, 292
verapamil hydrochloride, sustained-release, 292
verapamil hydrochloride **1,** 65
warfarin **2,** 96
Quinine,
    cyclosporine **2,** 351
    flecainide acetate **3,** 52
Radioactive iodine-131,
    metformin hydrochloride, 305
Ranitidine hydrochloride, parenteral,
    ethotoin, 115
    fosphenytoin sodium, parenteral, 115
    mephenytoin, 115
    phenytoin, 115
    warfarin, 79
Ranitidine hydrochloride, oral,
    ethotoin, 115
    fosphenytoin sodium, parenteral, 115
    mephenytoin, 115
    phenytoin, 115
    sucralfate **3,** 366
    warfarin, 79
Remifentanil hydrochloride,
    citalopram hydrobromide, 14
    pargyline hydrochloride, 14
    phenelzine sulfate, 14
    selegiline hydrochloride, 14
    tranylcypromine sulfate, 14
Reserpine,
    digitalis **3,** 267

ephedrine **2,** 169
halothane **3,** 170
imipramine **3,** 145
quinidine **3,** 64
thiopental sodium **2,** 39
Rifabutin,
acenocoumarol, 97
anisindione, 97
cyclosporine, 202
dicumarol, 97
digitoxin, 269
digoxin, 269
estradiol, 202
estradiol, transdermal, 202
ethinyl estradiol, 202
nicoumalone, 97
oral contraceptive agents, 202
oral contraceptives, low-dose, 202
phenindione, 97
warfarin, 97
Rifampin,
acenocoumarol, 97
aminosalicylic acid **4,** 201
anisindione, 97
chloramphenicol **2,** 176
chlorotrianisene, 202
clofibrate **3,** 202
clonidine hydrochloride **4,** 160
conjugated estrogens, 202
cyclosporine **1,** 202
dapsone **3,** 181
deslanoside, 269
diazepam **3,** 236
dicumarol, 97
diethylstilbestrol, 202
digitalis, 269
digitoxin **1,** 269
digoxin, 269
digoxin capsule, stabilized, 269
disopyramide phosphate **3,** 50
enalapril maleate **3,** 161
esterified estrogens, 202
estradiol, 202
estradiol, transdermal, 202
estriol, 202
estrogen, 202
estrone, 202
estropipate, 202
ethinyl estradiol, 202
glyburide **3,** 300
haloperidol **2,** 237
halothane **2,** 27
isoniazid **2,** 190
ketoconazole **2,** 194
mestranol, 202
methadone hydrochloride **2,** 16
metoprolol tartrate **2,** 255
mexiletine hydrochloride **3,** 56
nicoumalone, 97
nortriptyline hydrochloride **3,** 148
oral contraceptive agents **1,** 202

oral contraceptives, low-dose, 202
phenytoin **2,** 126
polyestradiol phosphate, 202
prednisolone **2,** 202
probenecid **4,** 203
quinestrol, 202
quinidine **2,** 64
theophylline **2,** 341
verapamil hydrochloride **2,** 66
warfarin **1,** 97
zidovudine **2,** 369
Rimiterol hydrobromide,
chloroform, 26
enflurane, 26
halothane, 26
methoxyflurane, 26
metoprolol tartrate, 260
timolol maleate, oral, 260
Ritodrine hydrochloride,
bupivacaine hydrochloride **2,** 24
glycopyrrolate **2,** 354
Rocuronium bromide,
amikacin sulfate, 40
bacitracin, 40
colistin sulfate, 40
demeclocycline hydrochloride, 40
doxycycline hyclate, parenteral, 40
doxycycline hydrochloride, 40
gentamicin sulfate, 40
kanamycin sulfate, oral, 40
kanamycin sulfate, parenteral, 40
lymecycline, 40
methacycline hydrochloride, 40
minocycline hydrochloride pellets, 40
minocycline hydrochloride, 40
minocycline, parenteral, 40
neomycin sulfate, oral, 40
neomycin sulfate, parenteral, 40
netilmicin, 40
oxytetracycline, 40
oxytetracycline, parenteral, 40
paromomycin sulfate, 40
polymyxin B sulfate, 40
polymyxin B sulfate, vaccine use, 40
rolitetracycline, injectable, 40
streptomycin sulfate, 40
tetracycline, 40
tetracycline hydrochloride, parenteral, 40
tobramycin, 40
Rolitetracycline, injectable,
alcuronium chloride, 40
digoxin, 282
digoxin capsule, stabilized, 282
ether, 25
gallamine triethiodide, 40
metocurine iodide, 40
mivacurium chloride, 40

pipecuronium bromide, 40
rocuronium bromide, 40
succinylcholine chloride, 40
tubocurarine chloride, 40
vecuronium bromide, 40
Salicylamide,
   methotrexate, 216
   methotrexate sodium, parenteral,
    216
Salmeterol hydroxynaphthoate,
   chloroform, 26
   enflurane, 26
   halothane, 26
   methoxyflurane, 26
   propranolol hydrochloride, 260
Salmeterol xinafoate,
   chloroform, 26
   enflurane, 26
   halothane, 26
   methoxyflurane, 26
   metoprolol tartrate, 260
   timolol maleate, oral, 260
Salsalate,
   methotrexate, 216
   methotrexate sodium, parenteral,
    216
Scopolamine, ophthalmic,
   digoxin, 280
Scopolamine, systemic,
   digoxin, 280
Secobarbital,
   acenocoumarol, 94
   anisindione, 94
   dicumarol, 94
   methoxyflurane **2,** 28
   nicoumalone, 94
   warfarin, 94
Selegiline hydrochloride,
   alfentanil hydrochloride, 14
   anileridine, 14
   buprenorphine hydrochloride, 14
   butorphanol tartrate, 14
   citalopram hydrobromide, 141
   codeine, 14
   dexfenfluramine hydrochloride,
    153
   dextromethorphan hydrobromide,
    14
   dezocine, 14
   difenoxin hydrochloride, 14
   dihydrocodeine bitartrate, 14
   diphenoxylate hydrochloride, 14
   fentanyl citrate, 14
   fluoxetine hydrochloride, 141
   fluvoxamine maleate, 141
   hydrocodone bitartrate, 14
   hydromorphone hydrochloride, 14
   levorphanol tartrate, 14
   meperidine hydrochloride, 14
   meptazinol, 14
   nalbuphine hydrochloride, 14

opium, 14
oxycodone, 14
oxymorphone hydrochloride, 14
paroxetine hydrochloride, 141
pentazocine, 14
phenoperidine hydrochloride, 14
propoxyphene, 14
remifentanil hydrochloride, 14
sertraline hydrochloride, 141
sufentanil citrate, 14
venlafaxine hydrochloride, 141
Sertraline hydrochloride,
   isocarboxazid, 141
   phenelzine sulfate, 141
   selegiline hydrochloride, 141
Sevoflurane,
   epinephrine, 26
Simvastatin,
   clarithromycin, 359
   erythromycin, 359
   erythromycin estolate, 359
   erythromycin ethylsuccinate, 359
   erythromycin gluceptate, 359
   erythromycin lactobionate, 359
   erythromycin stearate, 359
   grapefruit juice, 360
   nefazodone hydrochloride **3,** 366
   troleandomycin, 359
Sodium acetate,
   lithium, 238
Sodium bicarbonate,
   amphetamine **3,** 347
   flecainide acetate **2,** 53
   lithium, 238
   methotrexate **3,** 219
   tetracycline **4,** 206
Sodium bicarbonate, parenteral,
   lithium, 238
Sodium citrate,
   lithium, 238
Sodium lactate,
   lithium, 238
Sodium polystyrene sulfonate,
   magnesium hydroxide **2,** 361
Sodium salicylate,
   acenocoumarol, 76
   anisindione, 76
   ardeparin sodium, 76
   certoparin, 76
   dalteparin sodium, 76
   dicumarol, 76
   enoxaparin, 76
   heparin, 76
   methotrexate, 216
   methotrexate sodium, parenteral,
    216
   nicoumalone, 76
   tinzaparin sodium, 76
   warfarin, 76
Sodium thiosalicylate,
   methotrexate, 216

methotrexate sodium, parenteral, 216
Sotalol hydrochloride,
  epinephrine, 260
  insulin, 304
Spiramycin,
  astemizole, 184
  terfenadine, 184
  theophylline, 335
Spironolactone,
  aspirin **3,** 292
  captopril **3,** 292
  cholestyramine **2,** 170
  digoxin **2,** 281
  mitotane **3,** 221
  potassium acetate, 292
  potassium bicarbonate, 292
  potassium biphosphate, 292
  potassium chloride **1,** 292
  potassium citrate, 292
  potassium gluconate, 292
  potassium iodide, 292
  potassium iodide, prenatal
    multivitamin use, 292
  potassium perchlorate, 292
  potassium phosphate, 292
  potassium salicylate, 292
  potassium, salt unspecified, 292
  warfarin **3,** 97
Stanozolol,
  acenocoumarol, 90
  dicumarol, 90
  nicoumalone, 90
  warfarin, 90
Streptomycin sulfate,
  alcuronium chloride, 40
  ampicillin sodium, 185
  atracurium besylate, 40
  benethamine penicillin, 185
  bumetanide, 191
  bumetanide, injectable, 191
  carbenicillin disodium, 185
  cefprozil, 185
  ceftibuten dihyrate, 185
  cefuroxime, 185
  cephalexin, 185
  cephalothin sodium, 185
  doxacurium chloride, 40
  enflurane, 25
  ethacrynic acid, 191
  ethacrynic acid, injectable, 191
  ether, 25
  furosemide, 191
  furosemide, injectable, 191
  gallamine triethiodide, 40
  halothane, 25
  isoflurane, 25
  methoxyflurane, 25
  metocurine iodide, 40
  mivacurium chloride, 40
  moxalactam disodium, 185
  nitrous oxide, 25

pancuronium bromide, 40
penicillin G, 185
penicillin G benzathine, 185
penicillin G procaine, 185
penicillin V, 185
pipecuronium bromide, 40
piretanide, 191
rocuronium bromide, 40
succinylcholine chloride, 40
temocillin sodium, 185
ticarcillin disodium, 185
torsemide, injection, 191
torsemide, oral, 191
tubocurarine chloride, 40
vecuronium bromide, 40
Streptomycin sulfate, vaccine use,
  ceftibuten dihyrate, 185
Succinylcholine chloride,
  amikacin sulfate, 40
  bacitracin, 40
  cimetidine, oral **2,** 34
  colistin sulfate, 40
  cyclophosphamide **2,** 34
  demeclocycline hydrochloride, 40
  dexpanthenol **4,** 35
  diethylstilbestrol **2,** 35
  digoxin **2,** 281
  doxycycline hyclate, parenteral,
    40
  doxycycline hydrochloride, 40
  echothiophate iodide **2,** 35
  gentamicin sulfate, 40
  isoflurane **2,** 36
  kanamycin sulfate, oral, 40
  kanamycin sulfate, parenteral, 40
  lidocaine hydrochloride, systemic
    2, 36
  lymecycline, 40
  methacycline hydrochloride, 40
  metoclopramide hydrochloride **3,**
    36
  minocycline hydrochloride
    pellets, 40
  minocycline hydrochloride, 40
  minocycline, parenteral, 40
  neomycin sulfate, oral, 40
  neomycin sulfate, parenteral, 40
  neostigmine **2,** 37
  netilmicin, 40
  oxytetracycline, 40
  oxytetracycline, parenteral, 40
  paromomycin sulfate, 40
  polymyxin B sulfate, 40
  polymyxin B sulfate, vaccine use,
    40
  procainamide hydrochloride **3,** 37
  promazine hydrochloride **2,** 37
  rolitetracycline, injectable, 40
  streptomycin sulfate, 40
  tetracycline, 40
  tetracycline hydrochloride,

parenteral, 40
thiopental sodium **2,** 38
tobramycin, 40
trimethaphan camsylate **2,** 38
Sucralfate,
chlorpropamide **4,** 298
demeclocycline hydrochloride, 205
doxycycline hydrochloride, 205
ketoconazole **3,** 195
levothyroxine sodium **3,** 358
methacycline hydrochloride, 205
norfloxacin **2,** 199
oxytetracycline, 205
phenytoin **2,** 127
ranitidine hydrochloride, oral **3,** 366
tetracycline, 205
theophylline **3,** 342
warfarin **3,** 97
Sufentanil citrate,
isocarboxazid, 14
pargyline hydrochloride, 14
phenelzine sulfate, 14
selegiline hydrochloride, 14
tranylcypromine sulfate, 14
Sulfacytine,
methotrexate, 220
methotrexate sodium, parenteral, 220
warfarin, 98
Sulfadiazine,
cyclosporine **2,** 203
methotrexate, 220
methotrexate sodium, parenteral, 220
warfarin, 98
Sulfadoxine,
methotrexate, 220
methotrexate sodium, parenteral, 220
warfarin, 98
Sulfamerazine,
methotrexate, 220
methotrexate sodium, parenteral, 220
warfarin, 98
Sulfamethazine,
methotrexate, 220
methotrexate sodium, parenteral, 220
warfarin, 98
Sulfamethizole,
methotrexate, 220
methotrexate sodium, parenteral, 220
phenytoin **2,** 127
tolbutamide **2,** 308
warfarin, 98
Sulfamethoxazole,
methotrexate **1,** 220

methotrexate sodium, parenteral, 220
warfarin **1,** 98
Sulfapyridine,
methotrexate, 220
methotrexate sodium, parenteral, 220
warfarin, 98
Sulfasalazine,
ampicillin sodium **3,** 204
digoxin **2,** 282
folic acid **3,** 323
methotrexate, 220
methotrexate sodium, parenteral, 220
warfarin, 98
Sulfinpyrazone,
acetaminophen **3,** 4
aspirin **2,** 21
niacin, vitamin B3 **3,** 22
probenecid **4,** 22
verapamil hydrochloride **3,** 67
warfarin **1,** 98
Sulfisoxazole,
methotrexate, 220
methotrexate sodium, parenteral, 220
phenelzine sulfate **3,** 152
pimozide **3,** 152
thiopental sodium **2,** 39
warfarin, 98
Tacrine hydrochloride,
aminophylline **2,** 329
haloperidol **2,** 238
Tacrolimus,
erythromycin **2,** 367
fluconazole **2,** 367
nifedipine **3,** 368
Talbutal,
acenocoumarol, 94
dicumarol, 94
nicoumalone, 94
warfarin, 94
Tamoxifen citrate,
warfarin **2,** 98
Temafloxacin hydrochloride,
warfarin, 92
Temazepam,
diphenhydramine **2,** 250
Temocillin sodium,
amikacin sulfate, 185
gentamicin sulfate, 185
kanamycin sulfate, oral, 185
kanamycin sulfate, parenteral, 185
neomycin sulfate, oral, 185
neomycin sulfate, parenteral, 185
netilmicin, 185
paromomycin sulfate, 185
streptomycin sulfate, 185
tobramycin, 185
Terbinafine hydrochloride,

cyclosporine **2,** 204
nortriptyline hydrochloride **2,** 148
warfarin **2,** 99
Terbutaline sulfate,
   chloroform, 26
   enflurane, 26
   epinephrine, 26
   ether, 26
   halothane, 26
   methoxyflurane, 26
   metoprolol tartrate, 260
   timolol maleate, oral, 260
Terconazole,
   cyclosporine, 193
   fosphenytoin sodium, parenteral,
     119
   phenytoin, 119
Terfenadine,
   acetaminophen **2,** 4
   carbamazepine **3,** 108
   clarithromycin, 184
   erythromycin **1,** 184
   erythromycin estolate, 184
   erythromycin ethylsuccinate, 184
   erythromycin gluceptate, 184
   erythromycin lactobionate, 184
   erythromycin stearate, 184
   grapefruit juice **2,** 324
   itraconazole, 195
   ketoconazole **1,** 195
   spiramycin, 184
   troleandomycin, 184
Tertatolol hydrochloride,
   clonidine hydrochloride,
     transdermal, 160
   clonidine hydrochloride, 160
   epinephrine, 260
   insulin, 304
Testosterone,
   vecuronium bromide **3,** 43
Tetracycline,
   alcuronium chloride, 40
   aluminum carbonate, basic, 205
   aluminum hydroxide **1,** 205
   aluminum oxide, 205
   aluminum phosphate, 205
   attapulgite, 205
   bismuth subsalicylate, 205
   calcium acetate, 205
   calcium ascorbate, 205
   calcium carbonate, oral, 205
   calcium chloride, oral, 205
   calcium citrate, oral, 205
   calcium glubionate, oral, 205
   calcium glucoheptonate, 205
   calcium gluconate, oral, 205
   calcium glycerophosphate, oral,
     205
   calcium iodate, 205
   calcium lactate gluconate, 205
   calcium lactate, oral, 205

calcium lactobionate, oral, 205
calcium phosphate, oral, 205
calcium, oral salt unspecified, 205
carbonyl iron, 205
cimetidine, oral **3,** 205
dicalcium phosphate, 205
digoxin **1,** 282
digoxin capsule, stabilized, 282
dihydroxyaluminum, 205
doxacurium chloride, 40
ether, 25
ferric ammonium citrate, 205
ferrous fumarate, 205
ferrous gluconate, 205
ferrous glycine sulfate, 205
ferrous hydroxide polymaltose,
   205
ferrous ions, salt unspecified, 205
ferrous succinate, 205
ferrous sulfate **1,** 205
gallamine triethiodide, 40
iron dextran complex, 205
iron peptonized, 205
kaolin, 205
lithium **2,** 244
magaldrate, 205
magnesium aspartate, 205
magnesium carbonate, 205
magnesium chloride, oral, 205
magnesium citrate, 205
magnesium glucoheptonate, 205
magnesium gluconate, 205
magnesium hydroxide, 205
magnesium lactate, 205
magnesium oxide, 205
magnesium sulfate, 205
magnesium trisilicate, 205
magnesium, salt unspecified, 205
methoxyflurane **2,** 29
metocurine iodide, 40
mivacurium chloride, 40
oral contraceptive agents **2,** 206
pancuronium bromide, 40
pipecuronium bromide, 40
rocuronium bromide, 40
sodium bicarbonate **4,** 206
succinylcholine chloride, 40
sucralfate, 205
theophylline **3,** 342
thimerosal, ophthalmic **3,** 206
tubocurarine chloride, 40
vecuronium bromide, 40
warfarin **3,** 99
Tetracycline hydrochloride,
  parenteral,
   alcuronium chloride, 40
   digoxin, 282
   digoxin capsule, stabilized, 282
   ether, 25
   gallamine triethiodide, 40
   metocurine iodide, 40

mivacurium chloride, 40
pipecuronium bromide, 40
rocuronium bromide, 40
succinylcholine chloride, 40
tubocurarine chloride, 40
vecuronium bromide, 40
Tetrahydrozoline hydrochloride,
　furazolidone, 153
　isocarboxazid, 153
　pargyline hydrochloride, 153
　phenelzine sulfate, 153
　tranylcypromine sulfate, 153
Theophylline,
　allopurinol **2,** 331
　aluminum hydroxide **3,** 332
　aminoglutethimide **3,** 332
　caffeine **2,** 332
　carbamazepine **2,** 333
　cefaclor **3,** 333
　charcoal **1,** 333
　cimetidine hydrochloride,
　　parenteral, 334
　cimetidine, oral **1,** 334
　ciprofloxacin hydrochloride **2,**
　　335
　clarithromycin, 335
　disulfiram **2,** 335
　erythromycin **1,** 335
　erythromycin estolate, 335
　erythromycin ethylsuccinate, 335
　erythromycin gluceptate, 335
　erythromycin lactobionate, 335
　erythromycin stearate, 335
　fluvoxamine maleate **3,** 336
　furosemide **2,** 336
　halothane, 327
　hydrocortisone acetate, injectable
　　3, 336
　hydrocortisone sodium succinate
　　3, 337
　hydrocortisone sodium phosphate
　　3, 337
　hydrocortisone, oral/systemic **3,**
　　337
　influenza virus vaccine, split virion
　　3, 337
　influenza virus vaccine, whole
　　virion **3,** 337
　isoniazid **3,** 337
　ketoconazole **3,** 338
　lithium **2,** 245
　lomustine **3,** 215
　magnesium hydroxide **3,** 332
　methimazole **3,** 338
　mexiletine hydrochloride **2,** 338
　moricizine hydrochloride **2,** 339
　omeprazole **4,** 339
　phenobarbital **2,** 340
　phenytoin **2,** 340
　propafenone hydrochloride **2,** 340
　propranolol hydrochloride **2,** 341

pyrantel pamoate **2,** 341
rifampin **2,** 341
spiramycin, 335
sucralfate **3,** 342
tetracycline **3,** 342
ticlopidine hydrochloride **2,** 342
tobacco **1,** 343
troleandomycin, 335
verapamil hydrochloride **2,** 343
vidarabine **3,** 343
Thiabendazole,
　aminophylline **2,** 329
Thiamylal sodium,
　acenocoumarol, 94
　dicumarol, 94
　nicoumalone, 94
　warfarin, 94
Thiethylperazine maleate,
　guanethidine, 162
Thimerosal, ophthalmic,
　tetracycline **3,** 206
Thiopental sodium,
　acenocoumarol, 94
　dicumarol, 94
　midazolam hydrochloride **3,** 247
　morphine **3,** 38
　nicoumalone, 94
　probenecid **3,** 39
　reserpine **2,** 39
　succinylcholine chloride **2,** 38
　sulfisoxazole **2,** 39
　warfarin, 94
Thioproperazine mesylate,
　guanethidine, 162
Thioridazine hydrochloride,
　bromocriptine mesylate **2,** 250
　desipramine hydrochloride **2,** 138
　guanethidine, 162
　lithium **2,** 245
　phenylpropanolamine **2,** 226
　guanethidine, 162
Thiram, topical,
　alcohol, ethyl - oral/injectable, 311
Thyroglobulin,
　acenocoumarol, 100
　dicumarol, 100
　nicoumalone, 100
　warfarin, 100
Thyroid desiccated,
　acenocoumarol, 100
　anisindione, 100
　dicumarol, 100
　insulin **2,** 180
　nicoumalone, 100
　warfarin **1,** 100
Thyroid strong,
　acenocoumarol, 100
　anisindione, 100
　cholestyramine **2,** 368
　dicumarol, 100
　digoxin **2,** 282

ketamine hydrochloride **3,** 28
nicoumalone, 100
propranolol hydrochloride **2,** 264
warfarin, 100
Ticarcillin disodium,
  amikacin sulfate, 185
  gentamicin sulfate, 185
  kanamycin sulfate, oral, 185
  kanamycin sulfate, parenteral, 185
  neomycin sulfate, oral, 185
  neomycin sulfate, parenteral, 185
  netilmicin, 185
  paromomycin sulfate, 185
  streptomycin sulfate, 185
  tobramycin, 185
Ticlopidine hydrochloride,
  aluminum hydroxide **3,** 73
  cyclosporine **2,** 74
  magaldrate **3,** 73
  magnesium hydroxide **3,** 73
  phenytoin **2,** 127
  theophylline **2,** 342
Timolol maleate, ophthalmic,
  acetazolamide **3,** 264
  dexfenfluramine hydrochloride, 260
  dobutamine hydrochloride, 260
  dopamine hydrochloride, 260
  epinephrine, 260
  etafedrine hydrochloride, 260
  insulin, 304
  mazindol, 260
  metaraminol bitartrate, 260
  methoxamine hydrochloride, 260
  norepinephrine bitartrate, 260
  phenylephrine, 260
  prednisone **2,** 265
Timolol maleate, oral,
  albuterol sulfate, 260
  bitolterol mesylate, 260
  clonidine hydrochloride, transdermal, 160
  clonidine hydrochloride, 160
  dexfenfluramine hydrochloride, 260
  dobutamine hydrochloride, 260
  dopamine hydrochloride, 260
  eformoterol fumarate, 260
  epinephrine, 260
  etafedrine hydrochloride, 260
  ethylnorepinephrine hydrochloride, 260
  fenoterol hydrobromide, 260
  insulin, 304
  isoetharine, 260
  mazindol, 260
  metaproterenol sulfate, 260
  metaraminol bitartrate, 260
  methoxamine hydrochloride, 260
  pirbuterol acetate, 260
  procaterol hydrochloride, 260
rimiterol hydrobromide, 260
salmeterol xinafoate, 260
terbutaline sulfate, 260
Tinzaparin sodium,
  ardeparin sodium, 71
  certoparin, 71
  dalteparin sodium, 71
  enoxaparin, 71
  sodium salicylate, 76
Tioconazole,
  cyclosporine, 193
  fosphenytoin sodium, parenteral, 119
  phenytoin, 119
Tobacco,
  aminophylline, 343
  chlorpromazine hydrochloride **3,** 229
  diazepam **3,** 236
  gold sodium thiomalate **3,** 11
  heparin **3,** 73
  imipramine **3,** 146
  insulin **3,** 305
  mexiletine hydrochloride **3,** 56
  oxtriphylline, 343
  propranolol hydrochloride **2,** 264
  theophylline **1,** 343
  warfarin **4,** 100
Tobramycin,
  alcuronium chloride, 40
  amoxicillin, 185
  ampicillin sodium, 185
  azlocillin sodium, 185
  bacampicillin hydrochloride, 185
  benethamine penicillin, 185
  bumetanide, 191
  bumetanide, injectable, 191
  carbenicillin disodium, 185
  cefaclor, 185
  cefadroxil monohydrate, 185
  cefamandole nafate, 185
  cefazolin sodium, 185
  cefdinir, 185
  cefepime hydrochloride, 185
  cefmetazole sodium, 185
  cefonicid sodium, 185
  cefoperazone sodium, 185
  ceforanide, 185
  cefotaxime sodium, 185
  cefotetan disodium, 185
  cefoxitin sodium, 185
  cefpirome sulfate, 185
  cefpodoxime proxetil, 185
  cefprozil, 185
  ceftazidime, 185
  ceftibuten dihyrate, 185
  ceftizoxime sodium, 185
  ceftriaxone sodium, 185
  cefuroxime, 185
  cephalexin, 185
  cephalothin sodium, 185

cephapirin sodium, 185
cephradine, 185
cloxacillin sodium, 185
cyclacillin, 185
dicloxacillin, 185
doxacurium chloride, 40
enflurane, 25
ethacrynic acid, 191
ethacrynic acid, injectable, 191
ether, 25
flucloxacillin, 185
furosemide, 191
furosemide, injectable, 191
gallamine triethiodide, 39
halothane, 25
isoflurane, 25
methicillin sodium, 185
methoxyflurane, 25
metocurine iodide, 39
mezlocillin sodium, 185
miconazole nitrate **3,** 207
mivacurium chloride, 39
moxalactam disodium, 185
nafcillin sodium, 185
nitrous oxide, 25
oxacillin sodium, 185
pancuronium bromide, 39
penicillin G, 185
penicillin G benzathine, 185
penicillin G procaine, 185
penicillin V, 185
pipecuronium bromide, 39
piperacillin sodium, 185
piretanide, 191
rocuronium bromide, 39
succinylcholine chloride, 39
temocillin sodium, 185
ticarcillin disodium, 185
torsemide, injection, 191
torsemide, oral, 191
tubocurarine chloride, 39
vecuronium bromide, 40
Tocopherol, vitamin E,
 warfarin **2,** 101
Tolazamide,
 alcohol, ethyl - oral/injectable, 296
 doxepin hydrochloride **2,** 306
 feprazone, 182
 oxyphenbutazone, 182
 phenylbutazone, 182
Tolbutamide,
 alcohol, ethyl - oral/injectable, 296
 chloramphenicol **2,** 306
 diazoxide, oral **3,** 306
 dicumarol **2,** 307
 digoxin **3,** 283
 feprazone, 182
 fluconazole **3,** 307
 methyldopa **3,** 307
 oxyphenbutazone, 307
 phenylbutazone **1,** 307

 sulfamethizole **2,** 308
Torsemide, injection,
 amikacin sulfate, 191
 gentamicin sulfate, 191
 kanamycin sulfate, oral, 191
 kanamycin sulfate, parenteral, 191
 lithium, 239
 neomycin sulfate, oral, 191
 neomycin sulfate, parenteral, 191
 netilmicin, 191
 streptomycin sulfate, 191
 tobramycin, 191
Torsemide, oral,
 amikacin sulfate, 191
 gentamicin sulfate, 191
 kanamycin sulfate, oral, 191
 kanamycin sulfate, parenteral, 191
 lithium, 239
 neomycin sulfate, oral, 191
 netilmicin, 191
 streptomycin sulfate, 191
 tobramycin, 191
Tranylcypromine sulfate,
 alfentanil hydrochloride, 14
 amobarbital **3,** 313
 amphetamine, 184
 anileridine, 14
 atracurium besylate **3,** 153
 benzphetamine hydrochloride,
  153
 buprenorphine hydrochloride, 14
 butorphanol tartrate, 14
 citalopram hydrobromide, 141
 codeine, 14
 dexfenfluramine hydrochloride,
  153
 dextroamphetamine, 153
 dextromethorphan hydrobromide,
  14
 diethylpropion hydrochloride, 153
 difenoxin hydrochloride, 14
 dihydrocodeine bitartrate, 14
 diphenoxylate hydrochloride, 14
 dopamine hydrochloride, 153
 ephedrine, 153
 etafedrine hydrochloride, 153
 fenfluramine hydrochloride, 153
 fentanyl citrate, 14
 fluoxetine hydrochloride **1,** 141
 fluvoxamine maleate, 141
 hydrocodone bitartrate, 14
 hydromorphone hydrochloride, 14
 imipramine **2,** 146
 isometheptene, 153
 levodopa, 152
 levorphanol tartrate, 14
 mazindol, 153
 meperidine hydrochloride, 14
 mephentermine sulfate, 153
 meptazinol, 14
 metaraminol bitartrate, 153

methamphetamine hydrochloride, 153
methylphenidate hydrochloride, 153
nalbuphine hydrochloride, 14
naphazoline hydrochloride, 153
opium, 14
oxycodone, 14
oxymetazoline hydrochloride, 153
oxymorphone hydrochloride, 14
paroxetine hydrochloride, 141
pentazocine, 14
phendimetrazine tartrate, 153
phenmetrazine hydrochloride, 153
phenoperidine hydrochloride, 14
phentermine hydrochloride, 153
phenylephrine, 153
phenylpropanolamine **1,** 153
propranolol hydrochloride **4,** 153
pseudoephedrine, 153
remifentanil hydrochloride, 14
sufentanil citrate, 14
tetrahydrozoline hydrochloride, 153
tryptophan **3,** 154
venlafaxine hydrochloride, 141
xylometazoline hydrochloride, 153
Trazodone hydrochloride,
    digoxin **3,** 283
    fluoxetine hydrochloride **3,** 154
    phenytoin **3,** 128
    warfarin **3,** 100
Triamterene,
    amantadine hydrochloride **3,** 292
    cimetidine, oral **3,** 293
    indomethacin **2,** 293
    potassium acetate, 292
    potassium bicarbonate, 292
    potassium biphosphate, 292
    potassium chloride, 292
    potassium citrate, 292
    potassium gluconate, 292
    potassium iodide, 292
    potassium iodide, prenatal
        multivitamin use, 292
    potassium perchlorate, 292
    potassium phosphate, 292
    potassium salicylate, 292
    potassium, salt unspecified, 292
Triazolam,
    itraconazole, 250
    ketoconazole **1,** 250
Trichlormethiazide,
    diazoxide, oral **3,** 293
    lithium, 239
Tridihexethyl chloride,
    digoxin, 280
Triethylene thiophosphoramide,
    pancuronium bromide **3,** 33
Trifluoperazine hydrochloride,

guanethidine, 162
Triflupromazine hydrochloride,
    guanethidine, 162
Trihexyphenidyl hydrochloride,
    digoxin, 280
    levodopa **4,** 356
Trimeprazine tartrate,
    guanethidine, 162
Trimethaphan camsylate,
    succinylcholine chloride **2,** 38
Trimethoprim,
    cyclosporine **3,** 203
    dapsone **3,** 181
    digoxin **3,** 283
    methotrexate **1,** 220
    methotrexate sodium, parenteral, 220
    oral contraceptive agents **3,** 204
    phenytoin **2,** 128
    pimozide **3,** 152
    procainamide hydrochloride **3,** 60
    warfarin, 98
Trimipramine maleate,
    guanethidine, 162
Troglitazone,
    warfarin **3,** 101
Troleandomycin,
    astemizole, 183
    carbamazepine, 104
    cyclosporine, 182
    methylprednisolone **2,** 207
    oral contraceptive agents **2,** 207
    simvastatin, 359
    terfenadine, 184
    theophylline, 335
    warfarin, 82
Tromethamine,
    lithium, 238
Tryptophan,
    fluoxetine hydrochloride **3,** 142
    tranylcypromine sulfate **3,** 154
Tubocurarine chloride,
    amikacin sulfate, 39
    bacitracin, 39
    colistin sulfate, 39
    demeclocycline hydrochloride, 39
    doxycycline hyclate, parenteral, 39
    doxycycline hydrochloride, 39
    gentamicin sulfate **1,** 40
    kanamycin sulfate, oral, 39
    kanamycin sulfate, parenteral, 39
    ketamine hydrochloride **2,** 40
    lymecycline, 39
    methacycline hydrochloride, 39
    minocycline hydrochloride
        pellets, 39
    minocycline hydrochloride, 39
    minocycline, parenteral, 39
    morphine **2,** 40
    neomycin sulfate, oral, 39

neomycin sulfate, parenteral, 39
netilmicin, 39
oxytetracycline, 39
oxytetracycline, parenteral, 39
paromomycin sulfate, 39
polymyxin B sulfate, 39
polymyxin B sulfate, vaccine use, 39
propranolol hydrochloride **2,** 41
quinidine **2,** 41
rolitetracycline, injectable, 39
streptomycin sulfate, 39
tetracycline, 39
tetracycline hydrochloride, parenteral, 39
tobramycin, 39
Tyropanoate sodium, 57.4% iodine, metformin hydrochloride, 305
Valproic acid,
aluminum hydroxide **3,** 130
amitriptyline hydrochloride **3,** 130
aspirin **2,** 131
carbamazepine **2,** 131
chlorpromazine hydrochloride **3,** 131
cimetidine, oral **3,** 129
clonazepam **3,** 132
erythromycin **2,** 132
erythromycin ethylsuccinate **2,** 132
ethosuximide **3,** 110
felbamate **2,** 133
fluoxetine hydrochloride **3,** 133
isoniazid **3,** 133
lamotrigine **3,** 110
naproxen **3,** 130
phenobarbital **2,** 111
phenytoin **2,** 128
Vancomycin hydrochloride, gentamicin sulfate **3,** 187
Vecuronium bromide,
amikacin sulfate, 39
bacitracin, 39
colistin sulfate, 39
dantrolene sodium **3,** 42
demeclocycline hydrochloride, 39
doxycycline hyclate, parenteral, 39
doxycycline hydrochloride, 39
gentamicin sulfate, 39
kanamycin sulfate, oral, 39
kanamycin sulfate, parenteral, 39
lymecycline, 39
magnesium sulfate, parenteral **2,** 42
methacycline hydrochloride, 39
minocycline hydrochloride pellets, 39
minocycline hydrochloride, 39
minocycline, parenteral, 39
neomycin sulfate, oral, 39

neomycin sulfate, parenteral, 39
netilmicin, 39
oxytetracycline, 39
oxytetracycline, parenteral, 39
paromomycin sulfate, 39
piperacillin sodium **2,** 42
polymyxin B sulfate, 39
polymyxin B sulfate, vaccine use, 39
rolitetracycline, injectable, 39
streptomycin sulfate, 39
testosterone **3,** 43
tetracycline, 39
tetracycline hydrochloride, parenteral, 39
tobramycin, 39
verapamil hydrochloride **2,** 43
Venlafaxine hydrochloride,
cimetidine, oral **3,** 154
dexfenfluramine hydrochloride, 153
furazolidone, 141
isocarboxazid, 141
moclobemide, 141
pargyline hydrochloride, 141
phenelzine sulfate, 141
procarbazine hydrochloride, 141
selegiline hydrochloride, 141
tranylcypromine sulfate, 141
Verapamil hydrochloride pellets,
cyclosporine, 46
digitoxin, 284
digoxin, 284
digoxin capsule, stabilized, 284
quinidine, 292
Verapamil hydrochloride, sustained-release,
cyclosporine, 46
digitoxin, 284
digoxin, 284
digoxin capsule, stabilized, 284
quinidine, 292
Verapamil hydrochloride,
calcium gluconate, oral **2,** 65
carbamazepine **2,** 108
cyclosporine, 46
dantrolene sodium **2,** 65
digitoxin, 284
digoxin **1,** 284
digoxin capsule, stabilized, 284
etomidate **3,** 25
lithium **2,** 246
phenobarbital **3,** 66
prazosin hydrochloride **3,** 169
propranolol hydrochloride **2,** 66
quinidine **1,** 65
rifampin **2,** 66
sulfinpyrazone **3,** 67
theophylline **2,** 343
vecuronium bromide **2,** 43
Vidarabine,

allopurinol **3,** 208
theophylline **3,** 343
Vinblastine sulfate,
erythromycin **3,** 222
mitomycin **2,** 220
phenytoin **2,** 114
Vincristine sulfate,
digoxin **2,** 272
Vindesine sulfate,
warfarin **3,** 83
Vitamin A,
neomycin sulfate, oral **3,** 325
Vitamin A, prenatal multivitamin use,
neomycin sulfate, oral **3,** 325
Vitamin D2, prenatal multivitamin
use,
phenytoin **2,** 321
Vitamin D3, prenatal multivitamin
use,
aluminum hydroxide **2,** 320
Warfarin,
acarbose **2,** 74
acetaminophen **3,** 75
alcohol, ethyl - oral/injectable **3,**
75
allopurinol, 69
aloxiprin, 76
aminoglutethimide, 86
amiodarone hydrochloride **1,** 75
amobarbital, 94
aprobarbital, 94
ascorbic acid, vitamin C **4,** 76
aspirin **1,** 76
azathioprine sodium **2,** 77
azithromycin, 82
barbital, 94
bezafibrate, 80
butabarbital sodium, 94
butalbital, 94
butobarbitone, 94
calcium carbaspirin, 76
calcium carbimide, 81
cefamandole nafate **2,** 77
chloral hydrate **2,** 78
chlordiazepoxide **4,** 78
chlorthalidone **3,** 78
cholestyramine **2,** 79
cimetidine hydrochloride,
parenteral, 79
cimetidine, oral **1,** 79
cinoxacin, 92
ciprofloxacin hydrochloride, 92
cisapride **2,** 80
clarithromycin, 82
clofibrate **1,** 80
cyclosporine **3,** 80
danazol, 90
dextrothyroxine sodium, 100
diazoxide, oral **3,** 81
diflunisal, 76
diphenhydramine **4,** 81

dirithromycin, 82
disopyramide phosphate **3,** 81
disulfiram **1,** 81
enoxacin, 92
erythromycin **1,** 82
erythromycin estolate, 82
erythromycin ethylsuccinate, 82
erythromycin glucceptate, 82
erythromycin lactobionate, 82
erythromycin stearate, 82
ethacrynic acid **2,** 82
ethchlorvynol **2,** 83
ethylestrenol, 90
etoposide **3,** 83
etretinate **2,** 83
felbamate **2,** 84
fenofibrate, micronized, 80
feprazone, 94
flosequinan, 92
fluconazole **2,** 84
fluoxetine hydrochloride **3,** 85
fluoxymesterone, 90
gemfibrozil, 80
ginkgo **3,** 85
ginseng **3,** 85
glucagon **1,** 86
glucagon, recombinant, 86
glutethimide **1,** 86
griseofulvin **2,** 87
ibuprofen **2,** 87
ifosfamide **2,** 87
indomethacin **2,** 88
influenza virus vaccine, split
virion **3,** 88
isoniazid **3,** 88
levothyroxine sodium, 100
liothyronine sodium, 100
lomefloxacin hydrochloride, 92
lovastatin **2,** 89
magnesium hydroxide **4,** 89
menadiol sodium diphosphate
vitamin K4, 95
menadione, 95
mephobarbital, 94
meprobamate **3,** 90
methandrostenolone, 90
metharbital, 94
methohexital sodium, 94
methyltestosterone **1,** 90
methyprylon, 86
metronidazole, systemic **2,** 90
mitotane **2,** 91
moricizine hydrochloride **2,** 92
nafcillin sodium **2,** 92
nalidixic acid **1,** 92
neomycin sulfate, oral **3,** 93
norfloxacin, 92
nortriptyline hydrochloride **4,** 93
ofloxacin, 92
omeprazole **3,** 93
oxandrolone, 90

oxymetholone, 90
oxyphenbutazone, 94
pentobarbital sodium, 94
phenobarbital **1,** 94
phenylbutazone **1,** 94
phytonadione, vitamin K1 **1,** 95
primidone, 94
proguanil hydrochloride, 98
propafenone hydrochloride **2,** 95
propoxyphene **2,** 96
propranolol hydrochloride **2,** 96
propylthiouracil, 100
quinidine **2,** 96
ranitidine hydrochloride,
  parenteral, 79
ranitidine hydrochloride, oral, 79
rifabutin, 97
rifampin **1,** 97
secobarbital, 94
sodium salicylate, 76
spironolactone **3,** 97
stanozolol, 90
sucralfate **3,** 97
sulfacytine, 98
sulfadiazine, 98
sulfadoxine, 98
sulfamerazine, 98
sulfamethazine, 98
sulfamethizole, 98
sulfamethoxazole **1,** 98
sulfapyridine, 98
sulfasalazine, 98
sulfinpyrazone **1,** 98
sulfisoxazole, 98
talbutal, 94
tamoxifen citrate **2,** 98
temafloxacin hydrochloride, 92
terbinafine hydrochloride **2,** 99
tetracycline **3,** 99
thiamylal sodium, 94
thiopental sodium, 94
thyroglobulin, 100
thyroid desiccated **1,** 100
thyroid strong, 100
tobacco **4,** 100
tocopherol, vitamin E **2,** 101
trazodone hydrochloride **3,** 100
trimethoprim, 98
troglitazone **3,** 101
troleandomycin, 82
vindesine sulfate **3,** 83
Xipamide,
  lithium, 239
Xylometazoline hydrochloride,
  furazolidone, 153
  isocarboxazid, 153
  pargyline hydrochloride, 153
  phenelzine sulfate, 153
  tranylcypromine sulfate, 153
Zidovudine,
  acetaminophen **3,** 208
  acyclovir, oral **3,** 208
  atovaquone **2,** 368
  probenecid **2,** 209
  rifampin **2,** 369
Zolpidem tartrate,
  paroxetine hydrochloride **3,** 150
Zuclopenthixol,
  guanethidine, 162